D1761356

Textbook of Post-ICU Medicine:
The Legacy of Critical Care

Textbook of Post-ICU Medicine: The Legacy of Critical Care

Edited by

Robert D. Stevens, MD

Associate Professor of Anesthesiology Critical Care Medicine
Associate Professor of Neurology, Neurosurgery and Radiology
Johns Hopkins University School of Medicine
F.M. Kirby Center for Functional Brain Imaging, Kennedy Krieger Institute
Baltimore, Maryland, USA

Nicholas Hart, MBBS, BSc, PhD, MRCP, FFICM

Clinical & Academic Director, Lane Fox Respiratory Unit, St Thomas'
Hospital, Guy's & St Thomas' NHS Foundation Trust, London UK

Reader in Respiratory & Critical Care Medicine, Department of Asthma,
Allergy and Respiratory Science, Division of Asthma, Allergy and Lung
Biology, King's College London, London UK

Margaret S. Herridge, MSc, MD, FRCPC, MPH

Professor of Medicine, University of Toronto Critical Care and
Pulmonary Medicine Scientist, Toronto General Research Institute
University Health Network/Toronto General Hospital NCSB 11C–1180
Toronto, ON Canada

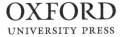

OXFORD
UNIVERSITY PRESS

UNIVERSITY PRESS

Great Clarendon Street, Oxford, OX2 6DP,
United Kingdom

Oxford University Press is a department of the University of Oxford.
It furthers the University's objective of excellence in research, scholarship,
and education by publishing worldwide. Oxford is a registered trade mark of
Oxford University Press in the UK and in certain other countries

Published in the United States of America by Oxford University Press
198 Madison Avenue, New York, NY 10016, United States of America

British Library Cataloguing in Publication Data
Data available

Library of Congress Control Number: 2014931564

ISBN 978–0–19–965346–1

Printed in Great Britain by
Clays Ltd, St Ives plc

Foreword

Over the last half century, critical care has made great advances towards preventing the premature deaths of many severely ill patients. The urgency, immediacy, and involved intimacy of the critical care team striving to correct acutely disturbed organ dysfunction meant that, for many years, physiological correction and ultimate patient survival alone was considered the unique measure of success. However, over the last quarter century, our survivor patients and their relatives have told us much more about what it means to have a critical illness. We work in an area of medicine where survival is a battle determined by tissue resilience, frailty, and the ability to recover, but this comes at a price. As our focus has moved beyond the immediate, we have learned about the 'legacy of critical care' and how having a critical illness impacts life after ICU through its consequential effects on physical and psychological function and the social landscape. This text explores how we can progress beyond simply saving a patient's life to how we can best help to recover the lives of patients and their family, following the ordeal of a critical illness.

This fundamental cultural change in how we perceive critical care as a specialty and where our measure of a successful outcome includes the quality of life restored has come about through the sound medical approach of listening to our patients and families, defining the problems, and carefully testing through research hypotheses as to causation and possible therapeutic benefit. It not only has changed how patients are considered and cared for after intensive care, but, through the detailed knowledge of how patients are affected by the consequences of the critical illness, it has fostered fundamental research to improve the care and therapies we use during their stay. As with all sound clinical advances, it has helped shed light on ill-informed dogma and helped re-focus the research agenda to ensure that the long-term legacies of a critical illness are equally considered. Immobility, oft considered of little consequence, is now recognized to be a significant pathological participant and contributor to disability. Amnesia, in short-term anaesthesia considered a benefit, has now a defined pathological significance, along with previously poorly recognized cognitive deficits and delusional experiences, all consequences of acute brain dysfunction. The family, often in the past merely a repository of information, are now recognized to play a much greater role in how patients recover and are themselves traumatized by the experience, so meriting help and support if they are to assist in rehabilitation.

Perhaps the purest achievement has been the bringing together of contributions not just from patients and their families, but from the wide breadth of professionals deeply involved in the care of the critically ill from across many continents. Not only have the doors of the intensive care unit been thrown open, but so too have the minds of those working for the best care of our patients. The reward of a visit some months later of a patient brought back from the brink of death is cherished by a critical care team. Added to this, the knowledge that our patients are now understanding what happened to them and they and their families are being given the help to recover their lives following the legacy of critical care is something of which our specialty should be justly proud. We cannot ignore the lessons we have learned, and this text hopefully will spur on the research and delivery of excellent care to the critically ill.

Richard D. Griffiths BSc. MD, FRCP, FFICM
Emeritus Professor of Medicine (Intensive care),
Musculoskeletal Biology,
Institute of Ageing & Chronic Disease,
Faculty of Health & Life Sciences,
University of Liverpool, UK.

Acknowledgements

Chapter 6

This work was supported by the US National Institutes of Health via K08, HL091249 and by the US Department of Veterans Affairs Health Services Research & Development Services via IIR 11–109.

Chapter 25

This work was funded in part by a grant from the Canadian Institutes of Health Research to Guy Trudel (MOP 77661).

Chapter 28

Dr Bagshaw is supported by a Canada Research Chair in Critical Care Nephrology and Clinical Investigator Award from Alberta Innovates–Health Solutions (formerly Alberta Heritage Foundation for Medical Research).

Chapter 34

This work was supported by the United States' National Institutes of Health via K23 HL74294.

Contents

Contributors

Neill K.J. Adhikari
Staff physician, Associate Scientist,
Department of Critical Care Medicine,
Sunnybrook Health Sciences Centre,
Sunnybrook Research Institute,
University of Toronto,
Toronto, Canada

Naeem A. Ali
Associate Professor
Division of Pulmonary, Allergy, Critical Care
and Sleep Medicine,
Wexner Medical Center at The Ohio State
University,
The Ohio State University
Columbus, USA

Derek C. Angus
Distinguished Professor and Mitchell P. Fink
Endowed Chair in Critical Care Medicine,
Professor of Critical Care Medicine, Medicine,
Health Policy and Management, and Clinical
and Translational Science,
The CRISMA Laboratory (Clinical Research,
Investigation, and Systems Modeling of Acute
Illness),
Department of Critical Care Medicine,
University of Pittsburgh,
Pittsburgh, USA

Sean M. Bagshaw
Associate Professor,
Division of Critical Care Medicine,
Faculty of Medicine and Dentistry,
University of Alberta,
Edmonton, Canada

Matthew Baldwin
Assistant Professor of Medicine,
Division of Pulmonary, Allergy, and Critical
Care Medicine,
Department of Medicine, College
of Physicians & Surgeons,

Columbia University,
New York, USA

Amelia Barry
Department of Medicine, Division of Physical
Medicine and Rehabilitation,
University of Ottawa,
The Ottawa Hospital—Rehabilitation Centre,
Ottawa, Canada

Gaëtan Beduneau
Medical Intensive Care Unit and Specialized
Weaning Unit,
University Hospital,
Rouen, France

Rinaldo Bellomo
Professor of Medicine,
Melbourne University;
Honorary Professor of Medicine,
Monash University;
Austin Health, Intensive Care Unit,
Department of Intensive Care,
Heidelberg, Australia

O. Joseph Bienvenu
Associate Professor of Psychiatry
and Behavioural Sciences,
Johns Hopkins University School
of Medicine,
Baltimore, USA

Stephen Brett
Consultant in Intensive Care Medicine,
Imperial College Healthcare NHS Trust,
London, UK

Laurent Brochard
Department of Critical Care,
St Michael's Hospital, Toronto and
Interdepartmental Division of Critical Care
Medicine,
University of Toronto,
Toronto, Canada

Lisa Burry
Clinician Scientist, Clinical Pharmacy Specialist,
Leslie Dan Faculty of Pharmacy,
University of Toronto,
Department of Pharmacy, Mount Sinai Hospital,
Toronto, Canada

Jill I. Cameron
CIHR New Investigator, Associate Professor,
Department of Occupational Science
and Occupational Therapy,
Graduate Department of Rehabilitation Science,
University of Toronto,
Toronto, Canada

Shannon S. Carson
Professor of Medicine and Chief,
Division of Pulmonary and Critical Care
Medicine,
University of North Carolina School of
Medicine,
Chapel Hill, USA

Nancy A. Collop
Professor of Medicine and Neurology,
Emory University School of Medicine,
Department of Medicine,
Division of Pulmonary, Allergy and Critical
Care Medicine,
Atlanta, USA

Christopher E. Cox
Associate Professor of Medicine,
Department of Medicine,
Division of Pulmonary and Critical Care
Medicine,
Duke University Medical Center,
Durham, USA

Benedict Creagh-Brown
Consultant Physician, Intensive Care
and Respiratory Medicine,
Chair, Surrey Peri-operative Anaesthesia and
Critical care collaborative Research (SPACeR)
Clinical Academic Group
Surrey, UK

Brian H. Cuthbertson
Chief and Professor of Critical Care,
Department of Critical Care Medicine,

Sunnybrook Health Sciences Centre, and
Department of Anaesthesia,
University of Toronto,
Toronto, Canada

Michele Dambrosio
Chief and Professor of Critical Care,
Department of Anesthesia and Critical
Care,
University of Foggia,
Foggia, Italy

Linda Denehy
Professor and Head,
Department of Physiotherapy,
Melbourne School of Health Sciences,
The University of Melbourne,
Melbourne,
Australia

Eva C. Diaz
Research Fellow,
University of Texas Medical Branch
at Galveston,
Galveston, USA

David Dyzenhaus
Professor of Law and Philosophy,
University of Toronto,
Toronto, Canada

Doug Elliott
Professor of Nursing,
University of Technology,
Sydney, Australia

E. Wesley Ely
Professor of Medicine and Critical Care,
Center for Health Services Research,
Associate Director of Aging Research,
Tennessee Valley, VA-GRECC,
Vanderbilt University Medical Center,
Nashville, USA

Christopher T. Erb
Postdoctoral Fellow,
Yale School of Medicine, Department
of Internal Medicine,
Section of Pulmonary, Critical Care,
and Sleep Medicine,
New Haven, USA

Vito Fanelli
Assistant Professor,
Department of Anesthesia and Critical
Care,
University of Turin,
Turin, Italy

Luca Fasano
Pulmonary and Critical Care Medicine,
Sant'Orsola Malpighi University Hospital,
Bologna, Italy

Celeste C. Finnerty
Associate Professor,
Department of Surgery, University of Texas
Medical Branch at Galveston,
Associate Director of Research,
Shriners Hospitals for Children-Galveston
Galveston, USA

Kevin M. Fischer
Clinical Assistant Professor of Medicine,
Division of Pulmonary and Critical Care
Medicine,
University of North Carolina School
of Medicine,
Chapel Hill, USA

Sinead Galvin
Consultant Anaesthetist,
Department of Anaesthesia and Critical
Care, Beaumont Hospital,
Dublin, Ireland

Vasiliki Gerovasili
Pulmonology Fellow,
First Critical Care Department,
National and Kapodistrian University
of Athens,
Athens, Greece

Neil J. Glassford
Research Fellow,
Austin Health, Department of Intensive Care
ANZIC-RC (Australian and New Zealand
Intensive Care Research Center)
Melbourne, Australia

Shannon L. Goddard
Staff Physician,
Department of Critical Care Medicine;

Sunnybrook Health Sciences Centre, and
Department of Anaesthesia,
University of Toronto,
Toronto, Canada

Rik Gosselink
Professor of Rehabilitation Sciences,
Faculty of Kinesiology and Rehabilitation
Sciences, Katholieke Universiteit Leuven,
Division of Respiratory Rehabilitation,
University Hospital Gasthuisberg,
Leuven, Belgium

Richard D. Griffiths
Emeritus Professor of Medicine (Intensive Care)
Musculoskeletal Biology
Institute of Ageing & Chronic Disease
Faculty of Health & Life Sciences
University of Liverpool
Liverpool, UK

Ziv Harel
Staff Physician, Assistant Professor,
Division of Nephrology, St. Michael's Hospital,
Department of Medicine, University
of Toronto,
Toronto, Canada

Stephen Harridge
Professor of Human & Applied Physiology,
and Director, Centre of Human & Aerospace
Physiological Sciences,
King's College London
London, UK

Greet Hermans
Associate Professor, Deputy Head of Clinic,
KU Leuven and Medical Intensive Care Unit,
University Hospitals Leuven,
Leuven, Belgium

David N. Herndon
Jesse H. Jones Distinguished Chair in Burn
Surgery, Professor, Departments of Surgery
and Pediatrics, University of Texas Medical
Branch at Galveston
Director of Burn Services and Director
of Research, Shriners Hospitals
for Children-Galveston,
Galveston, USA

Daren K. Heyland
Professor of Medicine,
Clinical Evaluation Research Unit,
Kingston General Hospital,
Department of Community Health
and Epidemiology,
Queen's University,
Department of Medicine,
Queen's University,
Kingston, Canada

Scott Hoff
Assistant Professor of Medicine,
Emory University School of Medicine,
Department of Medicine, Division of
Pulmonary, Allergy and Critical Care
Medicine,
Atlanta, USA

Karen Hoffman
Senior Occupational Therapist,
Trauma Sciences, Blizard Institute,
Queen Mary University of London
London, UK

José G.M. Hofhuis
Department of Intensive Care,
Gelre Hospitals,
Apeldoorn, Netherlands

Aluko A. Hope
Assistant Professor of Medicine,
Department of Medicine, Division of Critical
Care Medicine,
Albert Einstein College of Medicine of
Yeshiva University,
Bronx, USA

Ramona O. Hopkins
Psychology Department and Neuroscience
Center, Brigham Young University, Provo,
Department of Medicine, Pulmonary and
Critical Care Division,
Intermountain Medical Center,
Murray, USA

Catherine L. Hough
Associate Professor of Medicine,
Division of Pulmonary and Critical Care
Medicine, Harborview Medical Center,

University of Washington,
Seattle, USA

Stefano Italiano
Intensive Care Unit
Hospital Verge de la Cinta,
Tortosa, Spain

Theodore J. Iwashyna
VA Center for Clinical Management
Research,
Department of Internal Medicine, University
of Michigan,
Institute for Social Research, University
of Michigan,
Ann Arbor, USA

James C. Jackson
Assistant Professor of Allergy,
Pulmonary, and Critical Care Medicine,
Division of Allergy, Pulmonary, Critical Care
Medicine,
Center for Health Services Research,
Vanderbilt University School of Medicine,
Nashville, USA

Christina Jones
Nurse Consultant Critical Care Rehabilitation,
Honorary Reader,
Critical Care Unit, Whiston Hospital, Prescot,
Institute of Aging and Chronic Disease,
University of Liverpool,
Liverpool, UK

Jeremy M. Kahn
Associate Professor of Critical Care and
Health Policy and Management,
Clinical Research, Investigation and Systems
Modeling of Acute Illness (CRISMA) Center,
Department of Critical Care Medicine,
University of Pittsburgh School of
Medicine,
Department of Health Policy and
Management, University of Pittsburgh
Graduate School of Public Health,
Pittsburgh, USA

Stefan Kluge
Director of Division of Critical Care
Medicine,

Department of Intensive Care,
University Medical Center,
Hamburg, Germany

John P. Kress
Professor of Medicine, Director of Medical ICU,
Department of Medicine, Section of Pulmonary and Critical Care,
University of Chicago,
Chicago, USA

Nicola Latronico
Associate Professor of Anesthesia and Critical Care Medicine, and Director of the University Division and School of Specialty of Anesthesia and Critical Care Medicine,
University of Brescia, Spedali Civili,
Brescia, Italy

Eric Magalhaes
Physician,
General Intensive Care Unit, Raymond Poincaré Teaching Hospital,
University of Versailles Saint-Quentin en Yvelines,
Garches, France

Michael Marber
Professor of Cardiology,
The Rayne Institute, St Thomas' Hospital,
London, UK

Victoria McCredie
Staff Physician,
Department of Critical Care Medicine,
Sunnybrook Health Sciences Centre
Toronto, Canada

Robert C. McDermid
Clinical Professor,
Division of Critical Care Medicine, Faculty of Medicine and Dentistry,
University of Alberta,
Edmonton, Canada

Sangeeta Mehta
Research Director, Medical/Surgical ICU,
Associate Professor,
University of Toronto, Mount Sinai Hospital,
Toronto, Canada

Lucia Mirabella
Assistant Professor of Critical Care,
Department of Critical Care,
University of Foggia,
Foggia, Italy

Cheryl Misak
Professor of Philosophy,
University of Toronto,
Toronto, Canada

Hugh Montgomery
Professor of Intensive Care Medicine,
University College London, and
Whittington Hospital NHS Trust
London, UK

Marina Mourtzakis
Assistant Professor,
Department of Kinesiology,
University of Waterloo,
Waterloo, Canada

John Moxham
Professor of Respiratory Medicine,
Department of Respiratory Medicine,
King's College London,
London, UK

Serafim N. Nanas
Professor of Intensive Care Medicine,
First Critical Care Department,
National and Kapodistrian University of Athens
Athens, Greece

Stefano Nava
Respiratory and Critical Care,
Sant'Orsola Malpighi Hospital;
Alma Mater Studiorum,
University of Bologna,
Department of Specialistic, Diagnostic and Experimental Medicine (DIMES),
Bologna, Italy

Judith E. Nelson
Professor of Medicine,
Department of Medicine, Division of Pulmonary, Critical Care and Sleep Medicine,
Mount Sinai School of Medicine,
New York, USA

Sanjeev Noel
Postdoctoral Fellow,
Division of Nephrology, School of Medicine,
Johns Hopkins University,
Baltimore, USA

Simone Piva
Staff Physician,
University Division of Anesthesia and
Critical Care Medicine,
Section of Neuroanesthesia and Neurocritical
Care,
University of Brescia at Spedali Civili,
Brescia, Italy

Andréa Polito
Senior Intensivist,
Critical Care Department, Raymond Poincaré
Hospital,
Garches, France

Angelo Polito
Paediatric Anaesthesiology and Critical Care
Medicine Physician,
Cardiac Intensive Care Unit,
Bambino Gesù Children's Hospital IRCCS,
Rome, Italy

Zudin Puthucheary
Respiratory and Critical Care Consultant,
National University Hospital Singapore,
Singapore

Hamid Rabb
Professor and Vice Chairmen,
Department of Medicine, Division
of Nephrology, School of Medicine,
Johns Hopkins University,
Baltimore, USA

Gerrard Rafferty
Senior Lecturer in Human Physiology,
Department of Respiratory Medicine,
King's College London,
London, UK

V. Marco Ranieri
Department of Anesthesia and Critical Care
Medicine,
Università degli Studi di Torino,
Turin, Italy

Vanessa Raymont
Clinical Research Fellow,
Centre for Mental Health, Department
of Medicine,
Imperial College London,
London, UK

Mark M. Rich
Professor,
Department of Neuroscience, Cell Biology
and Physiology,
Wright State University,
Dayton, USA

Jean-Christophe M. Richard
Associate Professor,
Intensive Care Division, Anesthesiology,
Pharmacology and Intensive Care
Department, University Hospital,
School of Medicine, University of Geneva,
Geneva, Switzerland

Antoine G. Schneider
Research Fellow,
Austin Health, Intensive Care Unit,
Department of Intensive Care,
ANZIC-RC (Australian and New Zealand
Intensive Care Research Center)
Heidelberg Australia

Bernd Schönhofer
Professor
Klinikum Region Hannover,
Krankenhaus Oststadt-Heidehaus,
Department of Pulmonary and Intensive Care
Medicine,
Hannover, Germany

William D. Schweickert
Assistant Professor of Medicine,
Department of Medicine, Division of
Pulmonary, Allergy and Critical Care
Medicine,
University of Pennsylvania,
Philadelphia, USA

Nishant K. Sekaran
RWJF Clinical Scholars Program,
University of Michigan
Ann Arbor, USA

Tarek Sharshar
General Intensive Care Unit, Raymond
Poincaré Teaching Hospital, University of
Versailles Saint-Quentin en Yvelines,
Garches, France, and
Laboratory of Human Histopathology and
Animal Models,
Institut Pasteur,
Paris, France

Mark D. Siegel
Associate Professor, Director, Traditional
Internal Medicine Residency
Yale School of Medicine,
Department of Internal Medicine,
Section of Pulmonary, Critical Care,
and Sleep Medicine
New Haven, USA

Peter E. Spronk
Department of Intensive Care,
Gelre Hospitals,
Apeldoorn, Netherlands

Joerg Steier
Consultant Physician and Senior Lecturer
King's College London and King's Health
Partners, Lane Fox Respiratory Unit/Sleep
Disorders Centre,
St Thomas' Hospital, Guy's and St Thomas'
NHS Foundation Trust,
London, UK

Amanda Thomas
Clinical Specialist Physiotherapist,
Adult Critical Care Unit, The Royal London
Hospital,
London, UK

Guy Trudel
Professor of Medicine,
Faculty of Medicine,
Bone and Joint Research Laboratory,
University of Ottawa,

The Ottawa Hospital—Rehabilitation Centre,
Ottawa, Canada

Ching-Wei Tsai
Postdoctoral Fellow-STU,
Division of Nephrology, School of Medicine,
Johns Hopkins University,
Baltimore, USA

Kavitha Vimalesvaran
Research Fellow
The Rayne Institute, St Thomas' Hospital,
London, UK

Ron Wald
Staff Physician,
Division of Nephrology, St. Michael's Hospital,
Scientist, Li Ka Shing Knowledge Institute
of St. Michael's Hospital,
Assistant Professor,
Department of Medicine, University
of Toronto,
Toronto, Canada

Hannah Wunsch
Herbert Irving Assistant Professor of
Anesthesiology & Epidemiology,
Department of Anesthesiology, College of
Physicians & Surgeons, Columbia University,
Department of Epidemiology, Mailman
School of Public Health, Columbia
University,
New York, USA

Sachin Yende
Associate Professor/Director of CRISMA
Fellowship/Director of Clinical Epidemiology
Program,
The CRISMA Laboratory (Clinical Research,
Investigation, and Systems Modeling of Acute
Illness),
Department of Critical Care Medicine,
University of Pittsburgh,
Pittsburgh, USA

Abbreviations

Ab	antibody
ACE	angiotensin-converting enzyme
ACOS	Adult Respiratory Distress Syndrome Cognitive Outcomes Study
ACTH	adrenocorticotropic hormone
ACV	assist control ventilation
ADL	activities of daily living
ADP	adenosine diphosphate
AIDS	acquired immunodeficiency syndrome
AKI	acute kidney injury
ALDS	Academic Medical Center Linear Disability Score
ALI	acute lung injury
alkP	alkaline phosphatase
AMP	adenosine monophosphate
AMPK	AMP-activated protein kinase
ANP	atrial natriuretic peptide
APACHE	Acute Physiology and Chronic Health Evaluation
AQoL	assessment of quality of life
ARA	aldosterone receptor antagonist
ARB	angiotensin receptor blocker
ARDS	acute respiratory distress syndrome
ARF	acute renal failure; acute respiratory failure
ASV	adaptive support ventilation
ATICE	Assessment to Intensive Care Environment
ATP	adenosine triphosphate
BAMPS	bilateral, anterolateral magnetic phrenic nerve stimulation
BAN	body area network
BBB	blood-brain barrier
bd	twice daily
BDI	Beck Depression Inventory
bFGF	basic fibroblast growth factor
BIS	bispectral index
BMC	bone mineral content
BMD	bone mineral density

BMI	body mass index
BMSC	bone marrow stem cell
BNP	brain natriuretic peptide
BRC	brain reserve capacity
CAF	Comprehensive Assessment of Frailty
CAM-ICU	confusion assessment method for the ICU
CBF	cerebral blood flow
CBT	cognitive behavioural therapy
cc	cubic centimetre
CCFNI	Critical Care Family Needs Inventory
CCI	chronic critical illness
CES-D	Center for Epidemiologic Studies Depression (scale)
CFS	Clinical Frailty Scale
CGA	Comprehensive Geriatric Assessment
CGIC-PF	Clinical Global Impression of Change in Physical Frailty
cGy	centigray
CHF	congestive heart failure; chronic heart failure
CI	confidence interval
CIM	critical illness myopathy
CINM	critical illness neuromyopathy
CINMA	critical illness neuromuscular abnormality
CIP	critical illness polyneuropathy
CIPNM	critical illness polyneuromyopathy
CIT	conventional insulin therapy
CK	creatine kinase
CKD	chronic kidney disease
cm	centimetre
CMAP	compound muscle action potential
cmH_2O	centimetre of water
CMS	cervical magnetic stimulation
CNS	central nervous system
CO	cardiac output
CO_2	carbon dioxide
COPD	chronic obstructive pulmonary disease
CPAP	continuous positive airway pressure

CPM	continuous passive motion	ERS	European Respiratory Society
CRIMYNE	critical illness myopathy and/or neuropathy	ES	electrical stimulation
		ESR	erythrocyte sedimentation rate
CRP	C-reactive protein	ESRD	end-stage renal disease
CRRT	continuous renal replacement therapy	ETT	endotracheal tube
CSF	cerebrospinal fluid	FACTT	Acute Respiratory Distress Syndrome Clinical Trials Network Fluid and Catheter Treatment Trial
CSF-1	colony-stimulating factor 1		
CT	computed tomography		
CVO	circumventricular organ	FDR	false discovery rate
CVVH	continuous veno-venous haemofiltration	FI	Frailty Index
		FIM	Functional Independence Measure
CVVHDF	continuous veno-venous haemodiafiltration	FiO_2	fraction of inspired oxygen
		fMRI	functional magnetic resonance imaging
DASS	Depression, Anxiety, and Stress Scale	FS-ICU	Family Satisfaction in the ICU
dB	decibel	FSR	fractional synthetic rate
DC	dendritic cell	ft	foot
DEXA	dual-energy X-ray absorptiometry	g	gram
DIC	disseminated intravascular coagulation	GABA	gamma-aminobutyric acid
DIS	daily interruption of sedation	GC	glucocorticoid
dL	decilitre	GCS	Glasgow coma scale
DLCO	diffusing capacity for carbon monoxide	GFP	green fluorescence protein
DNA	deoxyribonucleic acid	GFR	glomerular filtration rate
DSM	Diagnostic and Statistical Manual of Mental Disorders	GH	growth hormone
		GLUT	glucose transporter
DTI	diffusion tensor imaging	GM-CSF	granulocyte-macrophage colony-stimulating factor
ECCM	extracellular collagen matrix		
ECG	electrocardiography	GP	general practitioner
ECHO	echocardiography	GWAS	genome-wide association studies
ECM	extracellular matrix	Gy	gray
EEF	eukaryotic elongation factor	HADS	Hospital Anxiety and Depression Scale
EEG	electroencephalogram	HCO_3^-	bicarbonate ion
EGF	epidermal growth factor	H & E	haematoxylin and eosin (stain)
eGFR	estimated glomerular filtration rate	HF	heart failure
EIF	eukaryotic initiation factor	HGF	hepatocyte growth factor
EM	electron microscopy	HHD	handheld dynamometry
EMDR	eye movement desensitization and reprocessing	HIF	hypoxia-inducible factor
		HIV	human immunodeficiency virus
EMG	electromyography	HO	heterotopic ossification
EMS	electrical muscle stimulation	HR	hazard ratio
EMT	epithelial-mesenchymal transition	HRQoL	health-related quality of life
EN	enteral nutrition	HSC	haematopoietic stem cell
EndoMT	endothelial-mesenchymal transition	Hz	hertz
EPO	erythropoietin	IADL	instrumental activity of daily living
EQ-5D	EuroQol-5D	ICD	International Classification of Disease
ERF	eukaryotic release factor	ICDSC	intensive care delirium screening checklist
ERK	extracellular signal regulated kinase		

ICF	International Classification of Functioning, Disability, and Health	mg	milligram
		MHC	myosin heavy chain
ICP	intracranial pressure	MI	myocardial infarction; motivational interviewing
ICU	intensive care unit		
ICUAW	ICU-acquired weakness	MIF	macrophage inhibitory factor
IES	Impact of Events Scale	min	minute
IES-R	Impact of Events Scale—Revised	MIP	maximal inspiratory pressure
IFN-γ	interferon gamma	miR	micro-RNA
Ig	immunoglobulin	mL	millitre
IGF-1	insulin-like growth factor-1	mm	millimetre
IHD	intermittent haemodialysis	mmHg	millimetre of mercury
IIT	intensive insulin therapy	mmol	millimole
IL	interleukin	MMP	metalloproteinase
IMV	invasive mechanical ventilation	MMV	mandatory minute ventilation
iNOS	inducible nitric oxide synthase	MODS	multiple organ dysfunction syndrome
IQ	intelligence quotient	MOF	multiple organ failure
I/R	ischaemia-reperfusion	MPB	muscle protein breakdown
IRF	inpatient rehabilitation facility	MPS	muscle protein synthesis
IRI	ischaemia-reperfusion injury	MRC	Medical Research Council
IRS-1	insulin receptor substrate 1	MRI	magnetic resonance imaging
IU	international unit	mRNA	messenger ribonucleic acid
IV	intravenous	ms	millisecond
IvIg	intravenous immunoglobulin	MSC	mesenchymal stem cell
IZ	infarct zone	mTOR	mammalian target of rapamycin
JNK	c-Jun N-terminal kinase	MV	mechanical ventilation
K$^+$	potassium ion	MVC	maximal voluntary contraction
kcal	kilocalorie	N	newton
kDa	kilodalton	Na$^+$	sodium ion
kg	kilogram	NAVA	neutrally adjusted ventilator assistance
kPa	kilopascal	NCS	nerve conduction studies
L	litre	NE	norepinephrine
LBM	lean body mass	NFκβ	nuclear factor kappa beta
LD	linkage disequilibrium	ng	nanogram
LDL	low-density lipoprotein	NHP	Nottingham Health Profile
LMA	laryngeal mask airway	NICE	National Institute for Health and Care Excellence
LPS	lipopolysaccharide		
LTAC	long-term acute care	NIH	National Institutes of Health
LV	left ventricular/ventricle	NIRS	near-infrared spectroscopy
lx	lux	NIV	non-invasive ventilation
m	metre	NIZ	non-infarcted zone
MAAS	Motor Activity Assessment Scale	NK	natural killer
MAP	mean arterial pressure	NKT	natural killer T (cell)
MAPK	mitogen-activated protein kinase	NMBA	neuromuscular blocking agent
MCS	mental health summary scale; mental component score	NMES	neuromuscular electrical stimulation
		nmol	nanomole

NNT	number to treat	PT	physical therapy
NO	nitric oxide	PTH	parathyroid hormone
NREM	non-rapid eye movement	PTS	post-traumatic stress
NSAID	non-steroidal anti-inflammatory drug	PTSD	post-traumatic stress disorder
		PTSS	post-traumatic symptom scale
NUTRIC	NUTrition Risk in the Critically ill (score)	QALY	quality-adjusted life year
		QoL	quality of life
NYHA	New York Heart Association	RANKL	receptor activator of nuclear transcription factor κB ligand
O_2	oxygen		
OA	osteoarthritis	RAS	renin-angiotensin system
OR	odds ratio	RASS	Richmond agitation and sedation scale
OT	occupational therapy	RBF	renal blood flow
P	probability	RCT	randomized controlled trial
$PaCO_2$	arterial partial pressure of carbon dioxide	REE	resting energy expenditure
		REM	rapid eye movement
PAI	plasminogen activator inhibitor	rhGH	recombinant human growth hormone
p-Akt	phosphorylated Akt	RICU	respiratory critical care unit
PaO_2	arterial partial pressure of oxygen	RNA	ribonucleic acid
PAV	proportional assist ventilation	RNS	reactive nitrogen species
PBW	predicted body weight	ROS	reactive oxygen species
PCS	physical health summary scale; physical component score; patient-controlled sedation	RRT	renal replacement therapy
		RSBI	rapid shallow breathing index
		s	second
PCT	procalcitonin	SAE	sepsis-associated encephalopathy
PD-1	programmed death 1	SaO_2	arterial oxygen saturation
PDGF	platelet-derived growth factor	SAPS	Simplified Acute Physiology Score
Pdi	diaphragm pressure	SARS	severe acute respiratory syndrome
PDS	Post-traumatic Diagnostic Scale	SBT	spontaneous breathing trial
PEEP	positive end-expiratory pressure	SCCM	Society of Critical Care Medicine
Pemax	maximal expiratory pressure	SCID	Structured Clinical Interview for DSM-IV
PET	positron emission tomography		
PFC	prefrontal cortex	SCN	suprachiasmatic nucleus
Pgas	gastric pressure	SD	standard deviation
PGHS	prostaglandin-H synthase	SEM	standard error of the mean
PICS	post-intensive care syndrome	SF-36	Short-form 36
PICS-F	post-intensive care syndrome-family	SIMV	synchronized intermittent mandatory ventilation
PI3K	phosphatidylinositol-3 kinase		
Pimax	maximal inspiratory pressure	Sir	silent information regulator
PMV	prolonged mechanical ventilation	SIRS	systemic inflammatory response syndrome
PN	parenteral nutrition		
Poes	oesophageal pressure	SLED	sustained low-efficiency dialysis
POLST	Physician Orders for Life Sustaining Treatment	SNAP	sensory nerve action potential
		SNF	skilled nursing facility
PRIS	propofol infusion syndrome	SNIP	sniff nasal inspiratory pressure
PSG	polysomnography	SNP	single nucleotide polymorphism
PSV	pressure support ventilation	SOFA	sequential organ failure

SpO$_2$	oxygen saturation		TwPdi	twitch Pdi
SWS	slow-wave sleep		TWEAK	TNF-related weak inducer of apoptosis
SWU	specialized weaning units			
TBI	traumatic brain injury		TwQ	quadriceps twitch response
TBSA-B	total body surface area burned		UK	United Kingdom
^{99m}Tc	technetium-99m		UPP	ubiquitin-proteasome pathway
TCR	T cell receptor		US	United States
TDT	transmission disequilibrium test		UTR	untranslated region
TEC	tubular epithelial cell		VAP	ventilator-associated pneumonia
TENS	transcutaneous electrical nerve stimulator		VAS	visual analogue scale
			VEGF	vascular endothelial cell growth factor
TGF	transforming growth factor			
TIMP	tissue inhibitor of metalloproteinase		VFD	ventilator-free day
TIR	timing it right		VICS	Vancouver Interaction and Calmness Scale
TKA	total knee arthroplasty			
TMS	transcranial magnetic stimulation		VIDD	ventilator-induced diaphragmatic dysfunction
TNF	tumour necrosis factor			
TNF-α	tumour necrosis factor alpha		VLPO	ventrolateral preoptic
Treg	regulatory T cell		VNTR	variable number of tandem repeats
TSH	thyroid-stimulating hormone		vs	versus
TST	total sleep time		WHO	World Health Organization
TTM	transtheoretical model		WHODAS II	WHO Disability Assessment Schedule II
TUG	Timed Up and Go (test)			
TwAP	adductor pollicis twitch tension		WOB	work of breathing
TwPaw	twitch airway pressure		YFP	yellow fluorescent protein
			ZDRS	Zung Depression Rating Scale

Part 1

Life after the ICU

Chapter 1

Introduction: Life after the ICU

Margaret S. Herridge

Surviving critical illness is not the happy ending that we imagined for our patients. No one really understood that saving someone's life in the intensive care unit (ICU) could cause harm and suffering for months or years to follow. A historic emphasis on mortality outcomes after critical illness could never have prepared us for the reality of the post-ICU experience, namely, long-term physical and neuropsychological dysfunction, ongoing health care utilization and incurred costs, and the risk of financial and mental health devastation of families. Forty-five years ago, Ashbaugh and colleagues published their landmark paper on the acute respiratory distress syndrome (ARDS)[1] and, although they did not realize this at the time, sparked the beginning of a movement to understand what happened to some of the sickest patients we care for in our critical care units.

The evolution of ICU outcomes work has progressed in a very systematic way over these past several decades. The initial outcome metric was physiologic, with countless studies evaluating cardiopulmonary function in samples of post-ARDS patients. This progressed to the study of generic health-related quality of life (HRQoL) which showed marked decrements in physical function without a clear understanding of contributing factors, but with the assumption that disability was the result of post-ARDS residual pulmonary disease. Next came an understanding that ARDS patients sustain important neurocognitive dysfunction and mood disorders. Subsequent in-person follow-up studies, employing exercise and functional measures, helped to identify muscle wasting and weakness as another central morbidity and determinant of compromised HRQoL.

Early outcomes work focused on ARDS but has now become generalized to include diverse populations of patients, organized into different clinical phenotypes with varied and distinct outcome patterns. Currently, there is an emerging spectrum of disability encompassing the younger and previously healthy, older patient with comorbid illness, the elderly with pre-existing functional disability, and the very long-term ventilated patient. We have moved away from simple cataloguing of morbidity to gaining a better understanding of ICU-based risk factors for long-term disability and initiating the generation of a hierarchy for competing risks associated with different ICU-based treatments. Current work is also focused on the link between clinical phenotype and molecular mechanisms of disease and the creation of individualized rehabilitation programmes, based on different vulnerabilities and risk. To embrace the notion of outcomes extending from epigenetics to family caregiver and patient mood disorders is a remarkable evolution in our approach and thinking.

This initial section of the text will help to orient the reader to the magnitude and burden of critical illness, its mortality, detailed morbidity, and costs. The central role of the family caregiver as outcome and risk modifier will be highlighted and further reinforced by personal essays from a wife and husband about their experiences after severe sepsis with multiple organ dysfunction. To understand how to make people better, we first need a description and proper framing of the issues that need to be addressed, and this introductory chapter will provide this essential context.

Reference

1 Ashbaugh DG, Bigelow DB, Petty TL Levine BE. Acute respiratory distress in adults. *Lancet* 1967; 2:319–23.

Chapter 2

Critical Illness and Long-Term Outcomes Worldwide

Neill K.J. Adhikari

Defining the worldwide burden of critical illness

Details of the global burden of various diseases, including cancer, cardiovascular disease, tuberculosis, and human immunodeficiency virus (HIV)/acquired immunodeficiency syndrome (AIDS), are available from web-based resources.[1] However, no reliable international comparative epidemiologic data on critical illness syndromes, such as ARDS, sepsis, and multiple organ dysfunction, are available. Similarly, although clinicians are better at appreciating complications of critical illness, including pulmonary dysfunction, weakness, impairment in activities of daily living (ADL), psychiatric disorders, cognitive decline, and an overall decrement in HRQoL,[2] epidemiologic data are limited and restricted to the US.

Several challenges impair the acquisition of detailed population-based data on critical illness and its sequelae. First, critical illness syndromes have no single diagnostic test, unlike serology for HIV or troponin for myocardial infarction. Definitions for sepsis,[3–5] nosocomial infections,[6,7] and ARDS[8,9] are derived by consensus bodies, subject to revision, and based on clinical, laboratory, radiologic, and physiologic criteria. Some definitions also lack reliability.[10,11] Psychiatric outcomes of critical illness are also syndrome-based, although ascertainment can be done by interviewers using standard assessment tools.[12] Second, compared with chronic diseases like cancer, asthma, and tuberculosis, critical illness syndromes have a relatively brief prodrome and high short-term mortality, which may be higher in countries with fewer ICU resources. This limits the number of prevalent cases available for study at any given time relative to chronic diseases. Sequelae in survivors, on the other hand, generally last months to years, and, therefore, cross-sectional methods should give more reliable data on the burden of disease. Third, critical illness is harder to study with existing administrative databases[13] than trauma or cardiovascular disease, because it is not defined by a procedure or well-captured by hospital coding. Population-based studies of non-mortality outcomes of critical illness have thus far been limited to the US and have linked cohort studies with ascertainment of cognitive[14,15] and functional[14] status to administrative databases to define exposures of ICU admission, critical illness (e.g. sepsis), or mechanical ventilation (MV). Finally, the epidemiology of critical **illness** and its sequelae depend on the availability and intensity of ICU resources, leading to the tautology that, without ICUs, there can be no critical illness or long-term consequences thereof. The epidemiology also depends on the intensity of other health services, since some critical illness is a side effect of other therapeutic interventions such as surgical procedures or bone marrow transplantation. Even mortality after critical illness reflects the interplay between a clinical decision to limit intensive care and the consequences of the disease.

Countries with the resources to provide organ transplantation, intensive chemotherapy for cancer, and surgery for cardiovascular disease in elderly patients with comorbid illness will have a higher burden of critical illness and morbidity in survivors associated with these conditions and treatments than those that do not. Although there is agreement that critical illness occurs outside of the ICU, research on critical illness, particularly internationally comparative epidemiology, generally occurs inside those walls. Observational studies comparing international practice have been conducted for sepsis,[16] nosocomial infection,[17,18] MV,[19,20] and end-of-life care[21] and have been used to generate severity of illness scores.[22,23] These studies were conducted in ICUs, using period prevalence or 'snapshot' data collection over short time periods. Although they show process and outcome differences among countries, they do not provide accurate population-based incidence data, as they lack a population denominator and complete case ascertainment within geographic areas. With a few exceptions,[20,24] these studies have not included data from the developing world.

Data on structure, case mix, care processes, and outcomes of critical care in low resource settings are restricted to descriptive studies suggesting limited intensive care beds, infrastructure, personnel, and equipment. Patients are thus admitted to ICUs with very high illness severity, and, not surprisingly, narrative reviews[25,26] and limited observational data[27,28] suggest that clinical outcomes are poor, owing, at least in part, to severe limitations of resources.[29,30] Maximizing the use of this scarce resource requires attention to regionalization and integration, based on prevailing local realities.[31] Studies on long-term morbidity following acute illness in the developing world have generally focused on children,[32–35] stroke,[36–38] and injury[39,40] and are limited to single centres, with few exceptions.[36,37]

As a prototype critical illness syndrome, observational studies of sepsis highlight these epidemiological challenges. Incidence, prevalence, and prognosis depend on whether the study design considers the measurement of population-based incidence or incidence among those treated in ICUs. Other important sources of bias include the duration of follow-up for patients admitted to hospital (one day vs the entire hospital stay), case definition, type of institution, study site (restricted to ICU or not), seasonal variability, and case mix.[41] US-based population studies, using administrative data, suggest a population-based incidence of 300 cases/100 000 person-years for severe sepsis[42] and 240 cases/100 000 person-years for sepsis.[43] When the setting is the ICU, most studies find a treated incidence of approximately ten cases per 100 ICU admissions.[44] Others have found a much higher incidence in settings with fewer ICU beds,[45,46] likely reflecting the admission of sicker patients or exclusion of low-risk patients for post-operative monitoring from the denominator.[16] Follow-up studies of sepsis have shown an increased risk of moderate to severe cognitive impairment and functional decline (measured by loss of ADL) after hospitalization for severe sepsis, compared to general hospital admissions.[14] Among patients over 65 receiving Medicare in the US, one study estimated that 637 867 (344 111) individuals had survived severe sepsis for at least 3 (5) years as of the end of 2008, with at least 106 311 (95% confidence interval (CI), 79 692–133 930) survivors with moderate to severe cognitive impairment and 476 862 (95% CI, 455 026–498 698) survivors with functional disability, requiring assistance with at least one activity or instrumental activity of daily living (IADL).[47] These effects may be primarily due to hospitalization for acute illness, rather than critical illness or MV per se,[15,48,49] similar to the increased risk of mortality in the 3 years following ICU discharge in the US among the elderly, which was driven by hospitalization, rather than ICU admission.[50]

Defining the population-based epidemiology of sequelae of critical illness therefore requires solutions to two problems. The first is to estimate the global burden of critical illness. Potential approaches and their challenges include:

1. Count the admissions to ICUs. Although this has the advantage of simplicity, variability in the availability of ICUs and the life support technologies they contain mean that case-mix and illness

severity will vary widely. In particular, this approach will seriously underestimate the incidence of critical illness in low- and middle-income countries. Comparisons among high-income countries are also challenging, as illustrated in a recent cohort study comparing characteristics and outcomes of medical admissions between the US and UK, where even standardized hospital mortality could not be reliably compared because of differences in discharge practices.[51]

2. Apply syndrome-specific data to the world population to generate very rough estimates of the global burden of critical illness syndromes (see Table 2.1). Of note, these estimates may underestimate the burden in developing countries, where a higher proportion of deaths are due to infection and injury, and assume that the age, gender, risk factor distributions, and critical care capacity are similar to the North American populations that generated the epidemiologic data. These latter assumptions are clearly flawed. Even in the developed world, epidemiologic data on ICU bed availability are sparse.

3. Estimate the burden of critical illness, using data on causes of death whose definitions are more standardized (e.g. from the Global Burden of Disease Project at http://www.who.int/topics/global_burden_of_disease/en/). This approach would model the burden of critical illness by adding together all deaths from acute causes, assuming that all patients who died had premortem critical illness, and an estimate of survivors of critical illness for each acute condition. For example, in high-resource countries, most patients with pneumonia or traumatic injuries leading to death would have been admitted to an ICU, and some multiple of the number of deaths would equal the number of survivors of critical illness. Using this framework, the most important causes of death to consider are those that arise from acute illness (e.g. acute infections, trauma, ischaemic heart disease); many chronic diseases (e.g. malignancy, hepatitis B and C) could be excluded. This burden could be estimated for each country and then compared to estimates of that country's critical care resources, including, e.g. the per capita number of acute hospital beds, intensive care beds with MV, and high dependency beds.

Even if the burden of critical illness can be quantified, the second challenge is to document the burden of sequelae of critical illness in survivors. Until these sequelae are more accurately coded in administrative data, cohort studies of survivors of critical illness with outcomes ascertainment, using culturally appropriate, translated, reliable, and valid instruments,[52] will be needed. Extrapolating population-based estimates of the burden of critical illness from the US to other parts of the world (akin to approach 2, discussed previously) is problematic for the reasons already discussed; in addition, the burden of post-critical illness morbidity likely differs in critically ill populations that are substantially younger than in the US. Younger critical illness survivors would be expected to have fewer comorbidities but may suffer substantial economic hardship if post-ICU morbidity prevents them from returning to previous employment.[53] The role of HIV coinfection, which is prevalent among septic patients in sub-Saharan Africa,[27] in modifying the trajectory of post-critical illness morbidity remains unexplored but has implications for patients, clinicians, and health policy makers.

These challenges imply that it may never be possible to define the global burden of critical illness or of its sequelae. Even the less ambitious goal of defining the global capacity to deliver critical care is difficult, given the lack of uniform definitions for an ICU bed, as illustrated in a study that found ≥5-fold variation in ICU bed availability among eight developed countries.[54] Nevertheless, meeting this goal is necessary to allocate health system resources, improve the quality of care for critically ill patients, and plan for unexpected surges (such as during a pandemic). Answering this question would also provide impetus for initiatives to improve the outcomes of acutely ill adults in low-resource settings such as the World Health Organization's (WHO) Integrated

Table 2.1 Rough estimates of global burden of critical illness by World Bank region*

World Bank region[a]	Population in 2004	Deaths (number x 1000 in 2004, % of total in region)[b]						Estimated potential burden of critical illness (annual number x 1000)[c]		
		Total	Infection	Maternal conditions	Malignant neoplasms	Cardiovascular diseases	Injuries	Patients mechanically ventilated	ARDS	Sepsis
High-income countries	949 818	8008	468 (5.8%)	1 (0.0%)	2146 (26.8%)	2978 (37.2%)	490 (9.8%)	2000–3000	170–820	2300–2800
East Asia and Pacific	1 892 113	14 000	1777 (12.7%)	44 (0.3%)	2284 (16.3%)	4439 (31.7%)	1678 (12.0%)	3900–5900	340–1600	4500–5700
Europe and Central Asia	476 096	5684	284 (5.0%)	3 (0.1%)	820 (14.4%)	3248 (57.1%)	604 (10.6%)	990–1500	85–410	1100–1400
Latin America and Caribbean	549 187	3499	474 (13.5%)	16 (0.4%)	543 (15.5%)	998 (28.5%)	407 (11.6%)	1100–1700	98–470	1300–1600
Middle East and North Africa	324 542	2114	299 (14.1%)	15 (0.7%)	181 (8.6%)	732 (34.6%)	281 (13.3%)	680–1000	58–280	780–970
South Asia	1 493 430	13 778	3993 (29.0%)	179 (1.3%)	954 (6.9%)	3438 (25.0%)	1476 (10.7%)	3100–4700	270–1300	3600–4500
Sub-Saharan Africa	749 269	11 662	6475 (55.5%)	269 (2.3%)	493 (4.2%)	1232 (10.6%)	847 (7.3%)	1600–2400	130–650	1800–2200
World	6 436 826	58 772	13 777 (23.4%)	527 (0.9%)	7424 (12.6%)	17 073 (29.0%)	5784 (9.8%)	13 000–20 000	1150–5500	15 000–19 000

[a] Regions include countries classified according to the World Bank income and geographic categories used in the Disease Control Priorities Project (details available at http://www.dcp2.org/pubs/GBD). World totals include some countries and territories not included in the World Bank regions.

[b] Infection includes categories of infectious and parasitic diseases and respiratory infections; maternal conditions include sepsis, haemorrhage, hypertensive disorders, obstructed labour, and abortions; cardiovascular diseases include rheumatic, ischaemic, hypertensive, and inflammatory diseases, and cerebrovascular diseases; injuries include both unintentional and intentional causes.

[c] These estimates are approximate. They are based on North American population-based estimates of the annual incidence of MV,[96,97] ARDS,[61,98] and sepsis[42] extrapolated to other regions, based on population. They assume that other regions have similar intensive care capacity, underlying risk factors for the outcomes listed, and age and sex distributions. These numbers can be best interpreted as the burden of critical illness, given capacity and population similar to North America.

Reprinted from *The Lancet*, 376, 9749, Adhikari NK et al., 'Critical care and the burden of critical illness in adults', pp. 1339–1346, Copyright 2010, with permission from Elsevier. Data on population and deaths are from the Global Burden of Disease Project, available at http://www.who.int/healthinfo/global_burden_disease/en/index.html.

Management of Adolescent and Adult Acute Illness guidelines.[55,56] A recent initiative to improve global surgical care that started with a study of the global burden of surgery[57,58] provides a model for this approach.

What global trends will affect the burden of critical illness and morbidities in survivors?

Several emerging trends all but guarantee that the demand for critical care services will increase, generating an increasing number of survivors.

Urbanization

More than half of the world's population now lives in an urban setting, a number that will only continue to rise (http://esa.un.org/unpd/wup/index.htm). As more people live in cities, their access to referral hospitals with critical care resources will rise. At the same time, increasing population density, especially in large slums, may enhance transmission of infectious diseases previously confined to rural areas, imposing additional demands on hospital care.[59] As recent pandemics have illustrated, critical care resources remain the last defence against death from large outbreaks of disease. This high population density would also be expected to magnify the impact of bioterrorism and natural disasters. An advantage of urbanization, however, is that higher population density should facilitate the provision of specialized critical care and rehabilitation services, since clinical expertise is concentrated in cities.[60]

Patient demographics

The prevalence of diseases and comorbid conditions that predispose to critical illness increases with age. As the rest of medicine advances, care has intensified for high-risk patients with multiple comorbidities (such as diabetes mellitus, chronic kidney disease (CKD), congestive heart failure, chronic obstructive pulmonary disease (COPD), and malignancy), compromised immune systems, and extreme old age. As these treatment boundaries are pushed, complications can be expected to increase. Assuming no effective treatment to prevent ALI, extrapolation of current US epidemiology suggests over 330 000 cases per year by 2030—a 50% increase over current numbers.[61] Parallel increases can be expected for sepsis[42] and MV.[62] Driven by this demographic reality, such demand may be particularly acute in the US, in which ICU utilization among hospitalized patients who die is very high (47% vs 10% in England), particularly among the elderly.[63]

The combination of an ageing population and relatively fewer young wage earners in developed countries will create a demand for critical care that cannot be fulfilled as it is currently delivered, even if economies recover. The inverted demographic pyramid in developed nations will be mirrored by a predominantly youthful population in many developing nations with high fertility rates and limited public health and critical care infrastructure. Although the latter trend has limited implications for critical care, given currently low ICU capacity in the developing world, the increase in burden of (largely untreated) critical illness from resultant conflicts and disasters seems inevitable, and projected political effects worldwide are profound.[64]

Hospital organization

Demand for intensivists' services will not only be driven by demographics, but also by their expanding role in hospitals. The number of ICU beds in US hospitals increased by 6.5% from 2000 to 2005, while other inpatient beds decreased by 4.2%, reflecting a prioritization of intensive care services.[65] Their role outside the ICU is increasing, as part of rapid response teams to assess acutely ill patients on general wards and prevent critical illness by early intervention[66] and in staffing follow-up clinics to screen for and treat post-critical illness complications,[67] although the effectiveness of these interventions is not established. Finally, regionalization of critical care services to high-volume centres,[68] if widely implemented, will increase requirements for critical care services at high-volume centres.

While most critical care services are organized with a trained intensivist managing the ICU, this model is not universal. Most studies exploring the effects of this model come from the US, the country with the most variation in intensive care delivery models. Available data suggest that intensivists improve patient outcomes,[69] possibly because they have the training and time commitment to provide care to very sick patients and their families or because they are able to manage the critical care team most effectively, but the question cannot be feasibly explored in randomized trials and the evidence from observational studies is not uniform.[70,71]

The overall effects of these and other decisions regarding hospital organization on the demand for critical care services acutely and after the episode of critical illness are unclear. Most appear to increase demand on a specialty with insufficient numbers and trainees,[72-74] although this mismatch between supply and demand is common to all specialties.[75] Potential solutions to this shortfall include training more intensivists, increased development and dissemination of guidelines and protocols, training of non-physician clinicians to substitute for intensivists, and telemedicine to allow experienced physicians and nurses to expand the geographic scope of their care (see Table 2.2).[76] For example, the WHO has developed two clinical training programmes to improve the technical capacity of non-specialist clinicians caring for critically ill adults in resource-limited settings. Training, based on the *Integrated Management of Adolescent and Adult Illness District Clinician Manual*, provides guidance on recognition, management, and monitoring of adults with severe respiratory distress and septic shock on medical wards.[56] *Critical Care Training for Management of Severe Influenza Infection* (available at http://influenzatraining.org/en/) teaches best practices for ICU clinicians, including safe MV. Both programmes complement evidence- and consensus-based recommendations; other short courses in general critical care have also been taught to non-specialists internationally.[77] Although disseminating knowledge to clinicians caring for severely ill patients is a worthy objective, the risk of extending approaches to critical care broadly accepted in high-resource settings to low-resource settings without evaluation must be acknowledged. For example, a recent randomized trial of fluid resuscitation strategies for febrile hypoperfused children in Africa provided a cautionary tale when it found excess short-term mortality with fluid boluses that are the standard of resuscitation in high-resource ICUs.[78] In contrast, although telemedicine-based approaches are conceptually attractive, they would require additional human and technological resources that may be feasible in middle- or high-income settings but would challenge the capacity of developing world health systems. The evidence that either telemedicine or the deployment of non-physicians as primary ICU clinicians is a safe and effective substitute for intensivist staffing is modest.

Wars, disasters, and pandemics

Natural and human-generated events generate acute and unpredictably large numbers of critically ill patients. Examples in the modern medical era have been rare; however, this situation may change if a pandemic of influenza or another virulent infection emerges to cause respiratory or other organ dysfunction. The 2003 outbreak of severe acute respiratory syndrome (SARS), mostly localized to East Asia[79,80] and Toronto, Canada,[81] highlighted challenges that would be amplified

Table 2.2 Strategies to address mismatch between demand for critical care and supply of intensivists

Strategy	Description	Comment
Train more intensivists	Increase number of trainees or offer incentives (shorter training, more pay)	Addressing intensivist shortage cannot be done in isolation from all physician specialties (see https://www.aamc.org/initiatives/fixdocshortage/)
Train other clinicians to provide intensive care	Training of non-intensivist physicians, nurses, or other clinical personnel to provide primary care for critically ill patients	Short courses for critical care training, incorporating evidence and expert opinion,[56,77] have been delivered to providers in many countries Limited evidence that non-physician providers provide safe care, compared to physician trainees[102]
Provide decision support to help intensivists provide better patient care more efficiently (adapted from [99])	Guideline: systematically developed statement, integrating current evidence Clinical pathway: comprehensive, stepwise, interdisciplinary care plan Protocol: set of sequential steps to standardize patient care Algorithm: set of instructions for particular issue, presented as series of decision points, with branches depending on patient status Order set: group of orders with common functional purpose, used for a specific patient[100]	Quality and clinical utility of tools are variable Knowledge translation interventions modestly improve processes of care for the critically ill[101] Tools based strictly on evidence-based guidelines may fail to cover common critical care crises (e.g. management of sudden desaturation in mechanically ventilated patients)
Telemedicine	Real-time exchange of patient information and direct interaction between bedside provider and geographically separated intensivist, facilitated by audio and video links	Potential to extend specialist coverage to units without it Implementation requires well-developed telecommunications infrastructure inside and outside the hospital Modest evidence of improved patient outcomes, but optimal telemedicine configuration unclear[76]

by a much broader pandemic: high illness severity of affected patients, stretched critical care resources diverted from general medical and high-risk elective surgical cases to look after SARS patients, transmission to health care workers, and high workload for remaining clinical staff.[82,83] Data from the 2009 pandemic of H1N1 influenza suggests that it caused serious illness and death in young, previously healthy persons, with a high burden of mechanically ventilated patients and deaths.[84–86]

Multiple ongoing wars, acts of terrorism, and the 2010 Haiti earthquake serve to remind us that both human-generated and natural disasters can quickly overwhelm local health care infrastructure in both developed and developing countries, even with mild to moderate numbers of casualties. Only recently has disaster management, including advanced planning for surge capacity, mobile critical care, triage and rationing, hospital resource management, and staffing, become an integrated part of critical care academic activity.[87,88] However, during times of war, systematic cluster household sampling indicates that most excess deaths, and by extension most demands for intensive care, do not arise from violence but from medical conditions arising from the breakdown of public health infrastructure (such as cholera) or lack of treatment of chronic disease due to interruption of pharmaceutical supplies.[89,90] In developing countries, these realities are aggravated by the presence of endemic diseases like trauma and HIV that represent a significant burden to healthcare systems.

Economics

The current economic slowdown will likely harm health care delivery in both developed and developing countries by decreasing government and donor expenditures, diverting household funds for health care to other essential expenditures, and increasing competition for government services as private insurance becomes less affordable.[91,92] Critically ill patients will not be spared, given that their care consumes between 0.5 and 1% of gross domestic product, at least in North America.[65] As the gross world product falls, the proportion consumed by health care in developed countries, and critical care specifically, will increase markedly, unless the demand for these services falls or can be delivered more cheaply. Health care funders facing these facts may focus spending on primary and preventive care. The current global recession and heightened disparities are highlighting decades-old questions: How effective is critical care? How **cost**-effective is critical care? How can we ration a service perceived to rescue lives in imminent risk of death?[93,94] Despite these realities, US clinicians perceive little or no resource restraints on their ability to deliver intensive care.[95]

Conclusion

To ascertain the worldwide demand for critical care and the burden of sequelae in survivors of critical illness, we need population-based estimates of critical illness (separate from the number of ICU beds), the resources available to care for it, and the morbidity among survivors. Detailed multi-country observational studies are likely to be required for suitably granular data on post-critical illness morbidity using common definitions. To ascertain the number of critically ill patients and acute care resources, modelling using existing administrative health databases would be more feasible and comprehensive. Such research would highlight the need of most of the world's critically ill patients for effective, feasible, and scaleable interventions to prevent and treat critical illness and its consequences.

Acknowledgement

Portions of this chapter, including Table 2.1, are reprinted from *The Lancet*, 376, 9749, Adhikari NK et al., 'Critical care and the burden of critical illness in adults', pp. 1339–1346, Copyright 2010, with permission from Elsevier.

References

1 **World Health Organization.** *Global health observatory.* (2013). Geneva: World Health Organization.

2 **Needham DM, Davidson J, Cohen H, et al.** Improving long-term outcomes after discharge from intensive care unit: report from a stakeholders' conference. *Crit Care Med* 2012;**40**:502–9.

3 **Bone RC, Balk RA, Cerra FB, et al.** Definitions for sepsis and organ failure and guidelines for the use of innovative therapies in sepsis. The ACCP/SCCM Consensus Conference Committee. American College of Chest Physicians/Society of Critical Care Medicine. *Chest* 1992;**101**:1644–55.

4 Levy MM, Fink MP, Marshall JC, et al. 2001 SCCM/ESICM/ACCP/ATS/SIS International Sepsis Definitions Conference. *Crit Care Med* 2003;**31**:1250–6.

5 Greenhalgh DG, Saffle JR, Holmes JH, et al. American Burn Association consensus conference to define sepsis and infection in burns. *J Burn Care Res* 2007;**28**:776–90.

6 Garner JS, Jarvis WR, Emori TG, et al. CDC definitions for nosocomial infections, 1988. *Am J Infect Control* 1988;**16**:128–40.

7 Calandra T, Cohen J. The international sepsis forum consensus conference on definitions of infection in the intensive care unit. *Crit Care Med* 2005;**33**:1538–48.

8 Bernard GR, Artigas A, Brigham KL, et al. The American-European Consensus Conference on ARDS. Definitions, mechanisms, relevant outcomes, and clinical trial coordination. *Am J Respir Crit Care Med* 1994;**149**:819–24.

9 The ARDS Definition Task Force. Acute respiratory distress syndrome: the Berlin definition. *JAMA* 2012;**307**:2526–33.

10 Villar J, Perez-Mendez L, Lopez J, et al. An early PEEP/F_1O_2 trial identifies different degrees of lung injury in patients with acute respiratory distress syndrome. *Am J Respir Crit Care Med* 2007;**176**:795–804.

11 Rubenfeld GD, Caldwell E, Granton J, et al. Interobserver variability in applying a radiographic definition for ARDS. *Chest* 1999;**116**:1347–53.

12 Homaifar BY, Brenner LA, Gutierrez PM, et al. Sensitivity and specificity of the Beck Depression Inventory-II in persons with traumatic brain injury. *Arch Phys Med Rehabil* 2009;**90**:652–6.

13 Wunsch H, Harrison DA, Rowan K. Health services research in critical care using administrative data. *J Crit Care* 2005;**20**:264–9.

14 Iwashyna TJ, Ely EW, Smith DM, et al. Long-term cognitive impairment and functional disability among survivors of severe sepsis. *JAMA* 2010;**304**:1787–94.

15 Ehlenbach WJ, Hough CL, Crane PK, et al. Association between acute care and critical illness hospitalization and cognitive function in older adults. *JAMA* 2010;**303**:763–70.

16 Vincent JL, Sakr Y, Sprung CL, et al. Sepsis in European intensive care units: results of the SOAP study. *Crit Care Med* 2006;**34**:344–53.

17 Vincent JL, Bihari DJ, Suter PM, et al. The prevalence of nosocomial infection in intensive care units in Europe. Results of the European Prevalence of Infection in Intensive Care (EPIC) Study. EPIC International Advisory Committee. *JAMA* 1995;**274**:639–44.

18 Bloemendaal AL, Fluit AC, Jansen WM, et al. Acquisition and cross-transmission of Staphylococcus aureus in European intensive care units. *Infect Control Hosp Epidemiol* 2009;**30**:117–24.

19 Esteban A, Anzueto A, Frutos F, et al. Characteristics and outcomes in adult patients receiving mechanical ventilation: a 28-day international study. *JAMA* 2002;**287**:345–55.

20 Esteban A, Ferguson ND, Meade MO, et al. Evolution of mechanical ventilation in response to clinical research. *Am J Respir Crit Care Med* 2008;**177**:170–7.

21 Sprung CL, Cohen SL, Sjokvist P, et al. End-of-life practices in European intensive care units: the Ethicus Study. *JAMA* 2003;**290**:790–7.

22 Knaus WA, Draper EA, Wagner DP, et al. APACHE II: a severity of disease classification system. *Crit Care Med* 1985;**13**:818–29.

23 Metnitz PG, Moreno RP, Almeida E, et al. SAPS 3–From evaluation of the patient to evaluation of the intensive care unit. Part 1: objectives, methods and cohort description. *Intensive Care Med* 2005;**31**:1336–44.

24 Rosenthal VD, Maki DG, Graves N. The International Nosocomial Infection Control Consortium (INICC): goals and objectives, description of surveillance methods, and operational activities. *Am J Infect Control* 2008;**36**:e1–12.

25 Towey RM, Ojara S. Intensive care in the developing world. *Anaesthesia* 2007;**62**(Suppl 1):32–7.

26 Dunser MW, Baelani I, Ganbold L. A review and analysis of intensive care medicine in the least developed countries. *Crit Care Med* 2006;**34**:1234–42.

27 Jacob ST, Moore CC, Banura P, et al. Severe sepsis in two Ugandan hospitals: a prospective observational study of management and outcomes in a predominantly HIV-1 infected population. *PLoS One* 2009;**4**:e7782.

28 Kwizera A, Dunser M, Nakibuuka J. National intensive care unit bed capacity and ICU patient characteristics in a low income country. *BMC Res Notes* 2012;**5**:475.

29 Baelani I, Jochberger S, Laimer T, et al. Availability of critical care resources to treat patients with severe sepsis or septic shock in Africa: a self-reported, continent-wide survey of anaesthesia providers. *Crit Care* 2011;**15**:R10.

30 Phua J, Koh Y, Du B, et al. Management of severe sepsis in patients admitted to Asian intensive care units: prospective cohort study. *BMJ* 2011;**342**:d3245.

31 Bhagwanjee S, Scribante J. National audit of critical care resources in South Africa—unit and bed distribution. *S Afr Med J* 2007;**97**:1311–4.

32 Abdullah JM, Kumaraswamy N, Awang N, et al. Persistence of cognitive deficits following paediatric head injury without professional rehabilitation in rural East Coast Malaysia. *Asian J Surg* 2005;**28**: 163–7.

33 Wilde JCH, Lameris W, van Hasselt EH, et al. Challenges and outcome of Wilms' tumour management in a resource-constrained setting. *Afr J Paediatr Surg* 2010;**7**:159–62.

34 Wandi F, Kiagi G, Duke T. Long-term outcome for children with bacterial meningitis in rural Papua New Guinea. *J Trop Pediatr* 2005;**51**:51–3.

35 Xu XJ, Tang YM, Song H, et al. Long-term outcome of childhood acute myeloid leukemia in a developing country: experience from a children's hospital in China. [Erratum appears in Leuk Lymphoma. 2011 Mar;52(3):544]. *Leuk Lymphoma* 2010;**51**:2262–9.

36 Kulesh SD, Kastsinevich TM, Kliatskova LA, et al. Long-term outcome after stroke in Belarus: the Grodno stroke study. *Stroke* 2011;**42**:3274–6.

37 Walker RW, Jusabani A, Aris E, et al. Post-stroke case fatality within an incident population in rural Tanzania. *J Neurol Neurosurg Psychiatry* 2011;**82**:1001–5.

38 Garbusinski JM, van der Sande MAB, Bartholome EJ, et al. Stroke presentation and outcome in developing countries: a prospective study in the Gambia. *Stroke* 2005;**36**:1388–93.

39 Gosselin RA, Coppotelli C. A follow-up study of patients with spinal cord injury in Sierra Leone. *Int Orthop* 2005;**29**:330–2.

40 Wal A. Long-term results of intramedullary pinning of forearm fractures in a developing country. *Aust N Z J Surg* 1997;**67**:622–4.

41 Angus DC, Pereira CA, Silva E. Epidemiology of severe sepsis around the world. *Endocr Metab Immune Disord Drug Targets* 2006;**6**:207–12.

42 Angus DC, Linde-Zwirble WT, Lidicker J, et al. Epidemiology of severe sepsis in the United States: analysis of incidence, outcome, and associated costs of care. *Crit Care Med* 2001;**29**:1303–10.

43 Martin GS, Mannino DM, Eaton S, et al. The epidemiology of sepsis in the United States from 1979 through 2000. *N Engl J Med* 2003;**348**:1546–54.

44 Linde-Zwirble WT, Angus DC. Severe sepsis epidemiology: sampling, selection, and society. *Crit Care* 2004;**8**:222–6.

45 Harrison DA, Welch CA, Eddleston JM. The epidemiology of severe sepsis in England, Wales and Northern Ireland, 1996 to 2004: secondary analysis of a high quality clinical database, the ICNARC Case Mix Programme Database. *Crit Care* 2006;**10**:R42.

46 Silva E, Pedro MA, Sogayar AC, et al. Brazilian Sepsis Epidemiological Study (BASES study). *Crit Care* 2004;**8**:R251–60.

47 Iwashyna TJ, Cooke CR, Wunsch H, et al. Population burden of long-term survivorship after severe sepsis in older Americans. *J Am Geriatr Soc* 2012;**60**:1070–7.

48 Iwashyna TJ, Netzer G, Langa KM, et al. Spurious inferences about long-term outcomes: the case of severe sepsis and geriatric conditions. *Am J Respir Crit Care Med* 2012;**185**:835–41.

49 Rubenfeld GD. Does the hospital make you older faster? *Am J Respir Crit Care Med* 2012;**185**:796–8.

50 Wunsch H, Guerra C, Barnato AE, et al. Three-year outcomes for Medicare beneficiaries who survive intensive care. *JAMA* 2010;**303**:849–56.

51 Wunsch H, Angus DC, Harrison DA, et al. Comparison of medical admissions to intensive care units in the United States and United Kingdom. *Am J Respir Crit Care Med* 2011;**183**:1666–73.

52 Wing JK, Babor T, Brugha T, et al. SCAN. Schedules for Clinical Assessment in Neuropsychiatry. *Arch Gen Psychiatry* 1990;**47**:589–93.

53 Herridge MS, Cheung AM, Tansey CM, et al. One-year outcomes in survivors of the acute respiratory distress syndrome. *N Engl J Med* 2003;**348**:683–93.

54 Wunsch H, Angus DC, Harrison DA, et al. Variation in critical care services across North America and Western Europe. *Crit Care Med* 2008;**36**:2787–9.

55 Crump JA, Gove S, Parry CM. Management of adolescents and adults with febrile illness in resource limited areas. *BMJ* 2011;**343**:d4847.

56 World Health Organization. *IMAI district clinician manual: hospital care for adolescents and adults: guidelines for the management of illnesses with limited resources.* (2011). Geneva: World Health Organization.

57 Haynes AB, Weiser TG, Berry WR, et al. A surgical safety checklist to reduce morbidity and mortality in a global population. *N Engl J Med* 2009;**360**:491–9.

58 Weiser TG, Regenbogen SE, Thompson KD, et al. An estimation of the global volume of surgery: a modelling strategy based on available data. *Lancet* 2008;**372**:139–44.

59 Alirol E, Getaz L, Stoll B, et al. Urbanisation and infectious diseases in a globalised world. *Lancet Infect Dis* 2011;**11**:131–41.

60 Gupta N, Zurn P, Diallo K, et al. Uses of population census data for monitoring geographical imbalance in the health workforce: snapshots from three developing countries. *Int J Equity Health* 2003;**2**:11.

61 Rubenfeld GD, Caldwell E, Peabody E, et al. Incidence and outcomes of acute lung injury. *N Engl J Med* 2005;**353**:1685–93.

62 Needham DM, Bronskill SE, Calinawan JR, et al. Projected incidence of mechanical ventilation in Ontario to 2026: preparing for the aging baby boomers. *Crit Care Med* 2005;**33**:574–9.

63 Wunsch H, Linde-Zwirble WT, Harrison DA, et al. Use of intensive care services during terminal hospitalizations in England and the United States. *Am J Respir Crit Care Med* 2009;**180**:875–80.

64 Jackson R, Howe N, with Strauss RaNK. *The graying of the great powers: demography and geopolitics in the 21st century.* Washington, DC: Center for Strategic and International Studies; 2008.

65 Halpern NA, Pastores SM. Critical care medicine in the United States 2000–5: an analysis of bed numbers, occupancy rates, payer mix, and costs. *Crit Care Med* 2010;**38**:65–71.

66 Winters BD, Pham JC, Hunt EA, et al. Rapid response systems: a systematic review. *Crit Care Med* 2007;**35**:1238–43.

67 Griffiths JA, Barber VS, Cuthbertson BH, et al. A national survey of intensive care follow-up clinics. *Anaesthesia* 2006;**61**:950–5.

68 Kahn JM, Goss CH, Heagerty PJ, et al. Hospital volume and the outcomes of mechanical ventilation. *N Engl J Med* 2006;**355**:41–50.

69 Pronovost PJ, Angus DC, Dorman T, et al. Physician staffing patterns and clinical outcomes in critically ill patients: a systematic review. *JAMA* 2002;**288**:2151–62.

70 Levy MM, Rapoport J, Lemeshow S, et al. Association between critical care physician management and patient mortality in the intensive care unit. *Ann Intern Med* 2008;**148**:801–9.

71 Rubenfeld GD, Angus DC. Are intensivists safe? *Ann Intern Med* 2008;**148**:877–9.

72 Angus DC, Kelley MA, Schmitz RJ, et al. Caring for the critically ill patient. Current and projected workforce requirements for care of the critically ill and patients with pulmonary disease: can we meet the requirements of an aging population? *JAMA* 2000;**284**:2762–70.

73 Robnett MK. Critical care nursing: workforce issues and potential solutions. *Crit Care Med* 2006;**34**(3 Suppl):S25–31.

74 Scribante J, Bhagwanjee S. National audit of critical care resources in South Africa—nursing profile. *S Afr Med J* 2007;**97**:1315–18.

75 Salsberg E, Grover A. Physician workforce shortages: implications and issues for academic health centers and policymakers. *Acad Med* 2006;**81**:782–7.

76 Wilcox ME, Adhikari NK. The effect of telemedicine in critically ill patients: systematic review and meta-analysis. *Crit Care* 2012;**16**:R127.

77 Joynt GM, Zimmerman J, Li TS, et al. A systematic review of short courses for nonspecialist education in intensive care. *J Crit Care* 2011;**26**:533.

78 Maitland K, Kiguli S, Opoka RO, et al. Mortality after fluid bolus in African children with severe infection. *N Engl J Med* 2011;**364**:2483–95.

79 Lee N, Hui D, Wu A, et al. A major outbreak of severe acute respiratory syndrome in Hong Kong. *N Engl J Med* 2003;**348**:1986–94.

80 Tsang KW, Ho PL, Ooi GC, et al. A cluster of cases of severe acute respiratory syndrome in Hong Kong. *N Engl J Med* 2003;**348**:1977–85.

81 Poutanen SM, Low DE, Henry B, et al. Identification of severe acute respiratory syndrome in Canada. *N Engl J Med* 2003;**348**:1995–2005.

82 Booth CM, Matukas LM, Tomlinson GA, et al. Clinical features and short-term outcomes of 144 patients with SARS in the greater Toronto area. *JAMA* 2003;**289**:2801–9.

83 Fowler RA, Lapinsky SE, Hallett D, et al. Critically ill patients with severe acute respiratory syndrome. *JAMA* 2003;**290**:367–73.

84 Dominguez-Cherit G, Lapinsky SE, Macias AE, et al. Critically ill patients with 2009 influenza A(H1N1) in Mexico. *JAMA* 2009;**302**:1880–7.

85 Kumar A, Zarychanski R, Pinto R, et al. Critically ill patients with 2009 influenza A(H1N1) infection in Canada. *JAMA* 2009;**302**:1872–9.

86 ANZIC Influenza Investigators, Webb SA, Pettilä V, et al. Critical care services and 2009 H1N1 influenza in Australia and New Zealand. *N Engl J Med* 2009;**361**:1925–34.

87 Christian MD, Hawryluck L, Wax RS, et al. Development of a triage protocol for critical care during an influenza pandemic. *CMAJ* 2006;**175**:1377–81.

88 Devereaux A, Christian MD, Dichter JR, et al. Summary of suggestions from the Task Force for Mass Critical Care summit, January 26–7, 2007. *Chest* 2008;**133**(5 Suppl):1S–7S.

89 Burnham G, Lafta R, Doocy S, et al. Mortality after the 2003 invasion of Iraq: a cross-sectional cluster sample survey. *Lancet* 2006;**368**:1421–8.

90 Coghlan B, Brennan RJ, Ngoy P, et al. Mortality in the Democratic Republic of Congo: a nationwide survey. *Lancet* 2006;**367**:44–51.

91 Horton R. The global financial crisis: an acute threat to health. *Lancet* 2009;**373**:355–6.

92 Marmot MG, Bell R. How will the financial crisis affect health? *BMJ* 2009;**338**:b1314.

93 Morgan A, Daly C, Murawski BJ. Dollar and human costs of intensive care. *J Surg Res* 1973;**14**:441–8.

94 Jonsen AR. Bentham in a box: technology assessment and health care allocation. *Law Med Health Care* 1986;**14**:172–4.

95 Ward NS, Teno JM, Curtis JR, et al. Perceptions of cost constraints, resource limitations, and rationing in United States intensive care units: results of a national survey. *Crit Care Med* 2008;**36**:471–6.

96 Carson SS, Cox CE, Holmes GM, et al. The changing epidemiology of mechanical ventilation: a population-based study. *J Intensive Care Med* 2006;**21**:173–82.

97 Needham DM, Bronskill SE, Sibbald WJ, et al. Mechanical ventilation in Ontario, 1992–2000: incidence, survival, and hospital bed utilization of noncardiac surgery adult patients. *Crit Care Med* 2004;**32**:1504–9.

98 Luhr OR, Antonsen K, Karlsson M, et al. Incidence and mortality after acute respiratory failure and acute respiratory distress syndrome in Sweden, Denmark, and Iceland. The ARF Study Group. *Am J Respir Crit Care Med* 1999;**159**:1849–61.

99 Sinuff T, Cook DJ. Guidelines in the intensive care unit. *Clin Chest Med* 2003;**24**:739–49.

100 O'Connor C, Adhikari NK, Decaire K, et al. Medical admission order sets to improve deep vein thrombosis prophylaxis rates and other outcomes. *J Hosp Med* 2009;**4**:81–9.

101 Sinuff T, Muscedere J, Adhikari NK, et al. Knowledge translation interventions for critically ill patients: a systematic review. *Crit Care Med* 2013;**41**:2627–40.

102 Gershengorn HB, Wunsch H, Wahab R, et al. Impact of nonphysician staffing on outcomes in a medical ICU. *Chest* 2011;**139**:1347–53.

Chapter 3

Mortality after Critical Illness

Matthew Baldwin and Hannah Wunsch

Introduction

The success of intensive care medicine has traditionally been gauged by the proportion of patients alive at hospital discharge or at day 28.[1-5] With technological advances, many critically ill patients now survive what were previously fatal illnesses,[6-8] in turn generating an enlarging population of ICU survivors. While some critical illness constitutes an acute event with minimal sequelae, we now recognize that a substantial proportion of patients are left in a state similar to a chronic disease, with increased risk of long-term morbidity and mortality. Understanding how critical illness may affect mortality after hospital discharge is important for measuring the true value of intensive care and fundamental to targeting both therapeutic and palliative interventions that will improve survival and/or quality of life (QoL) after critical illness. This chapter will: (1) examine the specific challenges of studying long-term mortality after critical illness, (2) review the current epidemiology, (3) describe the factors influencing death after critical illness, and (4) examine how measurements of frailty, disability, and comorbidity may aid in the development of reliable long-term mortality prediction models.

Challenges of studying mortality after critical Illness

Defining a population

Long-term studies of ICU populations either report death rates for all patients who are critically ill[9-17] or for subgroups that share clinical or therapeutic characteristics. Definitions of critical illness often use admission to an ICU as a proxy.[11,18] However, defining a group this way may either miss some critically ill patients who are cared for elsewhere[19] or include patients who may not have a particularly high severity of illness.[20] The alternative is to focus on one or more common subgroups of ICU patients such as those with severe sepsis,[21-24] ARDS,[25-29] prolonged mechanical ventilation (PMV),[10,30-34] or the elderly.[35-39] While studies of subgroups of patients provide important information regarding that specific patient population, the results may then not be applicable to other critically ill patients.

The majority of studies calculate long-term mortality from the time of ICU admission and include ICU patients who died in hospital.[12,13,17] However, more recent population-based studies have calculated long-term mortality from the date of hospital discharge among those who survived intensive care.[10,11,18] Given the high hospital mortality associated with most critically ill populations, the latter approach allows for a clearer assessment of post-hospitalization mortality. One must therefore use caution when comparing mortality across studies, since inclusion or exclusion of hospital deaths may substantially shift mortality estimates.

Choosing a control group

Ideally, when assessing the influence of critical illness on long-term risk of death, one could match ICU patients with controls to account for the impact of all factors, except the critical illness itself. But it is impossible to know whether this means critically ill patients should be compared with hospitalized controls who did not receive intensive care or non-hospitalized controls, as both options provide important information. Comparison with hospitalized patients may allow for better isolation of the severity of illness as a risk factor.[11,18] But comparison with the general population provides a better estimate of the total residual risk of death, compared to the 'average' person.[13,14,17,40,41] However, the reality is that unmeasured differences in comorbid disease between ICU patients and any control population may lead to residual confounding of the association between critical illness and long-term mortality.

Determining time of follow-up

Acute care discharge patterns have changed, with many more patients transferred at early stages to skilled care facilities, particularly in the US.[10] These patients who are discharged to skilled care are known to have much higher mortality in the weeks and months that follow, compared to patients who are discharged home.[10,18,42] Studies also demonstrate that increasing the number of discharges to skilled care by a small amount can artificially lower in-hospital mortality, further emphasizing the need for longer follow-up.[43,44] However, the preferred duration of long-term follow-up necessary to understand how patient outcomes may be related to the sequelae of critical illness is debatable.

Survivors of critical illness should ideally be followed until the gradient of their survival curve parallels that of a relevant control group (see Figure 3.1). But the exact length of time depends upon the specific types of critically ill patients studied and the chosen control group. Different

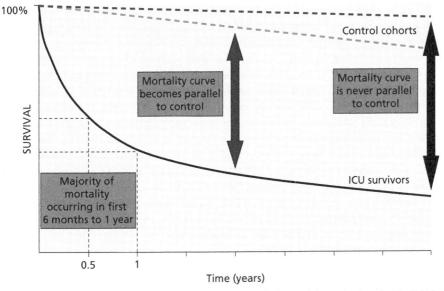

Fig. 3.1 Hypothetical survival curve for critically ill patients discharged from the hospital (solid black line), compared with possible control cohorts (dotted lines).

international consensus panels recommend using 3–6-month mortality as endpoints for clinical trials enrolling critically ill patients.[45,46] Recently published ICU studies on insulin therapy for hyperglycaemia in the ICU[47] and neuromuscular blocking agents (NMBAs) for early ARDS[48] adopted a 90-day (3-month) mortality endpoint. However, other studies suggest that even 3 months may be inappropriate for some critical illnesses that require prolonged hospitalization. For example, one-quarter of subjects enrolled in the ARDS Network study to assess the efficacy of corticosteroids were still hospitalized at 60 days.[49] While the optimum duration of follow-up after intensive care will vary by the specific research questions, the mechanisms and timing of the disease or treatment under study, and study design,[50] the time period chosen should ideally incorporate a length of time that captures a majority of the deaths that occur after hospital discharge.

The meaning of long-term mortality

Tracking and retaining subjects enrolled in any clinical investigation requires significant effort and financial resources. Death may be determined through direct follow-up with patients and families but is more often determined from administrative or government records. The majority of studies focused on long-term mortality assume that lower mortality is always the 'better' outcome.[18] However, some ICU survivors may prefer palliative over life-sustaining therapies.[51] Unfortunately administrative data often do not provide any information on patient preferences or decision making. We currently do not have any clear method to incorporate the quality of end-of-life care into our reporting of mortality as an outcome from critical illness.

Epidemiology of long-term mortality after intensive care

Population-based studies

Whether study populations are selected by country, age, intervention, or specific diagnosis, most investigations demonstrate that the majority of deaths after critical illness that do not occur in the hospital happen within 6 to 12 months after hospital discharge (see Figure 3.1).[10,12,13,15,17,18,41] A study of Medicare beneficiaries found that, among a 2.5% sample of elderly (age ≥ 65 years) patients who received intensive care, the risk of death after hospital discharge was concentrated during the first 6 months, especially among those who received MV or who were discharged to skilled-care facilities.[18] At 3 years after hospital discharge, ICU survivors had a slightly higher 3-year mortality (39.5%), compared with matched hospital controls (34.5%), and a substantially higher mortality, compared with general population controls (14.9%) (see Table 3.1).

A Canadian study attempted to distinguish the impact of critical illness on long-term mortality from the effect of hospital admission alone in a population of patients from British Columbia, Canada, between 1994 and 1996.[11] Whereas the US data were restricted to ICU survivors over the age of 65, the Canadian study examined ICU patients of all ages, including those who died in hospital (but did exclude neonates and pregnant women). This younger cohort of ICU survivors had 1- and 3-year mortality of only 10.8% and 17.0%, respectively. But mortality after ICU admission was still concentrated during the first year, remained significantly greater than general population controls through 3 years of follow-up, and was quantitatively similar to, but still significantly greater than, hospitalized controls after 3 years.

Multiple and single centre cohort studies

Smaller cohort studies consisting of general medical and surgical ICU patients show conflicting data regarding the length of time patients remain at an increased risk of death (see Table 3.1).

Table 3.1 Long-term mortality after admission to general intensive care units

Study type	Study period	n	Restrictions	Ages (years)	In-hospital mortality	Only ICU survivors[a]	Long-term mortality			
							1-year	3-year	5-year	Other
Population studies										
Wunsch (2010)[18]	2003	35 308	—	≥65	—	Yes	22%	40%	—	—
Kahn (2010)[10]	1997–2006	244 621	Discharge to long-term acute care	≥65	—	Yes	51%	—	—	—
Keenan (2002)[11]	1994–1996	27 103		>1	14%	Yes	11%	17%	—	—
Cohort studies of n >1000										
Dragsted (1991)[12]	1979–1983	1308		—	29%	No	42%	—	58%	—
Niskanen (1996)[17]	1987	12 180		≥15	19%	No	28%	32%	40%	—
Wright (2003)[13]	1985–1989	2104		≥16	21%[b]	No	36%	47%	55%	63%[c]
Williams (2008)[14]	1987–2002	19 921		≥16	11%	Yes	6.4%	—	31%	45%[d]
Kaufman (2009)[16]	1992–2000	3119	Medical and neurological ICU patients	—	34%	No	45%	—	—	—
Range					11–34%		6–51%	17–47%	31–58%	—

ICU, intensive care unit.

[a] Long-term mortality of ICU survivors was calculated from only those who survive to hospital discharge and excluded patients who died in hospital. Studies that did not calculate long-term mortality for ICU survivors instead calculated cumulative mortality that is defined as the cumulative percentage of patients dying after admission to ICU.

[b] ICU mortality; hospital mortality not reported.

[c] 9-year mortality.

[d] 15-year mortality.

Compared to age- and gender-matched general population controls, the mortality rate among ICU survivors in these studies remains elevated for anywhere from 2 to 15 years.[12-14,17,41] In a review of 19 cohort studies that measured mortality at least 1 year after hospital discharge from general ICUs, the case mix, demographic variables, and severity of illness varied widely.[15] Long-term mortality ranged from 26 to 63% at 1 year, 40–72% at 3 years, and 40–58% at 5 years. However, the majority of deaths after hospital admission with intensive care were still concentrated in the first year after discharge.

Factors influencing likelihood of death after critical illness

ICU admission diagnosis

Differences in case-mix and severity of illness between cohort studies likely explain most of the variation in reported long-term mortality. Studies of ICU subpopulations defined by specific critical illness diagnoses provide the most detailed information regarding mortality after critical illness. Some diagnostic categories are associated with only high short-term mortality, while others seem to confer an increased risk of death over a longer period of time (see Table 3.2a). Among general ICU cohort studies, patients with cardiovascular and trauma diagnoses usually have the best long-term survival, with mortality rates equalling that of the general population within 3 months to 2 years, while patients with cancer, respiratory failure, and neurological disorders tend to have higher rates of death for at least 5 years.[11,13,14,16,17]

Severe sepsis

Patients with severe sepsis[45] have an increased risk of death after hospital discharge for anywhere from 2 to 8 years when compared with general population controls.[13,21,23] In several studies of long-term mortality that included patients who died in hospital, approximately half of patients with severe sepsis were dead within 1 year,[23,52] and as many as 74% had died within 5 years after ICU admission.[22,23] Among 17 studies of ICU sepsis survivors who were discharged from the hospital, the weighted average 1-year mortality after hospital discharge was 23%, indicating that many patients die in the year after the infection has been treated[23] (see Table 3.2a).

Acute respiratory failure

In contrast with other critical illnesses, acute lung injury (ALI) and ARDS confer a substantial risk for in-hospital mortality, but surprisingly low risk for long-term mortality.

Cheung et al. observed an overall 2-year mortality of 49% among ARDS patients. But, among those who survived to hospital discharge, only 15% died in the subsequent 2 years.[26] These findings are supported by other cohort studies of ARDS survivors. One Canadian cohort reported 1- and 5-year mortalities among ARDS survivors of 12% and 19%, respectively,[27,28] and a US cohort, followed for 1 year, found that all of the deaths after hospital discharge (13%) had occurred by 6 months of follow-up[29] (see Table 3.2a).

These data are different from findings from general ICU cohorts that report increased mortality rates for at least 5 years among patients with respiratory disorders when compared to general population controls.[11,13,17] These general cohort studies of ICU patients include patients with acute-on-chronic respiratory failure, related to chronic lung disease and respiratory failure secondary to septic shock. Patients with chronic lung disease, such as COPD, tend to have poor long-term outcomes after critical illness. For example, one study of mechanically ventilated COPD patients found in-hospital, 1-year, and 5-year mortality

Table 3.2a Representative studies of long-term mortality of select ICU subgroups, based on diagnoses

	Type of study	Study period	Subgroup	n	ICU mortality	28-day or in-hospital mortality	Only ICU survivors[a]	Long-term mortality			
								1-year	2-year	3-year	5-year
Sepsis[b]											
Winters (2010)[23]	Review of 17 studies	1995–2009	All sepsis	33 482	–	–	Yes	7–43%	–	–	–
ARDS											
Herridge (2003)[27]	Multicentre cohort	1998–2002	ARDS	109	–	–	Yes	12%	–	–	–
Cheung (2006)[26]	Multicentre cohort	1998–2003	ARDS	109	40%	–	Yes	–	15%	–	–
Herridge (2011)[28]	Multicentre cohort	1998–2006	ARDS	109	–	–	Yes	–	–	–	19%
Angus (2001)[29]	Multicentre cohort	1996–1997	ARDS	200	–	31%	No	44%	–	–	–
Cancer											
Staudinger (2000)[56]	Single-centre cohort	1993–1999	All malignancies	414	47%	–	No	77%	–	–	–
			Solid tumour	174	35%	–	No	72%	–	–	–
			Leukaemia	127	43%	–	No	77%	–	–	–
			Lymphoma	75	51%	–	No	85%	–	–	–

Table 3.2a (continued) Representative studies of long-term mortality of select ICU subgroups, based on diagnoses

	Type of study	Study period	Subgroup	n	ICU mortality	28-day or in-hospital mortality	Only ICU survivors[a]	Long-term mortality			
								1-year	2-year	3-year	5-year
Kroschinsky (2002)[57]	Single-centre cohort	1995–2000	BMT	38	78%	–	No	95%	–	–	–
			All haematologic malignancies	104	44%	–	No	71%	–	–	–
Stroke											
Navarete (2003)[62]	Multicentre cohort	1999	Acute stroke	132	–	33%	No	54%	–	–	–
			Subarachnoid haemorrhage	28	–	32%	No	39%	–	–	–
			Intracerebral haemorrhage	77	–	37%	No	54%	–	–	–
			Ischaemic stroke	27	–	22%	No	66%	–	–	–
Golestanian (2009)[63]	Multicentre cohort	2000	Ischaemic stroke	8185[c]		21%	No	40%	–	–	–

ICU, intensive care unit; ARDS, acute respiratory distress syndrome; BMT, bone marrow transplant.

[a] Long-term mortality of ICU survivors was calculated from only those who survive to hospital discharge and excluded patients who died in hospital. Studies that did not calculate long-term mortality for ICU survivors instead calculated cumulative mortality that is defined as the cumulative percentage of patients dying after admission to ICU.

[b] Not all sepsis studies specify whether patients were treated in the ICU or on the general hospital floor.

[c] A total of 31 301 were in the entire study; however, only 8185 were admitted to the ICU.

rates of 25%, 39%, and 76%, respectively, demonstrating the radically different long-term patterns for these chronic lung disease patients, compared with patients diagnosed with ALI or ARDS.[53]

Cancer

Cancer patients admitted to the ICU also have higher mortality rates for at least 5 years when compared to general population controls.[13,17] However, the effect of the cancer cannot easily be separated from the impact of critical illness on long-term mortality. Over the past 30 years, treating cancer patients who become critically ill in the ICU has become widely accepted, as changes in patient selection criteria, new anti-cancer treatments, and better supportive care have decreased in-hospital mortality from over 80% to 30–60%.[54,55] Despite these short-term gains in survival, 1-year mortality remains high, ranging from 71% to 95%[56,57] (see Table 3.2a). Furthermore, patients with haematologic malignancies tend to have worse long-term survival than those with solid tumours.[11,13,16,58]

There are many other specific groups of patients, such as patients undergoing cardiac surgery[59–61] or with brain injury,[62,63] who are often cared for in specialty ICUs. All of these groups have been examined in detail with regard to both short- and long-term survival, with long-term prognosis clearly dependent on the specific diagnosis (see Table 3.2a).

ICU-related interventions

Mechanical ventilation

Often ICU patients are studied, not by a specific diagnosis, but based on interventions they receive when critically ill. In particular, patients are often grouped based on their need for MV and/or renal replacement therapy (RRT). Intensive care survivors who receive MV for any duration have a substantially higher long-term mortality rate, compared to either ICU patients who are not ventilated or other control groups. For example, the 3-year mortality of US patients aged ≥ 65 years who received MV was 58% vs 33% for hospitalized controls.[18] While smaller and older studies did not find a statistically significant association between MV and an increased long-term mortality in multivariable analyses,[64,65] a more recent larger study showed that MV is an independent predictor of poor long-term survival after adjusting for age, severity of illness, and comorbidities.[66]

Between 5 and 10% of patients who require MV for acute conditions progress to PMV,[33,67] which is defined differently across studies but often includes either MV for a specified duration (such as 21 days) and/or a tracheostomy.[68,69] One-year mortality of PMV patients has remained consistently poor over the past 15 years, ranging from 36% to 77%, with the majority of deaths occurring during the first 6 months after hospital discharge[10,33,34,70,71] (see Table 3.2b).

Age and premorbid functional status appear to be the strongest predictors of poor survival in PMV patients. Work by Carson et al. showed that patients older than 74, and patients older than 64 and functionally dependent before admission, had a 95% (95% CI 84–99%) 1-year mortality.[71] The same group also developed and externally validated a 1-year mortality prediction model for PMV.[72] Independent predictors of 1-year mortality were age ≥50 years, requirement of vasopressors, haemodialysis, and platelet count <150 000 on day 21 of MV.[73]

Renal replacement therapy

One-year mortality for patients with acute renal failure is well over 50%.[74] However, severe acute renal failure requiring RRT is most often secondary to poor renal perfusion related to problems, such as sepsis, cardiac surgery, or advanced liver disease, rather than primary glomerular

Table 3.2b Representative studies of long-term mortality of select ICU subgroups based on interventions

Study	Type of study	Study period	Subgroup	n	ICU mortality	28-day or in-hospital mortality	Only ICU survivors[a]	Long-term mortality			
								1-year	2-year	3-year	5-year
PMV											
Carson (1999)[71]	Single-centre cohort	1995–1996	PMV	133	–	–	Yes	77%	–	–	–
Engoren (2004)[33]	Single-centre cohort	1998–2000	Ventilation with tracheostomy	429	–	19%	Yes	36%	42%	–	–
Pilcher (2005)[34]	Single-centre cohort	1997–2000	PMV	153	–	27%	No	42%	–	53%	–
Kahn (2010)[10]	Population-based	2006	Age ≥65, PMV to LTAC	11 695	–	–	Yes	69%	–	–	–
RRT											
Chapman (2009)[78]	Multicentre cohort	1999–2004	Chronic haemodialysis	199	44%	–	Yes	–	44%	–	–
Morgera (2002)[76]	Single-centre cohort	1993–1998	Continuous RRT	979	–	69%	Yes	32%	–	–	50%
Bagshaw (2005)[75]	Population-based	1999–2002	Severe ARF needing RRT	240	50%	60%	No	64%	–	–	–

Table 3.2b (continued) Representative studies of long-term mortality of select ICU subgroups based on interventions

	Type of study	Study period	Subgroup	n	ICU mortality	28-day or in-hospital mortality	Only ICU survivors[a]	Long-term mortality			
								1-year	2-year	3-year	5-year
Ahlstrom (2005)[77]	Single-centre cohort	1998–2002	Severe ARF needing RRT	703	–	41%	No	57%	–	–	71%
Cardiovascular interventions											
Hannan (2005)[59]	Population-based	1997–2003	CABG	37212	–	1.75%	No	4–6%	5–8%	7–11%	–
Hannan (2008)[60]	Population-based	1997–2003	Stent implantation	22102	–	0.68%	No	5–9%	6–12%	9–16%	–
Lagercrantz (2010)[61]	Population-based	2004–2007	CABG and ICU length of stay >10 days	141	–	33%	No	38%	–	44%	48%

ICU, intensive care unit; PMV, prolonged mechanical ventilation; RRT, renal replacement therapy; LTAC, long-term acute care facility; ARF, acute renal failure; CABG, coronary artery bypass grafting.

[a] Long-term mortality of ICU survivors is calculated from only those who survive to hospital discharge and excludes patients who die in hospital. Studies that did not calculate long-term mortality for ICU survivors instead calculated cumulative mortality that is defined as the cumulative percentage of patients dying after admission to ICU.

disease.[74] Therefore, this high 1-year mortality is mostly attributable to the comorbid disease that predisposed to the critical illness.[74–77] In one study, chronic haemodialysis patients admitted to the ICU with multiple organ failure (MOF) had a 2-year mortality of 44%, but the survival curve of the patients admitted to the ICU paralleled that of the background population of haemodialysis patients within 1 month after hospital discharge.[78]

Effect of age

The elderly population is growing rapidly in developed countries, and patients aged 65 and older now make up more than half of all ICU admissions in the US.[79] Small cohort studies first reported that survival of ICU patients after hospital discharge was not affected by age.[35,37] More recent large cohort and population-based studies demonstrated that increasing age is an independent, albeit minor, predictor of long-term mortality after adjusting for severity of critical illness and chronic health status.[11,14,66,80] It is likely not advanced age per se, but other unmeasured factors associated with advanced age, that ultimately determine prognosis in elderly patients. In particular, poorer long-term outcomes in the elderly may reflect unmeasured premorbid functional disability and subclinical frailty that limit recovery after critical illness,[38] as well as decisions to receive less intensive courses of treatment.[39,81]

Causes of death

Epidemiology

Due to the challenges of follow-up, we know comparatively little about the relationship between critical illness and the subsequent cause of death. Three studies have specifically examined the cause of death among ICU survivors, but all are limited by their single-centre, retrospective cohort study design and the use of ICD-9 codes and diagnoses on death certificates to determine the cause of death.[82–84] Despite these limitations, these studies all suggest that ICU survivors who die from diagnoses related to their initial critical illness do so in the first 6 months to 1 year after hospital discharge.[82,84] Malignancy and chronic cardiovascular disease were the most frequently cited causes of death for ICU survivors in these studies, but this may reflect the fact that a majority of subjects were admitted to the ICU after cardiac or cancer-related surgery.[83,84]

Longitudinal studies of ICU survivors with PMV provide insight into both the cause and mechanism of death for the most debilitated survivors of critical illness. Most PMV patients develop chronic critical illness (CCI) which is characterized by protracted respiratory failure, its hallmark, and some combination of functional dependence due to profound weakness, endocrinopathy, poor nutrition, anasarca, and skin breakdown.[85] Chronically critically ill patients usually die from recurrent episodes of sepsis that lead to progressive multiorgan failure (MOF), regardless of the initial acute medical, surgical, neurologic, or cardiac critical illness.[86] Their enhanced susceptibility to infection likely results from barrier breakdown, exposure to virulent and resistant nosocomial pathogens, and impaired immunity that stems from the combined impact of comorbidities and the sequelae of critical illness.[87]

A growing number of studies suggest that mortality after critical illness for older (age ≥65 years) ICU survivors may also be due to repeat infections and sepsis. A repeat episode of pneumonia was the leading cause for hospital readmission and 90-day mortality among older patients hospitalized with community-acquired pneumonia (some of whom were treated in the ICU for respiratory failure and sepsis),[88,89] and infection and aspiration pneumonitis were the most common reasons for re-hospitalization of older individuals after acute stroke.[90] Future studies that prospectively follow ICU survivors should include careful ascertainment of causes of death.

Biologic mechanisms of increased long-term mortality

Sepsis-induced immunoparalysis

Both animal models and human studies suggest that severe sepsis can induce immunosuppression (also known as immunoparalysis), which in turn increases the risk for future episodes of sepsis and death.[91–93] Immunoparalysis, following prolonged severe sepsis, is mediated by multiple molecular mechanisms, leading to the depletion of lymphocytes and dendritic cells, decreased expression of the antigen-presenting complex HLA-DR, and increased expression of the negative costimulatory molecules programmed death 1 (PD-1) which prevents T cell proliferation, causing T cell inhibition (or 'exhaustion').[91] In addition to immunoparalysis, elevated pro-inflammatory markers, such as interleukin (IL)-6, that persist after treatment of pneumonia and sepsis have been associated with 1-year mortality, suggesting that some individuals may have lasting subclinical inflammation that impairs immunity and affects long-term mortality.[94]

Targeted immunostimulation trials in both mice and humans with severe sepsis have shown promising results. Mice treated with PD-1 inhibitors have improved survival with fungal infections and bacterial sepsis.[95] In a phase II trial, granulocyte-macrophage colony-stimulating factor (GM-CSF) was given to adults with severe sepsis or septic shock and low HLA-DR levels. GM-CSF restored markers of monocytic immunocompetence and was associated with lower MV time and hospital length of stay, and there were no noted side effects.[96] Future studies in animal and human models to further eludicate the mechanisms of sepsis-induced immunoparalysis and trials of immunoenhancing therapy that are tailored to the individual patient on the basis of biomarkers and/or clinical findings are needed.[91]

ICU-acquired weakness

ICU-acquired weakness (ICUAW) is a prevalent and long-lasting morbidity of critical illness that is due to critical illness polyneuropathy (CIP), critical illness myopathy (CIM), or a combination of the two.[97] While there is a range of functional outcomes related to disability from ICUAW, the severity and time to recovery appear to increase with decreased nerve and muscle reserve that is age- and/or comorbidity-related. Other factors that influence severity and recovery include having a critical illness due to sepsis and the duration of immobilization (i.e. the severity of critical illness).[98,99] ICU survivors who develop sustained ICUAW, rendering them bedbound or even dependent on MV, may be more likely to be exposed to multidrug-resistant pathogens, because they often require care in skilled-care facilities, and may be susceptible to recurrent infection due to decubital ulcers and ventilator-associated pneumonias,[86] both of which can lead to sepsis and death. While our understanding of the pathophysiologic process of CIM and CIP has increased in animal models, the temporal sequence of interaction is poorly described.[99] Future studies in animal models should focus on further elucidating the timing and mechanisms of CIM and CIP, which will in turn lead to the development of targeted therapies. Clinical studies in humans that correlate clinical evaluation and test findings with histopathology on muscle and nerve biopsies are needed to determine different phenotypes of ICUAW so that early clinical recognition, prevention, and treatment can be tailored to improve the disability that confers morbidity and mortality after critical illness.

Neuroendocrine changes and poor nutrition

Some ICU survivors of prolonged critical illness develop a catabolic state that persists after the critical illness resolves. These patients are most often chronically critically ill and have some combination of loss of skeletal muscle mass, increased adiposity, and anasarca.[86,100] They frequently have hypothalamic hypopituitarism, with blunting or loss of the pulsatile secretion of anterior pituitary hormones.[101] Impaired growth hormone (GH) and insulin-like growth factor-1 (IGF-1) activity and hypogonadotropism with low (and often undetectable) testosterone levels in men likely contribute to the wasting and catabolism.[100,102,103] Previous studies with oral anabolic agents and recombinant human GH (rhGH) in subjects with prolonged critical illness have shown negative results or have been associated with increased morbidity and mortality.[104,105] However, these hormones have not yet been specifically tested during the post-critical illness recovery phase when anabolism is critical.[106] Treatment with hypothalamic releasing factors is emerging as a promising means of correction of the abnormal neuroendocrine function that allows the body to adjust target hormone levels, as needed, to prevent overdose and toxicity.[101,107]

Observational studies of patients with CCI who rely on tube-fed enteral nutrition (EN) have shown that patients achieve only 43–68% of their daily nutritional goals.[108–110] While a recent study suggests no additional benefit for full vs trophic enteral feeds in the first week of acute critical illness,[111] longer-term underfeeding is common in PMV patients, is most often due to inadequate tolerance of feeds and frequent nil per os status for procedures or ventilator-weaning trials,[109] and has been associated with increased infectious complications and mortality.[112,113] Micronutrient deficiencies of vitamin D and glutamine are also prevalent among chronically critically ill patients[114,115] and may hinder protein synthesis and immunity after critical illness, leaving patients weaker and more susceptible to repeat infections. Little is known about the nutritional intake of ICU survivors without CCI who are discharged home or to a skilled-care facility.

Genetic variance

Finally, genetic variation may underpin the increased risk of death of some patients after critical illness. The majority of research to date has focused on examining the genetic polymorphisms in genes that control the inflammatory response to explain differing morbidity and mortality from sepsis. For example, polymorphisms in Toll-like receptor 1,[116] plasminogen activator inhibitor-1 (PAI-1),[117] and macrophage migration inhibitory factor[118] in patients with pneumonia and/or sepsis have been associated with increased susceptibility to repeat infection, organ dysfunction, and death. Future studies that aim to improve our understanding of genetic determinants of critical illness may improve risk stratification, allow individualized therapies, and provide insights into the biological mechanisms of disease.[119] However, conflicting results from early studies in the genetics of critical illness and more recent limitations in the predictive capacity of personal genome sequencing for common diseases have tempered the initial enthusiasm of using genetics to improve outcomes from critical care.[120,121] Well-designed genetic studies of larger cohorts are needed to improve our understanding of how genetics affect long-term mortality from critical illness.

Predicting mortality in survivors of critical illness

Severity of illness scores

Multiple severity of illness scores risk-stratify critically ill patients for short-term (hospital or 28-day) mortality.[58,122–124] The Acute Physiology and Chronic Health Evaluation (APACHE) II score is perhaps the most frequently used, particularly to describe the initial severity of critical illness in cohorts of ICU patients.[58] Several studies have examined how severity of illness scores, calculated at different times during the ICU admission, predict long-term mortality. In two different studies, the APACHE II score did not independently predict 1-year mortality in elderly patients (ages ≥75 or ≥80 years) who were admitted to the ICU.[125,126] The APACHE III score on the third day of an ICU stay appeared to have better discrimination in predicting 1-year mortality in persons aged 80 years and older, compared with scores calculated on ICU admission.[127] But, without the inclusion of other variables, it still remained a poor overall predictor of long-term mortality. Severity of illness calculated on the day of hospital discharge/admission to skilled care for debilitated ICU survivors also did not predict subsequent mortality, suggesting that these scores may need to be modified to incorporate more factors relevant to chronic, rather than acute, disease to be useful for long-term prediction.[128]

Comorbidity

Emerging research points to the evaluation of disability, comorbidity, and frailty in ICU survivors prior to hospital discharge as central to accurately predicting post-discharge mortality, regardless of diagnosis.[129] Comorbidity, defined as the total burden of illness unrelated to a patient's principal diagnosis, is often measured in ICU outcome studies with the Charlson comorbidity index.[130,131] Comorbidity is known to significantly heighten the risk of disability and long-term mortality, over and above the risk from individual disease.[132] Second only to age, the Charlson comorbidity index was found to contribute more to predicting long-term mortality in ICU survivors than the APACHE II score, ventilator days, vasopressor use, use of RRT, peak number of organ failures, and gender.[14,66] Mechanistically, comorbid conditions are both a risk factor for, and result of, critical illness. For example, patients with renal insufficiency are at increased risk for sepsis.[21] Renal insufficiency may worsen during an episode of severe sepsis, leading to a need for chronic dialysis, which in turn confers an even greater risk of infection and sepsis thereafter.[52] Hence, the interaction of comorbidity and critical illness may lead to a spiral of progressive debilitation that eventually ends in death.

Premorbid disability

Both premorbid disability and loss of functional independence immediately after critical illness were important independent predictors of mortality for 1 to 3 years after discharge in multiple studies.[18,125,126,133,134] However, premorbid disability is difficult to gather prospectively, and estimates are inherently susceptible to recall bias from the patient or surrogate.[135,136] Prospective assessment of functional status immediately prior to hospital discharge may be a more pragmatic and precise measurement that is still relevant to a patient's long-term prognosis. We need more research that prospectively examines the association between functional status at hospital discharge and long-term mortality in ICU survivors. Published studies examining discharge status are mostly limited to older adults hospitalized without critical illness.[137,138]

Frailty

Frailty is increasingly recognized as a unique domain of health status that can be a marker for decreased reserves and resultant vulnerability in older patients. It is an 'aggregate expression of risk, resulting from age- or disease-associated physiologic accumulation of sub-threshold decrements affecting multiple physiologic systems'.[139] While disability, comorbidity, and frailty are related, each is clinically important and can occur independently of the others.[139] For community-dwelling elders, frailty accurately predicts morbidity and mortality, independent of comorbidities and disability.[140] Evaluating frailty in ICU patients might help explain why some older patients recover better than expected and others fare far worse. For example, surrogate measures of frailty accounted for 30% of the predictive power of a 6-month mortality prediction model for older ICU survivors.[129]

Future research is needed to model frailty among debilitated survivors of critical illness. In addition to testing established frailty models,[140,141] collectively evaluating other cognitive, physiologic, and biochemical markers of frailty that have all been associated with poor long-term outcomes in ICU survivors, such as persistent delirium,[142] sarcopenia,[143–145] and IL-6,[94] may help stratify frailty severity and predict long-term mortality in this population.

Conclusion

Long-term mortality after critical illness varies widely as a function of the interaction between the acute critical illness, comorbid disease, pre-illness functional status, and physiologic reserve. Yet, for most groups of critically ill patients, the majority of deaths among ICU survivors occur during the first 6 to 12 months after hospital discharge, suggesting there may be a window for future studies and potential interventions to improve outcomes. Survival to hospital discharge must therefore no longer be an endpoint for success, but a beginning of a comprehensive evaluation of biochemical, physiologic, and cognitive markers that will be crucial to reliably predict long-term mortality and fundamental to targeting palliative and therapeutic interventions that will improve care after critical illness.

References

1 The Acute Respiratory Distress Syndrome Network. Ventilation with lower tidal volumes as compared with traditional tidal volumes for acute lung injury and the acute respiratory distress syndrome. *N Engl J Med* 2000;**342**:1301–8.

2 Bernard GR, Vincent JL, Laterre PF, et al. Efficacy and safety of recombinant human activated protein C for severe sepsis. *N Engl J Med* 2001;**344**:699–709.

3 Hebert PC, Wells G, Blajchman MA, et al. A multicenter, randomized, controlled clinical trial of transfusion requirements in critical care. Transfusion Requirements in Critical Care Investigators, Canadian Critical Care Trials Group. *N Engl J Med* 1999;**340**:409–17.

4 Van den Berghe G, Wilmer A, Hermans G, et al. Intensive insulin therapy in the medical ICU. *N Engl J Med* 2006;**354**:449–61.

5 Higgins TL, Teres D, Copes WS, Nathanson BH, Stark M, Kramer AA. Assessing contemporary intensive care unit outcome: an updated Mortality Probability Admission Model (MPM0-III). *Crit Care Med* 2007;**35**:827–35.

6 Spragg RG, Bernard GR, Checkley W, et al. Beyond mortality: future clinical research in acute lung injury. *Am J Respir Crit Care Med* 2010;**181**:1121–7.

7 Lerolle N, Trinquart L, Bornstain C, et al. Increased intensity of treatment and decreased mortality in elderly patients in an intensive care unit over a decade. *Crit Care Med* 2010;**38**:59–64.

8 Kvale R, Flaatten H. Changes in intensive care from 1987 to 1997 - has outcome improved? A single centre study. *Intensive Care Med* 2002;**28**:1110–16.

9 Wunsch H, Angus DC, Harrison DA, Linde-Zwirble WT, Rowan KM. Comparison of medical admissions to intensive care units in the United States and United kingdom. *Am J Respir Crit Care Med* 2011;**183**:1666–73.

10 Kahn JM, Benson NM, Appleby D, Carson SS, Iwashyna TJ. Long-term acute care hospital utilization after critical illness. *JAMA* 2010;**303**:2253–9.

11 Keenan SP, Dodek P, Chan K, et al. Intensive care unit admission has minimal impact on long-term mortality. *Crit Care Med* 2002;**30**:501–7.

12 Dragsted L. Outcome from intensive care. A five year study of 1,308 patients. *Dan Med Bull* 1991;**38**:365–74.

13 Wright JC, Plenderleith L, Ridley SA. Long-term survival following intensive care: subgroup analysis and comparison with the general population. *Anaesthesia* 2003;**58**:637–42.

14 Williams TA, Dobb GJ, Finn JC, et al. Determinants of long-term survival after intensive care. *Crit Care Med* 2008;**36**:1523–30.

15 Williams TA, Dobb GJ, Finn JC, Webb SA. Long-term survival from intensive care: a review. *Intensive Care Med* 2005;**31**:1306–15.

16 Kaufmann PA, Smolle KH, Krejs GJ. Short- and long-term survival of nonsurgical intensive care patients and its relation to diagnosis, severity of disease, age and comorbidities. *Curr Aging Sci* 2009;**2**:240–8.

17 Niskanen M, Kari A, Halonen P. Five-year survival after intensive care—comparison of 12,180 patients with the general population. Finnish ICU Study Group. *Crit Care Med* 1996;**24**:1962–7.

18 Wunsch H, Guerra C, Barnato AE, Angus DC, Li G, Linde-Zwirble WT. Three-year outcomes for Medicare beneficiaries who survive intensive care. *JAMA* 2010;**303**:849–56.

19 Simchen E, Sprung CL, Galai N, et al. Survival of critically ill patients hospitalized in and out of intensive care units under paucity of intensive care unit beds. *Crit Care Med* 2004;**32**:1654–61.

20 Zimmerman JE, Kramer AA. A model for identifying patients who may not need intensive care unit admission. *J Crit Care* 2010;**25**:205–13.

21 Quartin AA, Schein RM, Kett DH, Peduzzi PN. Magnitude and duration of the effect of sepsis on survival. Department of Veterans Affairs Systemic Sepsis Cooperative Studies Group. *JAMA* 1997;**277**:1058–63.

22 Weycker D, Akhras KS, Edelsberg J, Angus DC, Oster G. Long-term mortality and medical care charges in patients with severe sepsis. *Crit Care Med* 2003;**31**:2316–23.

23 Winters BD, Eberlein M, Leung J, Needham DM, Pronovost PJ, Sevransky JE. Long-term mortality and quality of life in sepsis: a systematic review. *Crit Care Med* 2010;**38**:1276–83.

24 Perl TM, Dvorak L, Hwang T, Wenzel RP. Long-term survival and function after suspected gram-negative sepsis. *JAMA* 1995;**274**:338–45.

25 Davidson TA, Rubenfeld GD, Caldwell ES, Hudson LD, Steinberg KP. The effect of acute respiratory distress syndrome on long-term survival. *Am J Respir Crit Care Med* 1999;**160**:1838–42.

26 Cheung AM, Tansey CM, Tomlinson G, et al. Two-year outcomes, health care use, and costs of survivors of acute respiratory distress syndrome. *Am J Respir Crit Care Med* 2006;**174**:538–44.

27 Herridge MS, Cheung AM, Tansey CM, et al. One-year outcomes in survivors of the acute respiratory distress syndrome. *N Engl J Med* 2003;**348**(8):683–93.

28 Herridge MS, Tansey CM, Matte A, et al. Functional disability 5 years after acute respiratory distress syndrome. *N Engl J Med* 2011;**364**:1293–304.

29 Angus DC, Musthafa AA, Clermont G, et al. Quality-adjusted survival in the first year after the acute respiratory distress syndrome. *Am J Respir Crit Care Med* 2001;**163**:1389–94.

30 Carson SS, Bach PB. The epidemiology and costs of chronic critical illness. *Crit Care Clin* 2002;**18**:461–76.

31 Schonhofer B, Euteneuer S, Nava S, Suchi S, Kohler D. Survival of mechanically ventilated patients admitted to a specialised weaning centre. *Intensive Care Med* 2002;**28**:908–16.

32 Combes A, Costa MA, Trouillet JL, et al. Morbidity, mortality, and quality-of-life outcomes of patients requiring > or =14 days of mechanical ventilation. *Crit Care Med* 2003;**31**:1373–81.

33 Engoren M, Arslanian-Engoren C, Fenn-Buderer N. Hospital and long-term outcome after tracheostomy for respiratory failure. *Chest* 2004;**125**:220–7.

34 Pilcher DV, Bailey MJ, Treacher DF, Hamid S, Williams AJ, Davidson AC. Outcomes, cost and long term survival of patients referred to a regional weaning centre. *Thorax* 2005;**60**:187–92.

35 Chelluri L, Pinsky MR, Donahoe MP, Grenvik A. Long-term outcome of critically ill elderly patients requiring intensive care. *JAMA* 1993;**269**:3119–23.

36 Chelluri L, Pinsky MR, Grenvik AN. Outcome of intensive care of the 'oldest-old' critically ill patients. *Crit Care Med* 1992;**20**:757–61.

37 Rockwood K, Noseworthy TW, Gibney RT, et al. One-year outcome of elderly and young patients admitted to intensive care units. *Crit Care Med* 1993;**21**:687–91.

38 de Rooij SE, Abu-Hanna A, Levi M, de Jonge E. Factors that predict outcome of intensive care treatment in very elderly patients: a review. *Crit Care* 2005;**9**:R307–14.

39 Boumendil A, Aegerter P, Guidet B. Treatment intensity and outcome of patients aged 80 and older in intensive care units: a multicenter matched-cohort study. *J Am Geriatr Soc* 2005;**53**:88–93.

40 Flaatten H, Kvale R. Survival and quality of life 12 years after ICU. A comparison with the general Norwegian population. *Intensive Care Med* 2001;**27**:1005–11.

41 Ridley S, Plenderleith L. Survival after intensive care. Comparison with a matched normal population as an indicator of effectiveness. *Anaesthesia* 1994;**49**:933–5.

42 Nasraway SA, Button GJ, Rand WM, Hudson-Jinks T, Gustafson M. Survivors of catastrophic illness: outcome after direct transfer from intensive care to extended care facilities. *Crit Care Med* 2000;**28**:19–25.

43 Kahn JM, Kramer AA, Rubenfeld GD. Transferring critically ill patients out of hospital improves the standardized mortality ratio: a simulation study. *Chest* 2007;**131**:68–75.

44 Hall WB, Willis LE, Medvedev S, Carson SS. The implications of long term acute care hospital transfer practices for measures of in-hospital mortality and length of stay. *Am J Respir Crit Care Med* 2012;**185**:53–57.

45 Levy MM, Fink MP, Marshall JC, et al. 2001 SCCM/ESICM/ACCP/ATS/SIS International Sepsis Definitions Conference. *Crit Care Med* **2003**;31:1250–6.

46 Angus DC, Carlet J. Surviving intensive care: a report from the 2002 Brussels Roundtable. *Intensive Care Med* 2003;**29**:368–77.

47 Finfer S, Chittock DR, Su SY, et al. Intensive versus conventional glucose control in critically ill patients. *N Engl J Med* 2009;**360**:1283–97.

48 Papazian L, Forel JM, Gacouin A, et al. Neuromuscular blockers in early acute respiratory distress syndrome. *N Engl J Med* 2010;**363**:1107–16.

49 Steinberg KP, Hudson LD, Goodman RB, et al. Efficacy and safety of corticosteroids for persistent acute respiratory distress syndrome. *N Engl J Med* 2006;**354**:1671–84.

50 Rubenfeld GD, Angus DC, Pinsky MR, Curtis JR, Connors AF, Jr, Bernard GR. Outcomes research in critical care: results of the American Thoracic Society Critical Care Assembly Workshop on Outcomes Research. The Members of the Outcomes Research Workshop. *Am J Respir Crit Care Med* 1999;**160**:358–67.

51 Fried TR, Bradley EH, Towle VR, Allore H. Understanding the treatment preferences of seriously ill patients. *N Engl J Med* 2002;**346**:1061–6.

52 Yende S, Angus DC. Long-term outcomes from sepsis. *Curr Infect Dis Rep* 2007;**9**:382–6.

53 Ai-Ping C, Lee KH, Lim TK. In-hospital and 5-year mortality of patients treated in the ICU for acute exacerbation of COPD: a retrospective study. *Chest* 2005;**128**:518–24.

54 Darmon M, Azoulay E. Critical care management of cancer patients: cause for optimism and need for objectivity. *Curr Opin Oncol* 2009;**21**:318–26.

55 Kress JP, Christenson J, Pohlman AS, Linkin DR, Hall JB. Outcomes of critically ill cancer patients in a university hospital setting. *Am J Respir Crit Care Med* 1999;**160**:1957–61.

56 Staudinger T, Stoiser B, Mullner M, et al. Outcome and prognostic factors in critically ill cancer patients admitted to the intensive care unit. *Crit Care Med* 2000;**28**:1322–8.

57 Kroschinsky F, Weise M, Illmer T, et al. Outcome and prognostic features of intensive care unit treatment in patients with hematological malignancies. *Intensive Care Med* 2002;**28**:1294–300.

58 Knaus WA, Draper EA, Wagner DP, Zimmerman JE. APACHE II: a severity of disease classification system. *Crit Care Med* 1985;**13**:818–29.

59 Hannan EL, Racz MJ, Walford G, et al. Long-term outcomes of coronary-artery bypass grafting versus stent implantation. *N Engl J Med* 2005;**352**:2174–83.

60 Hannan EL, Wu C, Walford G, et al. Drug-eluting stents vs. coronary-artery bypass grafting in multi-vessel coronary disease. *N Engl J Med* 2008;**358**:331–41.

61 Lagercrantz E, Lindblom D, Sartipy U. Survival and quality of life in cardiac surgery patients with prolonged intensive care. *Ann Thorac Surg* 2010;**89**:490–5.

62 Navarrete-Navarro P, Rivera-Fernandez R, Lopez-Mutuberria MT, et al. Outcome prediction in terms of functional disability and mortality at 1 year among ICU-admitted severe stroke patients: a prospective epidemiological study in the south of the European Union (Evascan Project, Andalusia, Spain). *Intensive Care Med* 2003;**29**:1237–44.

63 Golestanian E, Liou JI, Smith MA. Long-term survival in older critically ill patients with acute ischemic stroke. *Crit Care Med* 2009;**37**:3107–13.

64 Zaren B, Bergstrom R. Survival compared to the general population and changes in health status among intensive care patients. *Acta Anaesthesiol Scand* 1989;**33**:6–12.

65 Nunn JF, Milledge JS, Singaraya J. Survival of patients ventilated in an intensive therapy unit. *Br Med J* 1979;**1**:1525–7.

66 Ho KM, Knuiman M, Finn J, Webb SA. Estimating long-term survival of critically ill patients: the PREDICT model. *PLoS One* 2008;**3**:e3226.

67 Seneff MG, Zimmerman JE, Knaus WA, Wagner DP, Draper EA. Predicting the duration of mechanical ventilation. The importance of disease and patient characteristics. *Chest* 1996;**110**:469–79.

68 MacIntyre NR, Epstein SK, Carson S, Scheinhorn D, Christopher K, Muldoon S. Management of patients requiring prolonged mechanical ventilation: report of a NAMDRC consensus conference. *Chest* 2005;**128**:3937–54.

69 Cox CE, Carson SS, Lindquist JH, Olsen MK, Govert JA, Chelluri L. Differences in one-year health outcomes and resource utilization by definition of prolonged mechanical ventilation: a prospective cohort study. *Crit Care* 2007;**11**:R9.

70 Unroe M, Kahn JM, Carson SS, et al. One-year trajectories of care and resource utilization for recipients of prolonged mechanical ventilation: a cohort study. *Ann Intern Med* 2010;**153**:167–75.

71 Carson SS, Bach PB, Brzozowski L, Leff A. Outcomes after long-term acute care. An analysis of 133 mechanically ventilated patients. *Am J Respir Crit Care Med* 1999;**159**:1568–73.

72 Carson SS, Kahn JM, Hough CL, et al. A multicenter mortality prediction model for patients receiving prolonged mechanical ventilation. *Crit Care Med* 2012;**40**:1171–6.

73 Carson SS, Garrett J, Hanson LC, et al. A prognostic model for one-year mortality in patients requiring prolonged mechanical ventilation. *Crit Care Med* 2008;**36**:2061–9.

74 Bagshaw SM. The long-term outcome after acute renal failure. *Curr Opin Crit Care* 2006;**12**:561–6.

75 Bagshaw SM, Laupland KB, Doig CJ, et al. Prognosis for long-term survival and renal recovery in critically ill patients with severe acute renal failure: a population-based study. *Crit Care* 2005;**9**:R700–9.

76 Morgera S, Kraft AK, Siebert G, Luft FC, Neumayer HH. Long-term outcomes in acute renal failure patients treated with continuous renal replacement therapies. *Am J Kidney Dis* 2002;**40**:275–9.

77 Ahlstrom A, Tallgren M, Peltonen S, Rasanen P, Pettila V. Survival and quality of life of patients requiring acute renal replacement therapy. *Intensive Care Med* 2005;**31**:1222–8.

78 Chapman RJ, Templeton M, Ashworth S, Broomhead R, McLean A, Brett SJ. Long-term survival of chronic dialysis patients following survival from an episode of multiple-organ failure. *Crit Care* 2009;**13**:R65.

79 Angus DC, Shorr AF, White A, Dremsizov TT, Schmitz RJ, Kelley MA. Critical care delivery in the United States: distribution of services and compliance with Leapfrog recommendations. *Crit Care Med* 2006;**34**:1016–24.

80 Nierman DM, Schechter CB, Cannon LM, Meier DE. Outcome prediction model for very elderly critically ill patients. *Crit Care Med* 2001;**29**:1853–9.

81 Hanson LC, Danis M. Use of life-sustaining care for the elderly. *J Am Geriatr Soc* 1991;**39**:772–7.

82 Ridley S, Purdie J. Cause of death after critical illness. *Anaesthesia* 1992;**47**:116–19.

83 Mayr VD, Dunser MW, Greil V, et al. Causes of death and determinants of outcome in critically ill patients. *Crit Care* 2006;**10**:R154.

84 Hicks PR, Mackle DM. Cause of death in intensive care patients within 2 years of discharge from hospital. *Crit Care Resusc* 2010;**12**:78–82.

85 Nelson JE MD, Litke A, Natale DA, Siegel RE, Morrison RS. The symptom burden of chronic critical illness. *Crit Care Med* 2004;**32**:1527–34.

86 Nelson JE, Cox CE, Hope AA, Carson SS. Chronic critical illness. *Am J Respir Crit Care Med* 2010;**182**:446–54.

87 Kalb TH, Lorin S. Infection in the chronically critically ill: unique risk profile in a newly defined population. *Crit Care Clin* 2002;**18**:529–52.

88 Yende S, Angus DC, Ali IS, et al. Influence of comorbid conditions on long-term mortality after pneumonia in older people. *J Am Geriatr Soc* 2007;**55**:518–25.

89 Mortensen EM, Coley CM, Singer DE, et al. Causes of death for patients with community-acquired pneumonia: results from the Pneumonia Patient Outcomes Research Team cohort study. *Arch Intern Med* 2002;**162**:1059–64.

90 Kind AJ, Smith MA, Pandhi N, Frytak JR, Finch MD. Bouncing-back: rehospitalization in patients with complicated transitions in the first thirty days after hospital discharge for acute stroke. *Home Health Care Serv Q* 2007;**26**:37–55.

91 Hotchkiss RS, Opal S. Immunotherapy for sepsis--a new approach against an ancient foe. *N Engl J Med* 2010;**363**:87–9.

92 Otto GP, Sossdorf M, Claus RA, et al. The late phase of sepsis is characterized by an increased microbiological burden and death rate. *Crit Care* 2011;**15**:R183.

93 Benjamim CF, Hogaboam CM, Kunkel SL. The chronic consequences of severe sepsis. *J Leukoc Biol* 2004;**75**:408–12.

94 Yende S, D'Angelo G, Kellum JA, al. Inflammatory markers at hospital discharge predict subsequent mortality after pneumonia and sepsis. *Am J Respir Crit Care Med* 2008;**177**:1242–7.

95 Huang X, Venet F, Wang YL, Lepape A, Yuan Z, Chen Y, et al. PD-1 expression by macrophages plays a pathologic role in altering microbial clearance and the innate inflammatory response to sepsis. *Proc Natl Acad Sci USA* 2009;**106**(15):6303–8.

96 Meisel C, Schefold JC, Pschowski R, Baumann T, Hetzger K, Gregor J, et al. Granulocyte-macrophage colony-stimulating factor to reverse sepsis-associated immunosuppression: a double-blind, randomized, placebo-controlled multicenter trial. *Am J Respir Crit Care Med* 2009;**180**(7):640–8.

97 Stevens RD, Marshall SA, Cornblath DR, et al. A framework for diagnosing and classifying intensive care unit-acquired weakness. *Crit Care Med* 2009;**37**(10 Suppl):S299–308.

98 Schefold JC, Bierbrauer J, Weber-Carstens S. Intensive care unit-acquired weakness (ICUAW) and muscle wasting in critically ill patients with severe sepsis and septic shock. *J Cachexia Sarcopenia Muscle* 2010;**1**:147–57.

99 Batt J, Dos Santos CC, Cameron JI, Herridge MS. Intensive-care unit acquired weakness (ICUAW): clinical phenotypes and molecular mechanisms. *Am J Respir Crit Care Med* 2013;**187**:238–46.

100 Hollander JM, Mechanick JI. Nutrition support and the chronic critical illness syndrome. *Nutr Clin Pract* 2006;**21**:587–604.

101 Van den Berghe G. Novel insights into the neuroendocrinology of critical illness. *Eur J Endocrinol* 2000;**143**:1–13.

102 **Schulman RC, Mechanick JI.** Metabolic and nutrition support in the chronic critical illness syndrome. *Respir Care* 2012;**57**:958–77; discussion 77–8.

103 **Nierman DM, Mechanick JI.** Hypotestosteronemia in chronically critically ill men. *Crit Care Med* 1999;**27**:2418–21.

104 **Takala J, Ruokonen E, Webster NR, et al.** Increased mortality associated with growth hormone treatment in critically ill adults. *N Engl J Med* 1999;**341**:785–92.

105 **Bulger EM, Jurkovich GJ, Farver CL, Klotz P, Maier RV.** Oxandrolone does not improve outcome of ventilator dependent surgical patients. *Ann Surg* 2004;**240**:472–8; discussion 8–80.

106 **Mechanick JI, Nierman DM.** Gonadal steroids in critical illness. *Crit Care Clin* 2006;**22**:87–103, vii.

107 **Van den Berghe G, Baxter RC, Weekers F, et al.** The combined administration of GH-releasing peptide-2 (GHRP-2), TRH and GnRH to men with prolonged critical illness evokes superior endocrine and metabolic effects compared to treatment with GHRP-2 alone. *Clin Endocrinol (Oxf)* 2002;**56**:655–69.

108 **Kemper M, Weissman C, Hyman AI.** Caloric requirements and supply in critically ill surgical patients. *Crit Care Med* 1992;**20**:344–8.

109 **McClave SA, Sexton LK, Spain DA, et al.** Enteral tube feeding in the intensive care unit: factors impeding adequate delivery. *Crit Care Med* 1999;**27**:1252–6.

110 **Heyland D, Cook DJ, Winder B, Brylowski L, Van deMark H, Guyatt G.** Enteral nutrition in the critically ill patient: a prospective survey. *Crit Care Med* 1995;**23**:1055–60.

111 **Rice TW, Wheeler AP, Thompson BT, et al.** Initial trophic vs full enteral feeding in patients with acute lung injury: the EDEN randomized trial. *JAMA* 2012;**307**:795–803.

112 **Rubinson L, Diette GB, Song X, Brower RG, Krishnan JA.** Low caloric intake is associated with nosocomial bloodstream infections in patients in the medical intensive care unit. *Crit Care Med* 2004;**32**:350–7.

113 **Artinian V, Krayem H, DiGiovine B.** Effects of early enteral feeding on the outcome of critically ill mechanically ventilated medical patients. *Chest* 2006;**129**:960–7.

114 **Coeffier M, Dechelotte P.** The role of glutamine in intensive care unit patients: mechanisms of action and clinical outcome. *Nutr Rev* 2005;**63**:65–9.

115 **Nierman DM, Mechanick JI.** Bone hyperresorption is prevalent in chronically critically ill patients. *Chest* 1998;**114**:1122–8.

116 **Wurfel MM, Gordon AC, Holden TD, et al.** Toll-like receptor 1 polymorphisms affect innate immune responses and outcomes in sepsis. *Am J Respir Crit Care Med* 2008;**178**:710–20.

117 **Yende S, Angus DC, Ding J, et al.** 4G/5G plasminogen activator inhibitor-1 polymorphisms and haplotypes are associated with pneumonia. *Am J Respir Crit Care Med* 2007;**176**:1129–37.

118 **Yende S, Angus DC, Kong L, et al.** The influence of macrophage migration inhibitory factor gene polymorphisms on outcome from community-acquired pneumonia. *FASEB J* 2009;**23**:2403–11.

119 **Yende S, Kammerer CM, Angus DC.** Genetics and proteomics: deciphering gene association studies in critical illness. *Crit Care* 2006;**10**:227.

120 **Weiss KM, Terwilliger JD.** How many diseases does it take to map a gene with SNPs? *Nat Genet* 2000;**26**:151–7.

121 **Roberts NJ, Vogelstein JT, Parmigiani G, Kinzler KW, Vogelstein B, Velculescu VE.** The predictive capacity of personal genome sequencing. *Sci Transl Med* 2012;**4**:133ra58.

122 **Lemeshow S, Teres D, Klar J, Avrunin JS, Gehlbach SH, Rapoport J.** Mortality Probability Models (MPM II) based on an international cohort of intensive care unit patients. *JAMA* 1993;**270**:2478–86.

123 **Le Gall JR, Lemeshow S, Saulnier F.** A new Simplified Acute Physiology Score (SAPS II) based on a European/North American multicenter study. *JAMA* 1993;**270**:2957–63.

124 **Le Gall JR, Klar J, Lemeshow S, et al.** The logistic organ dysfunction system. A new way to assess organ dysfunction in the intensive care unit. ICU Scoring Group. *JAMA* 1996;**276**:802–10.

125 **Boumendil A, Maury E, Reinhard I, Luquel L, Offenstadt G, Guidet B.** Prognosis of patients aged 80 years and over admitted in medical intensive care unit. *Intensive Care Med* 2004;**30**:647–54.

126 Somme D, Maillet JM, Gisselbrecht M, Novara A, Ract C, Fagon JY. Critically ill old and the oldest-old patients in intensive care: short- and long-term outcomes. *Intensive Care Med* 2003;**29**:2137–43.

127 Teno JM, Harrell FE, Jr, Knaus W, et al. Prediction of survival for older hospitalized patients: the HELP survival model. Hospitalized Elderly Longitudinal Project. *J Am Geriatr Soc* 2000;**48** (5 Suppl):S16–24.

128 Carson SS, Bach PB. Predicting mortality in patients suffering from prolonged critical illness: an assessment of four severity-of-illness measures. *Chest* 2001;**120**:928–33.

129 Baldwin MR,Narain WR, Wunsch H et al. A prognostic model for six-month mortality in elderly survivors of critical illness. *Chest* 2013;**143**:910–19.

130 Needham DM, Scales DC, Laupacis A, Pronovost PJ. A systematic review of the Charlson comorbidity index using Canadian administrative databases: a perspective on risk adjustment in critical care research. *J Crit Care* 2005;**20**:12–19.

131 Charlson ME, Pompei P, Ales KL, MacKenzie CR. A new method of classifying prognostic comorbidity in longitudinal studies: development and validation. *J Chronic Dis* 1987;**40**:373–83.

132 Fried LP, Kronmal RA, Newman AB, et al. Risk factors for 5-year mortality in older adults: the Cardiovascular Health Study. *JAMA* 1998;**279**:585–92.

133 Bo M, Massaia M, Raspo S, et al. Predictive factors of in-hospital mortality in older patients admitted to a medical intensive care unit. *J Am Geriatr Soc* 2003;**51**:529–33.

134 Sligl WI, Eurich DT, Marrie TJ, Majumdar SR. Only severely limited, premorbid functional status is associated with short- and long-term mortality in patients with pneumonia who are critically ill: a prospective observational study. *Chest* 2011;**139**:88–94.

135 Granja C, Azevedo LF. When (quality of) life is at stake and intensive care is needed: how much can we trust our proxies? *Intensive Care Med* 2006;**32**:1681–2.

136 Rogers J, Ridley S, Chrispin P, Scotton H, Lloyd D. Reliability of the next of kins' estimates of critically ill patients' quality of life. *Anaesthesia* 1997;**52**:1137–43.

137 Walter LC, Brand RJ, Counsell SR, et al. Development and validation of a prognostic index for 1-year mortality in older adults after hospitalization. *JAMA* 2001;**285**:2987–94.

138 Espaulella J, Arnau A, Cubi D, Amblas J, Yanez A. Time-dependent prognostic factors of 6-month mortality in frail elderly patients admitted to post-acute care. *Age Ageing* 2007;**36**:407–13.

139 Fried LP, Ferrucci L, Darer J, Williamson JD, Anderson G. Untangling the concepts of disability, frailty, and comorbidity: implications for improved targeting and care. *J Gerontol A Biol Sci Med Sci* 2004;**59**:255–63.

140 Fried LP, Tangen CM, Walston J, et al. Frailty in older adults: evidence for a phenotype. *J Gerontol A Biol Sci Med Sci* 2001;**56**:M146–56.

141 Ensrud KE, Ewing SK, Taylor BC, et al. Comparison of 2 frailty indexes for prediction of falls, disability, fractures, and death in older women. *Arch Intern Med* 2008;**168**:382–9.

142 Pisani MA, Kong SY, Kasl SV, Murphy TE, Araujo KL, Van Ness PH. Days of delirium are associated with 1-year mortality in an older intensive care unit population. *Am J Respir Crit Care Med* 2009;**180**:1092–7.

143 Englesbe MJ, Patel SP, He K, et al. Sarcopenia and mortality after liver transplantation. *J Am Coll Surg* 2010;**211**:271–8.

144 Slinde F, Gronberg A, Engstrom CP, Rossander-Hulthen L, Larsson S. Body composition by bio-electrical impedance predicts mortality in chronic obstructive pulmonary disease patients. *Respir Med* 2005;**99**:1004–9.

145 Vestbo J, Prescott E, Almdal T, et al. Body mass, fat-free body mass, and prognosis in patients with chronic obstructive pulmonary disease from a random population sample: findings from the Copenhagen City Heart Study. *Am J Respir Crit Care Med* 2006;**173**:79–83.

Chapter 4

The Role of Long-Term Ventilator Hospitals

Jeremy M. Kahn

Introduction

ICU survivors pose an important problem for health systems worldwide.[1] Currently, an estimated 4 to 7 million ICU admissions occur in the US each year.[2] A majority of these patients will survive, requiring ongoing health care services due to the numerous physical, emotional, and neurocognitive sequelae of critical illness.[3] Of these survivors, between 5 and 10% develop CCI, a syndrome characterized by persistent organ failures and ongoing dependence on life support, including PMV.[4] Currently, over 100 000 individuals in the US require PMV each year, and this number is expected to rise as the population ages and demand for critical care increases.[5] Also fuelling this rise are recent medical advances in intensive care medicine that reduce ICU mortality. As more patients than ever survive intensive care, more will progress to CCI, rather than making an immediate full recovery. These patients consume a disproportionate amount of health care resources and experience significant morbidity and mortality after hospital discharge. Six-month survival is 40%, compared to 80% for all survivors of intensive care.[6]

Much of the current discussion surrounding the topic of critical illness recovery concerns **how** to care for ICU survivors, specifically the development and testing of evidence-based care strategies to speed organ system recovery and optimize QoL. However, an equally compelling issue concerns **where** to care for ICU survivors, specifically whether specific types of hospitals, or organizational and management strategies within acute care hospitals, may be associated with improved treatment and recovery. Indeed, the ICU is primarily designed to provide highly specialized acute care for patients at significant risk for imminent mortality. As such, it may not be the optimal care setting in which to attend to the special needs of patients in the convalescent phase of acute illness, even if they require ongoing life support.

Based on this consideration, hospitals and health systems have developed alternatives to the ICU for patients who are in the recovery phase of critical illness but still have persistent organ failures necessitating high acuity care. Among these ICU alternatives are 'step-down' units within acute care hospitals, skilled nursing facilities (SNFs) capable of providing MV or RRT, and specialized, long-term hospitals designed purely for patients with CCI. All of these models have theoretical benefits and drawbacks, but all play a unique, and potentially important, role in the spectrum of care for ICU survivors. This chapter will review the different critical illness recovery care models, discuss the theoretical clinical and financial implications of the different models, and highlight what role specialized hospitals for critical illness recovery might play in the future.

Care settings for critical illness recovery

Prior to the advent of specialized facilities for patients recovering from critical illness, those individuals that survived the acute episode of critical illness, but experienced PMV and other forms of CCI, continued to receive care in the ICU. This was because the ICU was the only health care setting capable of safely providing MV in patients with other complex care needs. Of course, MV at home was, and remains, a possibility; however, home MV is typically reserved for patients with respiratory failure due to chronic medical conditions, not patients recovering from acute respiratory failure.[7] Yet, caring for patients with CCI in the ICU has several drawbacks. The diversity of staff members in ICUs hinders the establishment of long-term relationships with patients, and it may be an inefficient use of scarce ICU resources. Consequently, hospitals, and later health systems, developed specialized areas to care for these patients (see Table 4.1).

At one end of the spectrum, these specialized areas take the form of 'step-down' units within acute care hospitals, which can provide higher intensity care than a traditional hospital ward but lack all the capabilities of an ICU. Step-down units are relatively common in countries like the UK, which have a relatively low number of ICU beds per capita and therefore must reserve them for the very sickest patients.[8] In other developed countries, step-down units are less common, although there are few data to indicate their exact prevalence. Nonetheless, they are still a relatively well-described location for care.[9] These units typically have lower nurse-to-patient ratios than traditional ICUs and lack the ability to provide some types of life support such as vasopressors, continuous RRT, or non-conventional modes of MV. However, they can provide traditional MV, especially weaning services for patients with prolonged ventilator dependence. Importantly, because these units are located within acute care hospitals, they can easily avail themselves of all the services of acute care hospitals. Patients can obtain radiographic studies, receive specialty consultations, and, if need be, can be rapidly transferred to a traditional ICU, should their condition deteriorate.

Rehabilitation hospitals and SNFs are another alternative site of care, especially in the US where these types of health care facilities are common. These hospitals provide specialized services for patients recovering from critical illness but usually cannot provide MV or other types of life support.[10,11] Consequently, they are reserved for patients who, although not yet ready to transition back to home, have been liberated from MV and are capable of participating in active physical therapy (PT) and other rehabilitation activities. Because, in most cases, these facilities do not provide MV, they are usually not considered alternatives to an acute care ICU. Still, they are likely to play an important role in the post-ICU care spectrum to the degree that they allow patients to continue a long trajectory of recovery outside the acute care hospital.

Table 4.1 Non-intensive care settings for patients with CCI

Category	Setting
Within acute care hospitals	Step-down units
Outside acute care hospitals, low capability	Rehabilitation hospitals Skilled nursing facilities
Outside acute care hospitals, high capability	Long-term acute care hospitals Weaning centres

Long-term acute care hospitals

In the US, another alternative to the ICU is the long-term acute care (LTAC) hospital.[12] The US government narrowly defines LTACs as acute care hospitals with a mean length of stay of at least 25 days.[13] By meeting this definition, LTAC hospitals operate under special reimbursement rules that allow them to profitably care for extremely high-cost patients with CCI. However, more broadly, LTAC hospitals can be defined as a hospital specifically designed to meet the needs of patients with CCI. Typically, this means that they can provide all of the services of an acute care ICU but in a less intense setting. Because they explicitly do not care for patients with extremely high severity of illness, they can provide more holistic care, including regular PT and occupational therapy (OT), in addition to prolonged ventilator care. LTACs in US originally rose in the 1950s as dedicated tuberculosis hospitals and only recently evolved into this more general role as hospitals for critical care recovery.

In contrast to ICUs, LTAC care is less intense and more geared toward long-term recovery than short-term survival. Nurse-to-patient ratios are more similar to step-down units than ICUs, and physician staffing is typically less intense.[14] Perhaps most importantly, LTACs typically employ standardized protocols for liberating patients from PMV.[15] Instead of the once-daily spontaneous breathing trial (SBT) which has become the norm in acute care ICUs,[16] LTACs more frequently employ weaning strategies that entail gradual reductions in pressure support and increasingly long periods of no ventilator support.[17] Many, if not all, LTAC patients on the ventilator have undergone tracheostomy and gastrostomy tube placement to facilitate the long-term respiratory and nutritional support necessary for this type of care.

United States LTACs

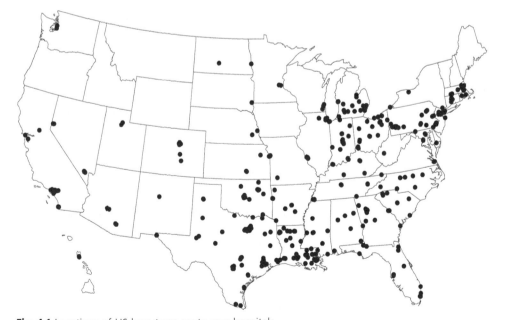

Fig. 4.1 Locations of US long-term acute care hospitals.

Data from Centers for Medicare and Medicaid Services Healthcare Cost Reporting Information System, 2006.

In part because of the increasing numbers of patients requiring PMV, LTACs have dramatically increased in number in the US. In the 10-year period between 1997 and 2006, the number of LTACs increased from 192 to 408, making them the fastest growing segment of acute care in the US.[18] Indeed, the number of traditional acute care hospitals declined during the same period.[19] The distribution of LTACs in the US is not homogenous (see Figure 4.1), with a greater number of LTACs in the southern and north-eastern areas of the country, compared to other areas. This variation has implications for utilization, as patients are more likely to be transferred to an LTAC for post-acute care if their admission hospital is in close proximity to an LTAC.[20]

Concomitant with the increase in the total number of LTACs is an increase in the number of patients receiving LTAC care. In Medicare, the US government-based health insurer for elderly Americans, the number of patients transferred to an LTAC after intensive care more than tripled from 1997 to 2006, from 13 732 to 40 352, at an annual total cost of $1.325 billion.[18] More and more frequently, the primary reason for admission was for liberation from MV, rather than non-ventilation convalescent care. In the period 1997–2000, only 16.4% of Medicare LTAC transfers received MV at the LTAC, while, in the period 2004–2006, this figure had increased to 29.8%.

Long-term acute care outside the US

Outside the US, LTAC-style care exists within dedicated weaning centres for patients with prolonged respiratory failure. In many cases, these hospitals pre-date the US LTAC model, having been established along with the advent of MV in response to the 1950s polio epidemic. Multiple countries have at least one, and sometimes more, of these centres, including the UK,[21] Canada,[22] Germany,[23] and Italy,[24,25] among others. These weaning centres are typically small hospitals but still possess the resources to care for patients requiring MV over the long term. Generally, weaning centres specialize not only in post-ICU rehabilitation and ventilator weaning, but also chronic respiratory failure, sleep disordered breathing, and neuromuscular disease, conditions analogous to post-ICU recovery in that they require a multidisciplinary approach to care. These conditions also all benefit from the judicious use of non-invasive ventilation (NIV), which may be best provided in regional centres of expertise.[26]

Long-term hospitals vs ICUs

There are a number of reasons why long-term hospitals, such as LTACs and weaning centres, may be either better or worse than traditional ICUs, both from a clinical and financial perspective (see Figure 4.2).

Long-term hospitals may improve clinical outcomes

Long-term hospitals may improve patient survival and functional outcomes after PMV through increased clinical experience with these types of patients. There are data to suggest that hospitals providing care for a high volume of patients receiving MV have improved outcomes, compared to patients at lower-volume hospitals.[27] Long-term hospitals might also improve outcomes through the use of multidisciplinary teams, protocolized weaning, and early mobilization, which are known to improve outcomes in short-stay ICUs.[28-30] These effects may be magnified in long-term hospitals which, as regional referral centres, care for a higher proportion of patients with PMV than traditional ICUs. Moreover, unlike traditional ICUs, LTAC hospitals are not burdened by the necessity to care for extremely high-acuity patients which may detract from the mission of providing coordinated long-term care.

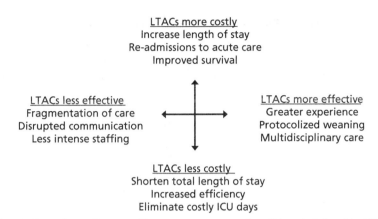

Fig. 4.2 Potential benefits and harms of long-term acute care (LTAC) hospitals in critical illness recovery.

Long-term hospitals may worsen clinical outcomes

Long-term hospitals may actually worsen clinical outcomes through several potential mechanisms. First, long-term hospitals are physically separate from traditional acute care hospitals, with different staff and clinicians. The resulting fragmentation of care creates the potential for communication deficits that may substantially disrupt continuity for these extremely complex patients (see Figure 4.3).[31,32] Second, since long-term hospitals typically have less intense nurse and physician staffing, compared to traditional ICUs, they may be less well equipped to handle physiological deterioration, airway emergencies, or other complications of CCI. Lower-intensity nurse and physician staffing is associated with higher mortality for critically ill patients, a relationship which may also exist in recovery after intensive care.[33,34]

Long-term hospitals may decrease health care costs

Long-term care hospitals could improve health care efficiency by decreasing the total duration of MV when compared to traditional ICUs. The duration of MV and length of stay are not tightly tied to costs in the ICU setting, at least in the short term,[35] but, over the long term, hospitals could scale back on resources and staff through reductions in length of stay, ultimately lowering costs.[36] Other mechanisms through which long-term hospitals could improve efficiency is through less intense staffing, leading to lower per-day costs than ICUs, and by caring for a high volume of mechanically ventilated patients, creating economies of scope and scale.[37]

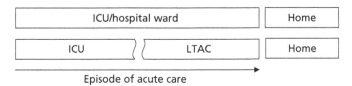

Fig. 4.3 Long-term hospitals fragment the episode of acute care.

Long-term hospitals may increase health care costs

Long-term care hospitals could also increase overall costs of care, particularly if they increase the overall length of stay. This might occur if communication deficits during the transition from short-stay hospital ICUs to LTACs lead to clinical fumbles and resulting complications, or if long-term hospitals are not able to successfully translate their experienced staff and weaning protocols into shorter lengths of stay. Costs could also increase if long-term hospitals improve patient survival, since patients who survive require more resources than if they had otherwise died.

To date, few clinical studies have directly compared patient outcomes between different types of hospitals. One-year survival for patients transferred to long-term hospitals for ventilator weaning is approximately 50%,[18] with many of these patients ultimately unable to wean from the ventilator.[38,39] Although, by some standards, these outcomes seem poor, without valid comparator groups, it is impossible to say whether long-term care hospitals offer clinical benefit. One US study in 1702 patients showed that patients transferred to an LTAC had similar 6-month survival and costs, compared to patients evaluated but not transferred.[40] Another US report echoed those findings, demonstrating that LTACs were of comparable efficacy, but potentially more costly, compared to acute care hospitals for similar patients.[41] Both studies were confounded by the selection inherent in long-term hospital admission—since long-term hospitals screen their patients for admission, they can potentially select for patients most likely to benefit. Ultimately, more research is needed to determine which specific patients may benefit from care in a long-term hospital outside the ICU.

Societal benefits

The presence of LTACs within a health system may have system-wide benefits, independent of the patients that actually receive care in them. These so-called 'spillover' effects are an important part of the equation in evaluating the role of LTACs in patients with CCI and can be both beneficial or harmful (see Table 4.2). On the beneficial side, the presence of LTACs in a community might have positive downstream effects by accepting long-stay patients in transfer and thus freeing up ICU beds for other patients. ICU beds are a scarce resource and, in the setting of constrained supply, must sometimes operate at peak capacity.[42] In turn, operating at peak capacity can result in deleterious effects such as premature ICU discharge[43] and delayed admission from emergency departments.[44] These negative consequences might be minimized if long-stay patients with chronic crucial illness could be transferred out of ICUs to LTACs, effectively increasing the number of available ICU beds. Freeing up ICU beds could also allow for more high-risk elective surgeries like cancer operations or coronary artery bypass grafting. In theory, the number of these procedures should be determined by societal norms, not by the availability of a post-operative ICU bed for recovery.[45] In this way, to the degree that health systems can use LTACs to provide

Table 4.2 Potential spillover effects of LTACs

Positive	Negative
Effective increase in ICU bed supply	Tolerance for CCI
Decreased emergency boarding	Fewer discussions with patients about their preferences at end of life
Decreased night-time ICU discharges	
Increased opportunity for elective surgery	Poor quality of end-of-life care

critical care to long-stay patients outside the ICU, LTACs might allow for more efficient use of existing ICU resources.[46]

Societal harms

The potential negative spillover effects of LTACs, paradoxically, also stem from the effective increase in ICU beds that may result from discharging long-stay patients out of the ICU. In this case, the existence of LTACs as an outlet for discharging long-stay patients may induce a tolerance of CCI among clinicians, who may be less likely to initiate end-of-life discussions in seriously ill patients if they know an LTAC is available as an alternative.[47] If the LTAC were not available, clinicians may feel more pressure to engage patients about their preferences for the end of life, potentially resulting in better palliative care.[48] Ultimately, critical care can be thought of as a contract between the patient and health system, wherein the patient seeks increased survival in exchange for some personal costs (in the form of discomfort) and some societal costs (in the form of resource use). Transitioning from intensive treatment to palliative care involves breaking that contract through the recognition that any potential survival advantage is no longer worth the costs.

This contract can also occur between patients and physicians, since physicians may view the failure to save a patient to be a personal failure, as sometimes occurs after high-risk surgeries.[49] To the degree that LTACs decrease the societal cost of critical care by making ICU beds less scarce and easing the physician's burden from a patient's death, they may less frequently force us to consider the human cost of prolonged critical care. Sometimes, this result may be beneficial if patients always want intense care at the end of life. Yet evidence suggests that this is not the case and that clinicians, at least in countries with ample ICU bed supply like the US, too infrequently offer palliative care as an option for patients.[50,51]

The role of reimbursement

Although the exact role of long-term hospitals in the health system can be evaluated, based on traditional issues of costs and effectiveness, the existence of these hospitals cannot be separated from their reimbursement. Different health systems reimburse long-term hospitals in different ways, creating financial incentives that can either encourage or discourage their use. This is especially true because, unlike traditional hospitals which must provide at least some care for any patient that shows up at the door, long-term hospitals have the unique ability to screen and select their patients, providing a mechanism for financial issues to enter into the decision surrounding admissions. Any discussion of these hospitals must therefore address issues of reimbursement, which can affect not only the ways in which they are used, but also the ways in which their outcomes are interpreted by the health care payers and policy makers.

LTAC reimbursement in the US

Reimbursement is essential to the LTAC discussion in the US, because the very existence of LTACs was born out of reimbursement policy. In the US, most payers, including the US government, reimburse hospitals for each patient by a fixed amount corresponding to that patient type's average cost in the region, a concept know as **prospective payment**.[52] Hospitals that can care for patients with lower costs than their prospective payment will earn money on that patient, while hospitals that care for patients at a higher cost than their prospective payment will lose money on that patient. When prospective payment was instituted in the US in the 1980s, LTACs were exempted on the idea that their case-mix is inherently different from traditional acute care hospitals. However, this unwittingly created a financial incentive for traditional hospitals to send patients to LTACs—patients with CCI are among the most resource-intensive patients in the hospital, and early discharge to an LTAC means that hospitals will lose less money. At the same time, LTACs are relatively profitable in the US, even after their own prospective payment system was implemented in 2002.[53] This means that financial incentives driving LTAC transfers work for both the sending and receiving hospital, while payers, such as the US government, must now pay for two hospitalizations instead of one.

These incentives were the primary driver behind LTAC growth in the US. This is not to say that LTACs are not clinically useful, only that their growth is due more to financial considerations than clinical considerations. The importance of these incentives is further evident in the idea of patient selection. In the US, health insurance status is among the strongest drivers of LTAC admission at the patient level: patients with commercial insurance are more likely to be transferred than patients with government insurance, and patients without health insurance essentially never go to LTACs.[54] Moreover, private, for-profit hospitals are more likely to send patients to LTACs than their non-profit counterparts.[20] Should LTAC-style care be beneficial to patients, then current reimbursement schemata create an unfortunate health disparity in which uninsured patients lack appropriate access.

Reimbursement outside the US

Many developed countries, even those with national health insurance programmes, reimburse hospitals, according to a prospective payment system, and so would face analogous financial issues regarding LTAC incentives. Other countries use a **capitated payment** system, in which hospitals receive a lump sum each year and must provide all their necessary care out of that amount. Under capitated payment, hospitals may or may not have an incentive towards early discharge.[55] There is a financial reward for efficiency, but only if the hospital is not responsible for the LTAC-related costs for those patients. In many capitated payment systems, the cost of weaning centre care is borne by the originating hospitals.[21] Since this care may or may not be less costly than the care provided in an ICU, hospitals must determine how frequently to refer patients, based on local conditions. Typically, weaning hospitals in these countries can still select patients for admission. The only potential drawback is that, since the weaning hospitals are reimbursed according to costs, they have no incentive to provide highly efficient care, potentially increasing the overall cost of care.

Conclusion

Regardless of how LTACs and weaning hospitals impact the care of patients in the post-ICU care period, they have become an important part of the health care landscape and are likely here to stay. Therefore, the primary goal in the coming years is not to determine whether or not they are a cost-effective method of post-ICU care, but how to use them most effectively and for the most societal good. As described in this chapter, there are reasons to hypothesize that LTACs have both positive and negative clinical effects, as well as positive and negative financial effects. And, even if clinically and financially neutral, they could provide important spillover benefits to society that justify their model of care, including increasing ICU bed availability for patients in need. These spillover benefits must be weighed against potential spillover harms, including an untoward tolerance for CCI that could prolong the dying process without improving net survival or QoL.

More patient-centred outcomes research is needed to further determine the optimal role of these hospitals in the health system. Moreover, this role will continue to evolve. Future advances will likely involve standardization of patient selection criteria for admission to an LTAC and better integration between acute care ICUs and weaning facilities that will allow for more seamless transitions with minimal disruption of care plans and miscommunication between providers.[56] If these advances proceed simultaneously, it will help to ensure that improved transitions do not lead to inappropriate use. Moreover, reimbursement reforms, including quality-based reimbursements, should be designed to maximize both appropriateness of transfer and quality of care. Finally, the evidence base should evolve to better guide care practices regarding ventilator weaning, sedation management, and PT. The practices that work well in ICUs may not work well in the long-term care setting.

In the meantime, clinicians caring for patients with CCI should be aware of these issues when considering referring a patient to an LTAC hospital or a weaning centre. Clinicians should investigate exactly what services those hospitals provide, determine in what way those services are different from a traditional ICU, engage patients and their families to discuss the implications of prolonged ventilator care, and verify that transfer to a long-term hospital is in keeping with the patients' preferences and values. In doing so, clinicians can help to ensure that long-term care hospitals provide minimal harm in the face of uncertain benefits.

References

1 Kahn JM, Angus DC. Health policy and future planning for survivors of critical illness. *Curr Opin Crit Care* 2007;**13**:514–18.

2 Halpern NA, Pastores SM, Thaler HT, Greenstein RJ. Changes in critical care beds and occupancy in the United States 1985–2000: differences attributable to hospital size. *Crit Care Med* 2006;**34**:2105–12.

3 Herridge MS. Long-term outcomes after critical illness: past, present, future. *Curr Opin Crit Care* 2007;**13**:473–5.

4 Nelson JE, Cox CE, Hope AA, Carson SS. Chronic critical illness. *Am J Respir Crit Care Med* 2010;**182**:446–54.

5 Carson SS, Bach PB. The epidemiology and costs of chronic critical illness. *Crit Care Clin* 2002;**18**: 461–76.

6 Douglas SL, Daly BJ, Gordon N, Brennan PF. Survival and quality of life: short-term versus long-term ventilator patients. *Crit Care Med* 2002;**30**:2655–62.

7 Wise MP, Hart N, Davidson C, et al. Home mechanical ventilation. *BMJ* 2011;**342**:d1687.

8 O'Dea J, Pepperman M, Bion J. Comprehensive Critical Care: a national strategic framework in all but name. *Intensive Care Med* 2003;**29**:341.

9 Criner GJ, Travaline JM. Transitional respiratory care and rehabilitation. *Curr Opin Crit Care* 1999;**5**:81.

10 Latriano B, McCauley P, Astiz ME, Greenbaum D, Rackow EC. Non-ICU care of hemodynamically stable mechanically ventilated patients. *Chest* 1996;**109**:1591–6.

11 Ambrosino N, Vianello A. Where to perform long-term ventilation. *Respir Care Clin N Am* 2002;**8**:463–78.

12 Eskildsen MA. Long-term acute care: a review of the literature. *J Am Geriatr Soc* 2007;**55**:775–9.

13 Carson SS. Know your long-term care hospital. *Chest* 2007;**131**:2–5.

14 Liu K, Baseggio C, Wissoker D, Maxwell S, Haley J, Long S. Long-term care hospitals under Medicare: facility-level characteristics. *Health Care Financ Rev* 2001;**23**:1–18.

15 MacIntyre NR, Epstein SK, Carson S, Scheinhorn D, Christopher K, Muldoon S. Management of patients requiring prolonged mechanical ventilation: report of a NAMDRC consensus conference. *Chest* 2005;**128**:3937–54.

16 Esteban A, Ferguson ND, Meade MO, et al. Evolution of mechanical ventilation in response to clinical research. *Am J Respir Crit Care Med* 2008;**177**:170–7.

17 Scheinhorn DJ, Hassenpflug MS, Votto JJ, et al. Post-ICU mechanical ventilation at 23 long-term care hospitals: a multicenter outcomes study. *Chest* 2007;**131**:85–93.

18 Kahn JM, Benson NM, Appleby D, Carson SS, Iwashyna TJ. Long-term acute care hospital utilization after critical illness. *JAMA* 2010;**303**:2253–9.

19 Halpern NA, Pastores SM. Critical care medicine in the United States 2000–5: an analysis of bed numbers, occupancy rates, payer mix, and costs. *Crit Care Med* 2010;**38**:65–71.

20 Kahn JM, Werner RM, Carson SS, Iwashyna TJ. Variation in long-term acute care hospital use after intensive care. *Med Care Res Rev* 2012;**69**:339–50.

21 Pilcher DV, Bailey MJ, Treacher DF, Hamid S, Williams AJ, Davidson AC. Outcomes, cost and long term survival of patients referred to a regional weaning centre. *Thorax* 2005;**60**:187–92.

22 Toronto Central Local Health Integration Network. *Long-term ventilation strategy development for Ontario*. Toronto: Ministry of Health and Long-Term Care; 2008.

23 Schonhofer B, Euteneuer S, Nava S, Suchi S, Kohler D. Survival of mechanically ventilated patients admitted to a specialised weaning centre. *Intensive Care Med* 2002;**28**:908–16.

24 Clini EM, Siddu P, Trianni L, Graziosi R, Crisafulli E, Nobile MT. Activity and analysis of costs in a dedicated weaning centre. *Monaldi Arch Chest Dis* 2008;**69**:55–8.

25 Carpene N, Vagheggini G, Panait E, Gabbrielli L, Ambrosino N. A proposal of a new model for long-term weaning: respiratory intensive care unit and weaning center. *Respir Med* 2010;**104**:1505–11.

26 Chandra D, Stamm JA, Taylor B, et al. Outcomes of noninvasive ventilation for acute exacerbations of chronic obstructive pulmonary disease in the United States, 1998–2008. *Am J Respir Crit Care Med* 2012;**185**:152–9.

27 Kahn JM, Goss CH, Heagerty PJ, Kramer AA, O'Brien CR, Rubenfeld GD. Hospital volume and the outcomes of mechanical ventilation. *N Engl J Med* 2006;**355**:41–50.

28 Kim MM, Barnato AE, Angus DC, Fleisher LA, Kahn JM. The effect of multidisciplinary care teams on intensive care unit mortality. *Arch Intern Med* 2010;**170**:369–76.

29 Girard TD, Kress JP, Fuchs BD, et al. Efficacy and safety of a paired sedation and ventilator weaning protocol for mechanically ventilated patients in intensive care (Awakening and Breathing Controlled trial): a randomised controlled trial. *Lancet* 2008;**371**:126–34.

30 Schweickert WD, Pohlman MC, Pohlman AS, et al. Early physical and occupational therapy in mechanically ventilated, critically ill patients: a randomised controlled trial. *Lancet* 2009;**373**:1874–82.

31 Coleman EA, Min SJ, Chomiak A, Kramer AM. Posthospital care transitions: patterns, complications, and risk identification. *Health Serv Res* 2004;**39**:1449–65.

32 White AC, Joseph B, Perrotta BA, et al. Unplanned transfers following admission to a long-term acute care hospital: a quality issue. *Chron Respir Dis* 2011;**8**:245–52.

33 Tarnow-Mordi WO, Hau C, Warden A, Shearer AJ. Hospital mortality in relation to staff workload: a 4-year study in an adult intensive-care unit. *Lancet* 2000;**356**:185–9.

34 Pronovost PJ, Angus DC, Dorman T, Robinson KA, Dremsizov TT, Young TL. Physician staffing patterns and clinical outcomes in critically ill patients: a systematic review. *JAMA* 2002;**288**:2151–62.

35 Kahn JM, Rubenfeld GD, Rohrbach J, Fuchs BD. Cost savings attributable to reductions in intensive care unit length of stay for mechanically ventilated patients. *Med Care* 2008;**46**:1226–33.

36 Rapoport J, Teres D, Zhao Y, Lemeshow S. Length of stay data as a guide to hospital economic performance for ICU patients. *Med Care* 2003;**41**:386–97.

37 Jacobs P, Rapoport J, Edbrooke D. Economies of scale in British intensive care units and combined intensive care/high dependency units. *Intensive Care Med* 2004;**30**:660–4.

38 Scheinhorn DJ, Hassenpflug MS, Votto JJ, et al. Ventilator-dependent survivors of catastrophic illness transferred to 23 long-term care hospitals for weaning from prolonged mechanical ventilation. *Chest* 2007;**131**:76–84.

39 Carson SS, Bach PB, Brzozowski L, Leff A. Outcomes after long-term acute care. An analysis of 133 mechanically ventilated patients. *Am J Respir Crit Care Med* 1999;**159**:1568–73.

40 Seneff MG, Wagner D, Thompson D, Honeycutt C, Silver MR. The impact of long-term acute-care facilities on the outcome and cost of care for patients undergoing prolonged mechanical ventilation. *Crit Care Med* 2000;**28**:342–50.

41   Medicare Payment Advisory Commission. Defining long term acute care hospitals. *Report to the Congress: new approaches in Medicare*. Washington, DC: MedPAC; 2004.

42 Terwiesch C, Diwas KC, Kahn JM. Working with capacity limitations: operations management in critical care. *Crit Care* 2011;**15**:308.

43 Goldfrad C, Rowan K. Consequences of discharges from intensive care at night. *Lancet* 2000;**355**: 1138–42.

44 Chalfin DB, Trzeciak S, Likourezos A, Baumann BM, Dellinger RP. Impact of delayed transfer of critically ill patients from the emergency department to the intensive care unit. *Crit Care Med* 2007;**35**:1477–83.

45 Truog RD, Brock DW, Cook DJ, et al. Rationing in the intensive care unit. *Crit Care Med* 2006;34: 958–63; quiz 971.

46 Hutchings A, Durand MA, Grieve R, et al. Evaluation of modernisation of adult critical care services in England: time series and cost effectiveness analysis. *BMJ* 2009;**339**:b4353.

47 Wunsch H, Linde-Zwirble WT, Harrison DA, Barnato AE, Rowan KM, Angus DC. Use of intensive care services during terminal hospitalizations in England and the United States. *Am J Respir Crit Care Med* 2009;**180**:875–80.

48 Lewis-Newby M, Curtis JR, Martin DP, Engelberg RA. Measuring family satisfaction with care and quality of dying in the intensive care unit: does patient age matter? *J Palliat Med* 2011;**14**:1284–90.

49 Schwarze ML, Bradley CT, Brasel KJ. Surgical 'buy-in': the contractual relationship between surgeons and patients that influences decisions regarding life-supporting therapy. *Crit Care Med* 2010;**38**:843–8.

50 Gries CJ, Curtis JR, Wall RJ, Engelberg RA. Family member satisfaction with end-of-life decision making in the ICU. *Chest* 2008;**133**:704–12.

51 Curtis JR, Engelberg RA, Wenrich MD, Shannon SE, Treece PD, Rubenfeld GD. Missed opportunities during family conferences about end-of-life care in the intensive care unit. *Am J Respir Crit Care Med* 2005;**171**:844–9.

52 Menke TJ, Ashton CM, Petersen NJ, Wolinsky FD. Impact of an all-inclusive diagnosis-related group payment system on inpatient utilization. *Med Care* 1998;**36**:1126–37.

53   Centers for Medicare and Medicade Services. Prospective payment for long-term care hospitals; proposed annual payment rate updates and policy changes; proposed rule. *Federal Register* 2004;**69**:4754–71.

54 Lane-Fall MB, Iwashyna TJ, Cooke CR, Benson NM, Kahn JM. Insurance and racial differences in long-term acute care utilization after critical illness. *Crit Care Med* 2012;**40**:1143–9.

55 Conrad D, Wickizer T, Maynard C, et al. Managing care, incentives, and information: an exploratory look inside the 'black box' of hospital efficiency. *Health Serv Res* 1996;**31**:235–59.

56 Kahn JM. The evolving role of dedicated weaning facilities in critical care. *Intensive Care Med* 2010;**36**:8–10.

Chapter 5

The Overlap of Palliative Care and Critical Illness

Aluko A. Hope and Judith E. Nelson

Introduction

As ICU survivors increase in number and investigators examine the experience of these patients and their families more fully, the lasting impact of critical illness is coming into clearer view.[1] Meanwhile, research continues to illuminate the discomforts and other difficulties that are often experienced during acute care of the critically ill. The same themes run throughout, from ICU admission to discharge and beyond. Patients are burdened by a broad range of physical and psychological symptoms,[2–7] along with impairments of function and cognition.[8–16] Families struggle with their own symptoms,[17–20] with the responsibility for making surrogate decisions,[21,22] and with caregiving strain.[23–25] The care plan becomes disconnected from the patients' own values and preferences and even from what is achievable. Continuity of care is undermined by the fragmentation across various venues and among multiple specialists. Attention to patients' and families' concerns is deferred.[26,27]

These patient and family needs are the focus of palliative care, which is both a medical specialty and an approach that can be integrated into the care of all patients facing serious and complex illness.[28–32] Specifically, palliative care comprises the following core elements: alleviation of symptom distress; communication about care goals; alignment of treatment with patients' values and preferences; transitional planning; and support for both patient and family throughout the illness trajectory.[33–35] At one time, palliative care was seen as simply a sequel to failed intensive care, its role restricted to the end of life, after the exhaustion of life-prolonging therapies. The broader relevance of palliative care is now reflected in practice recommendations that call for its integration into the care of all chronically or seriously ill patients with conditions that place them at increased risk for mortality and morbidity.[28–30]

In this chapter, we discuss ways in which effective integration of the core elements of palliative care during acute treatment of critical illness may help patients and families prepare more fully for the challenges to come in the days, months, and years after discharge from intensive care. We address palliative care approaches extending beyond the ICU. We include discussion of the particular problem of CCI, perhaps the most devastating legacy of critical illness, in which survival is severed from recovery and critical illness itself continues after ICU treatment. We also review the respective roles of palliative care specialists and other clinicians in providing palliative care for patients and their families across the trajectory of critical illness.

Narrowing the gap between expectations and outcomes: effective communication

Although the experience of ICU survivors and their families needs much more investigation, the data so far suggest that recovery from critical illness is often incomplete, with ongoing risks for increased mortality and morbidity.[36,37] Existing evidence also shows that few patients and families appreciate these risks, even after prolonged intensive care treatment.[12,26] More than a decade ago, Azoulay et al. documented that half of ICU families in a university-affiliated ICU, staffed by full-time critical care specialists, failed to comprehend even basic information about the patients' condition and prognosis at the time of acute treatment.[38] After an extended period of intensive care, most surrogates for patients who remain dependent on MV, and other life support, still lack knowledge of the nature and expected outcomes of prolonged critical illness.[12,26] For example, the vast majority of surrogates for chronically critically ill patients with recent tracheotomy, in one study, reported that they received no information about possible long-term functional dependency or prognosis for 1-year survival.[26] In a qualitative study, patients who survived treatment for CCI and their families perceived the placement of tracheotomy for ongoing MV as a positive development, associated with a favourable prognosis, only later to realize the grave implications of prolonged dependence on MV, including impaired function and cognition.[39] In another qualitative study, Cox et al. found that surrogates had high expectations for patients' 1-year survival, functional status, and QoL after PMV, whereas fewer than 10% of these patients were alive without major functional limitation at follow-up.[12] Although physicians were more realistic about these outcomes than surrogates, three-quarters of surrogates reported they had not discussed this information with the patient's physician.[12]

Evidence from family meetings in the ICU and other settings suggests that there are important opportunities to improve both the frequency and quality of communication by clinicians with patients and families,[27,40–42] which could help to align expectations more closely with outcomes and thereby contribute positively to the post-ICU experience. In a recent study of academic and community-based ICUs in different parts of the US, as late as 5 days after admission to the ICU, clinician meetings with families to address the patient's condition, prognosis, and care goals were documented in the medical record for fewer than 20% of patients.[42] Qualitative investigation of ICU family conferences and outpatient encounters has shown that physicians often miss opportunities to provide support, such as encouraging questions and other input from family, explaining the basics of surrogate decision making, attending to emotions that may otherwise overwhelm the ability of patients and families to absorb and integrate important information, and listening sensitively.[27,40,43] Physicians are also reluctant to provide specific prognostic information about critical illness and tend to avoid or inflate prognostic estimates,[21] although most surrogates of patients with critical illness understand and accept that physicians cannot prognosticate with certainty, and surrogates prefer to discuss expectations for outcomes, even if they are uncertain or unfavourable.[21,44] Physicians' fears that such discussions would extinguish hope or worsen emotional distress are lacking in empiric support.[21,44] The data do suggest, however, that patients with an overly optimistic understanding of their prognosis are more likely to choose non-beneficial treatments.[45,46]

Qualitative data obtained from surrogates for patients treated in ICUs indicate that timely, candid, compassionate discussion of expected outcomes is essential for emotional preparation, which is usually a slow and incremental process.[21,47,48] As explained by ICU surrogates who were interviewed in a rigorous study involving 179 such subjects, 'If you know something, you can think about it. You can discuss and you can prepare yourself emotionally.' 'You kind of go through all of those cycles of starting to accept something that's hard. I don't think you can do that in a short time. So, I think the sooner you have information, the better.'[21] Surrogates have also highlighted the value of early prognostic discussions in facilitating logistical and practical preparation and in solidifying the support of family members both for the patient and for themselves.[21] Families with inadequate information and unrealistic expectations experience anger, frustration, and disappointment as the burdens on surviving patients and the families themselves become clear.[39] Proactive discussion of expected decrements in physical and cognitive function after critical illness might help to mitigate these reactions. Just as early mobilization and attention to best practices for ventilator management and sedation in the ICU may be protective against longer-term sequelae, proactive and continuing emphasis on effective communication may help ICU survivors and their families to address future challenges.[49,50]

Expert opinion and qualitative investigations of clinician communication in ICUs and other care settings support specific approaches to improve the effectiveness of this communication. One recommended strategy, which is applicable across the trajectory of critical illness (including the post-ICU period) as well as of other serious conditions, is summarized as 'Ask–tell–ask.'[51] The clinician begins the discussion by asking patients or family members to describe their understanding of a situation (e.g. the patient's condition, status, and prognosis), including what they have been told by other clinicians, and asking permission to continue with the discussion. Thereafter, the clinician provides a concise update of the situation in layperson's terms, with sensitivity to differences in health literacy and cultural background. The family is then asked to summarize the discussion and bring forward any questions or concerns. Given the high prevalence of psychological distress for patients and families, both during and after ICU treatment,[17,18] the incorporation of empathic statements in clinician communication is also recommended as a way to help modulate emotions and thereby enhance cognitive processing of important clinical information.[43,52,53] The acronym 'NURSE.' abbreviates several effective strategies for communicating empathy explicitly: Name the emotion to make clear that it is recognized; express Understanding in an open and compassionate way; convey Respect for the person experiencing the emotion; provide assurance of Support; and Explore the emotional experience of the other person in greater depth.[43] Examples of 'NURSE' empathic statements are available as guides for clinicians.[43,54]

Spirituality—defined as the way in which people find meaning and purpose in life—may influence patients' and families' attitudes, expectations, decisions, and behaviour throughout the illness trajectory. Effective communication incorporates tolerance and respect for religious and spiritual beliefs. In one qualitative study of 50 surrogates of critically ill patients, spiritual beliefs led surrogates to express doubt about the accuracy of physician prognostication; 50% reported feeling that ICU outcomes were predetermined by God.[48] In another study, surrogates who, for spiritual reasons, doubted the physician's prediction of futility were more likely to request continued life support.[55] Studies of cancer patients suggest that failure to address spiritual concerns is associated with poorer health outcomes, increased end-of-life medical costs, decreased adherence to treatment plans, and lower ratings of care quality and patient satisfaction.[56,57] Tools exist for assessing spirituality in a patient encounter,[58–60] and guidance is available for approaching a patient or family with expectations of a miracle, or responding to a request for prayer or other spiritual ceremonies.[61,62]

As an adjunct to direct clinician communication, studies support the use of printed, online, or video informational materials about various aspects of the patient and family experience of critical illness.[63–65] One application of this approach is to provide a brochure that guides family preparation for a face-to-face conference with the clinical team; several templates for an 'ICU family meeting brochure' can be used or adapted for this purpose.[66,67] Another brochure has been developed and validated to provide information and prompt further discussion about CCI, including the potential long-term impact on the patient's cognition and function and burdens faced by families.[68] The Society of Critical Care Medicine (SCCM) also publishes a brochure entitled *What should I expect after leaving the ICU*, briefly addressing issues such as amnesia and several psychological sequelae of ICU care.[69] A growing body of work exploring the use of printed aids as well as video and newer technologies to educate and support decision making by patients and their families may have relevance across the critical illness trajectory.[65,70,71] As research continues to reveal more about the experience of the ICU survivor, new knowledge can be incorporated in such resources to help patients and their families anticipate and manage the ongoing challenges.

Aligning care with patient values and preferences: advance care planning

The typical patient with acute critical illness is too cognitively impaired to participate in planning for future care.[72,73] Among those whose critical illness becomes chronic, few have prepared an advance directive, and the vast majority have not even appointed a health care proxy to make surrogate decisions.[74] Recovery from critical illness, however, may provide an opportunity for advance care planning by the ICU survivor, who remains at medical risk. The patient who personally experienced intensive care therapy is better informed about its benefits and burdens and should have a stronger appreciation of the value of advance planning. However, data suggest that the specific preferences of individuals for future care need to be explored, since the impact of prior ICU treatment is variable and unpredictable,[75] treatment preferences are influenced by the likelihood of adverse outcomes, including not only death but also functional or cognitive impairment,[76] and preferences can change over time in relation to changing health states as well as other factors.[77,78]

Although the value of advance directives has been questioned, recent studies suggest that they are helpful in aligning care with patients' preferences and in supporting surrogates in decision making.[73–79] Silveira et al. found in a large observational study that, among older Americans who had prepared a living will stating a preference for or against 'all care possible under any circumstances in order to prolong life,' there was strong agreement between the stated preference and care given at the end of life; subjects who had requested all care possible were much more likely to receive it than those who had not requested such care, while those who had requested limited care or care focused on comfort were much more likely to receive that care than subjects who had not indicated a preference for it.[73] In addition, 90% of the appointed proxies reported that the patient's living will addressed most of the decisions they faced. Subjects who had designated a proxy were less likely to die in a hospital. In a randomized controlled interventional study, Detering et al.[79] showed that, compared to usual care, facilitation by trained non-medical staff of advance care planning by hospitalized adults 80 years of age or older was associated with concordance between patients' preferences and their treatment at the end of life, patient and family satisfaction, and lower levels of post-traumatic stress disorder (PTSD), anxiety, and depression among relatives of patients who died. Families in the intervention group were included in the planning discussions, thus enhancing their understanding of the patient's wishes and helping to lessen burdens of surrogate decision making.

Templates for written directives are available as models for use in formalizing the process of advance care planning through documentation of specific preferences; relevant legal requirements vary across states in the US.[80] With increasing use of electronic medical records, such directives can be made accessible across venues to the entire health care team. Preferences can also be incorporated in a preprinted order, specifying treatment instructions in the event of serious illness such as cardiopulmonary resuscitation, intravenous (IV) fluids, feeding tubes, and other interventions; the Physician Orders for Life-Sustaining Treatment (POLST) is an example of this approach, which has been effective in aligning care with stated patient preferences and in enhancing attention to palliative care goals.[81–83]

As has been observed, 'the ongoing challenge is to transform advance care planning from the act of signing a form to a process that begins by clarifying the patient's current health status, moves to elicitation of the goals of care, and then designates a proxy to work with clinicians in interpreting and implementing those goals.'[84] The advance directive is most valuable as a tool for initiating that process.[85,86] A discussion of values, including functional and cognitive states that make the patient's life worthwhile, provides the basic platform for establishing care goals in relation to the patient's condition, while, as previously highlighted, attention to the affect that may arise in planning for a future condition of incapacity and illness creates an empathic, patient-centred framework. Since specific decisions are difficult to anticipate, the appointment of a medical decision maker to address changing circumstances in real time is especially important in advance care planning, although the proxy may not be well informed as to the patient's wishes, unless these are directly discussed.[87] The emphasis must always remain on the process of communication between the patient, surrogate decision maker, and health care professionals.

Alleviating patient distress: symptom management

Relief of symptom distress is a core element of high-quality palliative care for all patients and a domain of key concern to patients who have been treated for critical illness and to their families.[33] Symptom data are of special interest for several reasons. Most important, interventions to promote patient comfort depend on a clear understanding of symptom frequency, intensity, and related levels of distress. Second, there is increasing evidence from a variety of clinical contexts, including critical illness, that physical and emotional symptom distress are associated with other unfavourable outcomes, including mortality, while regular assessment and effective management of symptoms are associated with physiologic stability, recovery, and rehabilitation.[88–90]

Although analgesia is an area of increasing clinical and research attention, performance improvement, and regulatory oversight in ICUs, evidence indicates that further progress is needed.[91] Puntillo showed over 20 years ago that, among patients interviewed after transfer from a surgical ICU, 70% recalled pain that 63% rated as moderate or severe.[4] Yet, just recently, Gelinas et al. found that 77% of patients transferred from cardiac surgery ICUs recalled pain, of whom 64% rated the pain as moderate or severe.[91] In a study of critically ill cancer patients receiving ICU care with a hospital mortality rate of over 50%, 56% of those who could self-report symptoms experienced moderate or severe pain.[3] Less evidence is available about other symptoms in diverse ICU patient groups, but data suggest that non-pain symptoms are also highly prevalent and distressing during critical illness.[5,92] Among a heterogeneous group of 171 ICU patients at high risk of hospital death (one-third actually died), 50–75% of multi-symptom assessments revealed patient reports of thirst, anxiety, and fatigue, and many patients also reported a range of other physical and psychological symptoms;[5] symptom intensity was highest for thirst. A study of 96 medical ICU patients who were mechanically ventilated for more than 24 hours and could respond to symptom assessment found that half experienced dyspnoea that was often intense and was strongly associated with anxiety.[92]

Patients who remain critically ill on a chronic basis have a heavy burden of symptoms.[2] In a prospective study of chronically critically ill patients with tracheotomy for continuing ventilator dependence after the ICU, three-quarters of those who could report symptoms in real time experienced ≥10 of 16 symptoms in the assessment tool.[2] Over 40% of the patients reported pain at the highest levels on the scale, and more than 60% reported psychological symptoms (sadness, worry, and nervousness) 'frequently' or 'almost constantly', along with other distressing physical and psychological symptoms. A subsequent prospective study of more than 300 patients transferred to an LTAC facility for further efforts to wean from MV found that more than 40% met criteria for a depressive disorder in the DSM-IV.[88] The duration of MV was twice as long for depressed patients, and they were three times more likely to remain ventilator-dependent as those without a depressive disorder.[88] Patients with depression were also more than twice as likely to die in the facility as those without depression, and this increased rate of mortality remained significant after controlling for age, comorbid illness, and other independent predictors of death.

The symptom experience of ICU survivors returning to the community is an important area for further investigation. In a qualitative study of ARDS survivors between 3 and 9 months after the ICU, patient reports of debilitating insomnia, fatigue, and pain were common, along with emotional lability, depression, and anxiety.[93] Longer-term follow-up of a larger cohort of ARDS patients in Canada has documented that, in addition to ongoing functional limitations and decrements in physical QoL, survivors of ARDS have psychological sequelae for as long as 5 years after the ICU.[94] At a median of 22 months post-discharge, one-third of survivors had moderate or severe depressive symptoms,[95] while, at 5-year follow-up, nearly 20% still reported such symptoms.[96] Half of the 5-year survivors reported at least one episode of depression, anxiety, or both, diagnosed by a physician between 2 and 5 years after the ICU, while more severe disturbances affected a small number of patients in the cohort.[94,97] Less information is available about symptom distress in other groups of ICU survivors. A systematic review of depression in general ICU survivors found that the median point prevalence of clinically significant depressive symptoms was 28% and that depression in the early post-ICU period predicted longer-term depressive symptoms.[98] A single-centre study in Australia found that, during a 6-month period of follow-up after ICU discharge, more than a quarter of survivors experienced chronic pain, with associated decrements in HRQoL.[99]

As the results of ongoing and future research are awaited, clinicians caring for patients during or after critical illness are encouraged to incorporate systematic assessment of both physical and psychological symptoms as part of comprehensive patient-centred care. For patients, such as those with CCI, who cannot self-report symptoms because of brain dysfunction and/or continuing endotracheal intubation, several objective tools are available to assess pain and dyspnoea (e.g. behavioural pain scale,[100] Critical Care Pain Observation Tool,[101] 'Assume pain present' approach,[102] and Respiratory Distress Observation Scale).[103] For patients who can respond to symptom assessment, palliative care researchers have developed simple, practical symptom measurement tools that avoid undue burden and provide sufficient information for clinical management. Examples that measure a diverse group of symptoms include the Condensed Form of the Memorial Symptom Assessment Scale,[104] which can be modified for use with critically ill patients,[2] and the Edmonton Symptom Assessment Scale.[105] Abbreviated instruments are also available to evaluate specific symptoms, such as pain,[106] dyspnoea,[107] or depression,[108] which are all prevalent in critically ill patients and worthy of assessment among survivors.[96] To date, no published studies have evaluated interventions to alleviate symptoms in the chronically critically ill or in survivors who recover but remain burdened by symptom distress. Until such data are available, evidence-based strategies for management of symptoms in other patient groups can be applied, with adaptations as appropriate for particular clinical circumstances.

Addressing unmet family needs: interdisciplinary support and transition planning

In the aftermath of critical illness, substantial evidence shows that emotional, physical, and practical burdens for families weigh heavily, even if the patient survives ICU treatment. The term post-intensive care syndrome, which describes 'new or worsening impairments in physical, cognitive, or mental health status arising after critical illness and persisting beyond acute care hospitalization', has been suggested as equally applicable to a family member or an ICU survivor.[109] Acute and post-traumatic stress (PTS) symptoms affect families as well as patients.[18,110–112] Depression is also prevalent in survivors' families, whether the patient is cared for at home or institutionalized.[25,113,114] For informal caregivers, emotional distress can be long-lasting; Cameron et al. found that informal caregivers for ARDS survivors experienced such distress as late as 2 years after the patients' discharge from hospital,[115] and qualitative research has captured themes of regret, exhaustion, isolation, and hopelessness, as expressed in caregivers' own words.[93] Among families of patients receiving MV for as little as 3 days, post-ICU decrements in physical health and HRQoL are common, as is the experience of role overload and burden that accumulate over time.[24,116] Informal caregivers who feel strained by this role are known to be at higher risk of mortality.[117] In addition, their personal and professional lives may be significantly disrupted. After 1 week or more in a surgical ICU, families, studied by Swoboda and Lipsett, were providing caregiving assistance for months, many leaving their paid employment and depleting savings.[23] Similarly, Van Pelt et al. documented that disruption in lifestyle and reduction in employment were common and persistent for informal caregivers of ICU survivors over a year of follow-up.[24]

More data are needed to define effective and cost-efficient interventions addressing these challenges, which are expected to mount as the population of critically ill patients and their informal caregivers continues to age and families are forced to accept an increasing share of non-institutional caregiving. Since burdens on caregivers may in turn limit patients' recovery and achievement of rehabilitative potential, such interventions are all the more important. Douglas et al. evaluated a disease management programme, in which an advanced practice nurse provided emotional support, care coordination, education, and case management services to ICU patients receiving MV and their caregivers for a total of 8 weeks before and after hospital discharge.[118] Compared to usual care, this intervention neither improved depression, burden, or physical health for caregivers nor lowered rates of patient readmission. The range of issues facing families suggests that interdisciplinary support is more likely to meet their ongoing needs, but research has yet to answer such key questions as: who the most appropriate members of such a team are; which components are essential to alleviate distress for families and enable them to support the patient's recovery; when the optimal time to initiate a programme of this kind is and what its duration should be; and how support for the family can be integrated and coordinated across various venues of care within a comprehensive framework of care for the ICU survivor. Studies of interventions for caregivers of other groups of chronically ill may be helpful in designing and evaluating strategies for supporting families of ICU survivors. Research needs to focus not only on further description of the experience, outcomes, and unmet needs of families after critical illness, and on appropriate interventions, but also on models for delivery that can be accommodated in a rapidly changing and increasingly cost-conscious health care environment.

Meeting palliative care needs: the role of expert consultants

Over the past decade, palliative care consultants have rapidly and steadily increased their presence in acute care hospitals in the US, and the field is also growing in other countries.[119,120] Today, 85% of hospitals with 300 or more beds and half of hospitals with at least 50 beds report a palliative care programme on the American Hospital Association's Annual Survey.[120] Qualified physicians can become certified by the American Board of Internal Medicine as subspecialists in palliative medicine through any of ten cosponsoring specialty boards. Palliative care nurses are certified by the National Board for Certification of Hospice and Palliative Nurses. Social workers at Bachelor's and Master's levels may also be credentialled as specialists in palliative care, while other integral members of palliative care specialty teams include pastoral care providers and psychologists.[35] Because 20% of dying patients in US hospitals have received intensive care during the final hospitalization,[121] much attention has been focused on involving palliative care specialists in the management of symptoms, discussions of care goals, transitional planning, and family support in the acute ICU setting.[122–124] A series of studies has documented benefits of palliative care consultation in the ICU, including reduction in length of stay, early identification of a dying trajectory with shortened time to patient-centred, comfort-focused treatment goals, and transfer of patients to lower-intensity care sites when appropriate.[122–124] Outside of ICUs, palliative care consultation for hospitalized patients has been associated with improvements across a range of domains, including symptom control, timely establishment of appropriate care goals, and efficient resource utilization.[125,126] Some hospitals or ICUs have developed 'trigger criteria' to engage palliative care specialists for patients at highest risk of death or severe functional or cognitive impairments.[32,122,124]

Programmes to extend interdisciplinary, non-hospice, specialist palliative care beyond the acute hospital into the community are still relatively few in number and have generally been targeted to patients with a life expectancy that is only slightly longer than the 6-month period used to determine hospice eligibility. At Kaiser Permanente in Southern California, a pioneering home-based palliative care programme was made available to patients (the most common diagnoses in the study cohort were COPD, congestive heart failure (CHF), and cancer) whose estimated life expectancy was approximately 1 year.[127] Patients could continue with restorative care and with care from their primary physician while also receiving visits from a palliative care physician on a team, including a nurse and social worker with expertise in symptom management and care coordination. Focusing on patients who died during the 2-year study period and comparing intervention patients to those receiving usual care, including home care for patients meeting Medicare-certified criteria of an acute condition, patients in the palliative care programme were more satisfied with their services and used less acute care or other institutional care, resulting in significantly lower costs. These benefits were subsequently confirmed in a randomized controlled two-state trial.[128] A broader patient group of COPD, CHF, and cancer patients with a life expectancy of 1 to 5 years were included in a randomized controlled study of outpatient palliative care consultation by Rabow et al.,[129] which was conducted within the general medicine practice of a university medical centre. Over a 1-year period, an interdisciplinary team, composed of physicians, a social worker, nurse, chaplain, psychologist, and others, provided recommendations to primary care physicians for the management of physical and psychological symptoms, spiritual care, social support, and advance care planning, together with case management, family caregiver support, and other services by non-physician team members in person and by telephone. Patients receiving this intervention reported greater improvements in some symptoms, but not others, and made fewer visits for primary care or urgent care, compared to control patients, while overall medical charges for the two groups were not significantly different. As the investigators observed, the effects of this intervention may have been limited by inconsistent implementation of the palliative care team's recommendations.[129]

Specialist palliative care is also provided to outpatients with cancer in supportive care or oncology clinics based in comprehensive cancer centres. In a retrospective study of a supportive care clinic, an interdisciplinary team, led by palliative medicine physicians, provided care for patients with advanced cancer, according to a standardized management plan comprising an initial consultative visit, followed by a subsequent evaluation within a month.[130] Distress from a range of physical and psychological symptoms decreased significantly over the period of follow-up.[130] A randomized controlled trial (RCT) evaluated the integration of palliative care with oncology care for patients with newly diagnosed metastatic lung cancer who visited an outpatient thoracic oncology clinic where specialists in palliative care attended to physical and psychosocial symptoms, establishing care goals, assisting patients with treatment decision making, and coordinating care.[131] Compared to patients receiving standard oncologic care alone, patients also receiving palliative care in this ambulatory setting had a better QoL and mood. In addition, the palliative care intervention was associated with longer survival, a secondary outcome of the study.

Conclusion

In the future, palliative care specialists may be more widely available to assist in the care of patients living in the community, including those who have survived intensive care but live on with symptom distress and significant impairments that affect the quality of their lives. For now, access to specialty palliative care is best sought during acute hospitalization where symptoms can be closely managed, goals of care can be addressed, advance care planning can be initiated, and preparations made for transition to other venues. The interface of hospital-based palliative care and critical illness has previously concentrated on the management of patients who are dying or expected to die despite intensive care, but an expanded role for palliative care is supported by ICU professionals and others who recognize the benefits of such care throughout critical illness for all patients and their families, regardless of prognosis.[31] Over time, this role might increasingly encompass contributions to the care of survivors of critical illness, including not only patients who remain institutionalized with CCI or other conditions of dependency, but also individuals returning to the community with less severe, but chronic, impairments. Even if specialists are available, however, attention to basic palliative care needs of patients and families is an ongoing responsibility for intensive care clinicians and others with primary responsibility for restorative care.[31,32] Ideally, all such clinicians will have sufficient knowledge and skill to manage basic needs but also have access to specialty-level palliative care services for more complex or refractory problems.

References

1 Desai SV, Law TJ, Needham DM. Long-term complications of critical care. *Crit Care Med* 2011;**39**:371–9.

2 Nelson JE, Meier DE, Litke A, Natale DA, Siegel RE, Morrison RS. The symptom burden of chronic critical illness. *Crit Care Med* 2004;**32**:1527–34.

3 Nelson JE, Meier DE, Oei EJ, et al. Self-reported symptom experience of critically ill cancer patients receiving intensive care. *Crit Care Med* 2001;**29**:277–82.

4 Puntillo KA. *Pain* experience of intensive care unit patients. *Heart Lung* 1990;**19**:525–33.

5 Puntillo KA, Arai S, Cohen NH, et al. Symptoms experienced by intensive care unit patients at high risk of dying. *Crit Care Med* 2010;**38**:2155–60.

6 Myhren H, Ekeberg O, Toien K, Karlsson S, Stokland O. Posttraumatic stress, anxiety and depression symptoms in patients during the first year post intensive care unit discharge. *Crit Care* 2010;**14**:R14.

7 Davydow DS, Gifford JM, Desai SV, Needham DM, Bienvenu OJ. Posttraumatic stress disorder in general intensive care unit survivors: a systematic review. *Gen Hosp Psychiatry* 2008;**30**:421–34.

8 Nelson JE, Tandon N, Mercado AF, Camhi SL, Ely EW, Morrison RS. Brain dysfunction: another burden for the chronically critically ill. *Arch Intern Med* 2006;**166**:1993–9.

9 Jackson JC, Hart RP, Gordon SM, et al. Six-month neuropsychological outcome of medical intensive care unit patients. *Crit Care Med* 2003;**31**:1226–34.

10 Jackson JC, Girard TD, Gordon SM, et al. Long-term cognitive and psychological outcomes in the awakening and breathing controlled trial. *Am J Respir Crit Care Med* 2010;**182**:183–91.

11 Iwashyna TJ, Ely EW, Smith DM, Langa KM. Long-term cognitive impairment and functional disability among survivors of severe sepsis. *JAMA* 2010;**304**:1787–94.

12 Cox CE, Martinu T, Sathy SJ, et al. Expectations and outcomes of prolonged mechanical ventilation. *Crit Care Med* 2009;37:2888–94; quiz 904.

13 van der Schaaf M, Dettling DS, Beelen A, Lucas C, Dongelmans DA, Nollet F. Poor functional status immediately after discharge from an intensive care unit. *Disabil Rehabil* 2008;**30**:1812–8.

14 van der Schaaf M, Beelen A, Dongelmans DA, Vroom MB, Nollet F. Functional status after intensive care: a challenge for rehabilitation professionals to improve outcome. *J Rehabil Med* 2009;**41**:360–6.

15 van der Schaaf M, Beelen A, Dongelmans DA, Vroom MB, Nollet F. Poor functional recovery after a critical illness: a longitudinal study. *J Rehabil Med* 2009;**41**:1041–8.

16 Girard TD, Jackson JC, Pandharipande PP, et al. Delirium as a predictor of long-term cognitive impairment in survivors of critical illness. *Crit Care Med* 2010;**38**:1513–20.

17 Pochard F, Azoulay E, Chevret S, et al. Symptoms of anxiety and depression in family members of intensive care unit patients: ethical hypothesis regarding decision-making capacity. *Crit Care Med* 2001;**29**:1893–7.

18 Anderson WG, Arnold RM, Angus DC, Bryce CL. Posttraumatic stress and complicated grief in family members of patients in the intensive care unit. *J Gen Intern Med* 2008;**23**:1871–6.

19 McAdam JL, Dracup KA, White DB, et al. Symptom experiences of family members of intensive care unit patients at high risk for dying. *Crit Care Med* 2010;**38**:1078–85.

20 McAdam JL, Dracup KA, White DB, et al. Psychological symptoms of family members of high-risk intensive care unit patients. *Am J Crit Care* 2012;**21**:386–94.

21 Apatira L, Boyd EA, Malvar G, et al. Hope, truth, and preparing for death: perspectives of surrogate decision makers. *Ann Intern Med* 2008;**149**:861–8.

22 Wendler D, Rid A. Systematic review: the effect on surrogates of making treatment decisions for others. *Ann Intern Med* 2011;**154**:336–46.

23 Swoboda SM, Lipsett PA. Impact of a prolonged surgical critical illness on patients' families. *Am J Crit Care* 2002;**11**:459–66.

24 Van Pelt DC, Milbrandt EB, Qin L, et al. Informal caregiver burden among survivors of prolonged mechanical ventilation. *Am J Respir Crit Care Med* 2007;**175**:167–73.

25 Douglas SL, Daly BJ. Caregivers of long-term ventilator patients: physical and psychological outcomes. *Chest* 2003;**123**:1073–81.

26 Nelson JE, Mercado AF, Camhi SL, et al. Communication about chronic critical illness. *Arch Intern Med* 2007;**167**:2509–15.

27 Curtis JR, Engelberg RA, Wenrich MD, Shannon SE, Treece PD, Rubenfeld GD. Missed opportunities during family conferences about end-of-life care in the intensive care unit. *Am J Respir Crit Care Med* 2005;**171**:844–9.

28 Lanken PN, Terry PB, Delisser HM, et al. An official American Thoracic Society clinical policy statement: palliative care for patients with respiratory diseases and critical illnesses. *Am J Respir Crit Care Med* 2008;**177**:912–27.

29 Truog RD, Campbell ML, Curtis JR, et al. Recommendations for end-of-life care in the intensive care unit: a consensus statement by the American College [corrected] of Critical Care Medicine. *Crit Care Med* 2008;**36**:953–63.

30 Selecky PA, Eliasson CA, Hall RI, Schneider RF, Varkey B, McCaffree DR. Palliative and end-of-life care for patients with cardiopulmonary diseases: American College of Chest Physicians position statement. *Chest* 2005;**128**:3599–610.

31 Nelson JE, Bassett R, Boss RD, et al. Models for structuring a clinical initiative to enhance palliative care in the intensive care unit: a report from the Improve Palliative Care in the ICU (IPAL-ICU) Project and the Center to Advance Palliative Care. *Crit Care Med* 2010;**38**:1765–72.

32 Weissman DE, Meier DE. Identifying patients in need of a palliative care assessment in the hospital setting: a consensus report from the Center to Advance Palliative Care. *J Palliat Med* 2011;**14**:17–23.

33 Nelson JE, Puntillo KA, Pronovost PJ, et al. In their own words: patients and families define high-quality palliative care in the intensive care unit. *Crit Care Med* 2010;**38**:808–18.

34 Clarke EB, Curtis JR, Luce JM, et al. Quality indicators for end-of-life care in the intensive care unit. *Crit Care Med* 2003;**31**:2255–62.

35 National Consensus Project for Quality Palliative Care. *Clinical practice guidelines for quality palliative care.* (2009). Available at: http://www.nationalconsensusproject.org/guideline.pdf (accessed 15 December 2012).

36 Desai SV, Law TJ, and Needham DM. Long-term complications of critical care. *Crit Care Med* 2011;**39**:371–9.

37 Needham DM, Davidson J, Cohen H, et al. Improving long-term outcomes after discharge from intensive care unit: report from a stakeholders' conference. *Crit Care Med* 2012;**40**:502–9.

38 Azoulay E, Chevret S, Leleu G, et al. Half the families of ICU patients experience inadequate communication with physicians. *Crit Care Med* 2000;**8**:3044–9.

39 Nelson JE, Kinjo K, Meier DE, Ahmad K, Morrison RS. When critical illness becomes chronic: informational needs of patients and families. *J Crit Care* 2005;**20**:79–89.

40 McDonagh JR, Elliott TB, Engelberg RA, et al. Family satisfaction with family conferences about end-of-life care in the intensive care unit: increased proportion of family speech is associated with increased satisfaction. *Crit Care Med* 2004;**32**:1484–7.

41 Teno JM, Fisher E, Hamel MB, et al. Decision-making and outcomes of prolonged ICU stays in seriously ill patients. *J Am Geriatr Soc* 2000;**48**:S70–S4.

42 Penrod JD, Pronovost PJ, Livote EE, et al. Meeting standards of high-quality ICU palliative care: Clinical performance and predictors. *Crit Care Med* 2012; **40**:1105–12.

43 Pollak KI, Arnold RM, Jeffreys AS, et al. Oncologist communication about emotion during visits with patients with advanced cancer. *J Clin Oncol* 2007;**25**:5748–52.

44 Wright AA, Zhang B, Ray A, et al. Associations between end-of-life discussions, patient mental health, medical care near death, and caregiver bereavement adjustment. *JAMA* 2008;**300**:1665–73.

45 Weeks JC, Cook EF, O'Day SJ, et al. Relationship between cancer patients' predictions of prognosis and their treatment preferences. *JAMA* 1998;**279**:1709–14.

46 El-Jawahr A, Podgurski LM, Eichler AF, et al. Use of video to facilitate end-of-life discussions with patients with cancer: a randomized controlled trial. *J Clin Oncol* 2010;**28**: 305–10.

47 Evans LR, Boyd EA, Malvar G et al. Surrogate decision-makers' perspectives on discussing prognosis in the face of uncertainty. *Am J Respir Crit Care Med* 2009;**179**:48–53.

48 Zier LS, Burack JH, Micco G, et al. Doubt and belief in physicians' ability to prognosticate during critical illness: the perspective of surrogate decision makers. *Crit Care Med* 2008;**36**:2341–7.

49 Scheunemann LP, McDevitt M, Carson SS, Hanson LC. Randomized, controlled trials of interventions to improve communication in intensive care: a systematic review. *Chest* 2011;**139**:543–54.

50 Schaefer KG, Block SD. Physician communication with families in the ICU: evidence-based strategies for improvement. *Curr Opin Crit Care* 2009;**15**:569–77.

51 Back AL, Arnold RM, Baile WF, Tulsky JA, Fryer-Edwards K. Approaching difficult communication tasks in oncology. *CA Cancer J Clin* 2005;**55**:164–77.

52 Selph RB, Shiang J, Engelberg R, Curtis JR, White DB. Empathy and life support decisions in intensive care units. *J Gen Intern Med* 2008;**23**:1311–17.

53 Back A, Arnold R, Tulsky J. *Mastering communication with seriously ill patients: balancing honesty with empathy and hope.* New York: Cambridge University Press;2009.

54 Krimshtein NS, Luhrs CA, Puntillo KA, et al. Training nurses for interdisciplinary communication with families in the intensive care unit: an intervention. *J Palliat Med* 2011;**14**:1325–32.

55 Zier LS, Burack JH, Micco G, et al. Surrogate decision makers' responses to physicians' predictions of medical futility. *Chest* 2009;**136**:110–17.

56 Puchalski CM. Spirituality in the cancer trajectory. *Ann Oncol* 2012;**23**(Suppl 3):49–55.

57 Balboni T, Balboni M, Paulk ME, et al. Support of cancer patients' spiritual needs and associations with medical care costs at the end of life. *Cancer* 2011;**117**:5383–91.

58 Anandarajah G, Hight E. Spirituality and medical practice: Using the HOPE questions as a practical tool for spiritual assessment. *Am Fam Physician* 2001;**63**:81–9.

59 Borneman T, Ferrell B, Puchalski CM. Evaluation of the FICA tool for spiritual assessment. *J Pain Sympt Manage* 2010;**40**:163–73.

60 Steinhauser KE, Voils CI, Clipp EC, et al. 'Are you at peace?': one item to probe spiritual concerns at the end of life. *Arch Intern Med* 2006;**166**:101–5.

61 Delisser HM. A practical approach to the family that expects a miracle. *Chest* 2009; **135**:1643–7.

62 Lo B, Kates LW, Ruston D, et al. Responding to requests regarding prayer and religious ceremonies by patients near the end of life and their families. *J Palliat Med* 2003;**6**:409–15.

63 Azoulay E, Pochard F, Chevret S, et al. Impact of a family information leaflet on effectiveness of information provided to family members of intensive care unit patients: a multicenter, prospective, randomized, controlled trial. *Am J Respir Crit Care Med* 2002;**165**:438–42.

64 Lautrette A, Darmon M, Megarbane B, et al. A communication strategy and brochure for relatives of patients dying in the ICU. *N Engl J Med* 2007;**356**:469–78.

65 McCannon JB, O'Donnell WJ, Thompson BT, et al. Augmenting communication and decision making in the intensive care unit with a cardiopulmonary resuscitation video decision support tool: a temporal intervention study. *J Palliat Med* 2012;**15**:1382–7.

66 Gay EB, Pronovost PJ, Bassett RD, Nelson JE. The intensive care unit family meeting: making it happen. *J Crit Care* 2009;**24**:629 e1–12.

67 The IPAL-ICU Project. *ICU family meeting guide.* Available at: http://ipal-live.capc.stackop.com/downloads/meeting-with-the-icu-team-a-guide-for-families.pdf (accessed 15 December 2012).

68 Carson SS, Vu M, Danis M, et al. Development and validation of a printed information brochure for families of chronically critically ill patients. *Crit Care Med* 2012;**40**:73–8.

69 Society of Critical Care Medicine. *What should I expect after leaving the ICU?* Available at: http://www.myicucare.org/Support_Brochures/Pages/AfterLeavingtheICU.aspx (accessed 15 December 2012).

70 Volandes AE, Paasche-Orlow MK, Mitchel SL, et al. Randomized controlled trial of a video decision support tool for cardiopulmonary resuscitation decision making in advanced cancer. *J Clin Oncol* 2013;**31**:380–6

71 Cox CE, Lewis CL, Hanson, LC, et al. Development and pilot testing of a decision aid for surrogates of patients with prolonged mechanical ventilation. *Crit Care Med* 2012;**40**:2327–34.

72 Smedira NG, Evans BH, Grais LS, et al. Withholding and withdrawal of life support from the critically ill. *N Engl J Med* 1990;**322**:309–15.

73 Silveira MJ, Kim SY, Langa KM. Advance directives and outcomes of surrogate decision making before death. *N Engl J Med* 2010;**362**:1211–18.

74 Camhi SL, Mercado AF, Morrison RS, et al. Deciding in the dark: advance directives and continuation of treatment in chronic critical illness. *Crit Care Med* 2009;**37**:919–25.

75 Danis M, Patrick DL, Southerland LI, Green ML. Patients' and families' preferences for medical intensive care. *JAMA* 1988;**260**:797–802.

76 Fried TR, Bradley EH, Towle VR, Allore H. Understanding the treatment preferences of seriously ill patients. *N Engl J Med* 2002;**346**:1061–6.

77 Fried TR, O'Leary J, Van Ness P, Fraenkel L. Inconsistency over time in the preferences of older persons with advanced illness for life-sustaining treatment. *J Am Geriatr Soc* 2007;**55**:1007–14.

78 Fried TR, Byers AL, Gallo WT, et al. Prospective study of health status preferences and changes in preferences over time in older adults. *Arch Intern Med* 2006;**166**:890–5.

79 Detering KM, Hancock AD, Reade MC, Silvester W. The impact of advance care planning on end of life care in elderly patients: randomised controlled trial. *BMJ* 2010;**340**:c1345.

80 Connections of the National Hospice and Palliative Care Organization. *Download your state's advance directives.* Available at: http://www.caringinfo.org/i4a/pages/index.cfm?pageid=3289 (accessed 15 December 2012).

81 POLST Paradigm Program. *Physician orders for life-sustaining treatment paradigm.* Available at: http://www.ohsu.edu/polst/ (accessed 15 December 2012).

82 Tolle SW, Tilden VP, Nelson CA, Dunn PM. A prospective study of the efficacy of the physician order form for life-sustaining treatment. *J Am Geriatr Soc* 1998;**46**:1097–102.

83 Lee MA, Brummel-Smith K, Meyer J, Drew N, London MR. Physician orders for life-sustaining treatment (POLST): outcomes in a PACE program. Program of All-Inclusive Care for the Elderly. *J Am Geriatr Soc* 2000;**48**:1219–25.

84 Gillick MR. Reversing the code status of advance directives? *N Engl J Med* 2010;**362**:1239–40.

85 Perkins HS. Controlling death: the false promise of advance directives. *Ann Intern Med* 2007;**147**:51–7.

86 Tulsky JA. Beyond advance directives: importance of communication skills at the end of life. *JAMA* 2005;**294**:359–65.

87 Shalowitz DI, Garrett-Mayer E, Wendler D. The accuracy of surrogate decision makers: a systematic review. *Arch Intern Med* 2006;**166**:493–7.

88 Jubran A, Lawm G, Kelly J, et al. Depressive disorders during weaning from prolonged mechanical ventilation. *Intensive Care Med* 2010;**36**:828–35.

89 Chang VT, Thaler HT, Polyak HT, Kornblith AB, Lepore JM, Portenoy RK. Quality of life and survival. *Cancer* 1998;**83**:173–9.

90 Covinsky KE, Kahana E, Chin MH, Palmer RM, Fortinsky RH, Landefeld CS. Depressive symptoms and 3-year mortality in older hospitalized medical patients. *Ann Intern Med* 1999;**130**:563–9.

91 Gelinas C, Fortier M, Viens C, Fillion L, Puntillo K. Pain assessment and management in critically ill intubated patients: a retrospective study. *Am J Crit Care* 2004;**13**:126–35.

92 Schmidt M, Demoule A, Polito A, et al. Dyspnea in mechanically ventilated critically ill patients. *Crit Care Med* 2011;**39**:2059–65.

93 Cox CE, Docherty SL, Brandon DH, et al. Surviving critical illness: acute respiratory distress syndrome as experienced by patients and their caregivers. *Crit Care Med* 2009;**37**:2702–8.

94 Herridge MS, Tansey CM, Matte A, et al. Functional disability 5 years after acute respiratory distress syndrome. *N Engl J Med* 2011;**364**:1293–304.

95 Adhikari NK, McAndrews MP, Tansey CM, et al. Self-reported symptoms of depression and memory dysfunction in survivors of ARDS. *Chest* 2009;**135**:678–87.

96 Adhikari NK, Tansey CM, McAndrews MP, et al. Self-reported depressive symptoms and memory complaints in survivors five years after acute respiratory distress syndrome. *Chest* 2011;**140**:1484–93.

97 Davydow DS, Desai SV, Needham DM, Bienvenu OJ. Psychiatric morbidity in survivors of the acute respiratory distress syndrome: a systematic review. *Psychosom Med* 2008;**70**:512–19.

98 Davydow DS, Gifford JM, Desai SV, Bienvenu OJ, Needham DM. Depression in general intensive care unit survivors: a systematic review. *Intensive Care Med* 2009;**35**:796–809.

99 Boyle M, Murgo M, Adamson H, Gill J, Elliott D, Crawford M. The effect of chronic pain on health related quality of life amongst intensive care survivors. *Aust Crit Care* 2004;**17**:104–6, 8–13.

100 Payen JF, Bru O, Bosson JL, et al. Assessing pain in critically ill sedated patients by using a behavioral pain scale. *Crit Care Med* 2001;**29**:2258–63.

101 Gelinas C, Harel F, Fillion L, Puntillo KA, Johnston CC. Sensitivity and specificity of the critical-care pain observation tool for the detection of pain in intubated adults after cardiac surgery. *J Pain Symptm Manage* 2009;**37**:58–67.

102 Herr K, Coyne PJ, Key T, et al. Pain assessment in the nonverbal patient: position statement with clinical practice recommendations. *Pain Manag Nurs* 2006;**7**:44–52.

103 Campbell ML, Templin T, Walch J. A Respiratory Distress Observation Scale for patients unable to self-report dyspnea. *J Palliat Med* 2010;**13**:285–90.

104 Chang VT, Hwang SS, Kasimis B, Thaler HT. Shorter symptom assessment instruments: the Condensed Memorial Symptom Assessment Scale (CMSAS). *Cancer Invest* 2004;**22**:526–36.

105 Bruera E, Kuehn N, Miller MJ, Selmser P, Macmillan K. The Edmonton symptom assessment system (ESAS): a simple method for the assessment of palliative care patients. *J Pall Care* 1991;**7**:6–9.

106 Melzack R. The short-form McGill Pain Questionnaire. *Pain* 1987;**30**:191–7.

107 Dorman S, Byrne A, Edwards A. Which measurement scales should we use to measure breathlessness in palliative care? A systematic review. *Palliat Med* 2007;**21**:177–91.

108 Chochinov HM, Wilson KG, Enns M, Lander S. 'Are you depressed?' Screening for depression in the terminally ill. *Am J Psych* 1997;**154**:674–6.

109 Needham DM, Davidson J, Cohen H, et al. Improving long-term outcomes after discharge from intensive care unit: Report from a stakeholders' conference. *Crit Care Med* 2012;**40**:502–9.

110 Azoulay E, Pochard F, Kentish-Barnes N, et al. Risk of post-traumatic stress symptoms in family members of intensive care unit patients. *Am J Respir Crit Care Med* 2005;**171**:987–94.

111 Paparrigopoulos T, Melissaki A, Efthymiou A, et al. Short-term psychological impact on family members of intensive care unit patients. *J Psychosom Res* 2006;**61**:719–22.

112 Jones C, Skirrow P, Griffiths RD, et al. Post-traumatic stress disorder-related symptoms in relatives of patients following intensive care. *Intensive Care Med* 2004;**30**:456–60.

113 Douglas SL, Daly BJ, O'Toole E, Hickman RL, Jr. Depression among white and nonwhite caregivers of the chronically critically ill. *J Crit Care* 2010;**25**:364 e11–19.

114 Im K, Belle SH, Schulz R, Mendelsohn AB, Chelluri L. Prevalence and outcomes of caregiving after prolonged (> or = 48 hours) mechanical ventilation in the ICU. *Chest* 2004;**125**:597–606.

115 Cameron JI, Herridge MS, Tansey CM, McAndrews MP, Cheung AM. Well-being in informal caregivers of survivors of acute respiratory distress syndrome. *Crit Care Med* 2006;**34**:81–6.

116 Choi J, Donahoe MP, Zullo TG, Hoffman LA. Caregivers of the chronically critically ill after discharge from the intensive care unit: six months' experience. *Am J Crit Care* 2011;**20**:12–22; quiz 3.

117 Schulz R, Beach SR. Caregiving as a risk factor for mortality: the Caregiver Health Effects Study. *JAMA* 1999;**282**:2215–9.

118 Douglas SL, Daly BJ, Kelley CG, O'Toole E, Montenegro H. Impact of a disease management program upon caregivers of chronically critically ill patients. *Chest* 2005;**128**:3925–36.

119 Goldsmith B, Dietrich J, Du Q, Morrison RS. Variability in access to hospital palliative care in the United States. *J Palliat Med* 2008;**11**:1094–102.

120 **Center to Advance Palliative Care.** *Growth of palliative care in US hospitals—2011 snapshot.* Available at: http://www.capc.org/news-and-events/releases/capc-growth-snapshot-2011.pdf (accessed 15 December 2012).

121 **Angus DC, Barnato AE, Linde-Zwirble WT, et al.** Use of intensive care at the end of life in the United States: An epidemiologic study. *Crit Care Med* 2004;**32**:638–43.

122 **Norton SA, Hogan LA, Holloway RG, Temkin-Greener H, Buckley MJ, Quill TE.** Proactive palliative care in the medical intensive care unit: effects on length of stay for selected high-risk patients. *Crit Care Med* 2007;**35**:1530–5.

123 **O'Mahony S, McHenry J, Blank AE, et al.** Preliminary report of the integration of a palliative care team into an intensive care unit. *Palliat Med* 2010;**24**:154–65.

124 **Campbell ML, Guzman JA.** Impact of a proactive approach to improve end-of-life care in a medical ICU. *Chest* 2003;**123**:266–71.

125 **Morrison RS, Penrod JD, Cassel JB, et al.** Cost savings associated with US hospital palliative care consultation programs. *Arch Intern Med* 2008;**168**:1783–90.

126 **Higginson IJ, Finlay I, Goodwin DM, et al.** Do hospital-based palliative teams improve care for patients or families at the end of life? J Pain Symptom Manage 2002;**23**:96–106.

127 **Brumley RD, Enguidanos S, Cherin DA.** Effectiveness of a home-based palliative care program for end-of-life. *J Palliat Med* 2003;**6**:715–24.

128 **Brumley R, Enguidanos S, Jamison P, et al.** Increased satisfaction with care and lower costs: results of a randomized trial of in-home palliative care. *J Am Geriatr Soc* 2007;**55**:993–1000.

129 **Rabow MW, Dibble SL, Pantilat SZ, McPhee SJ.** The comprehensive care team: a controlled trial of outpatient palliative medicine consultation. *Arch Intern Med* 2004;**164**:83–91.

130 **Yennurajalingam S, Urbauer DL, Casper KL, et al.** Impact of a palliative care consultation team on cancer-related symptoms in advanced cancer patients referred to an outpatient supportive care clinic. *J Pain Symptm Manage* 2011;**41**:49–56.

131 **Temel JS, Greer JA, Muzikansky A, et al.** Early palliative care for patients with metastatic non-small-cell lung cancer. *N Engl J Med* 2010;**363**:733–42.

Chapter 6

Patterns of Recovery after Critical Illness

Nishant K. Sekaran and Theodore J. Iwashyna

Introduction

As survival rates in the ICU increase[1] and the growing number of ICU survivors return to the community, further questions about what it means to live well after critical illness have become more apparent.[2] As critical care providers already know, and as patients and their loved ones come to understand, survival is a necessary, albeit insufficient, condition for living well after critical illness. Survivors suffer significant physical, cognitive, and psychological complications that are associated with the experience of critical illness.[3,4] In this chapter, we focus our discussion primarily on physical function among ICU survivors—what is known and not known with respect to physical decline and the recovery process. We aim to provide a conceptual overview and, in the process, help critical care providers to contextualize the problem and develop strategies for facilitating physical recovery among this at-risk patient population.

Conceptual approach

Current research indicates that critical illness survivors have higher rates of impaired physical function compared to matched population controls.[5] This research has not always proven that critical illness **caused** these declines; this lack of causal link does not detract from the reality that survivors of critical illness have unfulfilled long-term needs related to physical decline. Critical care providers and health care systems have a new opportunity—and arguably a professional obligation—to improve outcomes for survivors. Two conceptual tools will structure our discussion of injury and recovery: an understanding of the time course (see Figure 6.1), and an approach to classifying the types of outcomes in which we may be interested (see Table 6.1).

The phases of recovery over time are presented in Figure 6.1. Patients begin with a baseline trajectory of function. For many ICU patients, particularly older patients, there may have been a gradual decline in function during the years **before** critical illness. When critical illness strikes, a deep drop in functioning occurs during the acute illness and its inpatient care. There follows a period of gradual recovery and adaptation. This recovery can be quite pronounced. Of great relevance for this chapter is the duration of recovery. Work in geriatrics has suggested that there is continuing recovery of function until 18–24 months after acute general medical hospitalization.[6,7] Similarly prolonged time courses of recovery—certainly greater than a year—have been noted in older Spanish ICU patients with regard to geriatric syndromes[8] and in Canadian ARDS patients.[9] Once 1–2 years of recovery are completed, a new baseline level and trajectory are established. A full understanding of the dynamics of recovery—which we do not possess—would map the depth of the initial insult after critical illness; the slope, duration, and modifiability of recovery;

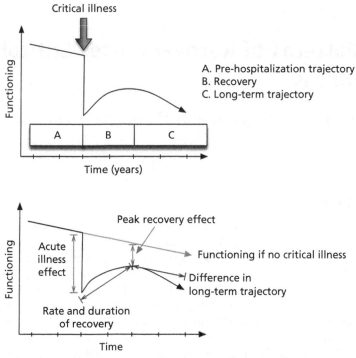

Fig. 6.1 Phases of recovery of critical illness, core model.
The top panel presents the basic model. A patient has some pre-illness rate of decline (period A). Critical illness occurs, leading to an acute decline in function. Over the next 1–2 years (period B), some degree of recovery of function occurs, until a new long-term steady state (period C) is obtained.
The bottom panel represents the distinct components of measuring the 'long-term effect' of a critical illness. There is the extent of acute loss of function, but also a long-term loss of function (that loss which persists despite peak recovery). Critical illness could also alter the long-term trajectory, compared to the pre-illness trajectory. An intervention might hasten the rate of recovery, change the peak recovery effect, and alter the long-term difference in trajectories.

the final level of the new steady state; and whether patients are set on a different trajectory after critical illness than they entered before. Each of these points might be amenable to distinct interventions.

Figure 6.1 represents a core model of injury and recovery after critical illness, but it is not the only model possible. More recently, Woon et al. presented fascinating data on trajectories of cognitive function between hospital discharge and 6 months followed.[10] They showed that many patients followed paths of transient decline, what we have termed a 'Big Hit' model[11] (see Figure 6.2). But, importantly, these authors showed two other trajectories to be present. First, they demonstrated the existence of a group of patients with no discernible injury—perhaps not unexpected but certainly overlooked. Second, they demonstrated the existence of a group of patients who appeared to be normal at discharge but who had significant cognitive impairment at 6-month follow-up. This group might be termed a 'progressive decline', a 'slow burn', or a 'late-injury' phenotype. These data are also consistent with a 'relapsing recurrent' trajectory, but Woon

Table 6.1 Integrating concepts from the ICF model and functional recovery to understand the long-term impact of ARDS, an illustrative example

ICF domain	Definition or presentation	Measures/evaluation	Acute illness	Rate and duration of recovery	Peak recovery	Long-term differences in trajectory
Tissue impairment	Problems in body function or structure					
Lung	Can present as difficulty with ventilator liberation	Pulmonary function tests and pulse oximetry	By definition of ARDS, profound difficulties in gas exchange, characterized by alveolar injury, hypoxaemia, and radiographic infiltrates	Median TLC, FEV$_1$, and FVC are 92%, 85%, and 80% of predicted within 6 months, respectively[63]	Return to normal or near-normal TLC and FVC, with deficits in DLCO (median 72% of predicted at 1 year);[63] lower recovery in more severe baseline lung injury for all domains[16]	The median predicted values of TLC, FEV$_1$, and FVC remain stable over a 5-year period among ARDS survivors (93, 84, and 85%, respectively)[9]
Nerve/muscle	Can present with limb weakness/ paresis or respiratory muscle weakness	Bedside examination Electrophysiologic testing and muscle biopsy	Prevalence of nerve and muscle impairments may be 46% within 1–2 weeks of MV; among these patients, 7.8% had CIP, 7.5% had CIM, 6.7% had mixed CIM/CIP, and 77.6% had unclassified neuromuscular abnormalities, according to the review criteria[23]	Among 15 survivors of critical illness in the Italian CRIMYNE study, 5/6 CIM patients recovered completely within 3–6 months, and 2/7 CIP or CIP/CIM patients recovered within 1 year[27]	Return to baseline function is possible, but its overall prevalence is unknown	Insufficient information about long-term tissue trajectory
Activity limitations	Difficulties that an individual may have in executing activities	6-minute walk test	ALI and poor mobility preclude reliable measurement	Median distance is 66% of predicted age-/sex-matched values at 1 year[9]	Median peak recovery is 76% of predicted age-/sex-matched values[9]	5-year trajectory ranges from 66 to 76% of predicted age-/sex-matched values; correlated with physical function and chronic comorbidities[9]

Table 6.1 (continued) Integrating concepts from the ICF model and functional recovery to understand the long-term impact of ARDS, an illustrative example

ICF domain	Definition or presentation	Measures/ evaluation	Acute illness	Rate and duration of recovery	Peak recovery	Long-term differences in trajectory
Participation restrictions	Problems that an individual may experience in actual life situations (related to fulfilment of social roles and expectations)	SF-36 Physical Function Score (PCS) ADLs IADLs	At hospital discharge, the SF-36 domains of physical function, role physical, social functioning, bodily pain, general health perceptions, and vitality were ≥20 points lower than age-/sex-matched population controls (at least moderate decr ease)[3]	Rate of recovery on SF-36 PCS is approximately 15 points over the first 2.5 years and were greater for younger age groups (<38 years and 38–52 years)[9] Early rehabilitation may facilitate the odds of returning to independent functional status 3-fold at ICU discharge[34]	Median physical function scores (SF-36, PFS) improve over the first 2.5 years and plateau, remaining 1 SD below age-/sex-matched population average[9]	Toronto ARDS cohort remained at 1 SD below average SF-36 PCS for at least 5 years[9], and trajectory appeared to remain stable
		Employment	N/A	In Toronto ARDS cohort, majority (65%) returned to work status at 2 years[9]	In Toronto ARDS cohort, 77% returned to work, with 94% returning to their original position; influenced by job demands, flexibility of work schedule, job re-training, and social support structures[9]	Long-term differences in trajectory are not known

Table 6.1 (continued) Integrating concepts from the ICF model and functional recovery to understand the long-term impact of ARDS, an illustrative example

ICF domain	Definition or presentation	Measures/ evaluation	Acute illness	Rate and duration of recovery	Peak recovery	Long-term differences in trajectory
HRQoL	• A multidimensional concept that includes self-reported measures of physical, mental, emotional, and social well-being	SF-36 Euro-Qual 5D (EQ-5D) Quality of Well-Being (QWB) Sickness Impact Profile (SIP)	• At hospital discharge, the SF-36 domains of physical function, role physical, social physical functioning, bodily pain, general health perceptions, and vitality were ≥20 points lower than age-/sex-matched population controls (at least moderate decrease)[3] • In some cohorts, 100% of ARDS survivors experienced cognitive problems in memory, attention, and concentration[64]	Majority of QoL improvement occurs within first 6 months, particularly in the physical, mental, and social functioning domains of the SF-36 Cognitive impairments may improve significantly within 1 year but not beyond; 78% may have deficits in at least one cognitive function, and 48% may have decreased mental processing speed[3,4]	Pooled domain-specific scores in physical function after 6 months remain 15–26 points below age-/sex-matched controls (moderate effect); mental health may[32]	• Average mental health trajectory may be comparable to age-/sex-matched controls over 5-year period; however, in the Toronto ARDS cohort, 50% of survivors exhibited depression within 2–5 years of follow-up[9] • Physical QoL including global strength and vitality, may remain significantly depressed (1 SD below age-/sex-matched population controls)[9]

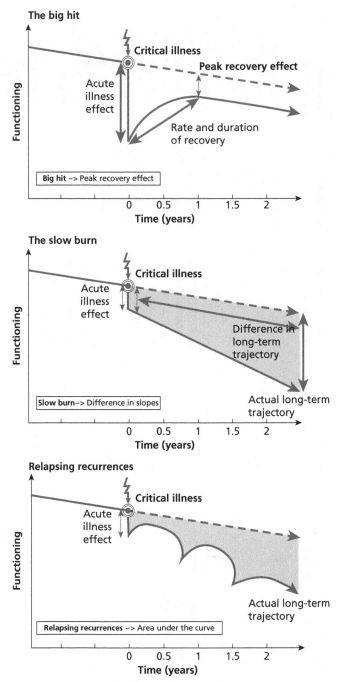

Fig. 6.2 Phases of recovery of critical illness, alternative models.
Prototypical trajectories of recovery. The upper grey line extending past critical illness is the counterfactual trajectory of functioning that would have occurred, had the patient not developed critical illness. Reproduced from Iwashyna TJ. Trajectories of recovery and dysfunction after acute illness, with implications for clinical trial design. *American Journal of Respiratory Critical Care Medicine*, 186(4):302–304, copyright 2012, with permission from the American Thoracic Society.

et al. lacked the temporal granularity to distinguish relapsing recurrence from progressive decline. Frustratingly, we do not yet have information about the relative frequencies of these trajectories across other populations or outcomes. This is despite the very different implication that these trajectories have for clinical trial design and prognostication. We have structured this review around the core model of the Big Hit but acknowledge an urgent need for more empirical research on the relative importance of other trajectories of recovery, and the determinants thereof.

The WHO's International Classification on Functioning, Disability and Health (ICF) provides a unifying framework for how critical illness affects physical function, how changes in physical function can impact the individual directly, and how critical care services may optimize both physical function and its effects on the longitudinal trajectories for survivors of critical illness. The ICF describes 'human functioning and disability as the product of a dynamic interaction between various health conditions and environmental and personal contextual factors.' The classification describes three major domains: (1) tissue **impairment**, which are 'problems in body function or structure such as a significant deviation or loss' (e.g. distortions in alveolar architecture and functional capacity in emphysema), (2) **activity limitation**, which are 'difficulties that an individual may have in executing activities' (e.g. an inability to lift an object), (3) **participation restrictions**, which are 'problems that an individual may experience in involvement in life situations' (e.g. an inability to fulfil personal care tasks or social participation). This conceptual approach has been highlighted by the US Institute of Medicine, who also note that it naturally extends to include (4) **QoL**.[11–13] The ICF also emphasizes that contextual elements, such as personal factors (e.g. age, gender, race) and environmental factors (e.g. community attitudes, patient-provider interactions), moderate the relationships within and particularly between domains.

We will structure our discussion in terms of the domains of the ICF and their changes over time. A summary is presented for patients with ARDS in Table 6.1, the medical critical illness for which we have the best information. Substantial research has been done, and this chapter does not seek to be a comprehensive review of all excellent articles; instead, we have chosen selectively to help illustrate key points.

Tissue impairment

Lung

ARDS is defined on the basis of profound acute changes in gas exchange. The underlying pathology of diffuse alveolar damage is well described and reviewed elsewhere.[14,15] As such, the extent of acute decline in lung function with ARDS is largely a result of the definition of the syndrome, rather than saying something intrinsic about tissue damage during critical illness. Indeed, impaired gas exchange is often one of the organ failures necessary to enter an ICU and thereby become 'critically ill' in the most common operational definition.

In contrast, the recovery of ARDS is not pre-specified by the definition and has been a subject of important study. ARDS survivors may have long-term radiographic abnormalities, including localized changes in non-dependent lung zones and fibrotic changes that may be related to ventilator-induced lung injury.[9] It was assumed that the long-term sequelae of ARDS would relate to this presumably irreversible fibrotic lung disease. Unexpectedly, changes in pulmonary architecture and function may result in persistent declines in the diffusing capacity for carbon monoxide (DLCO), but most pulmonary function abnormalities normalize within the first year.[16,17] The degree to which any residual pulmonary changes result in long-term changes in physical function or QoL is debated, but it is clear that enduring pulmonary problems is not the core problem of most survivors.[18-20] This illustrates several key points. First, the injuries most prominent in the ICU and the immediate post-ICU period may poorly predict the extent of recovery that is possible when sufficiently long follow-up is obtained. Second, the immediately obvious injuries in the acute stage may not be the major drivers of long-term problems. Third, long-term outcome studies, even of basic tissue impairment, can offer unexpected results that can reshape our understanding of a disease—as these results changed our understanding of the long-term outcomes of ARDS away from an initial lung-centred perspective to a neuromuscular focus.

Neuromuscular injury

The literature pertaining to impairments in nerve and muscle tissue evaluate heterogeneous patient samples with overlapping clinical conditions, particularly ARDS and sepsis. Nerve and muscle impairments often coexist, are not consistently defined in the literature, and are difficult to differentiate clinically. Given these considerations, the current state of our knowledge forces us to speak of 'critical illness' and 'neuromuscular injury'. Neuromuscular injury is often termed 'critical CIP and CIM'.[21,22] Yet these conditions often coexist, so other authors have argued for various more general nomenclatures.[23] This diversity reflects debate about whether the neurophysiologic manifestations or the clinical expression of the underlying tissue impairment is the primary frame of reference.[24] This echoes the tension between the appropriate roles for history and physical vs electromyography (EMG), nerve conduction studies (NCS), and muscle biopsies in evaluation.

Nerve and muscle impairments among the critically ill are thought to be common immediately after critical illness.[25] These impairments manifest as difficulty liberating from the ventilator and/or significant limb weakness or paresis that occur days or weeks after the onset of critical illness that has no identifiable alternative causes.[22] In a systematic review of 24 studies that evaluated 1421 critically ill patients, the prevalence rate of nerve or muscle impairments (classified as critical illness neuromyopathy or CINMA) was 46% (CI 43–49). The exact time of CINMA evaluation varied between the studies, but most occurred within 1–2 weeks of ICU admission or MV. The patients in this review were drawn from medical, surgical, and neurological ICUs who were receiving MV, were admitted for severe sepsis or septic shock, and/or had MOF. Individuals with prior neuromuscular disease were excluded from 20 studies in the review. Among the affected 46% of patients in the study, approximately 7.8% had CIP, 7.5% had CIM, 6.7% had mixed CIM/CIP, and 77.6% had unclassified neuromuscular abnormalities, according to the electrophysiologic review criteria in each study.[26] An important footnote highlighted by this review is that there is heterogeneity among studies with respect to specific criteria for CINMA and its subtypes.

To the extent that there is heterogeneity in the true neuromuscular outcomes among patients, it is not yet clear the extent to which this heterogeneity is a function of definition, patient diagnoses, ICU treatment practices, or other natural variability. The pathophysiology for nerve and muscle tissue impairments continues to be described, and most researchers believe that the injuries are mediated by metabolic, inflammatory, and bioenergetic derangements.[25] These diffuse injuries correspond to the diverse mechanisms of injury in ICU syndromes themselves.

At the tissue level, unlike in the lung, detailed information about **recovery** of the neuromuscular architecture is incomplete. Routine electrophysiologic testing and muscle biopsy are not commonly performed after discharge from the ICU; in studies when these data are available, the sample sizes are relatively small and prone to selection bias. In general, the limb and diaphragm weakness associated with CIP and CIM can persist for months to years, with CIP having a worse prognosis than CIM.[22] In a 1-year prospective follow-up of 15 Italian critical illness survivors with CIP or CIM at the time of ICU discharge, Guarneri and colleagues found that the five out of six CIM patients recovered completely (clinical exam, electrodiagnostic test) within 3–6 months, but only two out of seven patients with CIP or CIP/CIM recovered within 1 year.[27] Among the Toronto ARDS survivor cohort, the authors report that all of the patients reported lower functional status at 12 months, which they primarily attributed to global muscle atrophy, proximal weakness, and fatigue. In a small follow-up study from this cohort, Angel and colleagues evaluated neuromuscular function in 16 survivors who did not have frank paresis during their ICU course but noted functional limitations with abnormal motor examinations within 6–24 months after ICU discharge. They found that seven of 16 patients exhibited compressive mononeuropathies (electrodiagnostic testing was negative); of the four patients that agreed to muscle biopsy, all exhibited structurally non-specific changes.[28] Among these patients, no clear pattern emerged regarding the time course of recovery.

These tissue level injuries are of substantial interest; yet, physiologic impairments may not always correlate well with activity limitation or participation restrictions.[29] For example, a patient's cardiac ejection fraction will influence, but not determine, that patient's exercise capacity or mobility in daily life. Thus, we next turn to the patterns of recovery from disability after critical illness.

Activity limitation and participation restriction

The tissue impairments that are observed in critical illness have clear ramifications beyond the episode of care in the ICU. An emerging body of good-quality studies describes a consistent association between critical illness, activity limitations, and participation restrictions. Many of these longitudinal studies follow small samples over a period of time and examine the ways that these individuals differ from matched population controls. Besides the modest sample sizes, a major limitation of most of these cohort studies is the lack of, or potentially biased, information about the individual's capacities before the onset of critical illness.[30,31] We discuss some of the high-quality studies that describe the activity limitations and participation restrictions for patients with ARDS and sepsis, choosing findings for illustrativeness, rather than exhaustiveness.

ARDS

ARDS has served as a model paradigm for evaluating the long-term effects of critical illness, particularly given the substantial clinical heterogeneity and aetiologic overlap with other clinical conditions.[32,33] New activity limitations are quite common immediately after ARDS. In a cohort study of ARDS survivors, Hopkins and colleagues demonstrated that physical function and physical roles, measured by the SF-36 health outcomes questionnaire, were decreased by ≥75% (severe), compared to an age- and sex-matched population standard, at hospital discharge. In the control arm of Schweickert et al.'s randomized trial, evaluating early rehabilitation in patients undergoing MV (56% with an ARDS diagnosis), 65% were unable to return to independent functional status (independence in five ADLs and walking unassisted) at hospital discharge, even though all had been able to do so on enrolment.[34]

Recovery of physical function for patients with ARDS is slow and incomplete. In two separate studies of ARDS patients without non-pulmonary organ dysfunction or sepsis, Angus and colleagues found that a composite measure of physical function and related symptoms (Quality of Well-Being score) were significantly lower than normal population estimates and minimally different at 6 and 12 months.[35,36] In one of these studies, these scores were lower than cystic fibrosis control patients.[35] In a separate systematic review of 13 ARDS studies, Dowdy and colleagues found that physical function, measured using a variety of health instruments, including the SF-36, was persistently diminished for ARDS survivors, compared to matched population controls, across multiple studies.[32] The five studies that specifically used the SF-36 evaluated survivors at time points of 6 months post-discharge to 4 years and demonstrated comparable decrements of physical function scores across time, with an overall magnitude that was similar to reference patient populations with chronic systolic heart failure (15–26 points on average representing at least a moderate effect; effect on physical role impairment was even larger).[3,5,17,20,37,38] Although the samples in each study were relatively small, the scores were consistent across patients who were drawn from the US, Germany, and Canada.

Herridge et al.'s 5-year cohort analysis of ARDS survivors in Toronto, Canada has provided detailed observations about the rate and duration of recovery as well as the long-term trajectory for these patients. This cohort was relatively young (median age 44 years old) and had a low rate of chronic illness prior to acquiring ARDS primarily from pneumonia, sepsis, and trauma/burns. The authors supplemented SF-36 self-reported health outcomes with information from monthly patient diaries, detailed clinical assessments, pulmonary imaging and functional testing, caregiver interviews, and administrative health care records. Of significant interest is that, while pulmonary function largely recovered by 6–12 months, measures of physical function, including the 6-minute walk test and the physical function domains of the SF-36, were substantially lower than age- and sex-matched norms (76% of predicted and one standard deviation (SD) lower, respectively) for at least 5 years.[4] Younger patients (<52 years) and those with more rapid organ recovery seemed to have better physical recovery, although no patients reached the predicted age norms. Unexpectedly, features of the hospitalization, including length of stay, ventilator days, paralytic use, and glucocorticoid (GC) use, did not explain variation in the physical function scores.

The Toronto ARDS cohort sheds some light on the link between physical activity limitation and social participation. Most of the physical recovery in the cohort occurred within the first 2 years and then plateaued. While no patients exhibited demonstrable deficits on bedside muscle strength exams, almost all reported an inability to exercise vigorously or engage in physical activity at their pre-ARDS level. At 5 years, 77% of the respondents returned to work, with 94% returning to their original positions. This process was more gradual and required support from the employers, insurers, and research personnel—that is, these findings emphasize that changes in social disability (such as the ability to hold a job) are not simply the result of measurable tissue impairments, but rather of the interaction of those tissue injuries with the (modifiable) social world in which the patient lives and functions. Schelling and colleagues reported similar findings at approximately 5 years in a German cohort of ARDS survivors.[20]

An important feature of evaluating change in longitudinal studies is the ability to account for individual trajectories prior to the event of interest. Obtaining this information requires the ability to collect functional information on a random sample of patients, sometimes for a purpose other than the critical care study question of interest. Using data from a prospective, nationally representative, longitudinal cohort of Medicare beneficiaries (the Medicare Current Beneficiary Survey or MCBS), Barnato and colleagues evaluated the long-term impact of critical illness (defined as receiving MV) on disability in elder survivors of critical illness. The authors were able to: (1) obtain individual baseline values of pre-MV physical and cognitive functioning and (2) develop a comparison group of non-mechanically ventilated general hospitalizations. After controlling for the pre-critical illness functional trajectory and other clinical covariates, these data suggested a significant marginal increase in disability, on average, among those that received MV over a

4-year observation period. The study was not designed to evaluate the particular clinical details of the critical care condition nor the mechanism underlying the increased incidence of disability among this group but provides crucial scientific evidence that the disability effects after MV are not simply the result of 'selection' into respiratory failure by patients who were already disabled.[39] In fact, survivors of MV had similar pre-hospital disability and mobility scores, compared to the hospitalized group who did not receive MV. While these data have too coarse a timescale to map the recovery period, they do suggest enduring deficits after recovery.

Sepsis

Sepsis is a leading cause of ARDS, but far more common than ARDS. An emerging body of good quality literature suggests that the paradigm of altered long-term functional trajectory applies— perhaps to patients with severe sepsis, even if they do not require care in an ICU. In the acute setting, patients with sepsis can suffer significant declines in their overall physical functioning, with a prolonged and suboptimal recovery. Hofhuis and colleagues[40] assessed self-reported health measures using the SF-36 in a longitudinal cohort of Dutch sepsis patients before admission (through proxies) and at several time points up until 6 months after discharge. On average, the physical function and role physical domains of the SF-36 were lower at the time of ICU discharge, compared to baseline, recovered slightly over the ensuing 6 months but remained below the baseline. In comparison to a general Dutch population, the sepsis survivors were noted to have lower SF-36 scores, both pre-admission and at 6 months, which aligns with the common clinical intuition that disabled individuals may be at greater risk for sepsis. The authors strived to address the well-described measurement error associated with proxy reporting[30,31] by querying proxies within 72 hours of illness.[41] While measurement issues may persist, it is clear that researchers in this area are striving to be nuanced and rigorous.

In follow-up to this and other studies, a systematic review of 30 studies in the sepsis literature provides information about the rate and duration of recovery for this population. Winters and colleagues evaluated QoL scores in sepsis survivors beyond 3 months post-discharge. Like the study by Hofhuis et al., the authors found that physical function and role physical domains continued to be significantly diminished, compared to population norms at 6 months.[42] The authors were unable to disentangle the specific effects of sepsis from other comorbid ICU conditions such as ALI.

Information about the long-term trajectories of sepsis survivors is emerging. Iwashyna and colleagues evaluated the long-term cognitive and physical function in survivors of severe sepsis from a nationally representative cohort of older adults (the Health and Retirement Study). Similar to Barnato's MV study, the authors addressed the proxy or retrospective functional status reporting bias by including prospective reports of physical and cognitive functioning that were obtained before the onset of severe sepsis, and also developed a comparison group of non-sepsis general hospitalizations. The study cohort comprised older adults (mean age 76.9 years) who were hospitalized for severe sepsis. After adjusting for the baseline pre-sepsis functioning, the study indicated significantly higher incidence of cognitive decline and new physical functional limitations among sepsis survivors that were independent of a broad range of demographic and clinical characteristics. Patients without previous limitations developed 1.57 new physical limitations in their ADLs/ IADLs, and patients with some limitations at baseline developed a mean of 1.50 new limitations. Patients with some pre-sepsis limitations also had a statistically significant and clinically meaningful deterioration in their trajectory after severe sepsis, with continued increased rates of the development of yet further disability. The activity limitations and participation restrictions were spread over a wide range of activities and were applicable, irrespective of MV status. Similarly, the prevalence of moderate to severe cognitive impairment also increased. Among survivors, these changes persisted for at least 8 years and were robust to a variety of sensitivity analyses.[43]

Mechanisms of recovery for physical function

The problem of impaired physical function is hardly unique to critical care—indeed, it is integral to the clinical expertise of geriatrics and stroke care. These patient populations exhibit heterogeneity in the level and rate of transition between the multiple ICF domains. These disciplines have made progress in effectively dealing with impaired physical function in the context of acute illness. The research in these fields and the clinical models of health care delivery suggest that incorporating rehabilitative strategies into the acute care setting may improve care processes and clinical outcomes. Early experience in the ICU setting suggests that this may be the case.

For geriatric services, a key tool with well-substantiated positive effects is the Comprehensive Geriatric Assessment (CGA). The CGA has been defined as 'a multidimensional, interdisciplinary process to determine the medical, psychological, and functional capabilities of a frail elderly person in order to develop a coordinated and integrated care plan for treatment and long-term follow up.'[44] This process involves establishing a multidisciplinary care team and/or dedicated patient ward that can consistently carry out the (potentially complex) acute care and rehabilitative needs for patients. This model has been subjected to numerous randomized trials in the acute care hospital setting and has recently been summarized in a Cochrane systematic review and meta-analysis.[45,46] The main results indicate that CGA programmes facilitate independent living at home at both 6-month and 12-month follow-up (NNT = 17 and 33, respectively). Five studies evaluating the combined endpoints of death or functional deterioration (increased dependence) indicated a statistically significant benefit (NNT = 17). Studies that targeted CGA to the frailest patients showed stronger effects on the outcome of independent living (NNT ≈ 6)—a particularly promising finding for applying CGA-type interventions to the ICU. While this review captured the beneficial effect of CGA for geriatric patients presenting to acute care inpatient settings, questions remain about which patients should be targeted, when to initiate the programme (acute vs post-acute), and the intensity of outpatient follow-up. This structured, interdisciplinary approach to assessing and intervening on complex patients seems fundamentally complementary to current best ICU practice.

Similarly, for stroke patients, evidence from randomized trials demonstrates better process adherence and functional outcomes for specialized stroke units, compared to general wards, with specialist support in both the acute and rehabilitative phases.[47–49] A beneficial feature of these specialized wards includes high-fidelity functional assessment and earlier interventions to reduce progression across the dimensions of the ICF framework. Indredavik and colleagues assert that shorter time to mobilization/re-training was the most important factor for reducing 'bed-associated' complications, including pneumonia, venous thromboembolism, pressure ulcers, and orthostatic hypotension, while achieving favourable psychological and physical outcomes.[48]

In the present critical care context, there is little evidence examining the appropriate use or timing of validated physical function assessment tool specifically for critical care patients.[50] However, reasonable principles and rules of thumb can guide critical care providers in leading these assessments, using concepts that are highlighted in the ICF. A central emphasis in the ICF is on understanding the patient-environment interactions, particularly the functional capacity of a patient in their relevant environmental context. Performing these evaluations, particularly ADLs or IADLs, will require the assistance of non-physician providers, including physical and/or occupational therapists. These intensive evaluations—and the development of feasible remediation plans—are likely to be beyond the scope of traditional critical care practice and emphasize the need for multidisciplinary team-based care, efficient communications across multiple providers, and a streamlined integrated delivery system across a variety of health care settings. In a recent guideline for the rehabilitation of critical care patients, the National Institute for Health and Care Excellence (NICE) in the UK proposed that functional assessments be performed at multiple time points: during the critical care stay, before discharge from the ICU, after transfer to the hospital ward, before discharge to an out-of-hospital setting, and 2–3 months after critical care discharge.[50] The above data on the time course of recovery in both acute illness and critical illness suggest that even longer follow-up might be reasonable. The critical care health care delivery system should be designed to facilitate these evaluations and implement complementary management plans when handing off care to an integrated long-term follow-up system.

Indeed, there are some promising first steps. Recent efforts have focused on early mobility programmes that occur in the ICU itself, with greater integration of physical medicine and rehabilitation services into the daily workflow.[51–56] These interventions have coincided with an improved understanding of the neurologic complications of critical illness, including neuromuscular and cognitive complications, and the adverse iatrogenic effects of heavy sedation use.[57–59] The best currently available data supporting intensive ICU mobility interventions are currently applicable to a subset of ICU patients who are able to interact with hospital staff and demonstrate cardiopulmonary stability despite the need for MV.

Schweickert and colleagues performed an RCT that evaluated the efficacy of sedation interruption combined with PT/OT in a cohort of critically ill patients who were functionally independent at baseline. Intervention patients were more likely to be functionally independent at discharge (59% vs 35%, $P = 0.02$) and have lower rates of delirium and ventilator-free days (VFDs) at the 28-day follow-up, compared to individuals in the control arm who received interruption of sedation without early PT/OT.[34] The intervention was found to be safe and well tolerated. In the early PT/OT arm, the time from intubation to first PT/OT session was 1.5 days, compared to 7.4 days in the control arm. The patients in the intervention arm were more likely to be able to independently perform in each ADL at hospital discharge and, on average, reached activity milestones in nearly 50% of the time, compared to the control cohort. There have been important independent confirmations of evidence of benefit. Most prominently, in a prospective, non-randomized quality improvement study of early mobility therapy undertaken in the ICU, Morris and colleagues found that implementing an ICU mobility protocol that was carried out by a designating team of nurses and physical therapists increased the overall receipt of PT among assigned ICU patients and was associated with shorter hospital lengths of stay and post-discharge hospital readmission rates.[60,61]

Of interest was that the bedside strength measurements in the Schweickert trial were comparable for the two groups (MRC strength exam and hand dynamometry); the differences were concentrated in the activity limitation and participation restriction domains of the ICF, rather than the impairment domain. This suggests that actions in the ICU in the early recovery stage can set patients on a trajectory of more rapid recovery—adequately powered long-term follow-up is needed to determine whether this more rapid early recovery leads to better long-term plateau or (as the sceptical scientist must ask) whether it simply changes the dynamics of early recovery without changing the long-term level.

In contrast to the promising evidence for targeting early mobility therapy in the ICU for appropriate patients, recommending self-directed physiotherapy programmes as a part of a nurse-led intensive care follow-up for patients after ICU discharge appears to provide no marginal benefit, compared to 'usual care', in terms of QoL, efficacy, or cost effectiveness in a multicentre

RCT.[62] Further studies are still needed to determine the optimal timing and duration of physiotherapy interventions, the relative importance of mobility and strength-oriented (PT) vs adaptive-oriented (OT) therapy, and whether these programmes can optimize physical function and other QoL domains over the course of months and years. For the time being, it appears that rehabilitative interventions are best started in the ICU for patients in whom these efforts can be safely applied.

Conclusion

In this chapter, we have highlighted the prevalent and profound problem of impaired physical function among survivors of critical illness. We have used the conceptual tools of time course and the WHO's ICF to describe the patterns of physical decline and recovery that are associated with critical illness, particularly ARDS and sepsis. There is strong evidence to suggest that many survivors of critical illness experience deep declines in physical function that persist for months to years, recover slowly and incompletely, and leave an indelible imprint on individual well-being and social participation. Although, in some cases, there is insufficient information to prove a causal relationship between critical illness and limitations in ICF domains, critical care providers should not be dissuaded from striving to improve these adverse functional outcomes. Findings from the geriatric and stroke clinical arenas, and recent clinical evidence from the critical care literature, suggest that incorporating aspects of early rehabilitation into the acute care setting can be safely implemented and effectively improve functional outcomes in this vulnerable patient population.

References

1 **Erickson SE, Martin GS, Davis JL, Matthay MA, Eisner MD.** Recent trends in acute lung injury mortality: 1996–2005. *Crit Care Med* 2009;**37**:1574–9.

2 **Iwashyna TJ.** Survivorship will be the defining challenge of critical care in the 21st century. *Ann Intern Med* 2010;**153**:204–5.

3 **Hopkins RO, Weaver LK, Collingridge D, Parkinson RB, Chan KJ, Orme JF, Jr.** Two-year cognitive, emotional, and quality-of-life outcomes in acute respiratory distress syndrome. *Am J Respir Crit Care Med* 2005;**171**:340–7.

4 **Herridge MS.** Recovery and long-term outcome in acute respiratory distress syndrome. *Crit Care Clin* 2011;**27**:685–704.

5 **Davidson TA.** Reduced quality of life in survivors of acute respiratory distress syndrome compared with critically ill control patients. *JAMA* 1999;**281**:354–60.

6 **Boyd CM, Landefeld CS, Counsell SR, et al.** Recovery of activities of daily living in older adults after hospitalization for acute medical illness. *J Am Geriatr Soc* 2008;**56**:2171–9.

7 **Boyd CM, Ricks M, Fried LP, et al.** Functional decline and recovery of activities of daily living in hospitalized, disabled older women: the Women's Health and Aging Study I. *J Am Geriatr Soc* 2009;**57**:1757–66.

8 **Sacanella E, Perez-Castejon JM, Nicolas JM, et al.** Functional status and quality of life 12 months after discharge from a medical ICU in healthy elderly patients: a prospective observational study. *Crit Care* 2011;**15**:R105.

9 **Herridge MS, Tansey CM, Matte A, et al.** Functional disability 5 years after acute respiratory distress syndrome. *N Engl J Med* 2011;**364**:1293–304.

10 **Woon FL, Dunn C, Hopkins RO.** Predicting cognitive sequelae in survivors of critical illness with cognitive screening tests. *Am J Respir Crit Care Med* 2012;**186**:333–40.

11 Iwashyna TJ. Trajectories of recovery and dysfunction after acute illness, with implications for clinical trial design. *Am J Respir Crit Care Med* 2012;**186**:302–4.

12 Field MJ, Jette AM (eds). *The future of disability in America*. Washington, DC: National Academies Press (US); 2007.

13 Iezzoni LI, Freedman VA. Turning the disability tide: the importance of definitions. *JAMA* 2008;**299**:332–4.

14 Ware LB, Matthay MA. The acute respiratory distress syndrome. *N Engl J Med* 2000;**342**:1334–49.

15 Esteban A, Fernandez-Segoviano P, Frutos-Vivar F, et al. Comparison of clinical criteria for the acute respiratory distress syndrome with autopsy findings. *Ann Intern Med* 2004;**141**:440–5.

16 McHugh LG, Milberg JA, Whitcomb ME, Schoene RB, Maunder RJ, Hudson LD. Recovery of function in survivors of the acute respiratory distress syndrome. *Am J Respir Crit Care Med* 1994;**150**:90.

17 Herridge MS, Cheung AM, Tansey CM, et al. One-year outcomes in survivors of the acute respiratory distress syndrome. *N Engl J Med* 2003;**348**:683–93.

18 Heyland DK. Survivors of acute respiratory distress syndrome: relationship between pulmonary dysfunction and long-term health-related quality of life. *Crit Care Med* 2005;**33**:1549–56.

19 Orme J, Jr, Romney JS, Hopkins RO, et al. Pulmonary function and health-related quality of life in survivors of acute respiratory distress syndrome. *Am J Respir Crit Care Med* 2003;**167**:690–4.

20 Schelling G. Pulmonary function and health-related quality of life in a sample of long-term survivors of the acute respiratory distress syndrome. *Intensive Care Med* 2000;**26**:1304–11.

21 Latronico N, Fenzi F, Recupero D, et al. Critical illness myopathy and neuropathy. *Lancet* 1996;**347**:1579–82.

22 Latronico N, Bolton CF. Critical illness polyneuropathy and myopathy: a major cause of muscle weakness and paralysis. *Lancet Neurol* 2011;**10**:931–41.

23 Stevens RD, Marshall SA, Cornblath DR, et al. A framework for diagnosing and classifying intensive care unit-acquired weakness. *Crit Care Med* 2009;**37**(10 Suppl):S299–308.

24 Schweickert WD, Hall J. ICU-acquired weakness. *Chest* 2007;**131**:1541–9.

25 Hermans G, De Jonghe B, Bruyninckx F, Van den Berghe G. Clinical review: critical illness polyneuropathy and myopathy. *Crit Care* 2008;**12**:238.

26 Stevens RD, Dowdy DW, Michaels RK, Mendez-Tellez PA, Pronovost PJ, Needham DM. Neuromuscular dysfunction acquired in critical illness: a systematic review. *Intensive Care Med* 2007;**33**:1876–91.

27 Guarneri B, Bertolini G, Latronico N. Long-term outcome in patients with critical illness myopathy or neuropathy: the Italian multicentre CRIMYNE study. *J Neurol Neurosurg Psychiatry* 2008;**79**:838–41.

28 Angel MJ, Bril V, Shannon P, Herridge MS. Neuromuscular function in survivors of the acute respiratory distress syndrome. *Can J Neurol Sci* 2007;**34**:427–32.

29 Guyatt GH, Feeny DH, Patrick DL. Measuring health-related quality of life. *Ann Intern Med* 1993;**118**:622–9.

30 Scales DC. Difference in reported pre-morbid health-related quality of life between ARDS survivors and their substitute decision makers. *Intensive Care Med* 2006;**32**:1826–31.

31 Gifford JM, Husain N, Dinglas VD, Colantuoni E, Needham DM. Baseline quality of life before intensive care: a comparison of patient versus proxy responses. *Crit Care Med* 2010;**38**:855–60.

32 Dowdy DW, Eid MP, Dennison CR, et al. Quality of life after acute respiratory distress syndrome: a meta-analysis. *Intensive Care Med* 2006;**32**:1115–24.

33 Herridge MS, Angus DC. Acute lung injury—affecting many lives. *N Engl J Med* 2005;**353**:1736–8.

34 Schweickert WD, Pohlman MC, Pohlman AS, et al. Early physical and occupational therapy in mechanically ventilated, critically ill patients: a randomised controlled trial. *Lancet* 2009;**373**:1874–82.

35 Angus DC, Musthafa AA, Clermont G, et al. Quality-adjusted survival in the first year after the acute respiratory distress syndrome. *Am J Respir Crit Care Med* 2001;**163**:1389–94.

36 Angus DC, Clermont G, Linde-Zwirble WT, et al. Healthcare costs and long-term outcomes after acute respiratory distress syndrome: a phase III trial of inhaled nitric oxide. *Crit Care Med* 2006;**34**:2883–90.

37 McHorney CA, Ware JE, Jr, Raczek AE. The MOS 36-Item Short-Form Health Survey (SF-36): II. Psychometric and clinical tests of validity in measuring physical and mental health constructs. *Med Care* 1993;**31**:247–63.

38 Weinert CR. Health-related quality of life after acute lung injury. *Am J Respir Crit Care Med* 1997;**156**:1120–8.

39 Barnato AE, Albert SM, Angus DC, Lave JR, Degenholtz HB. Disability among elderly survivors of mechanical ventilation. *Am J Respir Crit Care Med* 2011;**183**:1037–42.

40 Hofhuis JGM, Spronk PE, van Stel HF, Schrijvers AJP, Rommes JH, Bakker J. The impact of severe sepsis on health-related quality of life: a long-term follow-up study. *Anesth Analg* 2008;**107**:1957.

41 Hofhuis JG, Spronk PE, van Stel HF, Schrijvers GJ, Rommes JH, Bakker J. The impact of critical illness on perceived health-related quality of life during ICU treatment, hospital stay, and after hospital discharge: a long-term follow-up study. *Chest* 2008;**133**:377–85.

42 Winters BD, Eberlein M, Leung J, Needham DM, Pronovost PJ, Sevransky JE. Long-term mortality and quality of life in sepsis: a systematic review. *Crit Care Med* 2010;**38**:1276–83.

43 Iwashyna TJ, Ely EW, Smith DM, Langa KM. Long-term cognitive impairment and functional disability among survivors of severe sepsis. *JAMA* 2010;**304**:1787–94.

44 Rubenstein LZ, Stuck AE, Siu AL, Wieland D. Impacts of geriatric evaluation and management programs on defined outcomes: overview of the evidence. *J Am Geriatr Soc* 1991;**39**:8S–16S; discussion 17S–18S.

45 Ellis G, Whitehead MA, O'Neill D, Langhorne P, Robinson D. Comprehensive geriatric assessment for older adults admitted to hospital. *Cochrane Database Syst Rev* 2011;**7**:CD006211.

46 Ellis G, Whitehead MA, Robinson D, O'Neill D, Langhorne P. Comprehensive geriatric assessment for older adults admitted to hospital: meta-analysis of randomised controlled trials. *BMJ* 2011;**343**:d6553.

47 Evans A, Perez I, Harraf F, et al. Can differences in management processes explain different outcomes between stroke unit and stroke-team care? *Lancet* 2001;**358**:1586–92.

48 Indredavik B, Bakke F, Slordahl SA, Rokseth R, Haheim LL. Treatment in a combined acute and rehabilitation stroke unit: which aspects are most important? *Stroke* 1999;**30**:917–23.

49 Langhorne P, Bernhardt J, Kwakkel G. Stroke rehabilitation. *Lancet* 2011;**377**:1693–702.

50 Tan T, Brett SJ, Stokes T. Rehabilitation after critical illness: summary of NICE guidance. *BMJ* 2009;**338**:b822.

51 Needham DM, Korupolu R, Zanni JM, et al. Early physical medicine and rehabilitation for patients with acute respiratory failure: a quality improvement project. *Arch Phys Med Rehabil* 2010;**91**:536–42.

52 Needham DM, Korupolu R. Rehabilitation quality improvement in an intensive care unit setting: implementation of a quality improvement model. *Top Stroke Rehabil* 2010;**17**:271–81.

53 Gosselink R, Bott J, Johnson M, et al. Physiotherapy for adult patients with critical illness: recommendations of the European Respiratory Society and European Society of Intensive Care Medicine Task Force on Physiotherapy for Critically Ill Patients. *Intensive Care Med* 2008;**34**:1188–99.

54 Hopkins RO, Spuhler VJ, Thomsen GE. Transforming ICU culture to facilitate early mobility. *Crit Care Clin* 2007;**23**:81–96.

55 Bailey P, Thomsen GE, Spuhler VJ, et al. Early activity is feasible and safe in respiratory failure patients. *Crit Care Med* 2007;**35**:139–45.

56 Needham DM. Mobilizing patients in the intensive care unit: improving neuromuscular weakness and physical function. *JAMA* 2008;**300**:1685–90.

57 Kress JP, Pohlman AS, O'Connor MF, Hall JB. Daily interruption of sedative infusions in critically ill patients undergoing mechanical ventilation. *N Engl J Med* 2000;**342**:1471–7.

58 **Ely EW, Truman B, Shintani A, et al.** Monitoring sedation status over time in ICU patients: reliability and validity of the Richmond Agitation-Sedation Scale (RASS). *JAMA* 2003;**289**:2983–91.

59 **Ely EW, Shintani A, Truman B, et al.** Delirium as a predictor of mortality in mechanically ventilated patients in the intensive care unit. *JAMA* 2004;**291**:1753–62.

60 **Morris PE, Goad A, Thompson C, et al.** Early intensive care unit mobility therapy in the treatment of acute respiratory failure. *Crit Care Med* 2008;**36**:2238–43.

61 **Morris PE, Griffin L, Berry M, et al.** Receiving early mobility during an intensive care unit admission is a predictor of improved outcomes in acute respiratory failure. *Am J Med Sci* 2011;**341**:373–7.

62 **Cuthbertson BH, Rattray J, Campbell MK, et al.** The PRaCTICaL study of nurse led, intensive care follow-up programmes for improving long term outcomes from critical illness: a pragmatic randomised controlled trial. *BMJ* 2009;**339**:b3723.

63 **Herridge MS, Cheung AM, Tansey CM, et al.** One-year outcomes in survivors of the acute respiratory distress syndrome. *N Engl J Med* 2003;**348**:683–93.

64 **Hopkins RO, Weaver LK, Pope D, Orme JF, Bigler ED, Larson LV.** Neuropsychological sequelae and impaired health status in survivors of severe acute respiratory distress syndrome. *Am J Respir Crit Care Med* 1999;**160**:50–6.

Chapter 7

Quality of Life after Critical Illness

José G.M. Hofhuis and Peter E. Spronk

Introduction

HRQoL is a relevant outcome measure for patients admitted to the ICU. In those patients, long-term outcomes of physical and psychological factors, functional status, and social interactions are becoming more and more important, both for doctors and nurses as well as for patients and their relatives.[1,2] Doctors and nurses want to know what a 'reasonable' QoL means to their patients. QoL is described as a 'unique personal perception'[3] and influenced by social, psychological, cultural, familial, relational, and individual factors. In HRQoL studies, in general as well as in critically ill patients, there is a paucity in the definitions clearly describing HRQoL. The QoL related to health, or HRQoL, does not take all dimensions of QoL into account but focuses on those dimensions that are influenced by the disease or its treatment. If specific populations in the ICU are examined, such as cardiac patients, a disease-specific instrument can be used to give information and comparisons. However, in the case of ICU patients with a multitude of different diagnoses, there is a need for generic outcomes that can be used across medical and surgical critically ill patients, as well as condition-specific ones.[4] The main reason for HRQoL research in critically ill patients is the lack of knowledge about the outcome of HRQoL in patients admitted to an ICU.

In this chapter, we will address several subjects, i.e. why measure HRQoL in critically ill patients; what do we mean with HRQoL; which HRQoL instruments are being used; how to score HRQoL before ICU admission; and what the impact of critical illness on HRQoL is, particularly in the elderly. We will also address the phenomenon of response shift in survivors from critically illness related to their perceived HRQoL.

Why measure HRQoL in critically ill patients?

Development of ICU technology has seen a rapid growth in the last decennium. This technology enables ICU staff to sustain and restore life of critically ill patients who otherwise would have died. In the past, survival alone was enough to justify all interventions, but the high costs make ICU staff more and more aware about the importance of measuring the QoL.[5] The costs of ICU treatment are high, and, frequently, a significant fraction of these costs are spent on patients with a poor prognosis and a large chance to die. It seems necessary to look at cost effectiveness and cost utility for developing guidelines in using ICU resources.[6,7] However, how do ICU patients feel and function? This information seems essential for making decisions at the bedside but is also important in the evaluation of the efficacy and efficiency of ICU interventions.[8] HRQoL investigation in critically ill patients can make a contribution to answering these questions of long-term prognosis.[8]

Definition and domains of HRQoL in critically ill patients

In HRQoL studies, in general as well as in critically ill patients, there is a lack of a clear framework for defining and describing HRQoL. One of the difficulties in HRQoL research is defining what is meant by HRQoL; there is no universally accepted definition. QoL, health status, functional status, and HRQoL are often used interchangeably in the literature.[9] Yet, each of these terms may reflect different aspects of an individual's well-being (see Figure 7.1).[8] This may lead to different measurement approaches and thus different results Measuring HRQoL is, in essence, evaluating the health status of individuals, both mental and physical, together with their own sense of well-being.[10] The WHO defines health as not only the absence of infirmity and disease, but also as a state of physical, mental, and social well-being.[11] By using this definition, we can define HRQoL, which can be divided into several dimensions, including physical, psychological, and social functioning. The physical domain contains items describing physical capacities of a patient and the physical complaints he or she has doing these activities like bathing or dressing, walking, climbing stairs, pushing a vacuum cleaner, biking, carrying groceries, or having pain. The psychological domain contains items describing psychological complaints like feeling depressed or anxious, or positive feelings like satisfaction, feeling full of energy, and happiness. The social domain contains items describing to what extent illness interfered with usual social activities with family, friends, neighbours, or groups. Besides that, patients can also give their overall opinion of the three domains. This overall opinion shows what the influence is of illness and the associated treatment on the current health of the patient.[11]

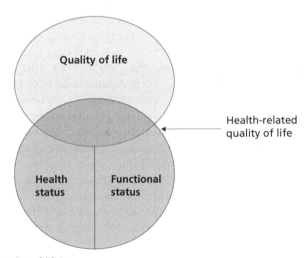

Fig. 7.1 What is quality of life?
The upper circle represents those aspects or domains that are of value to patients, as they influence their well-being or QoL. The lower circle represents health status measurement. The intersection of the two circles, the HRQoL, represents health status measurements that are of value to people.[107]

Reproduced from Heyland DK, Guyatt G, Cook DJ, Meade M, Juniper E, Cronin L, Gafni A. 'Frequency and methodologic rigor of quality-of-life assessments in the critical care literature'. *Critical Care Medicine*, 26(3): 591–8, copyright 1998, with permission from Wolters Kluwer and the Society of Critical Care Medicine.

HRQoL and utility measures in critically ill patients

Treatment of patients in the ICU is expensive, and the justification for ICU treatment has been questioned on clinical, ethical, and economic grounds.[6,12] HRQoL-measuring instruments (generic QoL questionnaires) provide descriptive information about individuals and are used when researchers wish to gain insight in the impact of illness and treatments on patients, but also in changes in the patient's health status over time. To incorporate differences in both quality and duration of survival, a unitary measure of outcome, the 'quality-adjusted life year' (QALY), has been introduced.[13] For example, a patient who gains 10 years of life, with a QoL of 60% of normal, has gained 6 QALYs. Thus, a disease causing only morbidity can be compared with diseases causing mortality. These utility measures, such as the EQ-5D,[14] Health Utilities Index,[15] and SF-6D[16] assign a single value from 0, representing death or worst health imaginable, to 1, representing optimal health. Combining the utility value with survival data allows an estimate of QALYs. Knowledge of outcome in terms of QALYs may potentially be used to assess the efficacy of treatment in the ICU.[13] Quality-adjusted survival integrates two of the most basic and important patient-valued and society-valued objectives: to prolong life and to preserve or enhance QoL. Viewed from this perspective, therapies that selectively improve the QoL of survivors could be as valuable as therapies that decrease mortality.[17]

Methods and description of measurement instruments used in critically ill patients

HRQoL measures in critically ill patients can be made longitudinally or cross-sectionally, with a focus on specific dimensions of health or disease, on economic utility, or on general health domains.[18] Evaluative instruments are suitable for assessing longitudinal changes in HRQoL within patients. A good measure is valid and reliable—it will measure what it aims to measure; the measure is consistent; it minimizes random errors, and the scale reflects the changes in its domains.[4] Instruments to measure HRQoL in critically ill patients can be divided in three groups: generic, disease-specific, and domain-specific questionnaires.[19] Generic instruments measure HRQoL relevant for each human being, independent of the clinical diagnosis. These instruments contain the physical, psychological, and social domains and can be used in patients with different diagnoses, disease stages, and treatments. This facilitates the comparison between clinical groups or with the general population. Domain-specific instruments measure the consequences of one part of health. These questionnaires are mostly used as a complement to the generic and disease-specific instruments. In 2002, a round-table conference recommended the Short-form 36 (SF-36) and EuroQol -5D (EQ-5D) as the most appropriate instruments for future research in intensive care (see Table 7.1).[20–22] Indeed, these two measures are the most commonly used instruments in the critically ill.

What makes a good HRQoL instrument in critically ill patients?

Several instruments measuring HRQoL have been used in ICU populations, both during and after ICU stay. The more global or generic instruments can be used but may be less responsive to changes in specific conditions.[8] As ICU patients have different admission diagnoses, there is a need for generic outcome measures that can be used across medical and surgical critically ill patients, as well as condition-specific ones.[4] An ideal generic instrument in ICU patients

Table 7.1 Generic instruments most commonly used to evaluate HRQoL in critically ill patients

Questionnaire	Purpose	Description	Concepts measured	Limitations/strengths
Short-form 36 (SF-36)	To measure general health status	36 items, grouped into eight scales and physical and mental component scores	Physical: physical functioning, role limitations, pain, and general health Mental: vitality, social, role limitations, and mental health transition	Well validated in critically ill patients and with population norms
EuroQol-5D (EQ-5D)	To assess state of health and preferences for 14 hypothetical health states	Five items assessed at three levels	Mobility, personal care, usual activities, pain/discomfort, and anxiety/depression	In critically ill patients less validated, may provide less information, and may be less discriminative than the SF-36
Nottingham Health Profile (NHP)	To measure general health status	Two-part questionnaire	First part: 38 statements related to six domains: physical mobility, pain, sleep, energy, emotional reactions, social isolation Second part: seven activities of daily life—occupation, housework, social activity, home life, sex life, hobbies, and holidays	Has been used in critically ill patients, especially in cardiac surgery patients. Internal consistency and sensitivity to change were better for the SF-36 than for the NHP

should be easy to administer, not present too great a burden for the patient, and yet be sensitive to modest changes in QoL.[23] It was recently recommended that either the EQ-5D or SF-36 should be used in critical care outcomes studies on the grounds that they are best suited to this setting.[20] The SF-36 is currently one of the most widely used generic questionnaire in critical care and may be appropriate for critical care patients.[23–26] The SF-36 is a questionnaire with 36 questions which comprise eight dimensions: physical functioning, social functioning, role limitation due to physical problems, role limitations due to emotional problems, general mental health, energy/vitality, bodily pain, and general health perceptions. The physical health summary scale (PCS) reflects physical functioning, physical role, pain, and general health. The mental health summary scale (MCS) reflects vitality, social functioning, emotional role, and mental health.[27] The shortened version of the SF-36 the SF-12 gives only the PCS and MCS, not the individual domains.[28] The shorter SF-12 improves efficiency in critically ill patients and lower costs. However, the SF-12 yields less precise scores, compared with the SF-36. Another generic questionnaire, designed to measure health outcomes and which is used in critically ill patients, was developed at European level: the EQ-5D.[29] The EQ-5D is a simple instrument, comprising two parts: the EQ-5D self-classifier, a self-reported description of health problems, according to a five dimensional classification, i.e. mobility, self-care, usual activities, pain/discomfort, and anxiety/depression; and the EQ-VAS, a self-rated health status, using a visual analogue scale (VAS) to record perceptions of the participant's own current overall health.[30] The EQ-5D requires significant less time to complete, compared with the SF-36. The SF-36 covers many more domains and is more precise. It seems important to make a choice, depending on the research questions and definition of the concept to be measured, on which instrument (HRQoL) or combination of instruments (HRQoL and disease-specific) or if a special instrument covering the specific problems of critically ill patients and HRQoL may be needed.

How to score HRQoL before ICU admission?

To assess the effects of critical illness and ICU treatment on HRQoL, measurements should be performed on admission to the ICU. However, this is rarely possible, as the patient's condition on admission usually limits the filling out of a questionnaire. Nevertheless, assessment of the HRQoL on admission provides valuable information that could support the intensivist in decisions on admission and treatment policies. As most of the patients cannot fill out questionnaires at the time of admission, proxies must frequently be used. However, can proxies provide useful information on HRQoL in critically ill patients? The literature concerning agreement between HRQoL assessment by patients and their relatives before ICU admission is not very conclusive. Some studies in critically ill patients reported moderate or good agreement between individual patients and their proxies, although lower levels of agreement may be reported for psychological or physical functioning.[31,32] Other groups have raised concerns of proxy estimations of HRQoL in populations with high disease severity.[33] Gifford et al. revealed in ALI patients, i.e. before hospital discharge, that proxy assessment had only fair to moderate agreement with patient assessment.[34]

However, when proxies are used to assess the patient's QoL, a significant and clinically relevant correlation is found between the patient's QoL and the assessment made by the proxy. In studies performed by our group, we found that proxies adequately reflect the patients' QoL on admission to the intensive care when the SF-36 questionnaire or the Academic Medical Center Linear Disability Score (ALDS) were used.[35,36] Rogers et al.[32] and Crispin et al.[23] showed that the use of proxies and the SF-36 reliably assessed the patient's QoL at time of discharge from the ICU. Also in specific subgroups, proxies using the SF-36 have been found to adequately reflect the patient's QoL.[24] However, in specific dimensions, especially in the area of mental well-being (role limitation due to emotional problems), agreement between patients and proxy is moderate. Others have reported similar results.[31,32,37–39] Relatives are more appropriate in their assessment of the physical characteristics than of psychological characteristics of the intensive care patient.[35]

Assessing the impact of critical illness on HRQoL in ICU patients

Patients recovering from critical illness may show persisting organ dysfunction that could impair functional status with an associated reduced HRQoL. Several reviews have investigated HRQoL in general ICU patients, sepsis patients, or patients with ARDS and reported that survivors have worse HRQoL, compared with matched general populations, at pre-admission[40,41] and follow-up.[40–43] Assessment of HRQoL in critically ill patients is complex and is usually only measured after ICU discharge. Several factors underscore the assessment of the patient's QoL. First, ICU patients with a low QoL on admission have higher hospital mortality and a worsened QoL following hospital discharge.[44–46] Cuthbertson et al.[47] showed that the pre-ICU admission PCS (physical component score) was significantly lower in non-survivors when compared to survivors. Wehler et al.,[48] using the SF-36 questionnaire, found that patients developing MOF had lower physical health scores on admission than non-MOF patients. At follow–up, MOF patients had lower scores in most areas of physical health than non-MOF patients, whereas domains of mental health did not differ between the two groups. These data underscore the importance of physical health, as assessed by QoL instruments, in surviving critical illness. Therefore, the benefit of ICU admission in patients with limited QoL could be limited. Second, knowledge of the QoL to be expected at discharge can be important for relatives, physicians, and nurses to value the appropriateness of additional interventions and/ or further treatment. Like other studies,[47,49] our group also found that HRQoL, at the time of discharge from the hospital, was impaired and that a gradual improvement occurred during follow-up, in some cases to pre-admission hospital levels, and have shown especially that a major part of recovery was already accomplished on discharge from the hospital.[50,51] In addition, a response shift, defined as the change in internal standards, values, or conceptualization of HRQoL,[52] may have caused an improvement in HRQoL during hospital admission. This could be because either the patients became accustomed to their illness or their expectations about their HRQoL had changed. Further studies would be needed to explore these mechanisms. Several investigators reported decreased pre-ICU admission HRQoL in surviving patients.[1,26,48,50] However, Cuthbertson et al.[47] showed that only pre-ICU admission physical scores were below values for the healthy population, whereas the mental scores were similar. Differences in inclusion criteria, case-mix, pre-ICU admission health status, comorbidity, social characteristics, individual coping capacity in patients from various geographical areas, and the assessment of pre-ICU admission HRQoL (prospectively vs retrospectively) may explain these differences.[53,54] Graf et al. used the SF-36 in medical ICU patients staying for >24 hours and found that physical and role emotional scores had deteriorated 1 month after ICU discharge but returned to baseline 9 months thereafter. In addition, they showed that the mental summary scale did not change during the investigational period.[1] Wehler et al. investigated patients with multiple organ dysfunction syndrome (MODS) and found that 83–90% of the survivors had regained HRQoL at 6 months after ICU discharge, although persistent deterioration was especially noted in the physical health domains.[48,55] Herridge et al. found that patients with ARDS have persistent functional limitation 1 year after being discharged from the ICU.[55] Others also have reported significant decreased HRQoL at follow-up.[56] Recently, in patients with COPD 6 years after ICU admission, Rivera-Fernandez found that survivors had a worse HRQoL, compared with pre-ICU admission.[57] In contrast, others reported the full recovery of all health dimensions to pre-ICU admission levels 9 months following ICU discharge; at 6 months after treatment, 73% of the patients considered their HRQoL to be the same as, or better than, it had been in the stable period before they were admitted.[58] However, in another recent study, 1 year after ICU discharge, patients had great limitations in physically related activities.[59] Orwelius et al. reported in their study that pre-existing disease was the most important factor for long-term HRQoL after critical illness.[1,60] Recently, Stricker et al reported that, 9 years after an ICU stay, the QoL may deteriorate for some individuals; however, overall QoL for most survivors remains acceptable and may even improve[61] (see Table 7.2; panels A, B, C).

Table 7.2 Panel A studies included in the paragraph: assessing the impact of critical illness on HRQoL in ICU patients

Studies	n	Follow-up time	Key findings
Goldstein et al. (1986)[44]	2213	Before and 1 year after ICU	Most survivors regained their pre-admission functional status, with 60% of the previously employed returning to work. However, even for hospital survivors, mortality was high and was related to prior functional status: active 7%, sedentary 20%, severely impaired 37%.
Yinnon et al. (1989)[46]	126	12 months after ICU	HRQoL in patients who survived longer than 6 months after ICU care was high and unimpaired when compared with their ratings before admission to the ICU. These findings indicate that HRQoL before admission is an important predictor of survival and that a high proportion of critically ill subjects whose HRQoL was relatively good before the episode requiring admission will be long-term survivors whose HRQoL is comparable to that preceding critical care.
Vasquez et al. (1992)[45]	606	Before and 12 months after ICU	12 months after ICU discharge, a patient's functional status, as measured by the HRQoL score, is influenced mostly by age and their HRQoL score at the time of ICU admission. While there is an overall decrease in the HRQoL score for survivors, admission and treatment in an ICU do not always result in deterioration of the HRQoL score.
Hurel et al. (1997)[54]	229	6 months after ICU discharge	HRQoL was fair at 6 months. There was a severe reduction in energy, sleep, and emotional reactions, whereas social isolation, pain, and physical handicap were infrequent. HRQoL was mainly a function of the diagnosis and severity of illness.
Ridley et al. (1997)[26]	166	Before and discharge from ICU	Patients who had suffered acute pathologies reported significant decreases in HRQoL, whilst other patients with pre-existing ill health reported significant improvement, with reduced pain and better mental health, vitality, and social function. This study suggests that HRQoL of most patients admitted to the ICU is not as good as in the normal population but does not deteriorate, except for those patients admitted after acute life-threatening events.
Flaatten et al. (2001)[56]	106	12 years after ICU	Two years after discharge, the survival of former ICU patients was significant less, compared with the normal population. HRQoL of the patients was significantly less 12 years after ICU, compared with the normal population.
Wehler et al. (2001)[49]	185	Before and 6 months after ICU	Six months after ICU, most survivors regained their pre-admission HRQoL. Pre-admission HRQoL, age, and severity of illness were most strongly associated with follow-up HRQoL.

Table 7.2 (continued) Panel B studies included in the paragraph: assessing the impact of critical illness on HRQoL in ICU patients

Studies	n	Follow-up time	Key findings
Wehler et al. (2003)[48]	318	Before and 6 months after ICU	MOF patients had a worse HRQoL than normal population. At 6 months after ICU, 83–90% had regained their previous HRQoL. MOF was the major determinant of poor physical health at follow-up but had no impact on mental health domains.
Graf et al. (2003)[1]	245	Before, 1 month, and 9 months after ICU	Physical and emotional role deteriorated after 1 month but returned to baseline thereafter. Notably, the mental health summary scale did not change during the course of the study, whereas the physical health summary scale consistently improved over time. Patients older than the median of 66 yers rated their physical functioning lower.
Herridge et al. (2003)[55]	109	At 3, 6, 12 months after ICU discharge	Three to 12 months after ICU discharge, HRQoL improved, especially physical role and physical functioning. At 12 months after ICU discharge, HRQoL was lower, except emotional role, compared with a normal population.
Cuthbertson et al. (2005)[47]	300	Before and 3, 6, 12 months after ICU	Mean physical score were below the population norm at all time points, but the mean mental scores were similar or higher than these population norms. Survivors showed a slow increase in physical HRQoL to premorbid levels at 12 months.
Orwelius et al. (2005)[60]	562	6 months after hospital discharge	Six months after discharge, HRQoL was significantly lower among patients than in the reference group. When comparisons were restricted to the previously healthy people in both groups, the observed differences were about halved, and, when the investigators compared the patients in the ICU who had pre-existing diseases with subjects in the reference group who had similar diseases, they found little difference in perceived HRQoL.
Capuzzo et al. (2006)[53]	618	At 90 days after admission ICU	Patients reported their general level of health to be better (33.8%), the same (31.1%), or worse (35.1%) in comparison with baseline. More than 60% of ICU patients report good recovery of their health 90 days after ICU admission, depending on their illness and circumstances of ICU admission.
Rivera-Fernandez et al. (2006)[57]	379	6 years after ICU	The 6-year mortality of patients with COPD requiring ICU admission was high. Mortality was mainly influenced by pre-ICU admission HRQoL. At 6 years, at least 15% were alive; survivors had a worse HRQoL, compared with pre-ICU admission, although three-quarters of them were self-sufficient.

Table 7.2 (continued) Panel C studies included in the paragraph: assessing the impact of critical illness on HRQoL in ICU patients

Studies	n	Follow-up time	Key findings
Hofhuis et al. (2008)[50]	451	Before, ICU discharge, hospital discharge, 3 and 6 months after ICU	Pre-ICU admission HRQoL in survivors was significantly worse, compared to the healthy population. HRQoL decreased in all dimensions during ICU stay, followed by a rapid improvement during hospital stay, gradually improving to near pre-ICU admission HRQoL at 6 months following ICU discharge. Physical functioning, general health, and social functioning remained significantly lower than pre-ICU admission values. Compared to the healthy Dutch population, ICU survivors had significantly lower HRQoL 6 months following ICU discharge.
Wildman et al. (2009)[58]	832	At 180 days after ICU	Of the respondents, 73% considered their HRQoL to be the same as, or better than, it had been in the stable period before they were admitted, and 96% would choose similar treatment again. Function during the stable pre-admission period was a reasonable indicator of function reported by those who survived 180 days.
van der Schaaf et al. (2009)[59]	255	1 year after ICU	54% of the patients had restrictions in daily functioning. Walking and social activities were most frequently restricted (30–60% of the patients). HRQoL was lower than the general Dutch population.
Stricker et al. (2011)[61]	334	9 years after ICU	Mortality was high 9 years after ICU stay. HRQoL may deteriorate for some individuals; however, overall HRQoL for most survivors remains acceptable and may even improve. Long-term outcome predictions made by caregivers during the ICU stay seem accurate.

Impact of critical illness on HRQoL in octogenerians

There is an increasing elderly population in the Western world. Therefore, the proportion of elderly patients admitted to the ICU will continue to increase as well. Consequently, the question of whether ICU admission is considered appropriate for octogenarians, with respect to the expected balance between burden of disease and life expectancy, becomes increasingly relevant for intensivists.[62] However, Bloumendil et al. concluded that it is impossible to define evidence-based recommendations for ICU admission in the elderly and recommended further studies that encompass HRQoL.[63] Beyond mortality, HRQoL is important to elderly patients and to the professionals taking care of them. One could also argue that the treatment of older patients is not always beneficial for the patients in terms of disease burden in relation to final outcome,[45] although several studies have reported good long-term HRQoL in the elderly.[64–69] Nevertheless, data reporting changes in HRQoL during hospital stay after ICU admission as a reflection of the burden of disease are lacking.[70,71] Moreover, it is unknown whether or not age has a strong impact on HRQoL in patients above 80 years. The decision to admit elderly patients, especially octogenarians, to the ICU is influenced by their clinical conditions[72] and evaluations of the benefit of admission to the ICU.[73]

In a single-centre study, Garrouste-Orgeas et al. showed that more than two-thirds of patients aged over 80 years were denied ICU admission.[62] Hence, when do-not-resuscitate orders are written for patients, they were written more quickly for older patients, regardless of prognosis, especially for those over the age of 75.[74] It is intriguing to evaluate the data supporting this approach. Recent studies have revealed that acute psychological impairment and diagnosis have much larger relative effects on prognosis than age per se.[75] Hospital mortality rates of patients aged ≥80 years are predominantly related to underlying disease, severity of illness, nosocomial infection, evolving organ dysfunction, and quality of care after discharge from the ICU.[76] The burden of disease should balance the benefits in the long term. Boumendil and colleagues[63] performed a review on the opportunity to admit elderly patients to the ICU and found that the majority of studies showed that older patients perceived their HRQoL not different from those of younger age,[65,69] and that it increases over time[65] despite a decrease in ADL.[67] The majority of the patients reported that their HRQoL remained unchanged or improved.[77] Compared with the general population, they reported worse HRQoL regarding isolation, emotional health, mobility, or physical function.[78] Their ADL status after hospitalization was unchanged, compared to baseline.[64,65] Only a small number of articles specifically addresses HRQoL in critically ill octogenarians. The observed decrease in HRQoL during critical illness, with gradual improvement thereafter, concurs with previous findings in critically ill patients.[1,50,51] Hennessy and colleagues performed a review of the literature on post-ICU outcomes of elderly patients.[79] Several studies showed improved or unchanged HRQoL and/or functional status. The majority of these studies reported good HRQoL and functional status post-ICU, although a change in conceptualization of HRQoL after critical illness was suggested.[79] Ridley and Wallace assessed HRQoL before and after ICU admission in older patients. However, they used a non-validated questionnaire and a retrospective baseline status assessment,[68] which makes this study difficult to compare to other studies. Eddleston and colleagues found that patients older than 65 years of age reported higher social functioning and emotional role limitation dimensions than younger patients.[80] Comparisons between different categories of elderly patients yielded similar results. Chelleri et al. compared patients aged 65–74 and aged ≥75 and found no differences in ADL, perceived HRQoL, or depression between the two elderly age groups.[64] In contrast, some studies showed worsened HRQoL and/or functional status.[45,67,69] Montuclard et al. showed in patients with ICU length of stay >30 days that independence in ADL had decreased significantly after admission to the ICU. However, only patients with an ICU length of stay >30 days were included in this study, limiting the interpretation of the results.[67] Linko et al. reported that, despite lower HRQoL compared to references values, the cost per hospital survivor and lifetime cost utility remained reasonable, regardless of age, disease severity, and type or duration of ventilation support.[81] Additionally, in a recent study of our group, we demonstrated in a prospective study that, after ICU admission, HRQoL of surviving octogenarians demonstrated a good recovery at 6 months after ICU discharge. Furthermore, we found that HRQoL in octogenerians was not significantly lower before ICU admission when compared to the matched general Dutch population. Patients discharged from the ICU showed a steady recovery to baseline values.[82]

Response shift in critically ill patients

Patients accommodate to their illness. An important mechanism in this adaptation process is called 'response shift' which involves internal standards, values, and the conceptualization of HRQoL. Response shift is the change in internal standards of values and of conceptualization and consequently in the perception of HRQoL.[52] This could be either because patients become accustomed to their illness or chronic disease or because their expectations about their HRQoL have changed. Cohen stated that coping was a crucial factor for QoL;[83] also patients' coping ability was found significantly positively correlated with QoL.[84] Recent research documents the presence and importance of response shifts in both treatment outcome research and longitudinal observations of HRQoL. Several studies suggest that patients make significant response shifts during treatments, i.e. in patients with cancer,[85,86] multiple sclerosis,[87] or pancreas-kidney transplants.[88] To our knowledge, no studies are performed to investigate response shift in critically ill patients. The question is whether we can measure response shift in critically ill patients. Response shift is not only important in longitudinal observations of HRQoL, but also in medical decision making. Lenert et al. used preference assessment methods common in cost effectiveness analysis to investigate interactions between preferences and health status. They found that patients in poor health status valued intermediate health status almost as much as near-normal states. Conversely, patients in good health valued intermediate states nearly as little as poor health states. Patients in poor physical and mental health tended to recalibrate their standards for comparing health states in a manner that downplayed current personal problems, and small gains were more valuable to disabled than to healthy persons.[89] To measure response shift, some investigators used the then-test. The then-test is a method that aims to measure change in reference values by comparison of a retrospective baseline measurement with a conventional baseline measurement.[86] In the then-test, which is conducted at follow-up, patients are asked to provide a renewed judgement about their HRQoL at the time of the conventional baseline measurement. If the then-test is completed with a concurrent follow-up measurement, it is assumed that the same reference value is used for both assessments. Comparing the then-test with a follow-up measurement has been proposed as a method to assess change in HRQoL over time, which is not confounded by change in reference values.[86] In conclusion, response shift is a phenomenon which is important and likely to be present but has rarely been investigated in critically ill patients.

HRQoL as a prognostic factor

It is difficult for doctors to predict whether a critically ill patient will survive intensive care treatment. Mortality in patients admitted to intensive care remains high.[90] An increasing number of in-hospital patients die in the ICU.[91] Consequently, ICU doctors must rely upon their clinical experience in their decision making. The predictive value of clinical experience in this regard is also limited.[92] Mortality is difficult to predict for an individual patient, because many factors determine survival from critical illness such as age, sex, acute physiological deterioration, and underlying illnesses. Several scoring systems aimed at predicting mortality have been developed that incorporate these factors. The APACHE II and III scores,[93,94] the Mortality Probability Model,[95] and the Simplified Acute Physiology score (SAPS)[96] are established examples. However, these scoring systems are only available after 24 hours of ICU admission, and they are highly specific (able to predict survival (specificity 90%)) but not very sensitive (less accurate in predicting death (sensitivity 50 to 70%)).[92] The advantages of using pre-admission HRQoL as a predictor of mortality are that it is easily obtained and available as soon as the patient, or a proxy (close family member) in the case of incapacity, can be questioned.

Can HRQoL be used as an indicator of final outcome? Several studies have addressed this question in dialysis patients,[97–99] coronary artery bypass graft surgery patients,[100] patients with CHF,[101] and those with advanced colorectal cancer.[102] Welsh and co-workers[103] found that baseline patient functional status, as assessed by care providers, is correlated with mortality after ICU admission. However, that study is hampered by several drawbacks. Although the investigators also focused on patients with an expected ICU stay longer than 48 hours, they included only 9% of all ICU patients, which may indicate at least some form of selection bias. In addition, it may be questionable to correlate HRQoL scores directly with APACHE II scores without making any attempt to correct for confounding by multivariate analysis. Also, hospital deaths were not included in their analysis, which makes it difficult to understand the relation between HRQoL before ICU admission and mortality during or after critical illness. More recently, Iribarren-Diarasarri et al. found that a patient's health status prior to ICU admission can be used as a prognostic factor to assess an individual's mid- to long-term prognosis and demonstrated a twofold higher risk for in-hospital and 1-year mortality.[104] A study of our group shows that pre-admission HRQoL, measured with either the one-item general health question or the complete SF-36, is as good at predicting survival/mortality in ICU patients as the APACHE II score.[105] Rivera-Fernandez and co-workers[106] demonstrated in a multicentre study that HRQoL before ICU admission is related to ICU mortality but that it contributes little to the discriminatory ability of the APACHE III prediction model and has little influence on ICU resource utilization, as indicated by length of stay in the ICU or therapeutic interventions. However, the number of surgical patients was only 24%, which is much lower than in a general ICU. In addition, the APACHE III score was used and related to a self-developed HRQoL questionnaire. Despite the differences that exist between these previous reports and our study,[105] their findings are generally in accordance with ours and indicate that estimation of HRQoL before ICU admission deserves more attention by those caring for critically ill patients.

Recommendations

Future studies should address the gaps which remain in our understanding of HRQoL. We suggest that studies should investigate the balance between feasibility of the HRQoL questionnaire and the complete coverage of all individually relevant variables. In addition, questionnaires regarding long-term HRQoL in critically ill patients in general do not take into account a region-religious background or are disease-specific, combined with several non-standardized generic variables. Therefore, follow-up studies should be done to develop and use a modified HRQoL questionnaire, including these variables. Our further recommendation would be to generate a standardized database which can be used for multicentre comparisons regarding knowledge and understanding of HRQoL in critically ill patients.

Conclusion

The demand for intensive care is on the rise and is expected to grow dramatically in the future. This increase is partly caused by a growing proportion of elderly admitted to hospitals, not only in the US, but in most developed countries. Recent advances in ICU medicine have resulted in a remarkable increase in the chance of survival for the critically ill patient admitted to an ICU. As a result, the traditional goal for ICU doctors and nurses to achieve a reduction in short-term mortality has been challenged. Assessment of HRQoL can improve the answers given by intensivists and nurses to questions raised by patients and relatives about future prospects. To get insight in issues related to the impact of ICU treatment on HRQoL, we should incorporate not only short-term outcomes, e.g. length of stay and mortality, but also long-term outcomes, measured using HRQoL for physical and psychological factors, functional status, and social interactions. A follow-up clinic evaluating ICU patients after hospital discharge may improve the speed and quality of recovery from critical illness.

References

1 Graf J, Koch M, Dujardin R, Kersten A, Janssens U. Health-related quality of life before, 1 month after, and 9 months after intensive care in medical cardiovascular and pulmonary patients. *Crit Care Med* 2003;**31**:2163–9.

2 Wu A, Gao F. Long-term outcomes in survivors from critical illness. *Anaesthesia* 2004;**59**:1049–52.

3 Gill TM, Feinstein AR. A critical appraisal of the quality of quality-of-life measurements. *JAMA* 1994;**272**:619–26.

4 Black NA, Jenkinson C, Hayes JA, et al. Review of outcome measures used in adult critical care. *Crit Care Med* 2001;**29**:2119–24.

5 Guyatt GH, Feeny DH, Patrick DL. Measuring health-related quality of life. *Ann Intern Med* 1993;**118**:622–9.

6 Cullen DJ. Results and costs of intensive care. *Anesthesiology* 1977;**47**:203–16.

7 Cullen DJ, Keene R, Waternaux C, Kunsman JM, Caldera DL, Peterson H. Results, charges, and benefits of intensive care for critically ill patients: update 1983. *Crit Care Med* 1984;**12**:102–6.

8 Heyland DK, Kutsogiannis DJ. Quality of life following critical care: moving beyond survival. *Intensive Care Med* 2000;**26**:1172–5.

9 Patrick DL, Bergner M. Measurement of health status in the 1990s. *Annu Rev Public Health* 1990;**11**:165–83.

10 Tian ZM, Miranda DR. Quality of life after intensive care with the sickness impact profile. *Intensive Care Med* 1995;**21**:422–8.

11 World Health Organization. *The first ten years of the World Health Organization*. Geneva: World Health Organization; 1958.

12 Weil MH, Weil CJ, Rackow EC. Guide to ethical decision-making for the critically ill: the three R's and Q.C. *Crit Care Med* 1988;**16**:636–41.

13 Kerridge RK, Glasziou PP, Hillman KM. The use of 'quality–adjusted life years' (QALYs) to evaluate treatment in intensive care. *Anaesth Intensive Care* 1995;**23**:322–31.

14 Brooks R. EuroQol: the current state of play. *Health Policy* 1996;**37**:53–72.

15 Feeny D, Furlong W, Boyle M, Torrance GW. Multi-attribute health status classification systems. Health Utilities Index. *Pharmacoeconomics* 1995;**7**:490–502.

16 Ware JE, Jr, Sherbourne CD. The MOS 36-item short-form health survey (SF-36). I. Conceptual framework and item selection. *Med Care* 1992;**30**:473–83.

17 Angus DC, Musthafa AA, Clermont G, et al. Quality-adjusted survival in the first year after the acute respiratory distress syndrome. *Am J Respir Crit Care Med* 2001;**163**:1389–94.

18 Garratt A, Schmidt L, Mackintosh A, Fitzpatrick R. Quality of life measurement: bibliographic study of patient assessed health outcome measures. *BMJ* 2002;**324**:1417.

19 Higginson IJ, Carr AJ. Measuring quality of life: using quality of life measures in the clinical setting. *BMJ* 2001;**322**:1297–300.

20 Angus DC, Carlet J. Surviving intensive care: a report from the 2002 Brussels Roundtable. *Intensive Care Med* 2003;**29**:368–77.

21 Ware JE. *Health survey manual and interpretation guide*. Boston: Medical Outcomes Trust; 1993.

22 Brazier J, Jones N, Kind P. Testing the validity of the Euroqol and comparing it with the SF-36 health survey questionnaire. *Qual Life Res* 1993;**2**:169–80.

23 Chrispin PS, Scotton H, Rogers J, Lloyd D, Ridley SA. Short Form 36 in the intensive care unit: assessment of acceptability, reliability and validity of the questionnaire. *Anaesthesia* 1997;**52**:15–23.

24 Heyland DK, Hopman W, Coo H, Tranmer J, McColl MA. Long-term health-related quality of life in survivors of sepsis. Short Form 36: a valid and reliable measure of health-related quality of life. *Crit Care Med* 2000;**28**:3599–605.

25 Khoudri I, Ali ZA, Abidi K, Madani N, Abouqal R. Measurement properties of the short form 36 and health-related quality of life after intensive care in Morocco. *Acta Anaesthesiol Scand* 2007;**51**:189–97.

26 Ridley SA, Chrispin PS, Scotton H, Rogers J, Lloyd D. Changes in quality of life after intensive care: comparison with normal data. *Anaesthesia* 1997;**52**:195–202.

27 Ware JE, Jr, Kosinski M, Bayliss MS, McHorney CA, Rogers WH, Raczek A. Comparison of methods for the scoring and statistical analysis of SF-36 health profile and summary measures: summary of results from the Medical Outcomes Study. *Med Care* 1995;33(4 Suppl):AS264–79.

28 Ware J Jr, Kosinski M, Keller SD. A 12-Item Short-Form Health Survey: construction of scales and preliminary tests of reliability and validity. *Med Care* 1996;**34**:220–33.

29 The EuroQol Group. EuroQol—a new facility for the measurement of health-related quality of life. *Health Policy* 1990;**16**:199–208.

30 Brooks R, Rabin RE, de Charro FT. *The measurement and validation of health status using EQ-5D: a European perspective.* Dordrecht: Kluwers Academic Publishers; 2003.

31 Capuzzo M, Grasselli C, Carrer S, Gritti G, Alvisi R. Quality of life before intensive care admission: agreement between patient and relative assessment. *Intensive Care Med* 2000;**26**:1288–95.

32 Rogers J, Ridley S, Chrispin P, Scotton H, Lloyd D. Reliability of the next of kins' estimates of critically ill patients' quality of life. *Anaesthesia* 1997;**52**:1137–43.

33 Scales DC, Tansey CM, Matte A, Herridge MS. Difference in reported pre-morbid health-related quality of life between ARDS survivors and their substitute decision makers. *Intensive Care Med* 2006;**32**:1826–31.

34 Gifford JM, Husain N, Dinglas VD, Colantuoni E, Needham DM. Baseline quality of life before intensive care: a comparison of patient versus proxy responses. *Crit Care Med* 2010;**38**:855–60.

35 Hofhuis J, Hautvast JL, Schrijvers AJ, Bakker J. Quality of life on admission to the intensive care: can we query the relatives? *Intensive Care Med* 2003;**29**:974–9.

36 Hofhuis JG, Dijkgraaf MG, Hovingh A, et al. The Academic Medical Center Linear Disability Score for evaluation of physical reserve on admission to the ICU: can we query the relatives? *Crit Care* 2011;**15**:R212.

37 Badia X, Diaz-Prieto A, Rue M, Patrick DL. Measuring health and health state preferences among critically ill patients. *Intensive Care Med* 1996;**22**:1379–84.

38 Rothman ML, Hedrick SC, Bulcroft KA, Hickam DH, Rubenstein LZ. The validity of proxy-generated scores as measures of patient health status. *Med Care* 1991;**29**:115–24.

39 Sprangers MA, Aaronson NK. The role of health care providers and significant others in evaluating the quality of life of patients with chronic disease: a review. *J Clin Epidemiol* 1992;**45**:743–60.

40 Dowdy DW, Eid MP, Sedrakyan A, et al. Quality of life in adult survivors of critical illness: a systematic review of the literature. *Intensive Care Med* 2005;**31**:611–20.

41 Winters BD, Eberlein M, Leung J, Needham DM, Pronovost PJ, Sevransky JE. Long-term mortality and quality of life in sepsis: a systematic review. *Crit Care Med* 2010;**38**:1276–83.

42 Dowdy DW, Eid MP, Dennison CR, et al. Quality of life after acute respiratory distress syndrome: a meta-analysis. *Intensive Care Med* 2006;**32**:1115–24.

43 Oeyen SG, Vandijck DM, Benoit DD, Annemans L, Decruyenaere JM. Quality of life after intensive care: a systematic review of the literature. *Crit Care Med* 2010;**38**:2386–400.

44 Goldstein RL, Campion EW, Thibault GE, Mulley AG, Skinner E. Functional outcomes following medical intensive care. *Crit Care Med* 1986;**14**:783–8.

45 Vazquez MG, Rivera FR, Gonzalez CA, et al. Factors related to quality of life 12 months after discharge from an intensive care unit. *Crit Care Med* 1992;**20**:1257–62.

46 Yinnon A, Zimran A, Hershko C. Quality of life and survival following intensive medical care. *Q J Med* 1989;**71**:347–57.

47 Cuthbertson BH, Scott J, Strachan M, Kilonzo M, Vale L. Quality of life before and after intensive care. *Anaesthesia* 2005;**60**:332–9.

48 Wehler M, Geise A, Hadzionerovic D, et al. Health-related quality of life of patients with multiple organ dysfunction: individual changes and comparison with normative population. *Crit Care Med* 2003;**31**:1094–101.

49 Wehler M, Martus P, Geise A, et al. Changes in quality of life after medical intensive care. *Intensive Care Med* 2001;**27**:154–9.

50 Hofhuis JG, Spronk PE, van Stel HF, Schrijvers GJ, Rommes JH, Bakker J. The impact of critical illness on perceived health-related quality of life during ICU treatment, hospital stay, and after hospital discharge: a long-term follow-up study. *Chest* 2008;**133**:377–85.

51 Hofhuis JG, Spronk PE, van Stel HF, Schrijvers AJ, Rommes JH, Bakker J. The impact of severe sepsis on health-related quality of life: a long-term follow-up study. *Anesth Analg* 2008;**107**: 1957–64.

52 Sprangers MA, Schwartz CE. Integrating response shift into health-related quality of life research: a theoretical model. *Soc Sci Med* 1999;**48**:1507–15.

53 Capuzzo M, Moreno RP, Jordan B, Bauer P, Alvisi R, Metnitz PG. Predictors of early recovery of health status after intensive care. *Intensive Care Med* 2006;**32**:1832–8.

54 Hurel D, Loirat P, Saulnier F, Nicolas F, Brivet F. Quality of life 6 months after intensive care: results of a prospective multicenter study using a generic health status scale and a satisfaction scale. *Intensive Care Med* 1997;**23**:331–7.

55 Herridge MS, Cheung AM, Tansey CM, et al. One-year outcomes in survivors of the acute respiratory distress syndrome. *N Engl J Med* 2003;**348**:683–93.

56 Flaatten H, Kvale R. Survival and quality of life 12 years after ICU. A comparison with the general Norwegian population. *Intensive Care Med* 2001;**27**:1005–11.

57 Rivera-Fernandez R, Navarrete-Navarro P, Fernandez-Mondejar E, Rodriguez-Elvira M, Guerrero-Lopez F, Vazquez-Mata G. Six-year mortality and quality of life in critically ill patients with chronic obstructive pulmonary disease. *Crit Care Med* 2006;**34**:2317–24.

58 Wildman MJ, Sanderson CF, Groves J, et al. Survival and quality of life for patients with COPD or asthma admitted to intensive care in a UK multicentre cohort: the COPD and Asthma Outcome Study (CAOS). *Thorax* 2009;**64**:128–32.

59 van der Schaff M, Beelen A, Dongelmans DA, Vroom MB, Nollet F. Functional status after intensive care: a challenge for rehabilitation professionals to improve outcome. *J Rehabil Med* 2009;**41**: 360–6.

60 Orwelius L, Nordlund A, Edell-Gustafsson U, et al. Role of preexisting disease in patients' perceptions of health-related quality of life after intensive care. *Crit Care Med* 2005;**33**:1557–64.

61 Stricker KH, Sailer S, Uehlinger DE, Rothen HU, Zuercher Zenklusen RM, Frick S. Quality of life 9 years after an intensive care unit stay: a long-term outcome study. *J Crit Care* 2011;**26**:379–87.

62 Garrouste-Org M, Timsit JF, Montuclard L, et al. Decision-making process, outcome, and 1-year quality of life of octogenarians referred for intensive care unit admission. *Intensive Care Med* 2006;**32**:1045–51.

63 Boumendil A, Somme D, Garrouste-Org M, Guidet B. Should elderly patients be admitted to the intensive care unit? *Intensive Care Med* 2007;**33**:1252–62.

64 Chelluri L, Pinsky MR, Grenvik AN. Outcome of intensive care of the 'oldest–old' critically ill patients. *Crit Care Med* 1992;**20**:757–61.

65 Chelluri L, Pinsky MR, Donahoe MP, Grenvik A. Long-term outcome of critically ill elderly patients requiring intensive care. *JAMA* 1993;**269**:3119–23.

66 Konopad E, Noseworthy TW, Johnston R, Shustack A, Grace M. Quality of life measures before and one year after admission to an intensive care unit. *Crit Care Med* 1995;**23**:1653–9.

67 Montuclard L, Garrouste-Org M, Timsit JF, Misset B, De Jonghe B, Carlet J. Outcome, functional autonomy, and quality of life of elderly patients with a long-term intensive care unit stay. *Crit Care Med* 2000;**28**:3389–95.

68 Ridley SA, Wallace PG. Quality of life after intensive care. *Anaesthesia* 1990;**45**:808–13.

69 Udekwu P, Gurkin B, Oller D, Lapio L, Bourbina J. Quality of life and functional level in elderly patients surviving surgical intensive care. *J Am Coll Surg* 2001;**193**:245–9.

70 de Rooij SE, Abu-Hanna A, Levi M, de Jonge E. Factors that predict outcome of intensive care treatment in very elderly patients: a review. *Crit Care* 2005;**9**:R307–14.

71 Solomon MZ, O'Donnell L, Jennings B, et al. Decisions near the end of life: professional views on life-sustaining treatments. *Am J Public Health* 1993;**83**:14–23.

72 Bayer AJ, Chadha JS, Farag RR, Pathy MS. Changing presentation of myocardial infarction with increasing old age. *J Am Geriatr Soc* 1986;**34**:263–6.

73 Chelluri L, Grenvik A, Silverman M. Intensive care for critically ill elderly: mortality, costs, and quality of life. Review of the literature. *Arch Intern Med* 1995;**155**:1013–22.

74 Hakim RB, Teno JM, Harrell FE Jr, et al. Factors associated with do-not-resuscitate orders: patients' preferences, prognoses, and physicians' judgments. SUPPORT Investigators. Study to Understand Prognoses and Preferences for Outcomes and Risks of Treatment. *Ann Intern Med* 1996;**125**:284–93.

75 Hamel MB, Davis RB, Teno JM, et al. Older age, aggressiveness of care, and survival for seriously ill, hospitalized adults. SUPPORT Investigators. Study to Understand Prognoses and Preferences for Outcomes and Risks of Treatments. *Ann Intern Med* 1999;**131**:721–8.

76 Castillo-Lorente E, Rivera-Fernandez R, Vazquez-Mata G. Limitation of therapeutic activity in elderly critically ill patients. Project for the epidemiological analysis of critical care patients. *Crit Care Med* 1997;**25**:1643–8.

77 Mahul P, Perrot D, Tempelhoff G, et al. Short- and long-term prognosis, functional outcome following ICU for elderly. *Intensive Care Med* 1991;**17**:7–10.

78 Sjogren J, Thulin LI. Quality of life in the very elderly after cardiac surgery: a comparison of SF-36 between long-term survivors and an age-matched population. *Gerontology* 2004;**50**:407–10.

79 Hennessy D, Juzwishin K, Yergens D, Noseworthy T, Doig C. Outcomes of elderly survivors of intensive care: a review of the literature. *Chest* 2005;**127**:1764–74.

80 Eddleston JM, White P, Guthrie E. Survival, morbidity, and quality of life after discharge from intensive care. *Crit Care Med* 2000;**28**:2293–9.

81 Linko R, Suojaranta-Ylinen R, Karlsson S, Ruokonen E, Varpula T, Pettila V. One-year mortality, quality of life and predicted life-time cost-utility in critically ill patients with acute respiratory failure. *Crit Care* 2010;**14**:R60.

82 Hofhuis JG, van Stel HF, Schrijvers AJ, Rommes JH, Spronk PE. Changes of health-related quality of life in critically ill octogenarians: a follow-up study. *Chest* 2011;**140**:1473–83.

83 Cohen C. On the quality of life: some philosophical reflections. *Circulation* 1982;**66**(Suppl. III):29–33.

84 Fok SK, Chair SY, Lopez V. Sense of coherence, coping and quality of life following a critical illness. *J Adv Nurs* 2005;**49**:173–81.

85 Hagedoorn M, Sneeuw KC, Aaronson NK. Changes in physical functioning and quality of life in patients with cancer: response shift and relative evaluation of one's condition. *J Clin Epidemiol* 2002;**55**:176–83.

86 Sprangers MA, Van Dam FS, Broersen J, et al. Revealing response shift in longitudinal research on fatigue—the use of the thentest approach. *Acta Oncol* 1999;**38**:709–18.

87 Schwartz CE, Coulthard-Morris L, Cole B, Vollmer T. The quality-of-life effects of interferon beta-1b in multiple sclerosis. An extended Q-TWiST analysis. *Arch Neurol* 1997;**54**:1475–80.

88 Adang EM, Kootstra G, Engel GL, van Hooff JP, Merckelbach HL. Do retrospective and prospective quality of life assessments differ for pancreas-kidney transplant recipients? *Transpl Int* 1998;**11**:11–15.

89 Lenert LA, Treadwell JR, Schwartz CE. Associations between health status and utilities implications for policy. *Med Care* 1999;**37**:479–89.

90 Knaus WA, Wagner DP, Zimmerman JE, Draper EA. Variations in mortality and length of stay in intensive care units. *Ann Intern Med* 1993;**118**:753–61.

91 Angus D, Ishizaka A, Matthay M, Lemaire F, Macnee W, Abraham E. Critical care in AJRCCM 2004. *Am J Respir Crit Care Med* 2005;**171**:537–44.

92 Consensus conference organised by the ESICM and the SRLF. Predicting outcome in ICU patients. *Intensive Care Med* 1994;**20**:390–7.

93 Knaus WA, Draper EA, Wagner DP, Zimmerman JE. APACHE II: a severity of disease classification system. *Crit Care Med* 1985;**13**:818–29.

94 Knaus WA, Wagner DP, Draper EA, et al. The APACHE III prognostic system. Risk prediction of hospital mortality for critically ill hospitalized adults. *Chest* 1991;**100**:1619–36.

95 Lemeshow S, Teres D, Klar J, Avrunin JS, Gehlbach SH, Rapoport J. Mortality Probability Models (MPM II) based on an international cohort of intensive care unit patients. *JAMA* 1993;**270**:2478–86.

96 Le Gall JR, Lemeshow S, Saulnier F. A new Simplified Acute Physiology Score (SAPS II) based on a European/North American multicenter study. *JAMA* 1993;**270**:2957–63.

97 Deoreo PB. Hemodialysis patient-assessed functional health status predicts continued survival, hospitalization, and dialysis-attendance compliance. *Am J Kidney Dis* 1997;**30**:204–12.

98 Kalantar-Zadeh K, Kopple JD, Block G, Humphreys MH. Association among SF36 quality of life measures and nutrition, hospitalization, and mortality in hemodialysis. *J Am Soc Nephrol* 2001;**12**:2797–806.

99 Lowrie EG, Curtin RB, LePain N, Schatell D. Medical outcomes study short form-36: a consistent and powerful predictor of morbidity and mortality in dialysis patients. *Am J Kidney Dis* 2003;**41**:1286–92.

100 Rumsfeld JS, MaWhinney S, McCarthy M Jr, et al. Health-related quality of life as a predictor of mortality following coronary artery bypass graft surgery. Participants of the Department of Veterans Affairs Cooperative Study Group on Processes, Structures, and Outcomes of Care in Cardiac Surgery. *JAMA* 1999;**281**:1298–303.

101 Konstam V, Salem D, Pouleur H, et al. Baseline quality of life as a predictor of mortality and hospitalization in 5,025 patients with congestive heart failure. SOLVD Investigations. Studies of Left Ventricular Dysfunction Investigators. *Am J Cardiol* 1996;**78**:890–5.

102 Maisey NR, Norman A, Watson M, Allen MJ, Hill ME, Cunningham D. Baseline quality of life predicts survival in patients with advanced colorectal cancer. *Eur J Cancer* 2002;**38**:1351–7.

103 Welsh CH, Thompson K, Long-Krug S. Evaluation of patient-perceived health status using the Medical Outcomes Survey Short-Form 36 in an intensive care unit population. *Crit Care Med* 1999;**27**:1466–71.

104 Iribarren-Diarasarri S, Izpuru-Barandiaran F, Munoz-Martinez T, et al. Health-related quality of life as a prognostic factor of survival in critically ill patients. *Intensive Care Med* 2009;**35**:833–9.

105 Hofhuis JG, Spronk PE, van Stel HF, Schrijvers AJ, Bakker J. Quality of life before intensive care unit admission is a predictor of survival. *Crit Care* 2007;**11**:R78.

106 Rivera-Fernandez R, Sanchez-Cruz JJ, Abizanda-Campos R, Vazquez-Mata G. Quality of life before intensive care unit admission and its influence on resource utilization and mortality rate. *Crit Care Med* 2001;**29**:1701–9.

107 Heyland DK, Guyatt G, Cook DJ, Meade M, Juniper E, Cronin L, Gafni A. Frequency and methodologic rigor of quality-of-life assessments in the critical care literature. *Crit Care Med* 1998;**26**:591–8.

Chapter 8

Costs and Resource Utilization in Prolonged Critical Illness

Christopher E. Cox

Introduction

Critical illness is an important and unique component of the health care system, as other chapters in this book have described. A general theme can be observed that many critically ill patients will survive and eventually recover the majority of their previous functional ability. However, as any clinician knows, there are long-stay outliers in this paradigm who may have an entirely different experience with critical illness. This challenging group has been identified, using terms such as PMV, CCI, or prolonged life support.[1] A range of definitions for these conditions exists as well, varying from as few as 2 days of ventilation to as long as 21 days of ventilation.[2]

Critical care delivery demands an enormous outlay of resources, owing to its staffing, technology, and pharmacological costs. Prolonged critical illness is even more costly because of the requirements for such expensive care that extend from long hospital stays to post-acute care facilities and beyond. In this chapter, the costs and resource utilization of patients with prolonged life support will be discussed within a context of both a patient-centred and a health policy framework.

Epidemiology of prolonged critical illness

In order to better understand the economic importance of prolonged critical illness, it is useful to first consider this phenomenon in epidemiological terms.

Prolonged critical illness includes approximately 7–10% of all ventilated patients, around 250 000 patients in the US alone.[2] The incidence of critical illness has been predicted to increase substantially because of the ageing of the population.[3] Because patients who receive prolonged life support are more likely to be older, it would be expected that the number of these patients would increase likewise. One group reported, using a state discharge database, that the number of tracheotomies per 1000 state residents was highest for those aged 65–84.[4] Another group, using the National Inpatient Sample/Health Care Utilization Project dataset, incorporating a historical annual growth rate of 5.5% and expected age-based population dynamics, forecast that the number of patients who receive PMV will more than double between 2005 and 2020 to over 600 000 persons.[5] Interestingly, others have reported that the incidence of PMV has in fact been increasing out of proportion to the provision of MV overall since the mid 1990s.[6]

Outcomes of prolonged critical illness

On average, patients who receive prolonged life support experience high short- and long-term mortality, significant functional disability, and diminished QoL.[1,7,8] Few recover their former health status. Notable exceptions are trauma patients, who tend to be younger and possess fewer chronic medical comorbidities.[8,9] Patients who experience particularly poor outcomes are the elderly and those who have shock, a dialysis requirement, or low platelet counts after 2 weeks of ventilation.[9,10]

An interesting phenomenon that has been observed in this population is the fact that hospital mortality for those who receive tracheotomy for prolonged respiratory failure may in fact be similar to, or even lower than, that experienced by ventilated patients overall. Of course, the denominator, from which the prolonged ventilation mortality rate is derived, does not include the sickest ventilated patients who die early in their course. There is also a selection bias, owing to physicians' estimation that only patients likely to experience relatively good survival will be referred for tracheotomy and continued efforts at weaning.

Although hospital mortality is typically 20–35% in most cohorts—a rate many intensivists may find reasonable—long-term survival is much less likely. Across various cohorts, 1-year survival ranges from 40 to 50%.[1] A particularly concerning mortality and disability trend emerges relatively early after hospital discharge, however. First, the risk of mortality remains high and may in fact increase after discharge. Using a time-varying, piecewise-constant non-proportional survival model, one group found that the risk of death for PMV patients, compared to other ventilated patients, increased substantially at 60–100 days post-discharge.[11] Second, there is an extremely high amount of hospital readmissions that occur within the first 3 months after discharge. One study reported that 65% of all readmissions during the first year after hospital discharge occurred during this time frame.[8] Because nearly 70% of all hospital survivors who received PMV are ultimately readmitted, significant resource utilization follows. Third, relatively few patients are observed to rectify newly acquired functional dependency by 3 months. And for those who still possess moderate to high functional disability at this time, it is unlikely that future recovery to a state of full independence is likely.[8] These observations help to inform the subsequent discussion of costs and resource utilization that follows.

Costs of prolonged critical illness

In health care economic discussions, costs are often divided into 'direct costs' and 'indirect costs'. Direct costs are those generally attributable to treatments, while indirect costs are those that are associated with illness-related losses productivity or well-being (see Figure 8.1).

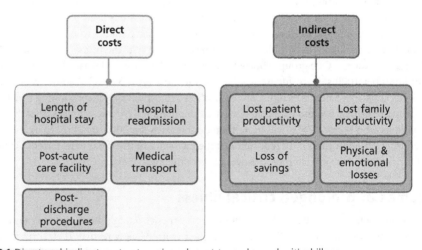

Fig. 8.1 Direct and indirect cost categories relevant to prolonged critical illness.

Acute care

Because hospital and ICU costs are closely related to length of stay,[12] the care of those with prolonged critical illness is often extremely expensive, compared to other hospitalized patients. In fact, hospital length of stay typically ranges from 30 to 50 days for these patients with ICU-level care usually comprising two-thirds of all hospital days.[1,8] As a result, average hospital costs have been reported for this group generally ranging from $100 000 to 250 000.[2,8,13,14]

Readmission to an acute care hospital after initial discharge from a similar facility is extremely common for members of this population, as described previously. In fact, the readmission rate is 50% greater than that reported for Medicare-paid hospital survivors of MV overall.[15] The primary reason for readmission is sepsis, which may require additional ICU- or step-down level care. Therefore, these are costly care episodes that add to cumulative resource utilization. The average contribution of readmissions to overall cost has been reported in one cohort study. These authors found that the average readmission cost $55 000 or approximately 25% of the index hospitalization.[8] It is worth noting that different methodologies were used to assign costs for each, likely underestimating the contribution of post-discharge costs. Specific risk factors for readmission in this population are not well described.

From an institutional perspective, there are also opportunity costs associated with the care of those with prolonged critical illness. Assuming ICUs are running at capacity, greater numbers of these chronically critically ill patients impair the inflow of those with acute critical illness or post-operative patients. Some hospitals with limited step-down resources may struggle with uninsured or underinsured patients who can leave the ICU but whose care needs exceed those found in a regular ward room. These patients are unlikely to be accepted for payment reasons by post-acute care facilities in transfer. Quantifying these costs is challenging.

Post-acute care

One unifying theme of PMV and CCI is the requirement for post-acute care facility-based management. Between 50 and 80% of hospital survivors of prolonged critical illness are transferred to a post-acute care facility at discharge.[2,8] The primary facility types include LTACs, SNFs, traditional nursing homes, and inpatient rehabilitation facilities (IRFs). The 5–10% of patients discharged home typically require paid home health care. To the onlooker, this may seem concerningly complicated. Indeed, there is much that is inconsistent, nebulous, and arcane about different facility types' admission criteria, needs assessment, quality indicators, and payment systems. Average costs per episode for these patients vary markedly by facility type, reflecting different levels of illness acuity, services provided, and the actual payment structure itself.[14]

Perhaps the most interesting facility type is the LTAC, the venue that counts PMV as its most common admission diagnosis. LTACs are the sole facility type in the US health care system that is defined by an average length of stay, rather than services provided or a specific patient type treated. Under the long-term care hospital prospective payment system, Medicare policy has set a lower fixed-loss outlier payment threshold than for acute care hospitals and also penalizes LTACs for discharging patients with a length of stay that is substantially less than the diagnostic group-related mean.[16] These facilities have doubled over the past two decades, with associated costs now totalling over $1.35 billion for post-critical care patients alone.[17] LTAC profit margins, 5.7% in 2009, have exceeded those of any other facility during the past few years.[18] The Centers for Medicare and Medicaid Services were in fact charged in the 2005 Deficit Reduction Act to reform post-acute care facility payments.[19] In addition to their high margins, LTACs have been criticized, because there is little evidence for their effectiveness in improving patient outcomes and of their lack of reporting of quality data. A recent report, using propensity score and multiple regression modelling techniques, found that costs were higher when patients with similar conditions were treated in long-term care hospitals, compared to acute care hospitals, though, in the case of ventilated patients, these differences were smaller than other diagnoses.[20] On the other hand, LTACs currently fill a need that acute care hospitals possess—a location to transfer long-stay, expensive, chronically critically ill patients. More research is urgently needed to understand the ideal role of LTACs and other post-acute care facilities in the care of these patients.

Long-term trajectories of care

It may be clear to the reader that examining the cumulative costs of care across venues may be instructive. One group that followed a cohort of patients from a single medical center over 1 year found that pathways patients experienced were complex. In this study, hospital survivors of PMV experienced a median of four separate transitions of care location after discharge and spent nearly 75% of all days alive in either a facility or receiving some type of paid health care assistance.[8] Total costs for the first year of care were over $300 000 on average.

Informal caregiving and family financial burden

The economic impact that critical illness imparts on patients, families, and society is perhaps the most poorly described and understood aspect of the experience. First, patients who work are removed from the workplace for months at a time. In contrast to populations, such as ALI, in which 78% of one cohort's members returned to work within 12 months, only 6% of PMV patients are able to do so.[8,21] Assuming 250 000 patients a year who spend 75% of their time in facilities or are too ill to work, there are nearly 50 million days lost from work. Second, family and friends all too often must quit their jobs or at least radically restructure their schedules to accommodate patients' frequent requirements for non-paid, informal caregiving assistance.[22] They also spend months alongside their loved ones in hospitals. Over 70% of patients with prolonged ventilation still require daily caregiving 1 year post-discharge.[23,24] This process strains family ties and is associated with stress, anxiety, and depression.[23,25,26]Using the metrics just described, it is entirely reasonable to estimate that the family members' lost productivity is similar to patients'. Some studies have demonstrated that nearly a third of families of the critically ill lose their entire life savings during the course of the illness.[27] Because critical illness more commonly occurs among those with lower incomes, these people are the least well prepared for financial strain. The experience of critical illness for family members deserves greater attention as a focus of research and health policy.

Economic analysis of prolonged critical illness

Although clinical care and research tends to be patient-centred in its orientation, it is useful to consider the case of prolonged critical illness from a societal perspective as well because of its notable cumulative resource demands on the health care system. This is particularly important for this patient population, because such a great proportion of patients are Medicare recipients.

The most intuitive analytic consideration in this context is whether or not the provision of prolonged life support is a good value for society. To make this a bit less subjective, defining value is important. Cost effectiveness analysis can be used to help to do so. Briefly, in a cost effectiveness analysis, you consider the ratio of the incremental cost difference of the two treatments with the incremental benefits in terms of effectiveness between the same treatments. Effectiveness is typically quantified as life years or life years that have been adjusted to reflect the average QoL in the population of interest. The resulting figure is the incremental cost effectiveness ratio or the assessment of relative value. By convention, an incremental cost effectiveness ratio less than $50 000–100 000 per QALY is seen as societally acceptable.[28]

There have been few cost effectiveness studies of prolonged critical illness. A conceptual challenge in analyses has been the validity of the comparator. One group found that, compared to withdrawal of ventilation and transitioning to comfort care, the provision of PMV cost $82 411 per QALY gained.[13] However, the incremental cost effectiveness ratio exceeded $100 000 per QALY gained for those aged 68 and above. Others, using the Study to Understand Patient Preferences and Treatments (SUPPORT) study database, have demonstrated that incremental cost effectiveness ratios exceeded $100 000 for patients with acute respiratory failure who possess greater than 50% likelihood of death at 2 months.[29] Using an outcome of costs per life saved, one group reported that the incremental costs of treating long-stay ICU patients, not describing ventilation status, was approximately $70 000.[30] Another group found higher costs within a surgical population for each life saved.[31]

Another unique metric is the concept of potentially ineffective care. This concept is defined as resource use in the upper 25th percentile of those with critical illness and survival for less than 100 days post-discharge.[32] Examined in one setting, 13% of ICU patients who fell into this category utilized 32% of all resources. When applied to a cohort of PMV patients, 22% ventilated for at least 4 days with tracheotomy placement met the criteria for potentially ineffective care, most of whom were 65 years of age or older.[11] In contrast, 41% of patients ventilated for 21 or more days met this definition. Although it is conceptually compelling to limit ineffective care to the critically ill, a danger in practice is that its pursuit could lead to the withholding of potentially beneficial care.[33]

Potential targets for improving quality and reducing costs

It is important to understand targets for improving outcomes and reducing costs, given the substantial costs and poor outcomes associated with the provision of prolonged life support. Currently, there are numerous areas on which further study will likely reveal key targets for future interventions (see Table 8.1).

Patient factors

Research has described some risk factors for PMV that are physiologic, socio-demographic, and disease-related. The overarching aim with the greatest effectiveness is likely to be the provision of high-quality critical care: early resuscitation, use of less harmful ventilation strategies, judicious management of sedation and assessment of readiness for extubation, and early mobilization.[34–37] Returning to the theme that length of stay is a serious patient-level cost-driver, strategies that emphasize care quality will likely have the highest return. On the other hand, some factors are non-modifiable such as the summative burden of chronic comorbid conditions, the acuity of the critical illness, and the patient's age. Whether or not these characteristics explain the majority of the chronic course of PMV is not clear.

Family and surrogate decision maker factors

Families are commonly placed in the difficult position of decision making for these critically ill patients—a decision that usually addresses end-of-life care. A sizable body of medical literature has clearly demonstrated that factors, such as sociocultural characteristics, language barriers, religiosity, health literacy and numeracy, and the extreme situational stress imparted by the critical

Table 8.1 Potentially modifiable targets for quality improvement and medical cost

Factors	Potential intervention	Possible influence on cost effectiveness
Patient factors	◆ Early resuscitation ◆ Non-harmful ventilation strategies ◆ Targeted sedation strategies ◆ Daily assessment for SBT readiness ◆ Early mobility programmes	◆ Reduce length of stay ◆ Attenuate need for post-acute care facility ◆ Improve QoL
Family member factors	◆ Early, intensive communication ◆ Decision support	◆ Enhanced patient-centred decisions ◆ Expedite decision making ◆ Reduce family member psychological distress
Physician factors	◆ Application of population-specific prediction models ◆ Communication skills training	◆ Reduce length of stay ◆ Enhanced patient-centred decisions ◆ Expedite decision making ◆ Reduce family member psychological distress
Health systems factors	◆ Foster partnership between acute and post-acute care facilities ◆ Align performance and reimbursement (incentivize quality, not quantity) ◆ Define post-acute care admission criteria	◆ Reduce length of stay ◆ Reduce costs of care

illness experience, represent potential barriers to timely, patient-centred decision making.[38–40] Surrogate decision makers greatly overestimate PMV recipients' long-term survival, functional independence, and QoL at the time ICU-based decision making is entertained.[22]

Physician factors

Physicians struggle with communication and decision making with families. They report reluctance to give bad news and also feel poorly prepared to prognosticate.[41] As a result, families commonly report that the quality of communication they experience in ICU settings is suboptimal.[39] With the development of a new 1-year survival predictive model for patients who have been ventilated for either 14 or 21 days, physicians now have a more reliable tool to help with clinical decision making.[9] Other interventions that could help physicians to engage in effective communication and shared decision making are needed.

Health system processes

The trajectories of care experienced by the average PMV patient highlight the need for acute and post-acute care providers to work more closely to achieve the best outcomes at the lowest cost. It seems inevitable that acute and post-acute care facilities will share accountability for the extended care (and costs) of this patient population. Such a partnership could force improved care behaviours, though how a shared culture of quality can be best constructed requires further collaborative research. Barriers to this partnership are present at many levels currently. For example, few facilities have access to these complicated patients' full medical records from other providers.

Also, the current reimbursement system serves to incent hospitals to transfer patients earlier to post-acute care facilities. Whether patients' rising illness severity over time simply serves to increase subsequent hospital readmission is unclear. Additionally, there are few measures of quality, care needs, and patient-centred outcomes that are transportable across acute and post-acute care venues. As described earlier, more precise admission criteria for different facility types are needed to guide providers and payers. Better evidence for the effectiveness of different post-acute care facilities, notably LTACs, is needed as well.

Conclusion

The care of patients with prolonged critical illness is extraordinarily expensive, compared to other hospitalized patients. These costs have likely been underestimated in the past, because post-discharge resource utilization was not incorporated in estimates. Although there may be non-modifiable socio-demographic and clinical factors associated with greater resource utilization, numerous other patient, family, physician, and health system factors exist that represent promising intervention targets for cost reduction.

References

1 Nelson JE, Cox CE, Hope AA, Carson SS. Chronic critical illness. *Am J Respir Crit Care Med* 2010;**182**: 446–54.

2 Carson SS, Bach PB. The epidemiology and costs of chronic critical illness. *Crit Care Clin* 2002;**18**: 461–76.

3 Angus DC, Kelley MA, Schmitz RJ, White A, Popovich J Jr. Current and projected workforce requirements for care of the critically ill and patients with pulmonary disease: can we meet the requirements of an aging population? *JAMA* 2000;**284**:2762–70.

4 Cox CE, Carson SS, Biddle AK. Cost-effectiveness of ultrasound in preventing femoral venous catheter-associated pulmonary embolism. *Am J Respir Crit Care Med* 2003;**168**:1481–7.

5 Zilberberg MD, de Wit M, Pirone JR, Shorr AF. Growth in adult prolonged acute mechanical ventilation: implications for healthcare delivery. *Crit Care Med* 2008;**36**:1451–5.

6 Cox CE, Carson SS, Holmes GM, Howard A, Carey TS. Increase in tracheostomy for prolonged mechanical ventilation in North Carolina, 1993–2002. *Crit Care Med* 2004;**32**:2219–26.

7 Carson SS, Bach PB, Brzozowski L, Leff A. Outcomes after long-term acute care. An analysis of 133 mechanically ventilated patients. *Am J Respir Crit Care Med* 1999;**159**:1568–73.

8 Unroe M, Kahn JM, Carson SS, et al. One-year trajectories of care and resource utilization for recipients of prolonged mechanical ventilation: a cohort study. *Ann Intern Med* 2010;**153**:167–75.

9 Carson SS, Kahn JM, Hough CL, et al. *Development and validation of a mortality prediction model for patients receiving at least 14 days of mechanical ventilation.* Poster presentation at the American Thoracic Society International Meeting, Denver; 2011.

10 Carson SS, Garrett J, Hanson LC, et al. A prognostic model for one-year mortality in patients requiring prolonged mechanical ventilation. *Crit Care Med* 2008;**36**:2061–9.

11 Cox CE, Carson SS, Hoff-Linquist JA, Olsen MA, Govert JA, Chelluri L. Differences in one-year health outcomes and resource utilization by definition of prolonged mechanical ventilation. *Crit Care* 2007;**11**:R9.

12 Chaix C, Durand-Zaleski I, Alberti C, Brun-Buisson C. A model to compute the medical cost of patients in intensive care. *Pharmacoeconomics* 1999;**15**:573–82.

13 Cox CE, Carson SS, Govert JA, Chelluri L, Sanders GD. An economic evaluation of prolonged mechanical ventilation. *Crit Care Med* 2007;**35**:1918–27.

14 MacIntyre NR, Epstein SK, Carson S, Scheinhorn D, Christopher K, Muldoon S. Management of patients requiring prolonged mechanical ventilation: report of a NAMDRC consensus conference. *Chest* 2005;**128**:3937–54.

15 Wunsch H, Guerra C, Barnato AE, Angus DC, Li G, Linde-Zwirble WT. Three-year outcomes for Medicare beneficiaries who survive intensive care. *JAMA* 2010;**303**:849–56.

16 Medpac. *Long-term care hospitals payment system.* (2008). Available at: http://www.medpac.gov/documents/MedPAC_Payment_Basics_08_LTCH.pdf (accessed 6 July 2009).

17 Kahn JM, Benson NM, Appleby D, Carson SS, Iwashyna TJ. Long-term acute care hospital utilization after critical illness. *JAMA* 2010;**303**:2253–9.

18 Medpac. *Long-term care hospital services.* (2011). Available at: http://www.medpac.gov/chapters/Mar11_Ch10.pdf.

19 Gage B. *Long-term care hospital project approach: Phase I.* (2005). Available at: http://www.cms.hhs.gov/LongTermCareHospitalPPS/Downloads/RTI_phaseI.pdf.

20 Kandilov AMG, Dalton K. *Utilization and payment effects of medicare referrals to long-term care hospitals: final report for the Centers for Medicare and Medicaid Services.* Research Triangle Park, NC; 2011.

21 Herridge MS, Cheung AM, Tansey CM, et al. One-year outcomes in survivors of the acute respiratory distress syndrome. *N Engl J Med* 2003;**348**:683–93.

22 Cox CE, Martinu T, Sathy SJ, et al. Expectations and outcomes of prolonged mechanical ventilation. *Crit Care Med* 2009;**37**:2888–94.

23 Van Pelt DC, Milbrandt EB, Qin L, et al. Informal caregiver burden among survivors of prolonged mechanical ventilation. *Am J Respir Crit Care Med* 2007;**175**:167–73.

24 Douglas SL, Daly BJ. Caregiving and long-term mechanical ventilation. *Chest* 2004;126:1387; author reply 1387–8.

25 Douglas SL, Daly BJ. Caregivers of long-term ventilator patients: physical and psychological outcomes. *Chest* 2003;**123**:1073–81.

26 Rossi Ferrario S, Zotti AM, Zaccaria S, Donner CF. Caregiver strain associated with tracheostomy in chronic respiratory failure. *Chest* 2001;**119**:1498–502.

27 Covinsky KE, Goldman L, Cook EF, et al. The impact of serious illness on patients' families. *JAMA* 1994;**272**:1839–44.

28 Neumann PJ, Rosen AB, Weinstein MC. Medicare and cost-effectiveness analysis. *N Engl J Med* 2005;**353**:1516–22.

29 Hamel MB, Phillips RS, Davis RB, et al. Are aggressive treatment strategies less cost-effective for older patients? The case of ventilator support and aggressive care for patients with acute respiratory failure. *J Am Geriatr Soc* 2001;**49**:382–90.

30 Heyland DK, Konopad E, Noseworthy TW, Johnston R, Gafni A. Is it 'worthwhile' to continue treating patients with a prolonged stay (>14 days) in the ICU? An economic evaluation. *Chest* 1998;**114**:192–8.

31 Fakhry SM, Kercher KW, Rutledge R. Survival, quality of life, and charges in critically III surgical patients requiring prolonged ICU stays. *J Trauma* 1996;**41**:999–1007.

32 Esserman L, Belkora J, Lenert L.Potentially ineffective care. A new outcome to assess the limits of critical care. *JAMA* 1995;**274**:1544–51.

33 Curtis JR, Rubenfeld GD. Aggressive medical care at the end of life. Does capitated reimbursement encourage the right care for the wrong reason? *JAMA* 1997;**278**:1025–6.

34 ARDS Network I. Ventilation with lower tidal volumes as compared with traditional tidal volumes for acute lung injury and the acute respiratory distress syndrome. The Acute Respiratory Distress Syndrome Network. *N Engl J Med* 2000;**342**:1301–8.

35 Girard TD, Kress JP, Fuchs BD, et al. Efficacy and safety of a paired sedation and ventilator weaning protocol for mechanically ventilated patients in intensive care (Awakening and Breathing Controlled trial): a randomised controlled trial. *Lancet* 2008;**371**:126–34.

36 **Rivers E, Nguyen B, Havstad S, et al.** Early goal-directed therapy in the treatment of severe sepsis and septic shock. *N Engl J Med* 2001;**345**:1368–77.

37 **Schweickert WD, Pohlman MC, Pohlman AS, et al.** Early physical and occupational therapy in mechanically ventilated, critically ill patients: a randomised controlled trial. *Lancet* 2009;**373**:1874–82.

38 **White DB, Curtis JR, Wolf LE, et al.** Life support for patients without a surrogate decision maker: who decides? *Ann Intern Med* 2007;**147**:34–40.

39 **Curtis JR, White DB.** Practical guidance for evidence-based ICU family conferences. *Chest* 2008;**134**:835–43.

40 **Wendler D, Rid A.** Systematic review: the effect on surrogates of making treatment decisions for others. *Ann Intern Med* 2011;**154**:336–46.

41 **Christakis NA, Iwashyna TJ.** Attitude and self-reported practice regarding prognostication in a national sample of internists. *Arch Intern Med* 1998;**158**:2389–95.

Chapter 9

Caring for the ICU Survivor: The Family Caregiver Burden

Christopher T. Erb and Mark D. Siegel

Introduction

More attention needs to be paid to the families of ICU survivors. Families play essential caregiving roles, supporting survivors' diverse and profound needs, often with insufficient outside help. Caregiving can be personally fulfilling, but many families suffer financially, physically, and emotionally. This chapter will review the burdens of caregiving and suggest ways to help ICU survivors' families.

Background

Forty-six million people (generally family members) provide informal (i.e. non-professional) supportive care to adults in the US—a role for which they are often untrained and unpaid.[1] Less has been written about caring for ICU survivors than for patients with chronic illnesses such as dementia.[2] Although most patients survive critical illness, few return directly home after discharge, especially following MV. Major functional decline is the rule.[3-10] In a large study of patients who had undergone more than 4 days of MV, only 15% returned directly home.[4] In another study, 75% of patients who had survived 2 months after at least 2 days of MV needed caregiver support.[11] Two years after discharge, 80% of ARDS survivors still need informal care.[12]

Unfortunately, insufficient systemic planning and infrastructure is in place to help survivors, much less their informal caregivers.[13] ICU survivors need help with countless physical, psychological, and cognitive problems, requiring many hours of attention and care per day.[11,12,14] The typical informal caregiver is a female spouse, although an array of relatives and friends may participate.[11,12,15,16] Caregiving occurs at home and at rehabilitation and extended care facilities, often for weeks, months, or years.[11,14] Although a potential source of satisfaction, an unremitting sense of responsibility can make caregiving an overwhelming job with physical, financial, and psychological costs.[17]

The benefits of caregiving

Caregiving can be rewarding.[12,18-23] Families may derive gratification from providing complex care, e.g. for patients who have undergone tracheostomy.[22] The ability to find meaning in caregiving may mitigate stress. Unfortunately, inadequate preparation to meet loved ones' physical, psychological, and technical needs can diminish benefit.

Certain factors correlate with a rewarding caregiving experience. In a study of caregivers for cancer patients, religious coping, social support, and lower educational levels were associated with benefit.[21] Better psychological adjustment correlated with more acceptance, a positive self-view, greater ability to appreciate life and new relationships, and less need to reprioritize. Negative adjustment correlated with less acceptance, more empathy for the patient, less positive change in self-view, and greater need to reprioritize. The authors suggested that interventions to help relatives accept their situation and find meaning in their roles could improve caregiver outcomes.

The burdens of caregiving

Caregivers for ICU survivors face countless physical, financial, and psychological challenges, including decreased employment, depression, sleeplessness, health problems, and lifestyle restrictions (see Figure 9.1; Table 9.1).[1,16,23,24] The risk of lifestyle disruption equates to rates in caregivers for Alzheimer's patients.[14] In one study, among caregivers for patients discharged after at least 7 days of MV, restrictions were more common when patients failed to return home or regain baseline function and included impaired ability to visit friends and pursue hobbies and recreation.[16] More than 20% of caregivers reported moderate or greater restrictions in nearly all areas of daily life. At 6 months, 20% had problems sleeping and eating. Caregivers were distressed by patients' pain and discomfort, helplessness, anxiety, sadness and depression, difficulty sleeping, waking others at night, nightmares, dangerous behaviours, argumentativeness, irritability, and complaining. Although lifestyle restrictions decreased with time, problem behaviour and caregiver distress did not. The authors suggested that caregivers might be helped by efforts to enhance coping, decrease social isolation, and improve patients' functional status.

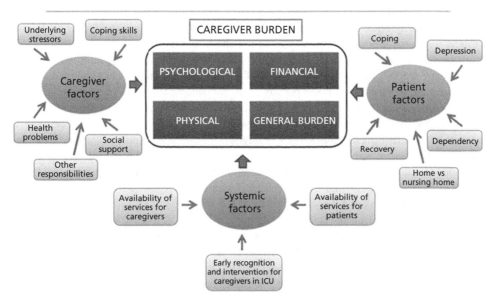

Fig. 9.1 Caregiver burden. Many factors contribute to the experience of burden by caregivers, such as underlying health problems or stressors, as well as a variety of other familial or professional responsibilities. There are also several factors, such as satisfaction with providing care to a loved one and well-developed social support networks, that may alleviate the burden. Patient factors that may increase the sense of burden among caregivers include the location where care is provided, the level of dependency, and whether the patient is showing signs of recovery. The relationship between caregiver burden and patient burden is bidirectional, such that worse burden in caregivers leads to worse burden in patients, and vice versa.

Table 9.1 The ICU caregiver burden: manifestations and risk factors

Burden	Typical manifestations
General	◆ Potentially overwhelming patient care responsibilities ◆ Lost personal/leisure time ◆ Social isolation
Physical	◆ Risk of multiple diseases, including mortality* ◆ Decreased attention to personal health ◆ Difficulty sleeping and eating
Financial	◆ Caregiving expenses ◆ Lost savings ◆ Lost or reduced work (patient and caregiver)
Psychological+	◆ Anxiety ◆ Depression ◆ PTSD ◆ Complicated grief ◆ Caregiving strain and fatigue

*Further details in text.
+Disorders generally identified, using screening tools to identify symptoms and patients at risk, not formal diagnoses.

Another group studied physical and psychological outcomes in caregivers 6 months after patients were hospitalized for more than 4 days of MV.[5] Caregiving was usually a new role, and subjects were predominantly female spouses and children, middle-aged, and employed. Only 30.1% of patients were discharged directly home; the rest went to a nursing home (40.4%), rehabilitation centre (26.5%), or another hospital (3%). Of those alive at 6 months, 21.9% were in a nursing home. Caregivers spent 4.9 hours per day caring for patients at home and 4.2 hours for those institutionalized. Forty-four per cent of caregivers for those at home got help from family and friends (mean 3 hours daily), whereas 85.7% of those institutionalized got help (3.7 hours daily).

Another study investigated burden in 71 caregivers 3 months after hospitalization.[2] Seventy-two per cent provided up to 40 hours and 19.6% over 60 hours of care weekly. Support services were used infrequently. Female spouses provided the most care, but males were burdened more, struggled more with caregiving, and needed more support. Caregiver burden correlated with a sense of filial obligation but not social support and self-efficacy.

Several patient, caregiver, and systems-related factors contribute to caregiver burden.[25] Strain is at least partly related to the responsibilities required. For example, those caring for patients with chronic respiratory failure must learn to suction and understand some technical aspects of ventilator management. In a study of 40 such caregivers, all showed a medium degree of strain (using a family strain questionnaire) persisting at 1 year.[23] Contributing factors included compromised leisure time and restricted social relationships. The most strain was felt by females and those caring for patients who had undergone tracheostomy less than 14 months before. Some wives reported disgust related to their partner's physical proximity. Caregivers desired ongoing education, even after months of caregiving. The relationship between caregiver burden and patient outcomes is likely bidirectional; factors contributing to patient disability likely exacerbate burden, and factors causing burden undermine patient well-being.

Increasing concern has focused on patients with CCI, a group needing weeks to months of ventilator support after acute illness.[26–28] In the US, more than 100 000 patients have CCI and the numbers are growing.[28] CCI patients do poorly: most are institutionalized for extended periods or permanently, with profound cognitive and functional disabilities.[26–28] Forty-eight to 68% die within a year, and less than 12% are alive and independent 1 year after becoming ill.[28] In one study, 61% of 1-year survivors needed daily caregiver assistance.[29] Forty-nine per cent of caregivers reported 'a lot' or 'severe' stress related to caregiving. Eighty-four per cent quit their jobs or altered their work schedule due to caregiving.[29] Patients' families often overestimate the likelihood that their loved one will survive CCI and return to independent breathing and function and go home.[26,28,29] Miscommunication between ICU staff and families fosters misunderstanding. Caregivers underestimate the intensity of support their relatives will need when consenting to tracheotomy.[26,29] The impact of such poor outcomes on caregivers' well-being merits further study.

Physical burdens

Data from non-ICU populations suggest that caregivers incur health risks, including immune dysfunction, cardiovascular disease, infections, delayed wound healing, faster cancer growth and chromosomal ageing, autoimmune disease, diabetes, metabolic syndrome, obesity, hypercho-lesterolaemia, depression, and early death[5,20,30] Chronic stress may contribute by impacting the sympathetic nervous system and hypothalamic-pituitary-adrenal axis.[20] In the elderly, biological vulnerability, combined with loss, prolonged distress, and the physical demands of caregiving, may play a role.[30] Decreased propensity to engage in preventive behaviours, such as exercise, personal health maintenance, and recreation, could contribute as well.

In the Caregiver Health Effects Study, approximately 400 elderly spousal caregivers were matched by age and gender to non-caregiving controls.[30] After adjusting for socio-demographic factors, prevalent disease, and subclinical cardiovascular disease, 4-year mortality was increased by 63% in caregivers experiencing strain.[30] Mortality was highest in those with prevalent disease and caregiver strain: 32.7% died during 4-year follow-up. Suggested mechanisms included insufficient time to rest or exercise, but limited sample size precluded analysing other potential factors.[30]

In a study of caregivers responsible for loved ones who had undergone more than 4 days of MV, 36.1% reported deteriorating health over 6 months.[5] Perceptions of poor health correlated with depression. Similar burdens have been noted in cancer patients' caregivers who may put the patient's needs before their own.[20] While many resources are available to help cancer caregivers, few exist for those of ICU survivors.

Financial burdens

Caregiver financial burden is difficult to measure, at least partly because caregiving time and energy are not clearly monetizable and because financial burden largely comes in the form of lost wages or reduced employment, rather than actual monetary outlays. However, caregivers clearly face financial strain. Contributing factors include the cost of caregiving, lost savings, and the inability of many patients and families to return to work.[8,10,29] In a study of survivors who required MV for at least 48 hours, only 28.7% of caregivers were working outside their caregiver role 2 months after discharge, and 30.3% discontinued or reduced paid work to provide care.[11] In another study, 14% reported at 1 year that they had stopped work to provide care.[14] In another report, almost half employed at study enrolment had reduced work hours, quit, or were fired because of caregiving.[31] In the SUPPORT study, which focused on seriously ill hospitalized adults, 31% of families lost most or all their savings and 29% lost their major source of income.[32] Loss of savings correlated with younger age, lower income, and poorer functional status. Caregivers are at particular risk for financial challenges indirectly related to the patient's health and not covered by health insurance.[32]

Psychological burdens

Many studies have considered the psychological disorders faced by bereaved ICU families,[33–35] but survivors' families experience a similar burden. Families suffer a range of disorders, including anxiety, depression, PTS, and, in those who lose a loved one, complicated grief.[10,11,14,34–39] Psychological trauma experienced in the ICU may predispose families to difficulty when burdened with caregiving.[34,40–43]

In a comprehensive review, Kentish-Barnes et al. described tools available to assess psychological burden.[43] Especially pertinent include assessments of family satisfaction (the Critical Care Family Needs Inventory (CCFNI), the Family Satisfaction in the ICU (FS-ICU), and the Critical Care Family Satisfaction Survey) and psychiatric disturbances (the Hospital Anxiety and Depression Scale (HADS) and the Impact of Events Scale (IES)). The HADS has been widely validated and used in the community to identify symptoms of anxiety and depression. The revised Impact of Events Scale (IES-R) can be easily administered by telephone and used to screen for PTSD. The American Medical Association has developed an easily accessible self-assessment tool to help caregivers to assess their own distress and need for interventions, including physician assessment, referral to support groups, or social services.[44] Although not expressly validated for ICU survivors' relatives, the tool could help identify caregivers needing care themselves.[44,45]

Psychological symptoms can diminish QoL and contribute to social isolation, marital discord, unemployment, and health problems.[46] Psychological morbidity undermines a relative's ability to care and interferes with patient recovery.[8,18,40,41,47,48] Fear for their loved ones' welfare can make some caregivers excessively protective.[48] Stress may be exacerbated by the fact that family members remember the ICU experience when loved ones do not.[48]

Davidson and colleagues recently introduced the concept of post-intensive care syndrome-family (PICS-F) to describe the psychological morbidity affecting families after the ICU, including acute stress disorder, PTSD, depression, and complicated grief.[18] PICS-F can last for years, and multiple risk factors have been described (see Box 9.1). Unfortunately, current practice is clearly insufficient to prevent PICS-F.

Prevalence and risk factors

Psychological symptoms are highly prevalent among families during the ICU stay, exceed the general population, and persist through discharge.[11,34,35,49] Up to 80% of family members experience at least one negative effect from a loved one's critical illness, including anxiety, depression, confusion, stress, frustration, guilt, and PTSD.[43] More study with larger sample sizes and better diagnostic tools is needed to identify the risk factors for psychological morbidity, particularly to clarify the relationship between patients' deficits and caregiver outcomes.[10,14] Attempts to relate psychological morbidity to the ICU stay and subsequent caregiving are confounded by insufficient baseline and longitudinal data.[12,14,24,41]

At ICU discharge or death, 73.4% of family members have symptoms of anxiety and 35.3% symptoms of depression.[35] Spouses are more likely to have symptoms than family members overall (82.9% vs 75.5%). Depression is more common when patients die (48.3%) but is also prevalent among family members of survivors (32.7%). Risk factors for anxiety include a high

Box 9.1 Risk factors for post-intensive care syndrome-family (PICS-F)[18]

Caregiver factors

- Female gender
- Young age
- Lower educational level
- Having a critically ill spouse
- Being the unmarried parent of a critically ill child
- Pre-existing anxiety and/or depression
- Family history of anxiety, depression, or severe mental illness
- Higher stress levels (e.g. related to death or high risk of death of a loved one)
- Presence at death
- Additional stressors
- Potentially protective factors
  - Ability to discuss feelings
  - Adequate social support
- Area of uncertainty: role of the family in decision making (discordance between the preferred and actual role likely contributes)

Patient factors

- Young age
- Unexpected illness
- Illness less than 5 years

ICU staff factors

- Providing incomplete information
- Failure of the family to find the physician comforting
- Potentially protective factors
  - Proactive end-of-life conferences and brochures
  - Beneficial communication and success in helping families of loved ones' to understand the patient's illness and their new caregiving role

Simplified Acute Physiology Score II (SAPS II), lower patient age, and being a spouse. Risk factors for depression include higher SAPS II, patient death, lower patient age, and having an ICU room with more than one bed. Spouses may be at particular risk because of their role as decision makers and responsibility for providing information to the medical team and sharing information with the rest of the family.

Forty-nine per cent of relatives have PTSD-related symptoms 6 months after an ICU stay.[24] Family psychological distress correlates with patient distress, raising concern that families may be too traumatized to address patients' needs. A major study described the prevalence and risk factors for PTS 90 days after discharge or death among 284 family members from 21 French ICUs.[34] Thirty-three per cent had symptoms of PTS. Higher rates were found in families who said information provided in the ICU was incomplete (48.4%), those who shared in decision making (47.8%), those whose relative died in the ICU (50%) or after an end-of-life decision (60%), and in those who shared in end-of-life decisions (81.8%). Other risk factors included female sex, being the patient's child, cancer in the ICU patient, and more severe acute illness. Severe PTS was associated with higher rates of anxiety and depression and diminished QoL. Unfortunately, only 25% of family members with PTS reaction were receiving medical care on follow-up. The potential contribution of stress related to caregiving at home was not addressed.

In a study of ARDS survivors, 31.9% of caregivers experienced emotional distress, which was higher than reported in a sample of American women.[12] Emotional distress correlated with higher rates of depressive symptoms in patients but not functional status. Other factors included disruption of personal lifestyle and lower levels of mastery (i.e. having a sense of control over one's life). Factors associated with psychological well-being and happiness included awareness of inner strengths as a consequence of caregiving, a greater sense of personal mastery, and social support.

Increasingly, studies have investigated the trajectory of caregivers' psychological symptoms. A study of 50 family members found anxiety in 42%, 21%, and 15% at ICU enrolment, 1 month, and 6 months afterwards.[36] Depression was found in 16%, 8%, and 6%. At 6 months, 35% had evidence of PTS, which, unlike other studies, was neither more common in bereaved than non-bereaved individuals nor was it associated with decision-making role preference, anxiety, or depression in the ICU. Psychological symptoms can persist for years: 5 years after ARDS, 27% of family members have mental health problems, including depression, anxiety, and PTSD.[8]

Depressive symptoms may decrease over time. In one study, among caregivers without depression at discharge, 78.6% remained that way 6 months later.[5] Of those mildly or moderately depressed, 62.5% and 57.9% improved at 6 months. Unfortunately, only 28.6% of those with severe symptoms at discharge improved. In another study, depression and caregiving burden were highest when patients were institutionalized as opposed to home.[15] Institutionalization was associated with a higher caregiver burden because of disrupted schedules, inadequate family support, and worse health. Burden and depression scores correlated. Depressive symptoms improved over time, but more than half of those with depression at discharge were depressed 2 months later. Importantly, caregiver variables, as opposed to patient variables, were the best predictors of depression after discharge. In a more recent study by the same group, depressive symptoms were common at discharge (75.5%) and decreased to a lower, but still substantial, rate 2 months later (43.3%).[31] Caregivers of patients institutionalized at 2 months were more likely to be depressed, compared to those caring for patients at home (odds ratio (OR) 2.75).

In one study, depression risk in caregivers at 2, 6, and 12 months after the patient underwent MV was 33.9, 30.8, and 22.8%.[14] The decrease over time was insignificant, and the patient's pre-ICU functional status did not impact risk. In a recent study, 90% of the caregivers of patients needing at least 4 days of MV had depressive symptoms on admission, 73% at discharge, and 61% 2 months later.[41] The authors identified two trajectories: one with high levels of depressive symptoms during ICU admission that remained high at 2 months, and another that was lower initially but subsequently fell. High trajectory subjects tended to be younger, female, and an adult child of the patient and reported financial difficulty and more health risk behaviours. Low trajectory subjects more commonly reported a religious background or preference.

One group used semi-structured qualitative interviews to explore the experience of caregivers during the year following ARDS in a family member.[50] Caregivers reported significant strain related to caregiving and frequent symptom minimization by patients. Caregivers also struggled with their loved ones' new cognitive deficits and cognitive fluctuation, lack of support after leaving the hospital, the need to balance childcare and work, the need to explain problems to children, distancing and stress in relationships, and feeling overwhelmed. Relatives felt unprepared for their loved ones' limitations, and the patient's psychological distress disrupted the family with life-changing repercussions.

A recent paper stands out for its use of premorbid data, allowing a more confident assessment of the impact of critical illness on outcomes. In a study of older Americans, Davydow et al. investigated how mortality, disability, premorbid depression, gender, and other factors impacted the risk of depressive symptoms after a spouse had sepsis.[47] Among wives, depressive symptoms increased from 20% a median 1.1 years before sepsis to 34% 1 year after; among husbands, symptoms increased from 17% to 25%. On logistic regression, the OR for developing depressive symptoms was 3.74 for wives, but no independent risk remained for husbands. However, the authors cautioned that a meaningful impact on husbands was not ruled out, given a relatively small sample size and because men may be less willing to report symptoms. Among wives, depressive symptoms were associated with more ADL limitations.

The degree to which caregivers develop psychological morbidity may correlate with related morbidity in patients.[19,24,46,51] Symptoms of PTSD in caregivers correlate with patients' symptoms.[37] Caregivers whose loved ones are institutionalized are more likely to have depressive symptoms and feel overloaded (defined as having negative attitudes or emotional reactions to caregiving) than when loved ones are home.[5]

Evidence for a relationship between functional dependency and caregiver psychological morbidity is mixed. Risk of depression correlates with time spent at home assisting with ADLs and instrumental ADLs (IADLs), although causality is unclear.[11] Discharge dependency and functional capacity inconsistently predict caregiver depressive symptoms.[41] Increased patient age and having paid help at home may correlate with depression but not functional dependency and cohabitation.[14] However, a subsequent study found no relationship between functional dependency and psychological outcomes, although an association between depressive symptoms in caregivers and patient male gender and tracheostomy was found.[1]

Baseline psychological morbidity appears to impact the risk of PTS, depression, and anxiety; in one study, trait anxiety was the most significant predictor of depressive reaction and the only predictor of PTSD symptoms on multivariable analysis.[52] Women and spouses appeared to be at highest risk for psychological distress. Another study examined the impact of demographic variables on the risk of depression in the caregivers of patients requiring at least 3 days of MV, interviewed 2 months after discharge.[31] Race had no impact. Depressive symptoms were more common and severe when patients were institutionalized than at home. Female caregivers and those with worse health were more likely to have depression. The authors suggested that increased mortality and worse functional status among institutionalized patients may contribute to depression and PTSD in caregivers. The authors noted that the Center for Epidemiologic Studies Depression (CES-D) technique used is relatively insensitive and could have led to an underestimate of the rates of depressive symptoms.[5,31]

Treatment and prevention of caregiver burden

A paucity of data makes it difficult to provide firm recommendations about the best approach to helping caregivers.[1,11,25,36,37,53,54] A better understanding of the factors contributing to caregiver burden would foster the development of effective interventions. Multidisciplinary support networks may help.[39] The high prevalence of caregiver symptoms suggests a need for screening in the primary care setting[36] as well as during the index ICU stay.[47] The patient's welfare clearly depends on the family's well-being.[40] Unfortunately, psychological morbidity may go unrecognized, leaving many patients and families to cope on their own.[37]

Suggestions to alleviate caregiver burden have included education, facilitating patient and caregiver adaptation and recovery, assisting the management of patients' psychiatric disorders, increasing availability of respite and home care, and improving access to social support (see Box 9.2).[12] Mastering understanding of the patient's illness could alleviate burden.[25] Jones et al. evaluated an informational programme targeted at patients and families in the hopes that it might reduce patient and caregiver stress.[24] A self-help manual was used for 6 weeks, beginning 1 week after the ICU, which provided information about recovery from critical illness, psychological information, and practical advice. Unfortunately, the intervention failed to reduce family member depression, anxiety, and PTSD-related symptoms. Another group studied the potential benefits of a disease management programme on physical and psychological outcomes in caregivers.[15] Although the intervention was unsuccessful, the authors suggested that the programme might need to be implemented for longer periods. Others have suggested that earlier interventions might prove helpful.[14]

Decisions, practice, and interventions within the ICU could prevent or ameliorate psychological morbidity.[40,55] The impact of reducing caregivers' symptoms in the ICU on subsequent psychological morbidity is uncertain.[56] Strategies designed to help families have been proposed,

---

Box 9.2 Potential strategies to improve caregiver outcomes

In the ICU

- Excellent communication
- Decrease environmental strain
- Include families in non-technical bedside care
- Information brochures
- Multidisciplinary support
- Screening family members for stress
- Assisting with referrals for family support
- Demonstrating caring by ICU team
- ICU diaries
- Thoughtful and compassionate decision making
- Preparation for post-ICU caregiving needs
- Facilitated sensemaking*

> **Box 9.2 Potential strategies to improve caregiver outcomes** *(continued)*
>
> ## Following discharge
>
> - Facilitate patient adaptation and recovery[+]
> - Multidisciplinary support networks (including friends and other family members)
> - Assist management of patients' psychiatric disorders
> - Improve caregiver education and mastery
> - Increase availability of respite and home care
> - Improve access to social support
> - Education to help caregivers to master understanding of patient's illness
> - ICU follow-up clinics?
> - Screen caregivers for stress
> - Promote caregiver coping skills
> - Decrease social isolation
>
> * See text for details.
> [+] Patient recovery and improvement, including the ability to return home, correlate with caregiver well-being.

including better communication and including loved ones in non-technical bedside care.[18] Information brochures, high-quality family meetings, and multidisciplinary support to address family members' needs and concerns could prove useful.[34,57,58]

Data on the relationship between psychological morbidity and interactions with the health care team and ICU environment are mixed.[34,36,49,57–59] A Norwegian study found no relationship between psychological distress 4–6 weeks after discharge and satisfaction with communication or support from friends, relatives, and the ICU team.[59] However, higher distress was associated with being unemployed, a higher degree of 'environmental strain' (related to noise and distress associated with seeing other patients and relatives), and being given less hope for improvement. Notably, this study was performed in a setting where satisfaction with communication and support was high and strain on relatives low.

Several important studies have suggested that efforts to improve communication mitigate subsequent morbidity, particularly among families facing a loved one's death.[34,58] For example, Lautrette et al. conducted an RCT of an intensive communication strategy, utilizing an information brochure on bereavement and a structured approach to family meetings. Family members in the intervention arm reported improved satisfaction and reduced symptoms of anxiety, depression, and PTSD.[58]

Regardless of patient outcome, the benefit of improved communication and helping families make sense of the ICU experience and their new roles warrants further study, as do other interventions such as support groups and ICU follow-up clinics.[18] Other practical interventions in the ICU which could help include screening for stress, making appropriate referrals, and demonstrating caring.[60]

Given their constant contact with families, nurses are well positioned to intervene.[61] One approach, termed 'facilitated sensemaking,' employs a multimodal approach to assisting families during a patient's ICU stay and is based on the concern that caregivers are frequently unprepared for their new roles—in part due to inadequate communication—and may have misconceptions about what is happening to their loved one.[61,62] Using this approach, nurses can help families make sense of the patient's condition and clinical course and help them to adapt to their new roles. Specific interventions include identifying and meeting the family's information needs, coaching them on how to visit and meet their own needs, providing support, and assigning or offering the opportunity for them to perform meaningful activities at the bedside. In a pilot study, a convenience sample of family members expressed satisfaction with this approach, but more work is needed to assess its value.[61,62]

There is growing interest in the use of ICU diaries to prevent or ameliorate PTS in patients and families.[46,51,63,64] Diaries may help patients and families make sense of the ICU experience.[51] Typical ICU diaries are maintained by ICU nurses, and sometimes other staff and family members, and contain written information about the patient's illness and ICU stay, using common, compassionate language. Photographs of the ICU, equipment, and of the patient and family prior to the illness may be included. A pilot study showed that diaries were associated with a lower incidence of new-onset PTS symptoms in relatives 3 months after the ICU stay.[46] The authors suggested that diaries could foster discussions between families and patients to help the latter understand their illness and treatment and also help relatives express feelings. Improving patient's emotional health could help caregivers too.[24,46]

In another study, diaries appeared to decrease avoidance and intrusion symptoms related to PTS 12 months after discharge.[63] Fewer relatives had severe PTS-related symptoms when diaries were used (31.7%) than before (80%) and after (67.6%). The authors suggested that diaries could counterbalance poor comprehension of information, inadequate time spent meeting with physicians, and family concerns that staff did not listen to them.

A recent grounded theory evaluation suggested that relatives used diaries to help patients' and their own recoveries.[64] Women valued diaries more than men, many of whom preferred to put the patient's illness behind them. The authors suggested that patients and families used diaries to help patients construct an illness narrative, necessitated in part by the absent, fragmented, and delusional memories typical of an ICU stay.

The ability to cope with caregiving may be as important, if not more important, than the severity of burden itself.[16,21,54] Johansson et al. studied coping methods used by caregivers managing ICU survivors, all of whom had required MV and were home at least 3 months.[42] Four main coping strategies were identified: 'volunteering' (i.e. finding it 'natural' to help a family member), 'accepting the situation' (i.e. taking on the responsibility out of a sense of humanity), 'modulating the situation' (i.e. transferring some of the caregiving burden to the community), and 'sacrificing oneself for the situation' (i.e. choosing to care for the patient despite a need for relaxation and time for themselves). Factors, such as the patient's psychological vulnerability, the relatives' physical and psychological function, and previous ICU experience, impacted strategies chosen. Clearly, more study is needed to better understand the coping methods used by survivors' families.

Many obstacles, including the patient's physical disability and decreased mobility, distance, and financial distress may make it difficult for caregivers to cope. A novel approach, using the telephone, suggests new ways to foster coping.[54] In a pilot study, investigators explored coping among ALI survivors and their informal caregivers and developed an ALI-specific coping skills training programme. Investigators sought to teach participants strategies to manage ALI-related emotional distress and physical symptoms and to teach caregivers to foster patients' coping skills.

Poor coping at baseline was found in patients and caregivers and correlated with depressive symptoms, anxiety, and PTSD. All 14 participants completed and supported the value of the intervention. Significant improvements were seen in HADS and post-traumatic symptom scale (PTSS) scores, especially among patients, and mean self-efficacy scores improved in patients and caregivers. Improved HADS and PTSS correlated with improved self-efficacy and adaptive coping styles. Additional research is needed to understand the factors that contribute to maladaptive coping and to determine if this relatively inexpensive, feasible, and well-tolerated intervention can be used on a larger scale to improve coping in patients and caregivers.

Conclusion

Crucial work over the past decade has shown that ICU survivors face overwhelming physical, psychological, and cognitive challenges. Survivors are critically dependent on informal care provided by family members to promote their well-being and recovery. Caring for the ICU survivor can be fulfilling for relatives, but the burdens of caregiving cannot be overstated. Caregiving imposes physical, financial, and psychological challenges that profoundly alter the lives of survivors' families. Recognition of these challenges has created a mandate for the critical care community to identify caregivers at risk and to develop and provide effective treatments, both within and beyond the ICU.

Additional research is needed to improve the quality and depth of support given to informal caregivers. Better tools are needed to identify those at risk of being overwhelmed. Similarly, a more nuanced understanding of the factors that contribute to effective coping and resiliency should help to guide interventions for families at risk. A deeper understanding of the way the specific features of a survivor's disability affects caregivers could guide planning for appropriate support. Finally, more study is needed to determine if provisions for respite and financial support for families would alleviate the burdens too many caregivers endure.

References

1 Van Pelt DC, Schulz R, Chelluri L, Pinsky MR. Patient-specific, time-varying predictors of post-ICU informal caregiver burden: the caregiver outcomes after ICU discharge project. *Chest* 2010;**137**:88–94.

2 Foster M, Chaboyer W. Family carers of ICU survivors: a survey of the burden they experience. *Scand J Caring Sci* 2003;**17**:205–14.

3 Herridge MS, Cheung AM, Tansey CM, et al. One-year outcomes in survivors of the acute respiratory distress syndrome. *N Engl J Med* 2003;**348**:683–93.

4 Zilberberg MD, Luippold RS, Sulsky S, Shorr AF. Prolonged acute mechanical ventilation, hospital resource utilization, and mortality in the United States. *Crit Care Med* 2008;**36**:724–30.

5 Douglas SL, Daly BJ. Caregivers of long-term ventilator patients. *Chest* 2003;**123**:1073–81.

6 Barnato AE, Albert SM, Angus DC, Lave JR, Degenholtz HB. Disability among elderly survivors of mechanical ventilation. *Am J Respir Crit Care Med* 2011;**183**:1037–42.

7 Iwashyna TJ. Survivorship will be the defining challenge of critical care in the 21st century. *Ann Intern Med* 2010;**153**:204–5.

8 Herridge MS, Tansey CM, Matte A, et al. Functional disability 5 years after acute respiratory distress syndrome. *N Engl J Med* 2011;**364**:1293–304.

9 Herridge MS. Long-term outcomes after critical illness: past, present, future. *Curr Opin Crit Care* 2007;**13**:473–5.

10 Wilcox ME, Herridge MS. Long-term outcomes in patients surviving acute respiratory distress syndrome. *Semin Respir Crit Care Med* 2010;**31**:55–65.

11 Im K, Belle SH, Schulz R, Mendelsohn AB, Chelluri L. Prevalence and outcomes of caregiving after prolonged (≥48 hours) mechanical ventilation in the ICU. *Chest* 2004;**125**:597–606.

12 Cameron JI, Herridge MS, Tansey CM, McAndrews MP, Cheung AM. Well-being in informal caregivers of survivors of acute respiratory distress syndrome. *Crit Care Med* 2006;**34**:81–6.

13 Kahn JM, Angus DC. Health policy and future planning for survivors of critical illness. *Curr Opin Crit Care* 2007;**13**:514–18.

14 Van Pelt DC, Milbrandt EB, Qin L, et al. Informal caregiver burden among survivors of prolonged mechanical ventilation. *Am J Respir Crit Care Med* 2007;**175**:167–73.

15 Douglas SL, Daly BJ, Kelley CG, O'Toole E, Montenegro H. Impact of a disease management program upon caregivers of chronically critically ill patients. *Chest* 2005;**128**:3925–36.

16 Choi J, Donahoe MP, Zullo TG, Hoffman LA. Caregivers of the chronically critically ill after discharge from the intensive care unit: six months' experience. *Am J Crit Care* 2011;**20**:12–23.

17 Rabow MW, Hauser JM, Adams J. Supporting family caregivers at the end of life. *JAMA* 2004;**291**: 483–91.

18 Davidson JE, Jones C, Bienvenu OJ. Family response to critical illness: postintensive care syndrome— family. *Crit Care Med* 2012;**40**:618–24.

19 Kleinpell R. Focusing on caregivers of the critically ill: beyond illness into recovery. *Crit Care Med* 2006;**34**:243–4.

20 Bevans M, Sternberg EM. Caregiving burden, stress, and health effects among family caregivers of adult cancer patients. *JAMA* 2012;**307**:398–403.

21 Kim Y, Schulz R, Carver CS. Benefit finding in the cancer caregiving experience. *Psychosom Med* 2007;**69**:283–91.

22 Scott LD, Arslanian-Engoren C. Caring for survivors of prolonged mechanical ventilation. *Home Health Care Management & Practice* 2002;**14**:122–8.

23 Rossi Ferrario S, Zotti AM, Zaccaria S, Donner CF. Caregiver strain associated with tracheostomy in chronic respiratory failure. *Chest* 2001;**119**:1498–502.

24 Jones C, Skirrow P, Griffiths RD, et al. Post-traumatic stress disorder-related symptoms in relatives of patients following intensive care. *Intensive Care Med* 2004;**30**:456–60.

25 Van Pelt D, Chelluri L, Schultz R, Pinsky M. Response. *Chest* 2010;**138**:1024–5.

26 Unroe M, Kahn JM, Carson SS, et al. One-year trajectories of care and resource utilization for recipients of prolonged mechanical ventilation: a cohort study. *Ann Intern Med* 2010;**153**:167–75.

27 Nelson JE, Tandon N, Mercado AF, Camhi SL, Ely EW, Morrison RS. Brain dysfunction: another burden for the chronically critically ill. *Arch Intern Med* 2006;**166**:1993–9.

28 Nelson JE, Cox CE, Hope AA, Carson SS. Chronic critical illness. *Am J Respir Crit Care Med* 2010;**182**:446–54.

29 Cox CE, Martinu T, Sathy SJ, et al. Expectations and outcomes of prolonged mechanical ventilation. *Crit Care Med* 2009;**37**:2888–94.

30 Schulz R, Beach SR. Caregiving as a risk factor for mortality. *JAMA* 1999;**282**:2215–19.

31 Douglas SL, Daly BJ, O'Toole E, Hickman RL. Depression among white and nonwhite caregivers of the chronically critically ill. *J Crit Care* 2010;**25**:364.e11–e19.

32 Covinsky KE, Goldman L, Cook EF, et al. The impact of serious illness on patients' families. *JAMA* 1994;**272**:1839–44.

33 Siegel MD, Hayes E, Vanderwerker LC, Loseth DB, Prigerson HG. Psychiatric illness in the next of kin of patients who die in the intensive care unit. *Crit Care Med* 2008;**36**:1722–8.

34 Azoulay E, Pochard F, Kentish-Barnes N, et al. Risk of post-traumatic stress symptoms in family members of intensive care unit patients. *Am J Respir Crit Care Med* 2005;**171**:987–94.

35 Pochard F, Darmon M, Fassier T, et al. Symptoms of anxiety and depression in family members of intensive care unit patients before discharge or death. A prospective multicenter study. *J Crit Care* 2005;**20**:90–6.

36 **Anderson WG, Arnold RM, Angus DC, Bryce CL.** Posttraumatic stress and complicated grief in family members of patients in the intensive care unit. *J Gen Intern Med* 2008;**23**:1871–6.

37 **Jones C, Griffiths RD.** Patient and caregiver counselling after the intensive care unit: what are the needs and how should they be met? *Curr Opin Crit Care* 2007;**13**:503–7.

38 **Needham DM, Davidson JD, Cohen HP, et al.** Improving long-term outcomes after discharge from intensive care unit: report from a stakeholders' conference. *Crit Care Med* 2012;**40**:502–9.

39 **Harvey MA.** The truth about consequences—post-intensive care syndrome in intensive care unit survivors and their families. *Crit Care Med* 2012;**40**:2506–7.

40 **Griffiths RD.** Rehabilitating the critically ill: a cultural shift in intensive care unit care. *Crit Care Med* 2012;**40**:681–2.

41 **Choi J, Sherwood PR, Schulz R, et al.** Patterns of depressive symptoms in caregivers of mechanically ventilated critically ill adults from intensive care unit admission to 2 months postintensive care unit discharge: a pilot study. *Crit Care Med* 2012;**40**:1546–53.

42 **Johansson I, Fridlund B, Hildingh C.** Coping strategies of relatives when an adult next-of-kin is recovering at home following critical illness. *Intensive Crit Care Nurs* 2004;**20**:281–91.

43 **Kentish-Barnes N, Lemiale V, Chaize M, Pochard F, Azoulay E.** Assessing burden in families of critical care patients. *Crit Care Med* 2009;**37**(10 Suppl):S448–56.

44 **American Medical Association.** *Caregiver self-assessment.* (2012). Available at: http://www.ama-assn. org/ama/pub/physician-resources/public-health/promoting-healthy-lifestyles/geriatric-health/ caregiver-health/caregiver-self-assessment.page?.

45 **Epstein-Lubow G, Gaudiano BA, Hinckley M, Salloway S, Miller IW.** Evidence for the validity of the American Medical Association's caregiver self-assessment questionnaire as a screening measure for depression. *J Am Geriatr Soc* 2010;**58**:387–8.

46 **Jones C, Backman C, Griffiths RD.** Intensive care diaries and relatives' symptoms of posttraumatic stress disorder after critical illness: a pilot study. *Am J Crit Care* 2012;**21**:172–6.

47 **Davydow DS, Hough CL, Langa KM, Iwashyna TJ.** Depressive symptoms in spouses of older patients with severe sepsis. *Crit Care Med* 2012;**40**:2335–41.

48 **Griffiths RD, Jones C.** Seven lessons from 20 years of follow-up of intensive care unit survivors. *Curr Opin Crit Care* 2007;**13**:508–13.

49 **Stevenson JE, Dowdy DW.** Thinking outside the box: Intensive care unit diaries to improve psychological outcomes in family members. *Crit Care Med* 2012;**40**:2231–2.

50 **Cox CE, Docherty SL, Brandon DH, et al.** Surviving critical illness: acute respiratory distress syndrome as experienced by patients and their caregivers. *Crit Care Med* 2009;**37**:2702–8.

51 **Jones C, Backman C, Capuzzo M, et al.** Intensive care diaries reduce new onset post traumatic stress disorder following critical illness: a randomised, controlled trial. *Crit Care* 2010;**14**:R168.

52 **Paparrigopoulos T, Melissaki A, Efthymiou A, et al.** Short-term psychological impact on family members of intensive care unit patients. *J Psychosom Res* 2006;**61**:719–22.

53 **Kulkarni HS.** Less-obvious predictors of post-ICU informal caregiver burden. *Chest* 2010;**138**:1024.

54 **Cox CE, Porter LS, Hough CL, et al.** Development and preliminary evaluation of a telephone-based coping skills training intervention for survivors of acute lung injury and their informal caregivers. *Intensive Care Med* 2012;**38**:1289–97.

55 **Herridge M, Cox C.** Linking ICU practice to long-term outcome. *Am J Respir Crit Care Med* 2012;**186**:299–300.

56 **McAdam JL, Dracup KA, White DB, Fontaine DK, Puntillo KA.** Symptom experiences of family members of intensive care unit patients at high risk for dying. *Crit Care Med* 2010;**38**:1078–85.

57 **Lautrette A, Ciroldi M, Ksibi H, Azoulay E.** End-of-life family conferences: rooted in the evidence. *Crit Care Med* 2006;**34**(11 Suppl):S364–72.

58 Lautrette A, Darmon M, Megarbane B, et al. A communication strategy and brochure for relatives of patients dying in the ICU. *N Engl J Med* 2007;**356**:469–78.

59 Myhren H, Ekeberg O, Stokland O. Satisfaction with communication in ICU patients and relatives: Comparisons with medical staffs' expectations and the relationship with psychological distress. *Patient Educ Couns* 2011;**85**:237–44.

60 Davidson JE. Time for a formal assessment, treatment, and referral structure for families of intensive care unit patients. *Crit Care Med* 2012;**40**:1675–6.

61 Davidson JE, Daly BJ, Agan D, Brady NR, Higgins PA. Facilitated sensemaking: a feasibility study for the provision of a family support program in the intensive care unit. *Crit Care Nurs Q* 2010;**33**:177–89.

62 Davidson JE. Facilitated sensemaking: a strategy and new middle-range theory to support families of intensive care unit patients. *Crit Care Nurse* 2010;**30**:28–39.

63 Garrouste-Orgeas M, Coquet I, Périer A, et al. Impact of an intensive care unit diary on psychological distress in patients and relatives. *Crit Care Med* 2012;**40**:2033–40.

64 Egerod I, Christensen D, Schwartz-Nielsen KH, Agard AS. Constructing the illness narrative: a grounded theory exploring patients' and relatives' use of intensive care diaries. *Crit Care Med* 2011;**39**:1922–8.

Chapter 10

Survival and Recovery: A Patient's Perspective

Cheryl Misak

Introduction

In 1998, I spent almost a month in an ICU with invasive group A *Streptococcus* infection and MOF, including severe ARDS.

By unlucky coincidence, I had got to the hospital very late. I had been to my general practitioner (GP) with some foot pain. When I awoke in the middle of the night, a few weeks later, with screaming pain in all my joints, she surmised that I might have some kind of arthritis. An appointment was made with a rheumatologist in a teaching hospital. The next day, I got the nasty 'flu' that my 6-year old had just recovered from, and I hunkered down with what I (and my GP) thought was an unfortunate double whammy. But, as I waited for my rheumatology appointment, I was in rapid decline. I should have realized that things were bad—that my kidneys were not functioning, for instance. With hindsight, I can see that my cognitive capacities were failing as well.

When I arrived at the rheumatologist's office, she took one look at me, put a blood pressure cuff around my arm, and declared that I had very little blood pressure. She called an ambulance to take me to the hospital's emergency room. They had a very difficult time getting a line in; my lungs failed, and I descended quickly into massive and MOF. Twice my husband was told that I wouldn't make it through the night. It was a roller coaster, but, in the end, I was what is charmingly called a 'big save.' I owe everything to those critical care physicians who worked night and day to secure my survival.

Much of the focus of this chapter is on what happens after that survival is secured—what happens when a patient leaves the ICU, with the intensivist's job apparently done. This topic must be an important one for intensivists. If it turned out, for instance, that they were very successful in getting their patients out the ICU door alive, only to find that some great number of them died in the coming weeks or had an astoundingly poor QoL in subsequent years, we would not count this as a success. Outcome measures, however, are thin on the ground and difficult to get a handle on. It is laudable that attempts like the systematic one found in this book are now being made.

Surviving

The critically ill undergo significant distress. Some of that is physical—pain, the intense discomfort that comes with ventilation, and extreme weakness. Some of that distress is mental. We know that ICU delirium is rampant in the critically ill patient population. This delirium has been (accurately in my view) described as 'nightmares often of a bizarre and extremely terrifying nature', hallucinations, and paranoid delusions—typically of a nurse or a doctor trying to rape, murder, or otherwise harm the patient.[1] I have suggested that what makes these phenomena especially terrifying and insidious is the fact that, unlike ordinary nightmares and more like paranoid delusions, they tend to occur in real time and to hook onto slices of external reality.[2] One takes an actual physician or nurse in the ICU, whips up a violent conspiracy theory around that person, and then has the conspiracy play itself out in the midst of actual conversations and medical procedures. It is the merging of reality and vicious invention that is most confusing and upsetting. One quite literally loses one's grip on what is true and what is false, because the true and the false are mixed together in one mess of experience.

I recently had an interesting external view on one of my worst delusions. After blowing out my knee on the tennis court, I had it reconstructed in the hospital at which I had been an ICU patient. One of the anaesthetists who had pulled me from death's door put in the spinal block. While I was waiting in pre-op, volume one of my thick file was sitting at my bedside, and I asked my anaesthetist if I could read it. It was a detailed account of my ICU stay, and one of the most interesting sections concerned my trying to effect what is quite gloriously understated in the literature as an 'unplanned extubation'.

The log makes it clear that things are going very badly—I'm in a psychotic state; my vital signs are plunging; my husband, who has for the first time in weeks been able to go home, is called; my brother is 'agitated'; and the writing is getting progressively more urgent and panicky. An anti-psychotic is dumped into me, which only makes things worse. Then, in capital letters, the following sentence appears: 'PATIENT IS TOLD THAT IF SHE RIPS THE TUBE OUT OF HER THROAT, <u>SHE WILL DIE</u>. PATIENT CEASES ATTEMPT TO SELF-EXTUBATE'.

What was going on in my mind at the time was the following. The physicians were having a drunken Christmas party (this was in April), at which they were being horribly abusive to the most vulnerable of the patients. They were parading us, naked, tied to our various machinery, through a gauntlet of verbal, physical, and sexual abuse. I was trying to escape.

To make my own attempt at understatement: being an ICU patient is not very pleasant. Indeed, as the relatively clear-headed thoughts started tumbling in after I returned to full consciousness, the following struck me forcibly. Dying is easy: it is the coming back that is unimaginably difficult. I was struck by the explicit and happy realization that it was highly unlikely that I would have to go through that again: another sinking into death was inevitable, but I would have to be horribly 'unlucky', I thought, to come back from it a second time.

Exiting the ICU

I was very anxious to get off the ventilator and then get out of the ICU. I was trying to cope with roving bouts of mental distress and harrowing psychotic episodes. It was still not clear to me whether certain of the nurses and physicians were trying to help me or kill me. It is no surprise that I wanted to get away from the scene of the imagined crimes. I lobbied my way off the ventilator and out of the ICU well before my physicians thought it desirable.

But, once I was moved to the ward, I found myself wishing I were back in the oasis of the ICU. My critical care physicians were busy hauling the next set of lives away from death's door. Save an occasional visit from one of the very special nurses, I was left in what seemed to me to be a precarious position. My room-mate and her biker friends were very loud, and the ward nurses were too busy to help me to the bathroom in the middle of the night. Indeed, they were irritated that I seemed not to know when the need was really upon me. It turns out that, if you have been catheterized for a month, the normal signals take a while to return.

It is hard to convey just how debilitated one is after an insult of this magnitude. When I regained consciousness, I was certain that it was only the ventilator mooring me to the bed and, once released from it, I would be able to get up and resume my life. But, when finally weaned, I could do precisely nothing. I was emaciated. Even sitting for a few minutes in a recovery chair, with all limbs fully supported, was near impossible. I spent much of that time marvelling at the discovery that one's lower leg muscles are very hard at work, even when on a footrest. It gives one a new appreciation of just what the body has to do to keep upright.

I lobbied to get myself out of the ward as well after just a couple of days, despite this too being thought not a wise idea. I very badly wanted to go home, and the physician into whose care I was moved said that I could leave only when I could walk from the bed to the door. I responded by insisting then and there to make the walk, with three people at my elbow, the room tilting and spinning around me, and my wasted legs somehow just managing the task. At the end, I felt like I had climbed Mt Everest.

I was allowed to leave. No doubt I was a difficult and strong-willed patient. I have written elsewhere on how problematic it is to take seriously the notion of patient autonomy in critical care medicine.[2,3] Perhaps my strong wishes should have been overridden. Nonetheless, I was on the way home, with all that entailed.

My husband was given strict instructions to take my temperature every few hours and to call an ambulance if it hit a certain degree or if one of a number of other things happened. But, apart from that, I was discharged into the hands of my very young and inexperienced GP. In an odd twist, my joints started to hurt, badly and symmetrically, a couple of weeks after I was released. The theory (translated into layman's language) is that my immune system was set on 'high' for a long time and did not reset itself perfectly. I rang the rheumatologist who had quite literally stopped me from dropping dead on her office floor, and she became the very effective manager of my health. Had I not had cause to reconnect with her, I would have been adrift, with countless issues to cope with, some serious and frightening.

Recovering

While every ICU patient of course will have a different profile, outcome studies are pouring in regarding the kinds of problems that travel along with those who have been critically ill.

Some of the problems have to do with the mind. It has been argued that ICU delirium of the kind I described previously 'may be as emotionally devastating as intraoperative awareness during anaesthesia'.[1] Both are associated with an elevated incidence of PTSD and depression in the weeks, and even years, after discharge.[4] Luckily, I had what I think of as only a whiff of PTS syndrome. Every time an ambulance went by, I was hit with a sinking feeling that all that **effort** would be expended to save one measly life. And, for a year after discharge, I had disrupted sleep. Every night, I fretted, half awake, half asleep, back in the ICU. These weren't nightmares, nor were they distressing. They were more like obsessive ruts from which I could not extract myself.

I was offered no heads-up about these phenomena when I was discharged and no follow-up either. It seems that this is a not-uncommon situation. Certainly, the steady stream of desperate emails I receive from ex-ICU patients (a paper of mine is posted on Wes Ely's Vanderbilt ICU Delirium website and comes up in internet searches on the topic) suggests to me that there are many survivors of critical illness, all over the world, who are not getting the counselling they need. My own emotional and psychological hangovers lasted for over a year and then went away entirely, perhaps helped by the fact that I started to write and give talks about ICU delirium. Other ex-ICU patients are far less lucky.

Some of the problems are mental in a different way. The last decade has produced many studies asserting that there is significant and long-lasting cognitive impairment after critical illness.

I have argued that it is very difficult to measure cognitive impairment in this patient population, given the potentially confounding factors of generalized weakness, depression, and PTSD. I have also argued that care must be taken not to generate destructive feedback loops in patients by suggesting to them that they are cognitively impaired.[5] Nonetheless, the brain is an organ, and it would be surprising if MOF had no impact on the brain. I certainly felt very 'fuzzy' for a long time, although it was hard to pull apart that fuzziness from all my other woes. This problem also dissipated after a year.

Other problems are more straightforwardly physical. There is growing evidence of systemic muscle injury in ventilated, critically ill patients.[6–8] This ICUAW is often disabling and long-lasting. To make matters worse, there is also evidence that the inability to engage in physical exercise might have negative effects on neurocognitive outcomes.[9,10]

There is also a significant amount of pain. Again, every patient's profile will differ. For my part, I had a troubling pain in my chest upon any upper body exercise. I felt that this must be simply due to scar tissue from the catheter that had gone into my heart. But the pain seemed to pull right from the heart—a worrying kind of sensation I had never experienced before. I had a crippling lung pain, again something not within the range of normal experience. And I had a vicious neuropathy. On the slightest bit of heat or exertion, a fire roared up my body, put out only by an application of ice.

The discharged ICU patient, I submit, is coping with rather a lot.

Rehabilitation and its obstacles

I took the rehabilitation project extremely seriously. I rejected the efforts of the physiotherapists I was referred to by my GP. They seemed not up to the task—they thought, for instance, that a transcutaneous electrical nerve stimulator (TENS) machine would, in a few weeks, sort out the neuropathy that was plaguing me. I could also see that the exercises they suggested were not going to be sufficient. Gentle range-of-motion exercise was not going to build up my absent muscle mass. I had run university track and had a lot of coaching as a tennis player, so I knew what kinds of pain one had to go through and could go through in order to strengthen oneself. I went through it as if I was training for the Olympics. I abandoned the TENS-wielding physiotherapists, got myself into a gym, connected up with serious personal trainers, and took freezing showers when the neuropathy clicked in.

There are countless obstacles in the way of rehabilitation. The various negative outcomes form themselves into a tightly woven cord of causal connections that provide an enormous disincentive to do what is necessary to get oneself back on the rails. We know that some patients never manage anything like a full recovery.[11] I will describe my own in an effort to bring those disincentives and obstacles into focus. I was back to work within weeks and, to the external world's eyes, functioning quite well. But, in fact, the road ahead was long and arduous. Indeed, although I have quite clearly made what anyone would count as a full recovery, I still find myself with an endless set of acute tendon issues, far above the normal for ageing athletes. This may well be a hangover, I'm told, of the syndrome that gets called ICUAW.

The neuropathy was a real barrier in the way of exercise. The drugs I was given to try to dampen it made me very sleepy—not something conducive to physical activity. I declined to take them and learned to tolerate the pain, which was on a slow, but downward, trajectory. I was grateful for any opportunity to exercise in cold water—running through the Maine surf, for instance, 2 months after discharge.

I also had lung pain whenever I tried to push myself. It was akin to the lung-bursting sensation when you post a best time in a middle-distance race. I was able to draw on that track experience and surmise that this was an acceptable kind of pain. But, after your lungs have been through severe ARDS and your heart has been racing at an unthinkable pace for weeks on end, you don't know for certain just what is dangerous and what is not. That is, it is not only the pain, etc. that gets in the way of rehabilitation, but also the worry about whether what you are doing is causing further damage to an already badly damaged body. Insecurity and anxiety abound about whether there might be permanent effects from having one's organs in acute decline and from having had a truly astounding radiation load of chest X-rays and computed tomography (CT) scans.

Generalized weakness and fatigue also stand in the way of rehabilitation. Eight months post-discharge, I was on sabbatical in Cambridge England where I attempted to take up my old sport—real tennis, the ancient and body-breaking game from which modern tennis evolved. I was, by this time, well on the road to recovery and back on the ordinary tennis court. But moving to more taxing activity was debilitating. I would return home from a game, unable to do anything but sit in the living room, with the walls pressing in on me. The fatigue was overwhelming. My English GP tutted and said that I was not listening to my body. But, after you've been critically ill, your body does not give you signals you can recognize, interpret, and understand. Your body speaks a foreign language for a long time.

Finally, the cognitive, emotional, and psychological troubles described previously do not produce an ideal state of mind in which to get off the couch and put some brutally hard work into physical rehabilitation. When one's normal life seems less vivid and less compelling than one's abnormal quasi-life in the ICU, energy and activity are not the natural upshots.

Intervening post-discharge

Much excellent work is being done on interventions within the ICU that might aid recovery, such as early mobilization and sedative interruption.[12,13] Although the evidence has yet to be gathered, it seems plausible, to say the least, that post-discharge interventions are also important. Indeed, this is the point I most want to make: If critically ill patients are to achieve something like a genuinely full recovery, significant and varied supports and interventions must be put in place after they leave the ICU. Patients need information, encouragement, and access to the experts.

Intensivists, I suggest, should be speaking to their patients about the need to rehabilitate, about how to do that safely, and about the obstacles likely to be faced in the particular circumstances. This encouragement is not always on offer once one leaves the ICU. I cannot count the number of times I had GPs and specialists at excellent teaching hospitals, on two continents, tell me that I seemed not to understand the severity of what had happened to me and that I must lower my expectations of what kind of recovery would be possible. The inclination to protect and to rest after such a traumatic and severe insult is natural. But the evidence is mounting that this is mistaken. Patients need to be encouraged to push themselves in the face of all sorts of apparent reasons to not do so.

There is, it seems, an ever-present tension for all those fine intensivists who care about what happens to their patients down the line. Patients leave the ICU with varied and significant comorbidities, with weakness, with the experience of having looked mortality in the eye, and with a great deal of uncertainty about how the future will unfold. How does an intensivist encourage the patient to push the boundaries of what seems possible, yet not set up the patient for failure? There is no easy answer to this question. But what can be said is that only by thinking through an appropriate approach, for each individual patient, is the intensivist likely to get it right. That is, there is a duty that must be shouldered by ICU physicians to start this conversation with each of their patients, for only they know what those patients have been through and only they know what the outcomes of their particular critical illness are likely to be.

It also seems clear that supports need to be made available for discharged ICU patients. When I had my knee reconstructed, I was immediately locked into an impressive regime of mandatory and closely supervised pre- and post- rehab. It seems rather curious that rehabilitative supports in place for knee surgery patients so significantly outstrip those in place for patients who suffer from the much more debilitating ICUAW and other serious problems post-critical illness. Perhaps there is a lesson to be learned from the orthopaedic surgeons. Patients should be given a roster of physiotherapists and physical trainers who have experience and knowledge about what is required; they should be told to put those supports in place immediately; they should be told to think of rehab, both physical and psychological, as critical and important.

All this leads, however, to another conundrum for intensivists. They are focused on the rather important job of saving critically endangered lives. It seems too much to ask that they follow their patients with their diverse, and perhaps less interesting, problems after discharge as well. But the hard fact is that the awareness of, and knowledge about, problems such as ICUAW reside largely within the critical care community. That community and its expertise needs to be somehow accessible to patients post-discharge.

Years after my own discharge, I was still experiencing residual breathlessness and wheezing when engaged in (very strenous) exercise. I was seen by a respirologist, who, after a CT scan and pulmonary function tests, told me that I was as recovered as I was going to be and that I should simply stop trying to do so much and aim so high. His resident slipped me the email address of another respirologist in town—one who was at the very forefront of work on ICU outcomes research. She advised me of the systemic muscle injuries suffered by ICU patients and suggested that my problem might be due to weak diaphragmatic muscles. (It has since been shown that PMV promotes significant diaphragmatic atrophy and contractile dysfunction.)[14,15]

I took myself to an excellent physical trainer and asked him to teach me how to breathe from the diaphragm and then push me hard on the treadmill. The results started to accrue quickly—after a few intense weeks, I could see some difference and at the end of the 12-week programme, the matter was entirely resolved. It felt like magic. But it was just the effect of highly specialized and intelligently delivered information by an intensivist who knew about outcomes.

Conclusion

I was lucky, not just in landing in one of the best ICUs in the country with first-rate physicians and nurses who went the extra mile for me. I was also lucky that in my baggage were decades of good health, sport and fitness, and education. That is, I entered the ICU with some markers of physiologic and cognitive reserve. The idea that such reserve is a principal determinant of outcomes is gaining traction (see Chapter 28).[16]

The idea raises some interesting and troubling questions. For one thing, the ability to measure reserve is in its infancy and it might stay there for a long time. But were we able to measure reserve and were we able to predict outcomes on the basis of such measurements, then such knowledge would have to be used with care. It has already been shown that physicians' predictions of the likely outcome for patients is correlated with the provision or withdrawal of life support, independent of the facts about the patient's severity of illness.[17] It does not take much imagination to see the moral problems that would flood in about predictions based on reserve. Are the uneducated to receive less life support than the educated? Are those who come in with excellent physiologic reserves to get special treatment?

The question of how to ensure that individuals have adequate physiologic and cognitive reserves (what we philosophers might call well-being) is one for public policy. So is the question of how to distribute scarce ICU resources. The job of critical care physicians includes participating in the latter public deliberation. But their primary job surely is to take their patients, with whatever reserves or deficits they have, and ensure the optimal outcome for each patient. That includes putting in place the structures and programmes that will help them to rehabilitate to the best state they can achieve.

The fact that something like genuinely full recoveries are possible, given the kinds of catastrophic medical events in question, is astounding and heartening. Helping patients to achieve them should be a core clinical aspiration of critical care medicine.

References

1 **Schelling G, Stoll C, Haller M,. et al.** Health-related quality of life and post-traumatic stress disorder in survivors of the acute respiratory distress syndrome. *Crit Care Med* 1998;**26**:651–9.

2 **Misak C.** ICU psychosis and patient autonomy: some thoughts from the inside. *J Med Philos* 2005; **30**:411–30.

3 **Misak C.** The critical care experience: a patient's view. *Am J Respir Crit Care Med* 2004;**170**:357–9.

4 **Jones C, Griffiths R, Humphris G, Skirrow P.** Memory, delusions, and the development of acute post-traumatic stress disorder-related symptoms after intensive care. *Crit Care Med* 2001;**29**:573–80.

5 **Misak C.** Cognitive dysfunction after critical illness: measurement, rehabilitation, and disclosure, *Crit Care* 2009;**13**:312.

6 **Herridge M, Cheung A, Tansey C, et al.** One-year outcomes in survivors of the acute respiratory distress syndrome *N Engl J Med* 2003;**348**:683–93.

7 **Schweickert WD, Hall J.** ICU acquired weakness. *Chest* 2007;**131**:1541–9.

8 **Stevens RD, Dowdy DW, Michaels RK, et al**, Neuromuscular dysfunction acquired in critical illness: a systematic review. *Int Care Med* 2007;**31**:157–61.

9 **Kramer AF, Colcombe SJ, McAuley E, Scalf PE, Erickson KI.** Fitness, aging, and neurocognitive function. *Neurobiol Again* 2005;**26**(Suppl 1):124–7.

10 **Colcombe SJ, Kramer AF, McAuley E, Ericson KI, Scalf P.** Neurocognitive aging and cardiovascular fitness: recent findings and future directions. *J Mol Neurosci* 2004;**24**:9–14.

11 **Barnato AE, Albert SM, Angus DC, Lave JR, Degenholtz HB.** Disability among elderly survivors of mechanical ventilation. *Am J Respir Crit Care Med* 2011;**183**:1037–42.

12 **Schweickert WD, Pohlman M, Pohlman AS, et al.** Early physical and occupational therapy in mechanically ventilated, critically ill patients: a randomized controlled trial. *Lancet* 2009;**373**:1874–82.

13 **Hough CL, Needham DM.** The role of future longitudinal studies in ICU survivors: understanding determinants and pathophysiology of weakness and muscular dysfunction. *Curr Opn Crit Care* 2007; **13**:489–96.

14 **Petrof BJ, Jaber S, Matecki S.** Ventilator-induced diaphragmatic dysfunction. *Curr Opin Crit Care* 2010; **16**:19–25.

15 **Powers SK, Kavazis AN, Levine S.** Prolonged mechanical ventilation alters diaphragmatic structure and function. *Crit Care Med* 2009;**37**:347–53.

16 **Stern Y.** Cognitive reserve in ageing and Alzheimer's disease. *Lancet Neurol* 2012;**11**:1006–12.

17 **Rocker G, Cook D, Sjokvist P, et al.** Clinician predictions of intensive care unit mortality. *Crit Care Med* 2004;**32**:1149–54.

Chapter 11

One Family's Perspective on the Legacy of Critical Illness

David Dyzenhaus

Introduction

I will, in this chapter, outline one family perspective on the legacy of critical illness. Since my experience in this regard has a seamless relationship with the experience of the actual illness, I will start with that.

Our story

On 1 April 1998, my wife Cheryl Misak was admitted to the ICU of St Michael's Hospital Toronto in a state of septic shock, the result of MOF. She was 38 years old and had, during the time I had known her, about 14 years, enjoyed excellent physical health. She is also one of the more psychologically robust people I know. When she became ill, we interpreted her illness as a bad flu; our 7-year-old son had had a Strep A infection the week or so before, and it turned out that Cheryl's infection was one of the lethal versions of Strep A.

But, while she was clearly feeling very unwell, she made little of it, other than taking to her bed and making only desultory attempts at eating. On the day she was admitted to the ICU, she was due to see a rheumatologist at one of our major teaching hospitals, as she had been suffering from severe pain in her joints just prior to her 'flu'. That morning, I realized that something more than flu was amiss with her, although she was insisting that she would be able to get on a plane later that day to attend a conference in the US.

I phoned our family physician and asked her whether I should call an ambulance and take Cheryl to emergency. Our family physician was young and inexperienced. She had seen Cheryl earlier that week when Cheryl had been so weak that she could hardly walk. But she advised me just to go to the appointment with the rheumatologist. Later that morning, desperate to talk to someone other than Cheryl, whom I did not want to worry with my concerns, I phoned my sister in South Africa and told her that I thought Cheryl was dying. I was in the middle of this conversation when a taxi arrived to take us to the hospital and I had to terminate it, as Cheryl was somehow proceeding out of the house and down the stairs of our porch.

Fortunately, the rheumatologist gave Cheryl a quick examination and summoned an ambulance to take her to the emergency department of St Michael's Hospital. An emergency department is a bewildering place, a flurry of noisy activity as health care workers rush to and fro, dealing with patients who range from those who can hardly move or speak to those who are raving in some drug- or alcohol-produced frenzy and so have to be physically restrained. It is thus very difficult to get any information. But I at least had the feeling that Cheryl now had help immediately at hand. I set about phoning my brother-in-law, who lives in Toronto, and various friends.

Our children, aged 7 and 5, were at school and daycare, and the rheumatologist had told me that Cheryl was 'very sick' and that I should not leave the hospital. So I had to set up childcare and was able to count on my brother-in-law being able to move into our house for a few days to take care of our children. I also phoned my parents-in-law, who live in Alberta, and told them that I might have to ask them to come to Toronto to help.

Admitted to the ICU

When Cheryl was admitted to the ICU, I felt better. The ICU is bewildering in its own way, but it is quiet, compared to the emergency room; activity there is constant but more measured, unless there is an emergency that requires significant activity around a patient.

That night, I did not sleep. I visited Cheryl frequently, and she seemed weak but cheerful. However, it was also clear that she was getting progressively weaker, and, in the early morning, the physicians told me that she would have to be intubated and anaesthetized, as her lungs were in a state of collapse, her kidneys had ceased to work, and her blood pressure had dropped alarmingly. I tried to get more information from them about the prognosis. But they were understandably reluctant to make predictions.

On the one hand, I knew that things were about as serious as they could be. This knowledge was confirmed to me when a woman in the ICU waiting room, whose very elderly father was living out his last hours in the ICU, threw her arms around me and burst into tears. She told me that she was a nurse and that, while she was very sad that her father had only hours to live, she felt more sorry for me, as my young wife was in the same position. I realized that her fellow nurses in the ICU had told her things that I was not privy to.

On the other hand, the obvious competence and kindness of the physicians and nurses gave me some sense of calm, and I had, throughout the 3 weeks that followed and a roller coaster ride that seemed to go more down than up, a faith that, if anyone could survive this episode, it would be Cheryl. I maintained this faith, even as she swelled to the point where she was unrecognizable, except for her eyebrows.

Over these 3 weeks, I had as much help as it is possible to have in this kind of situation. My parents-in-law came, as did my two sisters from South Africa and the UK. Our friends and relations in Toronto, as well as a group of neighbours, helped in various ways. I often wondered, during this time and since, how it would have been possible to manage if I had not been able to count so completely on so many people or on an employer (we are both academics at the University of Toronto) who was, in general, prepared to do everything possible to help.

During this time, I had no clear sense of what was happening with Cheryl. Even though the ICU is a much calmer place most of the time than an emergency department, the physicians are extraordinarily busy. They do not have the time to tend to the needs of the anxious relatives in the ICU waiting room. I found that the best source of information and comfort was the nurse who was charged with looking after Cheryl. But it was also clear to me that interrogating either the physicians or the nurses was largely unproductive. Sometimes, they just did not have answers. At other times, it was clear that they thought that that the answers they had were not good for me to know, and they might well have been right, as irrational hope is all that sustains one in these circumstances.

When Cheryl started to improve gradually, I became convinced that she would make a complete recovery. Although the physicians intimated that things could be very different, they did not know Cheryl, and so did not know that she regards life's obstacles as problems that require speedy and determined resolution. However, just what that resolution would be was a complete mystery, and, as far as I can recall, we were not offered any clues as to how to solve it.

Discharge from the ICU

When Cheryl had recovered sufficiently to be taken off the ventilator and sent to the general ward for a couple of days, and then finally home, I was, of course, immensely relieved. But I also felt stranded. Cheryl emerged from the blimpish caricature of herself during the worst period as a stick-thin person with wasted, indeed, ravaged muscles, and lungs that were barely functioning. She was so weak that it was difficult to imagine that it would be long before something happened that would force a return to hospital. And the only concrete advice we had was that, if she spiked a temperature, she should go to emergency.

Quite what happened during the first 6 or so weeks after Cheryl returned home is almost a complete blur to me, whereas I recall the 3 weeks of the ICU with great clarity. I know that I must have been juggling tending to Cheryl, who is not the easiest person in the world to tend to, with tending to our children, as those who had so generously dropped their lives to help us went back to their own concerns.

In retrospect, I know that Cheryl, in a way before she was capable of doing so, began, bit by bit, to push herself both physically and cognitively along the path to recovery. I mentioned that she is difficult to tend to for a reason. Cheryl hates feeling helpless so does not like the kind of attention that one gets when one is in fact helpless. It is that character trait that I firmly believe made it possible for her to recover in the way that she did. She addressed her recovery like a marathon runner, setting out her training schedule, preparing to go through the various 'walls' that would seem to impede progress. She did, as we have learned over the years, precisely what she had to do but which no one had told us that she should do.

It seems obvious that we would have been better off both if we could have had the benefit of being told on her release from hospital what it is that she had to do and if we had some ongoing monitoring and advice during her recovery. But I often wonder, just as I wonder how people manage without supportive family and friends, what difference such information and help can make if one does not have the character trait that permits one to surmount what seem, with good reason, to be insurmountable obstacles. Nevertheless, it is clear that such information and help should be given. It seems irrational that, after all of the work that dedicated physicians and nurses put into saving someone's life, when they do in fact succeed, more is not done after the patient leaves the ICU to make the most of their success.

Conclusion

Our story has a happy ending. Other than the fact that Cheryl was left with rheumatoid arthritis, she did make a complete recovery. Our children have barely any memory of this time. Cheryl's parents remain shaken to this day, and I vastly underestimated at that time that I summoned them across Canada to come and help me just how traumatic it is for a parent to contemplate the death of a child.

I was not unaccustomed to hospitals, illness, and death at the time Cheryl fell ill, as both my parents were deceased. My mother had chronic arthritis from the age of 3, and that and associated problems meant that she was in and out of hospital, including ICUs, until she died at the age of 55, and my father had died at the age of 67 of lung cancer. However, the experience of watching as my wife seemed to be slipping away was profoundly unsettling in a way that my experience with my parents was not. I am still sometimes seized with a sense of panic in regard to Cheryl, for example, when she travels by plane without me. In some way, our family is even closer because of this experience. A sense of the fragility of life is not a bad thing when one is generally very well off. However, there is no way that the experience is one that one can be grateful for.

In our neighbourhood, we know someone quite well whose sister's teenaged son died at the time Cheryl was ill after contracting the same kind of infection. The legacy for our neighbour's sister is clearly one of complete devastation. And there must be many states in between our happy one and that.

Part 2

Chronic Organ Dysfunction Following Critical Illness

Chapter 12

Introduction: Chronic Organ Dysfunction Following Critical Illness

Greet Hermans

General ICU management and technical organ support treatment have dramatically improved over the last decades. This resulted in the survival of patients who suffered from severe illness with failure of multiple organs systems during their ICU stay. The initial wave of enthusiasm, triggered by increased survival, has been tempered by a growing number of reports on hampered recovery of various organ systems after ICU stay.

Intubation and MV are part of daily ICU practice. If the patient suffered from ARDS, pulmonary dysfunction up to 1 year after the acute event is common although, most often, not even the major function limiting factor in these patients. The majority of ventilated patients will be easily weaned, but a subgroup will experience difficult weaning and receive PMV. Tracheostomy is a procedure frequently performed in these cases. Some patients may remain ventilator-dependent and are transferred to long-term care facilities. A substantial amount of these patients will eventually be weaned, but significant mortality stands in this group and removal of tracheostomy or endotracheal tubes (ETTs) may result in local complications. These include tracheal stenosis and vocal cord dysfunction. Troublesome scars may remain in the neck. A small subset of persisting ventilator-dependent patients may need home ventilation. This requires extensive supportive home care and therefore is not an obvious decision.

Reperfusion strategies and mechanical and pharmacological support also clearly improved survival, following acute myocardial injury. These survivors, however, have a clearly increased risk for further cardiovascular events and chronic heart failure. Some of them may be transplant candidates, but the majority will have impaired functional status and long-term survival. Surviving an episode of acute kidney injury (AKI) is also associated with long-term increased mortality. Whether this relationship is causal is unclear. Increased incidence of CKD and end-stage renal failure is clearly present in these patients. After burn injury, patients may be confronted with scars that may cause functional loss and disability. They may suffer from persisting pain and loss of sensitivity. In addition, altered appearance may cause psychological problems.

This transition of patients to a stage of persisting organ dysfunction may have major impact on the individual patient's physical and mental health status, as it may contribute to decreased functional capacity and decreased QoL. It poses a burden on the patient's family. It also involves a persisting increased hazard of long-term mortality. It represents a financial burden to society due to utilization of health care resources and costs and by affecting re-incorporation of the survivors in the professionally active society. Understanding the incidence and impact of persisting organ dysfunction as well as risk factors for its development are the first steps towards developing strategies for prevention and organizing optimal care for these patients. In the following chapter, the relevant aspects will be discussed.

Chapter 13

Chronic Multiple Organ Dysfunction

Kevin M. Fischer and Shannon S. Carson

Introduction

Advances in intensive care have led to a large and growing group of patients who survive the initial phase of critical illness but cannot be weaned from intensive therapies. They develop one or often multiple organ dysfunctions as a result of their acute illness or injury, and these can be layered on top of chronic pre-existing conditions. They can remain dependent upon life-sustaining therapies, such as MV, RRT, vasopressors or inotropes, enteral or parenteral feeding, and IV antibiotics, for weeks or months. This condition of chronic multiple organ dysfunction is frequently referred to as CCI. This is not merely a continuation of acute illness but a discrete syndrome of physiologic abnormalities and metabolic dysfunction.[1] The protective physiologic adaptations intended for surviving an acute illness or injury are not well suited for a prolonged critical event.[2] These derangements serve to slow or preclude recovery in CCI.[3]

The group of patients with CCI is large and growing. At any one time, there are an estimated 100 000 such patients in the US alone, at a cost of $20 billion per year.[4,5] With an ageing population and increasing rates of MV, this figure is projected to grow. Among all ICU patients requiring MV, 5–10% will progress to CCI.[6-8] Patients who are at the highest risk of developing CCI are the elderly with multiple comorbidities, although all age groups can be affected. In a study of 260 patients who required 21 days or more of MV at five geographically diverse tertiary care centre ICUs, the mean age was 55 ± 17; 41% were female, with an average of one comorbid condition and diverse admitting diagnoses.[9] Risk factors for proceeding from acute critical illness to CCI include: ARDS, sepsis, shock, and MOF syndrome.[10] Although many conditions, including ALI, end-stage COPD, and end-stage CHF, can lead to PMV, progression to chronic multiple organ dysfunction, or CCI, is usually associated with severe systemic inflammatory conditions. In addition to dependence on life-sustaining therapies, clinical features of CCI include profound weakness, distinctive neuroendocrine changes, increased vulnerability to infection, brain dysfunction, skin breakdown, nutritional deficiencies, and significant symptom burden (see Figure 13.1).[1] As a result of persistent multiple organ dysfunctions, these patients have significant long-term functional and cognitive limitations, require a high level of informal caregiver assistance, and have a high mortality rate.[11-16] This chapter will summarize the clinical features of chronic multiple organ dysfunction and how those features relate to patient outcome. The discussion will focus on organ dysfunction other than ALI, as this is presented elsewhere in this text.

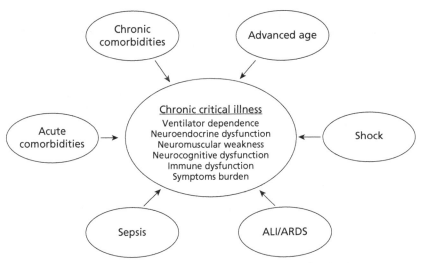

Fig. 13.1 Conceptual framework for the syndrome of CCI. Risk factors for developing CCI include age, acute and chronic comorbidities, sepsis, ALI/ARDS, and shock. The hallmark of CCI is prolonged ventilator dependence; however, CCI is a clinical syndrome, encompassing multiple characteristic organs and systems.

Clinical features of chronic multiple organ dysfunction

Neuroendocrine changes

The neuroendocrine stress response is a dynamic process, involving multiple hormonal alterations, with distinct features in the acute and chronic phase of critical illness.[17–19] The neuroendocrine changes in acute critical illness work to shift energy and resources from anabolic to catabolic pathways, in order to support vital organ function and acute inflammation.[20] Prolonged critical illness results in a fall in neuroendocrine hormone levels, leading to decreased target organ function, prolonged catabolism, and impaired anabolism. The pronounced catabolic state that ensues leads to muscle atrophy, loss of lean body mass (LBM), increased adiposity, and anasarca, which together impede recovery from critical illness.[21]

At the onset of critical illness, cortisol levels are increased through the actions of increased adrenocorticotropic hormone (ACTH) release, which in turn is influenced by corticotropin-releasing hormone, cytokines, and the noradrenergic system. Hypercortisolism acutely shifts carbohydrate, fat, and protein metabolism, so that energy is available to vital organs and anabolism is delayed.[17] In CCI, ACTH levels fall; however, cortisol remains elevated in most patients, leading to prolonged catabolism and impaired healing. Cortisol levels remain elevated despite low ACTH due to input from other unknown peripheral sources. Pregnenolone, which is a precursor to cortisol and androgens, is preferentially diverted to cortisol production, leading to androgen deficiency and resultant muscle wasting, impaired anabolism, and impaired wound healing.[20] Eventually though, as critical illness progresses, cortisol levels often drop in a condition called adrenal exhaustion.[22] The resultant relative hypocortisolism of CCI affects nearly every organ and system, increasing morbidity and mortality. Many authors recommend replacement of corticosteroids when adrenal insufficiency is demonstrated; however, there is considerable debate regarding timing and interpretation of testing as well as therapeutic regimens required.[23,24]

During acute critical illness, there are changes in peripheral thyroid hormone metabolism and availability. Peripheral conversion of T4 to T3 is impaired, leading to low T3. There is often failure of thyroid-stimulating hormone (TSH) to appropriately increase in the face of low T3, suggesting impaired feedback in the hypothalamic-pituitary-thyroid axis during critical illness. Decreased TSH initially leads to further decreased thyroid hormone action, which teleologically acts to conserve energy and resources required to survive acute illness.[20] As patients progress to CCI, there is a loss of pulsatile TSH secretions, producing continued hypothyroidism. Chronic hypothyroidism leads to neuropsychiatric changes, fluid retention, oedema, relative hypothermia, decreased ventilator drive, gastrointestinal hypomotility, anaemia, glucose intolerance, and malabsorption.[20] When and how to replace thyroid hormone in critical illness is debated.[25]

In critical illness, pulsatile and interpulsatile GH levels initially rise. In addition, IGF-1 levels are low as a function of peripheral resistance to GH.[17] The fall in IGF-1, coupled with the rise in GH, augments the lipolytic and insulin-antagonizing effects of GH while inhibiting the anabolic effect of IGF-1.[26] As acute critical illness progresses to prolonged critical illness around day 7–10, there is a marked decrease in pulsatile and interpulsatile GH levels, leading to even lower IGF-1 levels. These changes persist, leading to worsening of the catabolic state in CCI. The blunted GH secretion of prolonged critical illness in noted in both males and females, but the pulsatile GH levels are more disorderly in men, with a differential decrease in testosterone levels.[27] It is unclear how these abnormalities impact sexual function in survivors. Up to 44% of survivors of critical illness report sexual dysfunction, but it is difficult to dissociate the endocrine abnormalities from other issues, including underlying comorbidities and vascular abnormalities, medications, and psychosocial issues.[28,29] In one small study, sexual dysfunction in survivors was associated with PTSD symptoms and not age, gender, or length of ICU stay.[30]

Bone metabolism is profoundly affected during critical illness. In as early as the first 24 hours of critical illness, bone turnover is markedly elevated.[31] Furthermore, it appears that bone formation is also impaired in critical illness.[32] Therefore, in critical illness, bone resorption is accelerated and skeletal reparative mechanisms are inhibited.[33] The cause of ICU-related metabolic bone disease is multifactorial, and high-turnover bone loss cannot downregulate until the stress of critical illness has dissipated. Factors involved in the bone disease of critical illness include the effects of particular cytokines, prolonged immobilization, catabolic hormone excess, medications used in the ICU, and vitamin D deficiency.[33] The combined effect of bone loss and inhibited repair places survivors of critical illness at higher risk of fracture. Several studies have demonstrated that markers of bone resorption can be decreased with IV bisphosphonate, but it is unclear if this will result in a decreased risk of fracture.[34–36]

Neuromuscular changes

ICUAW affects a large number of patients admitted to the ICU.[37] ICUAW may occur within 3 days of the onset of septic shock and within 10 days of the onset of systemic inflammatory response syndrome (SIRS).[38–40] ICUAW is an acquired muscular weakness that includes myopathy, neuropathy, neuromuscular transmission defects, or any combination of these. This weakness prolongs weaning from MV and impairs physical rehabilitation, as it affects both limb and respiratory muscles.[41] Definitive ICU risk factors for ICUAW include sepsis, SIRS, renal replacement, hyperglycaemia, and MOF, while the role of corticosteroids, NMBAs, and benzodiazepines is less certain.[42] ICUAW occurs in 60% of ARDS patients, 70% of SIRS patients, and 100% of patients with SIRS and multiorgan dysfunction.[41] The gold standard for diagnosis of ICUAW is EMG and muscle biopsy; however, the clinical utility of these tests is not known. A clinical scoring system for the diagnosis of ICUAW, called the Medical Research Council (MRC) sum score, is mainly used for research purposes and is rather non-specific.[43]

ICUAW is composed of CIP, CIM, or a combination of the two, called CINM.[44] CIP is a disorder of peripheral motor nerve axonal dysfunction. Autopsy studies of patients with CIP show degeneration of motor and sensory nerves that supply the limbs and respiratory system.[45] The pathophysiology of CIP is unclear, and several theories have been advanced, including sepsis-related disturbances in microcirculation due to inflammatory cytokines, hyperglycaemia and oedema, as well as possible direct cytokine-related injury to peripheral nerves.[41] CIM is an acute primary myopathy whose spectrum extends from pure functional impairment, with normal histology, to atrophy and necrosis.[46] The pathophysiology of CIM is complex, involving metabolic, inflammatory, and bioenergetic alterations.[41] The long-term prognosis may be better for patients with CIM, compared to patients with CIP.[47]

Prevention and treatment of ICUAW have largely been supportive until recently. There is evidence to support new approaches to prevent ICUAW. Early mobilization of ventilated patients has been shown to prevent the onset and limit the severity of muscle wasting in one study where patients began receiving PT and OT within 72 hours of MV.[48] In two other studies, early mobilization of mechanically ventilated patients was associated with decreased length of hospital stay.[49,50] Intensive insulin therapy (IIT), with a target blood glucose range of 80–110 mg/dL, was shown to reduce the incidence of CIP/CIM in two recent studies of medical ICU patients.[51,52] The role of corticosteroids and neuromuscular blockers in ICUAW remains controversial. Early studies suggested that both are risk factors; however, more recent data bring this into question.[53] The impact of corticosteroids may be manifest through hyperglycaemia, which could be modulated by better glucose control through insulin therapy.[54] Neuromuscular blockers may have minimal risk when used in smaller doses and for shorter periods of time.[55,56] A bundled-care approach may provide the best method of preventing ICUAW. The ABCDE bundle includes systematic, spontaneous awakening and breathing coordination, attention to the choice of sedation, delirium monitoring, and early mobility and exercise.[57] Lastly, electrical muscle stimulation (EMS) may preserve muscle mass of critically ill patients.[58,59]

The impact of ICUAW in survivors of prolonged critical illness might depend on each patient's baseline functional capabilities and degree of physiologic reserve. Although age has not been conclusively determined to be an independent risk factor for developing ICUAW,[42,43] it could impact recovery. Younger patients who were in good health and fully functional prior to illness may have a greater degree of functional reserve and rehabilitation capacity.[60] Older patients or patients with severe chronic comorbidities may have less rehabilitation potential, especially as they are more susceptible to intervening medical complications and hospital readmissions.[61] In a recent longitudinal study of physical function in elderly patients experiencing critical illness, patients with the highest degree of physical dysfunction, following critical illness, had already been on a trajectory of declining function leading up to their acute illness. It is also important to consider how lasting physical dysfunction might impact the QoL in survivors. Patients with higher levels of prior function may have more difficulty adapting psychologically to abrupt changes in their condition than patients with more limited baseline function.

Immunologic changes and infection

Infections are the leading cause of mortality in CCI and contribute greatly to morbidity.[62] Infection is associated with difficulty weaning from MV, as fever and hypermetabolism increase ventilator demand.[63] The sepsis syndrome also induces mitochondrial dysfunction in the muscles of the diaphragm, further impairing ventilator weaning.[64,65] Patients undergoing acute and chronic critical care face the 'triple threat' of risk of infection: barrier breaches such as indwelling catheters and skin breakdown, exposure to virulent and multiple drug-resistant pathogens in the care environment, and the proposed syndrome of 'immune exhaustion' from critical illness and underlying comorbidities.[62]

Barrier breaches are common in critical illness. Decubitus ulcers form breaks in the skin barrier that are difficult to treat due to impaired wound healing and poor nutritional status of CCI patients. Iatrogenic barrier breaches are common and include IV catheters, urinary drainage catheters, nasogastric tubes, and tracheotomy sites. IV catheters and urinary drainage catheters may become colonized, leading to introduction of pathogens. Nasogastric tubes are associated with sinusitis and may be associated with aspiration events.[62,66] Patients undergoing PMV often have increased secretions, colonized lower respiratory tract, endotracheal and glottis mucosal inflammation, and impaired mucociliary clearance, all of which may enhance the risk of infection.[67]

Chronically critically ill patients are exposed to, and colonized with, virulent and multidrug-resistant organisms in both the acute care and long-term care facilities. Frequently encountered organisms include meticillin-resistant *Staphylococcus aureus*, vancomycin-resistant *Enterococcus*, Gram-negative enteric organisms, *Candida* species, and *Clostridium difficile*.[10,63,68] These organisms may be transmitted patient-to-patient or caregiver-to-patient. Once colonization occurs, nosocomial pathogens can replace normal flora and contaminate indwelling devices, making them difficult to eradicate.

The cumulative effects of critical illness and underlying comorbidities lead to impaired host defence. Following the initial 'cytokine storm' in the first few days of sepsis, a state of immunosuppression develops, potentially increasing the risk of new infection in patients with prolonged critical illness.[69] Further, in the course of prolonged critical illness, the patient may develop 'immune exhaustion', a proposed term to describe 'the potentially disabling effects of depleted, dysfunctional, or inhibited immune resources that may impair defence against pathogens'.[62] A prolonged critical illness leads to accumulation of other debilities which hamper the immune response to infection, including nutritional deficiency, micronutrient deficiency, protein depletion, and mitochondrial dysfunction. Current strategies to limit inflammatory response in sepsis have not clearly demonstrated improved outcomes.[70–72] It is unclear if an overly exuberant immune response to infection is the main driver of poor outcomes or if later sepsis-induced immune suppression is to blame. Some postulate that targeted pro-inflammatory interventions may be beneficial in sepsis, which would change the current paradigm of anti-inflammatory therapy for sepsis.[69]

Prevention and treatment of infections in acute and chronic critical care have been well studied. Multiple studies have demonstrated successful efforts to reduce the incidence of catheter-related bloodstream infections, ventilator-associated pneumonia (VAP), drug-resistant organism transmission, *Clostridium difficile* infections, and catheter-associated urinary tract infections.[73–82] Process of care should be systematized to maximize the use of essential preventive measures such as hand hygiene, isolation, removal of unnecessary indwelling devices, judicious use of antibiotics, and best practices for maintaining skin integrity.[83] Indeed, guidelines for the prevention of infection have been released.[84–89] When infection is suspected, source identification and control should focus first on possible line sepsis, pneumonia, and *Clostridium difficile* colitis, which account for the majority of infections.[62]

Neurocognitive and psychiatric dysfunction

High rates of neurocognitive dysfunction during and following critical illness have been observed.[13,90–94] This dysfunction may persist for months to years and may be permanent, impacting

QoL, the ability to return to work, and overall functional ability.[95] Delirium and coma are common in the acute and chronic phase of critical illness; however, more subtle dysfunction, including executive function, memory, and attention, are also frequently observed. Even in the absence of delirium, ICU patients frequently display neurocognitive dysfunction in both acute illness and during recovery. In one study of 30 non-sedated, non-delirious patients with more than 6 days of MV, 100% had impaired executive function and 67% had impaired memory during their acute illness; at 2-month follow-up, 50% had impaired executive function and 31% had impaired memory.[91] The mechanism of neurocognitive impairment is not entirely understood but likely includes repeat episodes of delirium, hypoxia, hypotension, glucose dysregulation, metabolic derangements, inflammation, and the effects of sedatives and narcotics.[95–97] These factors may more greatly impact patients with pre-existing vulnerabilities, including mild cognitive impairment, dementia, or prior traumatic brain injury (TBI).[95] Premorbid cognitive dysfunction alone though does not account for the high rates of post-ICU cognitive dysfunction. Two recent large prospective cohort studies with premorbid and post-ICU cognitive assessment show critical illness as an independent risk factor for developing dementia or other cognitive dysfunction when controlled for premorbid cognitive function.[93,94]

Psychological disorders, including depression, anxiety, and PTSD, occur frequently after critical illness. Depression has been reported in 25–58% of survivors of critical illness.[98,99] Critical illness has been shown to be an independent risk factor for developing depression in one cohort study with premorbid and post-ICU depression assessments.[100] Anxiety has been reported in 23–41% of ICU survivors.[101,102] PTSD has been reported in 5–63% of ICU survivors.[103,104] Risk factors related to developing depression and anxiety include length of ICU stay, length of MV, premorbid psychiatric disease, higher body mass index (BMI), surgical ICU admission, maximum organ failure score, and mean benzodiazepine dose.[96] Risk factors for PTSD include the development of delusional memories and sedative use.[105] Potential mechanisms for psychiatric disorders in ICU survivors include organ dysfunction, medications, pain, sleep deprivation, elevated cytokines, stress-related activation of the hypothalamic-pituitary axis, hypoxaemia, and neurotransmitter dysfunction due to brain injury.[96]

There is little known about the prevention and treatment of neurocognitive and neuropsychiatric dysfunction in ICU survivors. Depression, anxiety, and PTSD were all decreased in patients who had daily interruption of sedatives (DIS) in one study.[102] Avoidance of benzodiazepines reduces the incidence of delirium in acute ICU patients, but it is not yet known if this will reduce the prevalence or prolonged duration of brain dysfunction. In another study, patients given a prospectively collected diary of their ICU stay at 1 month following discharge decreased the incidence of new-onset PTSD.[106] The study authors hypothesize that lack of complete and factual memories of ICU stay may be important in the development of PTSD, and, by providing these facts, patients are less likely to develop PTSD.

Symptom burden

Physical and psychological symptoms are common among patients with CCI. Nelson and colleagues surveyed a cohort of 50 patients requiring tracheostomy for failure to wean in a respiratory care unit.[15] These patients were elderly (median age 73) and ethnically diverse, with most patients living at home prior to admission (86%) with multiple comorbid medical conditions. The average length of stay for these patients prior to respiratory care unit admission was 15 days. Of the included patients, 28% were too physically or cognitively impaired to respond to the survey and one can only speculate about their symptom burden. Of the patients able to respond to the survey, there was a high symptom burden; 90% of patients reported symptoms, with an average of 8.6 symptoms per patient. Pain at the highest level of distress was reported in 44% of the patients. High levels of psychological symptoms, including sadness, worry, or nervousness, were reported in 60% of patients. Ninety per cent of patients reported high levels of distress due to difficulties in communicating. Other common symptoms included thirst, nausea, insomnia, dyspnoea, fatigue, hunger, dry mouth, and lack of appetite.

Very little systematic evidence exists about the treatment of symptoms in CCI or whether symptom treatment affects outcomes. Nelson and colleagues argue that symptom experience is an independent predictor of important outcomes in other patient groups, with higher symptom burden associated with greater mortality.[15] Reduction in symptom burden may promote favourable outcomes, including physiologic stability and efficient resource utilization.

Outcomes

The constellation of multiple organ dysfunctions in chronically critically ill patients makes them vulnerable to new complications and hampers recovery. One-year mortality is 50–60%,[6,9,11,61,107] and age and number of ongoing organ dysfunctions are strong independent risk factors for long-term mortality.[9] Functional outcomes and QoL in this population are also poor due, in part, to high rates of physical dysfunction.[6,12,61,108,109] One study demonstrated that most patients also suffer from severe cognitive dysfunction following PMV.[13] The severe physical and cognitive dysfunction which accompanies CCI results in prolonged institutionalization for hospital survivors.[61] Patients undergo an average of four transitions in institutional care during the year after discharge from their index hospitalization.

As patients (and therefore surrogates) gain more autonomy in decision making, clinicians will need to improve processes to communicate prognosis and treatment options in CCI in order to align goals of care with patient values. Qualitative studies indicate that surrogate decision makers wish to hear information on long-term prognosis, but this information is usually not provided.[13] A recently validated mortality prediction model[9] can assist clinicians with estimates of long-term survival, but other interventions are necessary to improve communication of that information. Assistance from clinicians trained in communication, such as palliative care physicians, or innovations, such as electronic decision aids, may be useful, and these innovations are currently under study in the CCI population.

Conclusion

Chronic multiple organ dysfunction is not merely a continuation of acute illness but a discrete syndrome of diverse physiologic abnormalities and metabolic dysfunction. There has been increased recognition of this syndrome among health care providers, and efforts to prevent and treat components of this syndrome have shown some success. However, given its complex nature, no single intervention can likely prevent or treat this syndrome. Comprehensive and systematic programmes will need to be designed and implemented, involving bundled best-practice interventions, in order to lessen the incidence of and treat the consequences of chronic multiple organ dysfunction.

References

1 **Nelson JE, Cox CE, Hope AA, Carson SS.** Chronic critical illness. *Am J Respir Crit Care Med* 2010;**182**:446–54.

2 Cooper Z, Bernacki RE, Divo M. Chronic critical illness: a review for surgeons. *Curr Probl Surg* 2011;**48**:12–57.

3 Nierman DM, Nelson DE. Chronic critical illness. *Crit Care Clin* 2002;**18**:xi–xii.

4 Cox CE, Carson SS, Holmes GM, Howard A, Carey TS. Increase in tracheostomy for prolonged mechanical ventilation in North Carolina, 1993–2002. *Crit Care Med* 2004;**32**:2219–26.

5 Zilberberg MD, de Wit M, Pirone JR, Shorr AF. Growth in adult prolonged acute mechanical ventilation: implications for healthcare delivery. *Crit Care Med* 2008;**36**:1451–5.

6 Engoren M, Arslanian-Engoren C, Fenn-Buderer N. Hospital and long-term outcome after tracheostomy for respiratory failure. *Chest* 2004;**125**:220–7.

7 Seneff MG, Zimmerman JE, Knaus WA, Wagner DP, Draper EA. Predicting the duration of mechanical ventilation. The importance of disease and patient characteristics. *Chest* 1996;**110**:469–79.

8 Wagner DP. Economics of prolonged mechanical ventilation. *Am Rev Respir Dis* 1989;**140**:S14–18.

9 Carson SS, Kahn JM, Hough CL, et al. A multicenter mortality prediction model for patients receiving prolonged mechanical ventilation. *Crit Care Med* 2011;**40**:171–6.

10 Estenssoro E, Reina R, Canales HS, et al. The distinct clinical profile of chronically critically ill patients: a cohort study. *Crit Care* 2006;**10**:R89.

11 Cox CE, Carson SS, Lindquist JH, Olsen MK, Govert JA, Chelluri L. Differences in one-year health outcomes and resource utilization by definition of prolonged mechanical ventilation: a prospective cohort study. *Crit Care* 2007;**11**:R9.

12 Combes A, Costa MA, Trouillet JL, et al. Morbidity, mortality, and quality-of-life outcomes of patients requiring >or = 14 days of mechanical ventilation. *Crit Care Med* 2003;**31**:1373–81.

13 Nelson JE, Tandon N, Mercado AF, Camhi SL, Ely EW, Morrison RS. Brain dysfunction: another burden for the chronically critically ill. *Arch Intern Med* 2006;**166**:1993–9.

14 Hope AA, Morrison RS, Du Q, Nelson J. Predictors of long-term brain dysfunction after chronic critical illness. *Am J Respir Crit Care Med* 2010;**181**:A6713.

15 Nelson JE, Meier DE, Litke A, Natale DA, Siegel RE, Morrison RS. The symptom burden of chronic critical illness. *Crit Care Med* 2004;**32**:1527–34.

16 Van Pelt DC, Milbrandt EB, Qin L, et al. Informal caregiver burden among survivors of prolonged mechanical ventilation. *Am J Respir Crit Care Med* 2007;**175**:167–73.

17 Van den Berghe G. Neuroendocrine pathobiology of chronic critical illness. *Crit Care Clin* 2002;**18**:509–28.

18 Vanhorebeek I, Langouche L, Van den Berghe G. Endocrine aspects of acute and prolonged critical illness. *Nat Clin Pract Endocrinol Metab* 2006;**2**:20–31.

19 Van den Berghe G, de Zegher F, Bouillon R. Clinical review 95: acute and prolonged critical illness as different neuroendocrine paradigms. *J Clin Endocrinol Metab* 1998;**83**:1827–34.

20 Mechanick JI, Brett EM. Endocrine and metabolic issues in the management of the chronically critically ill patient. *Crit Care Clin* 2002;**18**:619–41.

21 Hollander JM, Mechanick JI. Nutrition support and the chronic critical illness syndrome. *Nutr Clin Pract* 2006;**21**:587–604.

22 Zaloga GP, Marik P. Hypothalamic-pituitary-adrenal insufficiency. *Crit Care Clin* 2001;**17**:25–41.

23 Cooper MS, Stewart PM. Adrenal insufficiency in critical illness. *J Intensive Care Med* 2007;**22**:348–62.

24 Patel GP, Balk RA. Systemic steroids in severe sepsis and septic shock. *Am J Respir Crit Care Med* 2011;**185**:133–9.

25 Farwell AP. Thyroid hormone therapy is not indicated in the majority of patients with the sick euthyroid syndrome. *Endocr Pract* 2008;**14**:1180–7.

26 Vanhorebeek I, Van den Berghe G. The neuroendocrine response to critical illness is a dynamic process. *Crit Care Clin* 2006;**22**:1–15.

27 Van den Berghe G, Baxter RC, Weekers F, Wouters P, Bowers CY, Veldhuis JD. A paradoxical gender dissociation within the growth hormone/insulin-like growth factor I axis during protracted critical illness. *J Clin Endocrinol Metab* 2000;**85**:183–92.

28 Griffiths J, Waldmann C, Quinlan J. Sexual dysfunction in intensive care survivors. *Br J Hosp Med (Lond)* 2007;**68**:470–3.

29 Somers KJ, Philbrick KL. Sexual dysfunction in the medically ill. *Curr Psychiatry Rep* 2007;**9**:247–54.

30 Griffiths J, Gager M, Alder N, Fawcett D, Waldmann C, Quinlan J. A self-report-based study of the incidence and associations of sexual dysfunction in survivors of intensive care treatment. *Intensive Care Med* 2006;**32**:445–51.

31 Shapses SA, Weissman C, Seibel MJ, Chowdhury HA. Urinary pyridinium cross-link excretion is increased in critically ill surgical patients. *Crit Care Med* 1997;**25**:85–90.

32 Van den Berghe G, Van Roosbroeck D, Vanhove P, Wouters PJ, De Pourcq L, Bouillon R. Bone turnover in prolonged critical illness: effect of vitamin D. *J Clin Endocrinol Metab* 2003;**88**:4623–32.

33 Hollander JM, Mechanick JI. Bisphosphonates and metabolic bone disease in the ICU. *Curr Opin Clin Nutr Metab Care* 2009;**12**:190–5.

34 Via MA, Potenza MV, Hollander J, et al. Intravenous ibandronate acutely reduces bone hyperresorption in chronic critical illness. *J Intensive Care Med* 2012;**27**:312–18.

35 Klein GL, Wimalawansa SJ, Kulkarni G, Sherrard DJ, Sanford AP, Herndon DN. The efficacy of acute administration of pamidronate on the conservation of bone mass following severe burn injury in children: a double-blind, randomized, controlled study. *Osteoporos Int* 2005;**16**:631–5.

36 Nierman DM, Mechanick JI. Biochemical response to treatment of bone hyperresorption in chronically critically ill patients. *Chest* 2000;**118**:761–6.

37 Lorin S, Nierman DM. Critical illness neuromuscular abnormalities. *Crit Care Clin* 2002;**18**:553–68.

38 Tepper M, Rakic S, Haas JA, Woittiez AJ. Incidence and onset of critical illness polyneuropathy in patients with septic shock. *Neth J Med* 2000;**56**:211–14.

39 Garnacho-Montero J, Madrazo-Osuna J, Garcia-Garmendia JL, et al. Critical illness polyneuropathy: risk factors and clinical consequences. A cohort study in septic patients. *Intensive Care Med* 2001;**27**:1288–96.

40 Tennila A, Salmi T, Pettila V, Roine RO, Varpula T, Takkunen O. Early signs of critical illness polyneuropathy in ICU patients with systemic inflammatory response syndrome or sepsis. *Intensive Care Med* 2000;**26**:1360–3.

41 Hermans G, De Jonghe B, Bruyninckx F, Van den Berghe G. Clinical review: critical illness polyneuropathy and myopathy. *Crit Care* 2008;**12**:238.

42 Stevens RD, Dowdy DW, Michaels RK, Mendez-Tellez PA, Pronovost PJ, Needham DM. Neuromuscular dysfunction acquired in critical illness: a systematic review. *Intensive Care Med* 2007;**33**:1876–91.

43 De Jonghe B, Sharshar T, Lefaucheur JP, et al. Paresis acquired in the intensive care unit: a prospective multicenter study. *JAMA* 2002;**288**:2859–67.

44 Stevens RD, Marshall SA, Cornblath DR, et al. A framework for diagnosing and classifying intensive care unit-acquired weakness. *Crit Care Med* 2009;**37**(10 Suppl):S299–308.

45 Zochodne DW, Bolton CF, Wells GA, et al. Critical illness polyneuropathy. A complication of sepsis and multiple organ failure. *Brain* 1987;**110**:819–41.

46 Latronico N, Shehu I, Seghelini E. Neuromuscular sequelae of critical illness. *Curr Opin Crit Care* 2005;**11**:381–90.

47 Guarneri B, Bertolini G, Latronico N. Long-term outcome in patients with critical illness myopathy or neuropathy: the Italian multicentre CRIMYNE study. *J Neurol Neurosurg Psychiatry* 2008;**79**:838–41.

48 Schweickert WD, Pohlman MC, Pohlman AS, et al. Early physical and occupational therapy in mechanically ventilated, critically ill patients: a randomised controlled trial. *Lancet* 2009;**373**:1874–82.

49 **Morris PE, Goad A, Thompson C, et al.** Early intensive care unit mobility therapy in the treatment of acute respiratory failure. *Crit Care Med* 2008;**36**:2238–43.

50 **Needham DM, Korupolu R, Zanni JM, et al.** Early physical medicine and rehabilitation for patients with acute respiratory failure: a quality improvement project. *Arch Phys Med Rehabil* 2010;**91**:536–42.

51 **Van den Berghe G, Schoonheydt K, Becx P, Bruyninckx F, Wouters PJ.** Insulin therapy protects the central and peripheral nervous system of intensive care patients. *Neurology* 2005;**64**:1348–53.

52 **Hermans G, Wilmer A, Meersseman W, et al.** Impact of intensive insulin therapy on neuromuscular complications and ventilator dependency in the medical intensive care unit. *Am J Respir Crit Care Med* 2007;**175**:480–9.

53 **Stevens RD, Dowdy DW, Michaels RK, Mendez-Tellez PA, Pronovost PJ, Needham DM.** Neuromuscular dysfunction acquired in critical illness: a systematic review. *Intensive Care Med* 2007;**33**:1876–91.

54 **Hermans G, Wilmer A, Meersseman W, et al.** Impact of intensive insulin therapy on neuromuscular complications and ventilator dependency in the medical intensive care unit. *Am J Respir Crit Care Med* 2007;**175**:480–9.

55 **Hermans G, De Jonghe B, Bruyninckx F, Van den Berghe G.** Interventions for preventing critical illness polyneuropathy and critical illness myopathy. *Cochrane Database Syst Rev* 2009;**1**:CD006832.

56 **Papazian L, Forel JM, Gacouin A, et al.** Neuromuscular blockers in early acute respiratory distress syndrome. *N Engl J Med* 2010;**363**:1107–16.

57 **Morandi A, Brummel NE, Ely EW.** Sedation, delirium and mechanical ventilation: the 'ABCDE' approach. *Curr Opin Crit Care* 2011;**17**:43–9.

58 **Gerovasili V, Stefanidis K, Vitzilaios K, et al.** Electrical muscle stimulation preserves the muscle mass of critically ill patients: a randomized study. *Crit Care* 2009;**13**:R161.

59 **Gerovasili V, Tripodaki E, Karatzanos E, et al.** Short-term systemic effect of electrical muscle stimulation in critically ill patients. *Chest* 2009;**136**:1249–56.

60 **Kress JP, Herridge MS.** Medical and economic implications of physical disability of survivorship. *Semin Respir Crit Care Med* 2012;**33**:339–47.

61 **Unroe M, Kahn JM, Carson SS, et al.** One-year trajectories of care and resource utilization for recipients of prolonged mechanical ventilation: a cohort study. *Ann Intern Med* 2010;**153**:167–75.

62 **Kalb TH, Lorin S.** Infection in the chronically critically ill: unique risk profile in a newly defined population. *Crit Care Clin* 2002;**18**:529–52.

63 **Scheinhorn DJ, Hassenpflug MS, Votto JJ, et al.** Ventilator-dependent survivors of catastrophic illness transferred to 23 long-term care hospitals for weaning from prolonged mechanical ventilation. *Chest* 2007;**131**:76–84.

64 **Callahan LA, Supinski GS.** Sepsis induces diaphragm electron transport chain dysfunction and protein depletion. *Am J Respir Crit Care Med* 2005;**172**:861–8.

65 **Galley HF.** Oxidative stress and mitochondrial dysfunction in sepsis. *Br J Anaesth* 2011;**107**:57–64.

66 **Desmond P, Raman R, Idikula J.** Effect of nasogastric tubes on the nose and maxillary sinus. *Crit Care Med* 1991;**19**:509–11.

67 **Ahmed QA, Niederman MS.** Respiratory infection in the chronically critically ill patient. Ventilator-associated pneumonia and tracheobronchitis. *Clin Chest Med* 2001;**22**:71–85.

68 **Poutsiaka DD.** Antimicrobial resistance in the chronically critically ill patient. *Clin Chest Med.* Mar 2001;**22**:87–103, viii.

69 **Boomer JS, To K, Chang KC, et al.** Immunosuppression in patients who die of sepsis and multiple organ failure. *JAMA* 2011;**306**:2594–605.

70 **Annane D, Bellissant E, Bollaert PE, et al.** Corticosteroids in the treatment of severe sepsis and septic shock in adults: a systematic review. *JAMA* 2009;**301**:2362–75.

71 **Mullard A.** Drug withdrawal sends critical care specialists back to basics. *Lancet* 2011;**378**:1769.

72 Angus DC. The search for effective therapy for sepsis: back to the drawing board? *JAMA* 2011;**306**:2614–15.

73 Pronovost P, Needham D, Berenholtz S, et al. An intervention to decrease catheter-related blood-stream infections in the ICU. *N Engl J Med* 2006;**355**:2725–32.

74 Bouadma L, Deslandes E, Lolom I, et al. Long-term impact of a multifaceted prevention program on ventilator-associated pneumonia in a medical intensive care unit. *Clin Infect Dis* 2010;**51**:1115–22.

75 Berenholtz SM, Pham JC, Thompson DA, et al. Collaborative cohort study of an intervention to reduce ventilator-associated pneumonia in the intensive care unit. *Infect Control Hosp Epidemiol* 2011;**32**:305–14.

76 Munoz-Price LS, De La Cuesta C, Adams S, et al. Successful eradication of a monoclonal strain of Klebsiella pneumoniae during a K. pneumoniae carbapenemase-producing K. pneumoniae outbreak in a surgical intensive care unit in Miami, Florida. *Infect Control Hosp Epidemiol* 2010;**31**:1074–7.

77 Munoz-Price LS, Hayden MK, Lolans K, et al. Successful control of an outbreak of Klebsiella pneumoniae carbapenemase-producing K. pneumoniae at a long-term acute care hospital. *Infect Control Hosp Epidemiol* 2010;**31**:341–7.

78 Ray A, Perez F, Beltramini AM, et al. Use of vaporized hydrogen peroxide decontamination during an outbreak of multidrug-resistant Acinetobacter baumannii infection at a long-term acute care hospital. *Infect Control Hosp Epidemiol* 2010;**31**:1236–41.

79 Climo MW, Sepkowitz KA, Zuccotti G, et al. The effect of daily bathing with chlorhexidine on the acquisition of methicillin-resistant Staphylococcus aureus, vancomycin-resistant Enterococcus, and healthcare-associated bloodstream infections: results of a quasi-experimental multicenter trial. *Crit Care Med* 2009;**37**:1858–65.

80 Ratnayake L, McEwen J, Henderson N, et al. Control of an outbreak of diarrhoea in a vascular surgery unit caused by a high-level clindamycin-resistant Clostridium difficile PCR ribotype 106. *J Hosp Infect* 2011;**79**:242–7.

81 Titsworth WL, Hester J, Correia T, et al. Reduction of catheter-associated urinary tract infections among patients in a neurological intensive care unit: a single institution's success. *J Neurosurg* 2012;**116**:911–20.

82 Nerandzic MM, Cadnum JL, Pultz MJ, Donskey CJ. Evaluation of an automated ultraviolet radiation device for decontamination of Clostridium difficile and other healthcare-associated pathogens in hospital rooms. *BMC Infect Dis* 2010;**10**:197.

83 Carasa M, Polycarpe M. Caring for the chronically critically ill patient: establishing a wound- healing program in a respiratory care unit. *Am J Surg* 2004;**188**(1A Suppl):18–21.

84 Cohen SH, Gerding DN, Johnson S, et al. Clinical practice guidelines for Clostridium difficile infection in adults: 2010 update by the Society for Healthcare Epidemiology of America (SHEA) and the infectious Diseases Society of America (IDSA). *Infect Control Hosp Epidemiol* 2010;**31**:431–55.

85 Smith PW, Bennett G, Bradley S, et al. SHEA/APIC Guideline: infection prevention and control in the long-term care facility. *Am J Infect Control* 2008;**36**:504–35.

86 O'Grady NP, Alexander M, Burns LA, et al. Guidelines for the prevention of intravascular catheter-related infections. *Am J Infect Control* 2011;**39**(4 Suppl 1):S1–34.

87 Gould CV, Umscheid CA, Agarwal RK, Kuntz G, Pegues DA. Guideline for prevention of catheter-associated urinary tract infections 2009. *Infect Control Hosp Epidemiol* 2010;**31**:319–26.

88 Siegel JD, Rhinehart E, Jackson M, Chiarello L. Guideline for isolation precautions: preventing transmission of infectious agents in health care settings. *Am J Infect Control* 2007;**35**(10 Suppl 2):S65–164.

89 Coffin SE, Klompas M, Classen D, et al. Strategies to prevent ventilator-associated pneumonia in acute care hospitals. *Infect Control Hosp Epidemiol* 2008;**29**(Suppl 1):S31–40.

90 Ely EW, Inouye SK, Bernard GR, et al. Delirium in mechanically ventilated patients: validity and reliability of the confusion assessment method for the intensive care unit (CAM-ICU). *JAMA* 2001;**286**:2703–10.

91 Jones C, Griffiths RD, Slater T, Benjamin KS, Wilson S. Significant cognitive dysfunction in non-delirious patients identified during and persisting following critical illness. *Intensive Care Med* 2006;**32**:923–6.

92 Jackson JC, Hart RP, Gordon SM, et al. Six-month neuropsychological outcome of medical intensive care unit patients. *Crit Care Med* 2003;**31**:1226–34.

93 Ehlenbach WJ, Hough CL, Crane PK, et al. Association between acute care and critical illness hospitalization and cognitive function in older adults. *JAMA* 2010;**303**:763–70.

94 Iwashyna TJ, Ely EW, Smith DM, Langa KM. Long-term cognitive impairment and functional disability among survivors of severe sepsis. *JAMA* 2010;**304**:1787–94.

95 Hopkins RO, Jackson JC. Long-term neurocognitive function after critical illness. *Chest* 2006;**130**:869–78.

96 Jackson JC, Mitchell N, Hopkins RO. Cognitive functioning, mental health, and quality of life in ICU survivors: an overview. *Crit Care Clin* 2009;**25**:615–28.

97 Hopkins RO, Suchyta MR, Snow GL, Jephson A, Weaver LK, Orme JF. Blood glucose dysregulation and cognitive outcome in ARDS survivors. *Brain Inj* 2010;**24**:1478–84.

98 Hopkins RO, Weaver LK, Collingridge D, Parkinson RB, Chan KJ, Orme JF, Jr. Two-year cognitive, emotional, and quality-of-life outcomes in acute respiratory distress syndrome. *Am J Respir Crit Care Med* 2005;**171**:340–7.

99 Cheung AM, Tansey CM, Tomlinson G, et al. Two-year outcomes, health care use, and costs of survivors of acute respiratory distress syndrome. *Am J Respir Crit Care Med* 2006;**174**:538–44.

100 Davydow DS, Russo JE, Ludman E, et al. The association of comorbid depression with intensive care unit admission in patients with diabetes: a prospective cohort study. *Psychosomatics* 2011;**52**:117–26.

101 Kapfhammer HP, Rothenhausler HB, Krauseneck T, Stoll C, Schelling G. Posttraumatic stress disorder and health-related quality of life in long-term survivors of acute respiratory distress syndrome. *Am J Psychiatry* 2004;**161**:45–52.

102 Kress JP, Gehlbach B, Lacy M, Pliskin N, Pohlman AS, Hall JB. The long-term psychological effects of daily sedative interruption on critically ill patients. *Am J Respir Crit Care Med* 2003;**168**:1457–61.

103 Griffiths J, Fortune G, Barber V, Young JD. The prevalence of post traumatic stress disorder in survivors of ICU treatment: a systematic review. *Intensive Care Med* 2007;**33**:1506–18.

104 Myhren H, Ekeberg O, Stokland O. Health-related quality of life and return to work after critical illness in general intensive care unit patients: a 1-year follow-up study. *Crit Care Med* 2010;**38**:1554–61.

105 Jones C, Griffiths RD, Humphris G, Skirrow PM. Memory, delusions, and the development of acute posttraumatic stress disorder-related symptoms after intensive care. *Crit Care Med* 2001;**29**:573–80.

106 Jones C, Backman C, Capuzzo M, et al. Intensive care diaries reduce new onset post traumatic stress disorder following critical illness: a randomised, controlled trial. *Crit Care* 2010;**14**:R168.

107 Carson SS, Garrett J, Hanson LC, et al. A prognostic model for one-year mortality in patients requiring prolonged mechanical ventilation. *Crit Care Med* 2008;**36**:2061–9.

108 Douglas SL, Daly BJ, Gordon N, Brennan PF. Survival and quality of life: short-term versus long-term ventilator patients. *Crit Care Med* 2002;**30**:2655–62.

109 Chelluri L, Im KA, Belle SH, et al. Long-term mortality and quality of life after prolonged mechanical ventilation. *Crit Care Med* 2004;**32**:61–9.

Chapter 14

Prolonged Respiratory Insufficiency and Ventilator Dependence in the ICU

Gaëtan Beduneau, Jean-Christophe M. Richard, and Laurent Brochard

Introduction

Single or multiple attempts to discontinue MV are part of the process referred to as weaning from MV, which may account for about 40% of the total time spent on MV.[1] Over the last two decades, an abundant literature on this topic has permitted a better understanding of the pathophysiological issues driving weaning and extubation difficulties.[2] Cumulative evidence has highlighted that a daily systematic evaluation of the patients' readiness to breathe spontaneously can help to reduce weaning duration and that a gradual, systematic decrease in ventilatory support may not be needed.[3–5] Management of sedation has also emerged as a key consideration for any strategy aiming to test spontaneous breathing readiness. Sedation interferes directly or indirectly with the weaning process because of the frequent occurrence of drug accumulation and of prolongation of sedation after having stopped sedative or analgesic medications.[6–9] In this context, several studies have investigated the benefit of weaning strategies or protocols, based on a systematic breathing trial associated with or without a specific management of sedation.[10–12] What researchers and clinicians meant by protocols has not been universally defined, however, and various results of protocols have been reported. Results of observational studies have shown that a majority of patients (50–80%) can be separated from their ventilator after the first SBT attempt.[4,5] Nevertheless, these studies also showed that a significant percentage of patients do not succeed on their first SBT. This group of patients poses specific problems and may benefit from targeted investigations for the diagnosis and treatment of the cause of weaning failure. Finally, an even smaller proportion of patients recovering from catastrophic illness and/or having severe underlying comorbidities require a very long time before being separated from the ventilator, either in the ICU or in specialized units. The outcome of this last group of patients is usually poor.[13,14]

New weaning classification

Based on these observations, a recent international consensus conference proposed to categorize patients in the weaning process into three groups, according to the pace and length of the weaning process.[15] Although arbitrary, this classification interestingly challenges the classical conception of the weaning process, as discussed hereafter (see Table 14.1).

Simple weaning

Patients successfully separated from the ventilator after the first SBT (and usually extubated) correspond to the first group referred to as '**simple weaning**'. This group represents approximately

Table 14.1 Specific objectives, proposals for management, and reasons for prolongation of MV, according to the recent weaning classification

	Objectives	Proposals	Reasons for prolongation of MV
Group 1: simple weaning	– To identify possible weaning readiness – To perform an SBT** in case of possible weaning readiness	– Systematic detection of weaning readiness (early screening) – Sedation management – SBT (30–120 min) – Automatic mode for weaning (SmartCare®)	– Oversedation – Excessive ventilatory support – Inadequate ventilator settings – Metabolic alkalosis – Use of SIMV+
Group 2: difficult weaning	– To identify and treat reversible causes of failure – To resume SBT as soon as possible	– Cardiac echography – Respiratory mechanics assessment – Consider NIV to prevent reintubation – Cuff leak test before extubation – Early mobilization – Measurements of natriuretic peptides as biomarker	– Glottic oedema – Fluid overload – Left cardiac dysfunction – Increased airway secretions – Ventilator-acquired pneumonia – CINM*** – Delirium-anxiety
Group 3: prolonged weaning	– To detect 'chronic critically ill patients'	– Consider specialized weaning unit – Consider tracheotomy – Progressive reduction in ventilatory support – Progressive reduction of the tracheotomy cannula diameter – Mobilization – Multidisciplinary approach	– Central neurological disease – Previous severe chronic respiratory or cardiac insufficiency – Chronic respiratory insufficiency – Severe denutrition – CINM – Depression

* Weaning readiness: the physician considers that a reasonable probability of weaning success exists.

** Spontaneous breathing trial. Either low pressure support with ZEEP ('SBT equivalent') or T-piece trial

*** CINM, critical illness neuromyopathy.

+ SIMV, synchronized intermittent mandatory ventilation

Data from Boles JM, Bion J, Connors A, et al. Weaning from mechanical ventilation. *Eur Respir J* 2007;29:1033–56.

50–80% of all patients who require MV and undergo the weaning process. The clinical challenge in this group is to assess their readiness to be separated from the ventilator by performing an SBT as early as possible and obviously as soon as they are able to sustain spontaneous ventilation. Screening their ability to breathe alone is therefore the key issue, and screening indexes like the rapid shallow breathing index[16] are valuable in this perspective.[17] Clinical trials have shown that the SBT may be performed either on pressure support ventilation (PSV), with 7–8 cmH$_2$O, with no positive end-expiratory pressure (PEEP) ('SBT equivalent'), or while breathing spontaneously through a T tube.[18,19] Evidence suggests that a significantly greater number of patients are able to succeed with PSV.[18,20,21] This suggests that the T tube trial may slightly underestimate weaning readiness or, in contradistinction, that the PSV test may expose the patient to a slightly higher risk of reintubation. In some patients, the amount of support provided by the pressure level may underestimate the risk of extubation. This has not been strictly demonstrated, but the implications are that the choice of technique used may be influenced by the patient undergoing testing. In any case, breathing through a T-piece is more challenging than using PSV[21] and accurately reproduces the work of breathing (WOB) that the patient will have to sustain after extubation, especially in the first few hours.[22] A formal approach with holding sedation (or avoiding sedation when possible), and followed by an SBT, may be an efficient strategy to manage this group of patients.[12] Another possible approach described in the literature is the use of a special automated system, initially called NeoGanesh and commercialized later as SmartCare®, which has been developed by researchers to serve as an automatic ventilation and weaning technique. It has been specifically designed to automatically detect readiness to breathe spontaneously and to subsequently send an incentive to the clinician.[23–25] Clinical trials have shown that this automatic system is able to perform either as well as or better than a formal clinically driven weaning protocol, even when applied in a context of high nurse-patient ratio.[26–28] Compared to usual practice, the system has the ability to significantly reduce the time on MV while maintaining the patient's respiratory pattern in a comfortable range. The relatively good results of such automated systems are probably explained, in part, by its ability to work 24 hours per day and 7 days a week.

Difficult weaning

Patients who fail the first SBT and require up to three SBTs or up to 7 days from the first attempt to be successfully extubated comprise the second group referred to as '**difficult weaning**'. Reversible causes of weaning failure should be scrutinized in this subgroup of patients, in whom cardiac failure or fluid overload is frequently observed as a cause of weaning difficulties. Several studies have demonstrated that cardiac decompensation can cause and explain weaning failure[29,30] and that fluid overload is a frequent contributor to failure to tolerate disconnection from the ventilator or extubation.[31,32] For this reason, there has been recent interest in using cardiac biomarkers as predictors of weaning failure.[33–35] A recent RCT showed that a strategy based on brain natriuretic peptide (BNP) measurement immediately before the SBT to help guide diuretic administration significantly increased the number of patients who succeeded in the SBT trial, thus significantly reducing the weaning time.[36] Systematic extubation, followed by NIV, has also been proposed as an alternative to continuation of conventional MV for patients belonging to this 'difficult weaning' group. This last approach, however, seems most promising for patients with COPD and sustained hypercapnia.[37,38] The results of studies addressing this question remain conflicting,[39] however, and NIV cannot be firmly recommended in these settings.

Prolonged weaning

The third group is referred to as '**prolonged weaning**' and includes a small proportion of patients, defined as requiring more than three weaning attempts or 7 days to be separated from the ventilator. At this stage of prolonged weaning, the vast majority of these patients have already been tracheotomized to facilitate their global and ventilatory management. The concept of patients with CCI emerged in the last decade from cohort studies and can be applied to many of these patients.[40] The long duration of MV usually reported in this subgroup of patients has led to the development of specialized weaning units (SWUs).[41]

Epidemiological data according to the weaning classification

To what extent the outcome differs between the three above-mentioned groups is a clinically important question that has been addressed by several recent studies. The first prospective study describing the distribution of the different weaning categories and their corresponding outcome was carried out in one centre in Vienna Austria by Funk et al.[42] and included slightly more than 250 medical-surgical patients. Distribution of simple, difficult, and prolonged weaning corresponded to 59%, 26%, and 14% of patients, respectively, arriving at the stage of weaning from MV. Mortality was highest in the third group, i.e. patients with prolonged weaning, compared to simple and difficult weaning. This last finding has been confirmed subsequently in several other observational studies. In addition to looking at the outcome of different weaning groups, Sellares et al. tried to determine the predictors associated with increased risk for prolonged weaning in a Spanish respiratory ICU.[43] They prospectively enrolled around 200 patients classified as follows: simple weaning 40%, difficult weaning 40%, prolonged weaning 20%. Increased heart rate and $PaCO_2$ during SBT were independently associated with prolonged weaning, whereas hypercapnia during the SBT and the need to reintubate predicted a decrease in 90-day survival. One should note that the patients enrolled in this study were mostly ventilated in the context of chronic respiratory disease, thus modifying the expected outcome on MV, compared to a non-specialized ICU. As observed in the Austrian study, the mortality of the prolonged weaning group was significantly higher, compared to simple and difficult weaning. Similarly, the duration of MV was longer in this third group, but, as mentioned in the accompanying editorial, this result was expected, according to the definition.[44] In an observational study by Tonnelier et al., prolonged weaning represented 30% of patients and was associated with a higher mortality in the ICU, though not after 1 year.[45] Most of these findings were corroborated by the largest cohort to date, reported by Penuelas et al.[46] This study was a second analysis of a large international cohort study on mechanically ventilated patients.[1] The authors found that prolonged weaning concerned only 6% of the total population. Again, mortality was found to be significantly higher in this subgroup of patients, while outcome did not differ in difficult weaning, compared to simple weaning patients. The conclusions of these four studies confirm the absence of a mortality difference between the first two groups, i.e. simple and prolonged weaning, suggesting that there is a large overlap between these two populations. Patients responding to simple and difficult weaning definitions may represent a single group, in which the staging (groups 1 and 2) depends on the time at which the first SBT is performed as well as the method used to assess readiness to breathe spontaneously. In the last study, SBT was performed either with PEEP and pressure support or disconnection from the ventilator (T-piece trial), and more than 25% of patients were ventilated with synchronized intermittent mandatory ventilation. These irregularities may have interfered with weaning definition and duration. Finally, an important concern regarding the new definition is the lack of precise timing at which sedation is stopped, which can markedly affect the assessment of spontaneous ventilation readiness.

Muscle weakness and prolonged weaning

General muscle weakness and respiratory muscle weakness are a common problem in ICU patients. No study has specifically focused on the best approach to separate weak patients from the ventilator, and these patients most likely fall into the difficult and prolonged weaning groups. After awakening, following sedation cessation, ICU-acquired paresis seems to occur in about 30% of patients after PMV.[47] It may affect the respiratory muscles, potentially leading to weaning difficulties, although precise data on this are lacking. However, ICU-acquired paresis has been shown to be associated with prolonged weaning.[48] De Jonghe and co-workers reanalysed a prospective cohort of 95 patients who were enrolled in an incidence and risk factor study of ICU-acquired paresis after 7 or more days of MV in five ICUs.[47] They looked at variables associated with a pro-longed weaning duration; variables were entered into a multivariable Cox proportional-hazards model to identify the independent variables that influenced the duration of weaning from MV. ICU-acquired paresis and the presence of COPD were both independent predictors of prolonged weaning. The probability of remaining on MV after awakening was 2.4 times greater for patients with paresis (95% CI 1.4–4.2) and 2.7 times greater for patients with COPD (95% CI 1.6–4.5). In patients with paresis but without COPD, the median duration of weaning was 3.5 days longer than in patients who did not have either paresis or COPD. More recently, the same investigators also showed that respiratory and limb muscle strengths were both altered after 1 week of MV, using maximal inspiratory and expiratory pressures and vital capacity as markers of respiratory muscle function.[49] Respiratory muscle weakness was associated with delayed extubation and prolonged ventilation, and septic shock was a contributor to respiratory weakness. Other risk factors include prior administration of steroids alone or combined with muscle relaxants (ARDS, severe acute asthma attack).

Searching for diaphragm fatigue as a cause of weaning failure in patients with COPD, Laghi and co-workers[50] measured the contractile response of the diaphragm to phrenic nerve stimulation in 16 patients being weaned from MV. The nine patients who failed the trial experienced a greater respiratory load and developed greater diaphragmatic effort than did the seven weaning-success patients. No patient, however, developed a decrease in transdiaphragmatic twitch pressure, elic-ited by phrenic nerve stimulation, as an indicator of fatigue. Seven of the nine weaning-failure patients had a tension-time index of the respiratory muscles (product of the mean pressure developed by the duty cycle) above the threshold reported to lead to task failure and fatigue.[51] Physicians probably reinstituted MV before the occurrence of fatigue, which explains why it could not be observed. Patients display clinical manifestations of respiratory distress for a substantial time before they would develop fatigue, and clinicians reinstitute MV before fatigue has time to develop. In all patients, however, a striking finding was the fact that the transdiaphragmatic pressure twitches, measured under phrenic nerve stimulation, were much lower than predicted, even compared to severe COPD patients at rest. This indicated that muscle weakness is a frequent occurrence, at least in patients with COPD, and is likely to contribute to weaning difficulties.

Phrenic nerve injury secondary to heart surgery may also cause severe diaphragmatic dysfunc-tion responsible for prolonged duration of MV, ventilator-associated complications, and difficult weaning.[52,53]

The results of these different studies suggest that patients with muscle weakness, and especially respiratory muscle weakness, may often belong to the category of difficult, and sometimes pro-longed, weaning.

Prevention of muscle weakness while on MV

Because muscle weakness may greatly influence the duration of MV and weaning, every effort should be made to prevent muscle wasting and atrophy of the respiratory muscles.[54] ICU-acquired polyneuromyopathy is difficult to prevent, although some factors may be modified. They include early recognition and treatment of infection, limited use of steroids,[47] NMBAs,[55] glucose control with insulin administration,[56] and early mobilization.[57,58]

Levine and co-workers[59] recently published data illustrating that mechanically ventilated patients are at risk for an additional mechanism of respiratory muscle weakness—muscle atrophy. These investigators obtained biopsies of the costal diaphragms from 14 brain-dead organ donors.

The patients exhibited diaphragmatic inactivity and had received MV for 18–69 hours. They also obtained intraoperative biopsies of the diaphragms of eight control patients undergoing thoracic surgery for suspected lung cancer. Histologic measurements revealed marked diaphragmatic atrophy in the brain-dead patients. Compared with the control group, the mean cross-sectional areas of muscle fibres were decreased by more than 50%. The cross-sectional area of fibres of the pectoralis major, a muscle not affected by MV, was equivalent in the two groups. Thus, the diaphragmatic atrophy experienced by the brain-dead patients was not part of some generalized muscle-wasting disorder. Biochemical and gene expression studies suggest that the atrophy resulted from oxidative stress, leading to muscle protein degradation. They concluded that 18–69 hours of complete diaphragmatic inactivity and MV produced marked diaphragmatic atrophy as a result of increased oxidative stress, leading to the activation of protein degradation pathways. This was recently confirmed by a second study of very similar design, showing that MV triggers autophagy of the diaphragm.[60]

These data confirmed in patients the results of numerous experimental studies performed in various animal species.[61–65] Interestingly, Sassoon and co-workers showed that the use of assist-control ventilation was able to partially avoid the effects of a 3-day period of controlled MV on disuse atrophy of the diaphragm in rabbits.[66] They concluded that preserving diaphragmatic contractions during MV attenuates the force loss induced by complete inactivity. This was also shown in a large animal model over a period of 3 days of MV.[67] This supports an important argument to use assisted modes of ventilation, allowing some degree of spontaneous breathing from the initiation of MV or whenever possible.

The ventilator-dependent patient

Patients who become dependent upon their ventilator in the ICU represent a new category. They survive their ICU stay after having experienced a catastrophic illness and cannot be fully separated from MV.

In the US, over 100 000 patients each year fall into this category, and this figure is expected to increase, thanks to intensive care therapeutic progress and to the changes in patients profiles (more elderly patients admitted, more comorbidities). Although this group represents fewer than 10% of the whole ICU patients, they require a disproportionally high number of ICU days, accounting for 40% of ICU expenditures. Reduction of the long periods spent in the ICU or on MV may facilitate a reduction in costs incurred by these patients.[68–70]

Recent studies confirm that prolonged weaning is associated with a higher mortality, longer stay in the ICU, and longer duration of MV.[46] Furthermore, ICU may be lacking the necessary organization and specialized staff to care for prolonged weaning patients.[41]

For three decades, SWUs have been developed because of the high cost and the potentially poor progress made by these patients in a classical ICU ward.[41,71,72] These units were started to be able to offer patients better and more specifically adapted care to meet their needs, together with cost savings related to reduced nurse-to-patient ratio, monitoring, and technical equipment. These units also facilitate more efficient use of critical care resources by increasing the availability of acute ICU beds.[6] Typically, these SWUs offer expertise in prolonged weaning and specialized multidisciplinary teams composed of clinicians, physiotherapists, nurses, nutritionists, and psychotherapists. The use of a standardized therapist-driven protocol, an adapted area with a focus on sleep quantity and quality, resources for rehabilitation, and a specific programme geared to restore functional independence comprise these programmes.[73]

In two of the main publications on this topic, Scheinhorn et al.[13,14] report data on 1419 consecutive ventilator-dependent patients enrolled in a 1-year period in 23 SWUs in the US. These descriptive publications give important insights into the characteristics of these patients, their premorbid diagnoses, and the procedures performed during SWU hospitalization. In these reports, the median patient age was almost 72 years, median duration of MV in ICU prior to admission was 25 days, and median length of stay in SWU was 40 days. The number of premorbid diagnoses averaged 2.6 per patient (hypertension in 47%, COPD in 42%), and a medical illness led to ventilator dependency in 61% of patients. Infections were the most frequent complications treated in SWU. Furthermore, a large number of patients received PT (85%) and needed procedures such as CT scan (25%) or bronchoscopy (15%). Overall, these patients require considerable medical interventions and treatments.

Almost all SWU patients were tracheotomized for a median of 2 weeks prior to admission. Recent studies[74–76] have demonstrated that performing a tracheotomy does not alter outcome in terms of mortality or duration of MV. It is generally acknowledged, however, that performing a tracheotomy on these ventilator-dependent patients permits a reduced WOB and makes mobilization, nursing, swallowing, oral nutrition, and speech much easier.[77,78]

In the above-mentioned study, Scheinhorn et al. also report that the median time to wean was 15 days,[13] 54% had weaning success, 21% had persistence of ventilator dependence, and 25% of patients died. Furthermore, the disposition of patients who were alive and discharged from the SWU were as follows: home for 29%, a new stay in acute hospital for 19%, and rehabilitation or 'extended-care facilities' for 49%. One year after discharge, 30% of patients were alive. This cohort study illustrates what prolonged weaning patients may need in terms of human and technical resources. In a recent study in five Italian respiratory ICUs, Polverino and al.[79] observed that their outcomes have progressively worsened over the last 15 years, with a reduction in their weaning success from 87% to 66% and was likely explained by the admission of more severely ill patients to these units. Although ventilatory management is important, no specific protocol has been demonstrated to outperform other strategies in this patient group.[80] Interestingly, a lot of attention needs to be paid to the decannulation protocol; for instance, decannulation can greatly interfere with the patient's work of breathing,[81] and it is important to wait until the appropriate time before removing the cannula. To our knowledge, only a single publication has outlined a step-by-step clinical flowchart for weaning these patients from tracheotomy.[82]

Conclusion

Proper selection of patients admitted to weaning units is very important. Most patients suffer mainly from respiratory failure but with important sequelae of their prolonged ICU stay (more than 21 days in the North American models) such as renal insufficiency, skin lesions, major loss of autonomy, or depression.[83,84] Several studies incorporate a majority of COPD patients,[79] whereas others[14,71] include patients who developed their MV dependence due to a large spectrum of medical or surgical diagnoses. The presence of ICUAW is rarely detailed. A sufficient level of consciousness and ability to actively participate in rehabilitation programmes is necessary to accommodate participation in physiotherapy programmes and to optimize and accelerate functional recovery from muscle injury and disuse.[73] From the current literature, for tracheostomized and difficult-to-wean COPD patients, increasing periods of spontaneous breathing T-piece trials or decreasing levels of pressure support appear to be equally effective.[80] Since a greater number of 'chronically critically ill patients' now survive catastrophic illness, they have a global worsening in clinical outcomes where weaning difficulty is only one of many issues to be addressed. Given their compromised organ reserve, it is imperative that difficult-to-wean patients should have a clear delineation of objectives, means, and organization at the time of admission, and this resource should be reserved for those with some recovery or rehabilitative potential. For example, Carpene et al.[85] proposed an original model of organization made up by two levels: first, a respiratory ICU and, second, a weaning centre for unweaned patients.

A strong association between depressive disorders or PTSD and prolonged weaning from MV has also been demonstrated recently.[83,84] This aspect of care must be prioritized and may be easier to administer in an SWU setting where the treatment may be more readily delivered in a more humane and personal setting.

There are some potential risks associated with such units. A dedicated weaning unit could lead physicians to lessen their efforts to wean patients while waiting for the transfer in the SWU; it could also reduce their commitment to address prognosis and engage in end-of-life issues. This would paradoxically cause increasing overall costs.[86]

In order to understand the risks and the advantages of SWUs, further studies are urgently needed, which incorporate patient-centred short and longer-term outcomes, so that it is clear who benefits from this specialized care.

References

1 Esteban A, Ferguson ND, Meade MO, et al. Evolution of mechanical ventilation in response to clinical research. *Am J Respir Crit Care Med* 2008;**177**:170–7.

2 Tobin MJ. Remembrance of weaning past: the seminal papers. *Intensive Care Med* 2006;**32**:1485–93.

3 Ely EW, Baker AM, Dunagan DP, et al. Effect on the duration of mechanical ventilation of identifying patients capable of breathing spontaneously. *N Engl J Med* 1996;**335**:1864–9.

4 Brochard L, Rauss A, Benito S, et al. Comparison of three methods of gradual withdrawal from ventilatory support during weaning from mechanical ventilation. *Am J Respir Crit Care Med* 1994;**150**:896–903.

5 Esteban A, Frutos F, Tobin MJ, et al. A comparison of four methods of weaning patients from mechanical ventilation. Spanish Lung Failure Collaborative Group. *N Engl J Med* 1995;**332**:345–50.

6 Heffner JE. A wake-up call in the intensive care unit. *N Engl J Med* 2000;**342**:1520–2.

7 Kress JP, Pohlman AS, O'Connor MF, Hall JB. Daily interruption of sedative infusions in critically ill patients undergoing mechanical ventilation. *N Engl J Med* 2000;**342**:1471–7.

8 Strøm T, Martinussen T, Toft P. A protocol of no sedation for critically ill patients receiving mechanical ventilation: a prospective randomised trial. *Lancet* 2010:**375**: 475–80.

9 Brochard L. Sedation in the intensive-care unit: good and bad? *Lancet* 2008;**371**:95–7.

10 Kollef MH, Shapiro SD, Silver P, et al. A randomized, controllet trial of protocol-directed versus physician-directed weaning from mechanical ventilation. *Crit Care Med* 1997;**25**:567–74.

11 Krishnan JA, Moore D, Robeson C, Rand CS, Fessler HE. A prospective, controlled trial of a protocol-based strategy to discontinue mechanical ventilation. *Am J Respir Crit Care Med* 2004;**169**:673–8.

12 Girard TD, Kress JP, Fuchs BD, et al. Efficacy and safety of a paired sedation and ventilator weaning protocol for mechanically ventilated patients in intensive care (Awakening and Breathing Controlled trial): a randomised controlled trial. *Lancet* 2008;**371**:126–34.

13 Scheinhorn DJ, Hassenpflug MS, Votto JJ, et al. Post-ICU mechanical ventilation at 23 long-term care hospitals: a multicenter outcomes study. *Chest* 2007;**131**:85–93.

14 Scheinhorn DJ, Hassenpflug MS, Votto JJ, et al. Ventilator-dependent survivors of catastrophic illness transferred to 23 long-term care hospitals for weaning from prolonged mechanical ventilation. *Chest* 2007;**131**:76–84.

15 Boles JM, Bion J, Connors A, et al. Weaning from mechanical ventilation. *Eur Respir J* 2007;**29**:1033–56.

16 Yang KL, Tobin MJ. A prospective study of indexes predicting the outcome of trials of weaning from mechanical ventilation. *N Engl J Med* 1991;**324**:1445–50.

17 Tobin MJ, Jubran A. Variable performance of weaning-predictor tests: role of Bayes' theorem and spectrum and test-referral bias. *Intensive Care Med* 2006;**32**:2002–12.

18 Esteban A, Alia I, Tobin MJ, et al. Effect of spontaneous breathing trial duration on outcome of attempts to discontinue mechanical ventilation. Spanish Lung Failure Collaborative Group. *Am J Respir Crit Care Med* 1999;**159**:512–18.

19 Foronda FK, Troster EJ, Farias JA, et al. The impact of daily evaluation and spontaneous breathing test on the duration of pediatric mechanical ventilation: a randomized controlled trial. *Crit Care Med* 2011;**39**:2526–33.

20 Ezingeard E, Diconne E, Guyomarc'h S, et al. Weaning from mechanical ventilation with pressure support in patients failing a T-tube trial of spontaneous breathing. *Intensive Care Med* 2006;**32**:165–9.

21 Cabello B, Thille AW, Roche-Campo F, Brochard L, Gomez FJ, Mancebo J. Physiological comparison of three spontaneous breathing trials in difficult-to-wean patients. *Intensive Care Med* 2010;**36**:1171–9.

22 Straus C, Louis B, Isabey D, Lemaire F, Harf A, Brochard L. Contribution of the endotracheal tube and the upper airway to breathing workload. *Am J Respir Crit Care Med* 1998;**157**:23–30.

23 Dojat M, Brochard L, Lemaire F, Harf A. A knowledge-based system for assisted ventilation of patients in intensive care units. *Int J Clin Monit Comput* 1992;**9**:239–50.

24 Dojat M, Harf A, Touchard D, Laforest M, Lemaire F, Brochard L. Evaluation of a knowledge-based system providing ventilatory management and decision for extubation. *Am J Respir Crit Care Med* 1996;**153**:997–1004.

25 Dojat M, Harf A, Touchard D, Lemaire F, Brochard L. Clinical evaluation of a computer-controlled pressure support mode. *Am J Respir Crit Care Med* 2000;**161**:1161–6.

26 Lellouche F, Mancebo J, Jolliet P, et al. A multicenter randomized trial of computer-driven protocolized weaning from mechanical ventilation. *Am J Respir Crit Care Med* 2006;**174**:894–900.

27 Rose L, Presneill JJ, Johnston L, Cade JF. A randomised, controlled trial of conventional versus automated weaning from mechanical ventilation using SmartCare/PS. *Intensive Care Med* 2008;**34**:1788–95.

28 Schadler D, Engel C, Elke G, et al. Automatic control of pressure support for ventilator weaning in surgical intensive care patients. *Am J Respir Crit Care Med* 2012;**185**:637–44.

29 Jubran A, Mathru M, Dries D, Tobin MJ. Continuous recordings of mixed venous oxygen saturation during weaning from mechanical ventilation and the ramifications thereof. *Am J Respir Crit Care Med* 1998;**158**:1763–9.

30 Lemaire F, Teboul JL, Cinotti L, et al. Acute left ventricular dysfunction during unsuccessful weaning from mechanical ventilation. *Anesthesiology* 1988;**69**:171–9.

31 Khamiees M, Raju P, DeGirolamo A, Amoateng-Adjepong Y, Manthous CA. Predictors of extubation outcome in patients who have successfully completed a spontaneous breathing trial. *Chest* 2001;**120**: 1262–70.

32 Frutos-Vivar F, Ferguson ND, Esteban A, et al. Risk factors for extubation failure in patients following a successful spontaneous breathing trial. *Chest* 2006;**130**:1664–71.

33 Chien JY, Lin MS, Huang YC, Chien YF, Yu CJ, Yang PC. Changes in B-type natriuretic peptide improve weaning outcome predicted by spontaneous breathing trial. *Crit Care Med* 2008;**36**:1421–6.

34 Grasso S, Leone A, De Michele M, et al. Use of N-terminal pro-brain natriuretic peptide to detect acute cardiac dysfunction during weaning failure in difficult-to-wean patients with chronic obstructive pulmonary disease. *Crit Care Med* 2007;**35**:96–105.

35 Mekontso-Dessap A, de Prost N, Girou E, et al. B-type natriuretic peptide and weaning from mechanical ventilation. *Intensive Care Med* 2006;**32**:1529–36.

36 Mekontso Dessap A, Roche-Campo F, Kouatchet A, et al. Natriuretic peptide-driven fluid management during ventilator weaning: a randomized controlled trial. *Am J Respir Crit Care Med* 2012; **186**:1256–63.

37 **Nava S, Ambrosino N, Clini E, et al.** Noninvasive mechanical ventilation in the weaning of patients with respiratory failure due to chronic obstructive pulmonary disease. A randomized, controlled trial. *Ann Intern Med* 1998;**128**:721–8.

38 **Ferrer M, Esquinas A, Arancibia F, et al.** Noninvasive ventilation during persistent weaning failure: a randomized controlled trial. *Am J Respir Crit Care Med* 2003;**168**:70–6.

39 **Girault C, Bubenheim M, Abroug F, et al.** Noninvasive ventilation and weaning in patients with chronic hypercapnic respiratory failure: a randomized multicenter trial. *Am J Respir Crit Care Med* 2011;**184**:672–9.

40 **Nelson JE, Cox CE, Hope AA, Carson SS.** Chronic critical illness. *Am J Respir Crit Care Med* 2010;**182**: 446–54.

41 **Scheinhorn DJ, Chao DC, Stearn-Hassenpflug M, LaBree LD, Heltsley DJ.** Post-ICU mechanical ventilation: treatment of 1,123 patients at a regional weaning center. *Chest* 1997;**111**:1654–9.

42 **Funk GC, Anders S, Breyer MK, et al.** Incidence and outcome of weaning from mechanical ventilation according to new categories. *Eur Respir J* 2010;**35**:88–94.

43 **Sellares J, Ferrer M, Cano E, Loureiro H, Valencia M, Torres A.** Predictors of prolonged weaning and survival during ventilator weaning in a respiratory ICU. *Intensive Care Med* 2011;**37**:775–84.

44 **Laghi F.** Stratification of difficulty in weaning. *Intensive Care Med* 2011;**37**:732–4.

45 **Tonnelier A, Tonnelier JM, Nowak E, et al.** Clinical relevance of classification according to weaning difficulty. *Respir Care* 2011;**56**:583–90.

46 **Penuelas O, Frutos-Vivar F, Fernandez C, et al.** Characteristics and outcomes of ventilated patients according to time to liberation from mechanical ventilation. *Am J Respir Crit Care Med* 2011;**184**:430–7.

47 **De Jonghe B, Sharshar T, Lefaucheur JP, et al.** Paresis acquired in the intensive care unit: a prospective multicenter study. *JAMA* 2002;**288**:2859–67.

48 **De Jonghe B, Bastuji-Garin S, Sharshar T, Outin H, Brochard L.** Does ICU-acquired paresis lengthen weaning from mechanical ventilation? *Intensive Care Med* 2004;**30**:1117–21.

49 **De Jonghe B, Bastuji-Garin S, Durand MC, et al.** Respiratory weakness is associated with limb weakness and delayed weaning in critical illness. *Crit Care Med* 2007;**35**:2007–15.

50 **Laghi F, Cattapan SE, Jubran A, et al.** Is weaning failure caused by low-frequency fatigue of the diaphragm? *Am J Respir Crit Care Med* 2003;**167**:120–7.

51 **Bellemare F, Grassino A.** Effect of pressure and timing of contraction on human diaphragm fatigue. *J Appl Physiol* 1982;**53**:1190–5.

52 **Diehl JL, Lofaso F, Deleuze P, Similowski T, Lemaire F, Brochard L.** Clinically relevant diaphragmatic dysfunction after cardiac operations. *J Thoracic Cardiovasc Surg* 1994;**107**:487–98.

53 **Lerolle N, Guerot E, Dimassi S, et al.** Ultrasonographic diagnostic criterion for severe diaphragmatic dysfunction after cardiac surgery. *Chest* 2009;**135**:401–7.

54 **Hermans G, De Jonghe B, Bruyninckx F, Van den Berghe G.** Interventions for preventing critical illness polyneuropathy and critical illness myopathy. *Cochrane Database Syst Rev* 2009;1:CD006832.

55 **Segredo V, Caldwell JE, Matthay MA, Sharma ML, Gruenke LD, Miller RD.** Persistent paralysis in critically ill patients after long-term administration of vecuronium. *N Engl J Med* 1992;**327**:524–8.

56 **van den Berghe G, Wouters P, Weekers F, et al.** Intensive insulin therapy in the critically ill patients. *N Engl J Med* 2001;**345**:1359–67.

57 **Needham DM.** Mobilizing patients in the intensive care unit: improving neuromuscular weakness and physical function. *JAMA* 2008;**300**:1685–90.

58 **Schweickert WD, Pohlman MC, Pohlman AS, et al.** Early physical and occupational therapy in mechanically ventilated, critically ill patients: a randomised controlled trial. *Lancet* 2009;**373**:1874–82.

59 **Levine S, Nguyen T, Taylor N, et al.** Rapid disuse atrophy of diaphragm fibers in mechanically ventilated humans. *N Engl J Med* 2008;**358**:1327–35.

60 **Hussain SN, Mofarrahi M, Sigala I, et al.** Mechanical ventilation-induced diaphragm disuse in humans triggers autophagy. *Am J Respir Crit Care Med* 2010;**182**:1377–86.

61 Decramer M, Gayan-Ramirez G. Ventilator-induced diaphragmatic dysfunction: toward a better treatment? *Am J Respir Crit Care Med* 2004;**170**:1141–2.

62 Gayan-Ramirez G, Testelmans D, Maes K, et al. Intermittent spontaneous breathing protects the rat diaphragm from mechanical ventilation effects. *Crit Care Med* 2005;**33**:2804–9.

63 Le Bourdelles G, Viires N, Boczkowski J, Seta N, Pavlovic D, Aubier M. Effects of mechanical ventilation on diaphragmatiq contractile properties in rats. *Am J Respir Crit Care Med* 1994;**149**:1539–44.

64 Jaber S, Sebbane M, Koechlin C, et al. Effects of short vs. prolonged mechanical ventilation on antioxidant systems in piglet diaphragm. *Intensive Care Med* 2005;**31**:1427–33.

65 Sassoon CS, Caiozzo VJ, Manka A, Sieck GC. Altered diaphragm contractile properties with controlled mechanical ventilation. *J Appl Physiol* 2002;**92**:2585–95.

66 Sassoon CS, Zhu E, Caiozzo VJ. Assist-control mechanical ventilation attenuates ventilator-induced diaphragmatic dysfunction. *Am J Respir Crit Care Med* 2004;**170**:626–32.

67 Jung B, Constantin JM, Rossel N, et al. Adaptive support ventilation prevents ventilator-induced diaphragmatic dysfunction in piglet: an in vivo and in vitro study. *Anesthesiology* 2010;**112**:1435–43.

68 Dasta JF, McLaughlin TP, Mody SH, Piech CT. Daily cost of an intensive care unit day: the contribution of mechanical ventilation. *Crit Care Med* 2005;**33**:1266–71.

69 Kahn JM. The evolving role of dedicated weaning facilities in critical care. *Intensive Care Med* 2010;**36**: 8–10.

70 Gracey DR, Hardy DC, Koenig GE. The chronic ventilator-dependent unit: a lower-cost alternative to intensive care. *Mayo Clin Proc* 2000;**75**:445–9.

71 Gracey DR, Naessens JM, Viggiano RW, Koenig GE, Silverstein MD, Hubmayr RD. Outcome of patients cared for in a ventilator-dependent unit in a general hospital. *Chest* 1995;**107**:494–9.

72 Gracey DR, Viggiano RW, Naessens JM, Hubmayr RD, Silverstein MD, Koenig GE. Outcomes of patients admitted to a chronic ventilator-dependent unit in an acute-care hospital. *Mayo Clin Proc* 1992; **67**:131–6.

73 Ambrosino N, Venturelli E, Vagheggini G, Clini E., Rehabilitation weaning and physical therapy strategies in chronic critically ill patients. *Eur Respir J* 2012;**39**:487–92.

74 Blot F, Similowski T, Trouillet JL, et al. Early tracheotomy versus prolonged endotracheal intubation in unselected severely ill ICU patients. *Intensive Care Med* 2008;**34**:1779–87.

75 Terragni PP, Antonelli M, Fumagalli R, et al. Early vs late tracheotomy for prevention of pneumonia in mechanically ventilated adult ICU patients: a randomized controlled trial. *JAMA* 2010;**303**:1483–9.

76 Trouillet JL, Luyt CE, Guiguet M, et al. Early percutaneous tracheotomy versus prolonged intubation of mechanically ventilated patients after cardiac surgery: a randomized trial. *Ann Intern Med* 2011;**154**: 373–83.

77 Diehl JL, El Atrous S, Touchard D, Lemaire F, Brochard L. Changes in the work of breathing induced by tracheotomy of ventilator-dependent patients. *Am J Respir Crit Care Med* 1999;**159**:383–8.

78 Nieszkowska A, Combes A, Luyt CE, et al. Impact of tracheotomy on sedative administration, sedation level, and comfort of mechanically ventilated intensive care unit patients. *Crit Care Med* 2005;**33**: 2527–33.

79 Polverino E, Nava S, Ferrer M, et al. Patients' characterization, hospital course and clinical outcomes in five Italian respiratory intensive care units. *Intensive Care Med* 2010;**36**:137–42.

80 Vitacca M, Vianello A, Colombo D, et al. Comparison of two methods for weaning patients with chronic obstructive pulmonary disease requiring mechanical ventilation for more than 15 days. *Am J Respir Crit Care Med* 2001;**164**:225–30.

81 Chadda K, Louis B, Benaissa L, et al. Physiological effects of decannulation in tracheostomized patients. *Intensive Care Med* 2002;**28**:1761–7.

82 Ceriana P, Carlucci A, Navalesi P, et al. Weaning from tracheotomy in long-term mechanically ventilated patients: feasibility of a decisional flowchart and clinical outcome. *Intensive Care Med* 2003;**29**:845–8.

83 **Jubran A, Lawm G, Duffner LA, et al.** Post-traumatic stress disorder after weaning from prolonged mechanical ventilation. *Intensive Care Med* 2010;**36**:2030–7.

84 **Jubran A, Lawm G, Kelly J, et al.** Depressive disorders during weaning from prolonged mechanical ventilation. *Intensive Care Med* 2010;**36**:828–35.

85 **Carpene N, Vagheggini G, Panait E, Gabbrielli L, Ambrosino N.** A proposal of a new model for long-term weaning: respiratory intensive care unit and weaning center. *Respir Med* 2010;**104**:1505–11.

86 **Subbe CP, Criner GJ, Baudouin SV.** Weaning units: lessons from North America? *Anaesthesia* 2007;**62**:374–80.

Chapter 15

The Long-Term Outcomes of Acute Kidney Injury

Ron Wald and Ziv Harel

Introduction

Acute kidney injury (AKI) is a common complication of critical illness, with important implications for short-term morbidity and mortality. Recent studies, using contemporary staging
systems, indicate that 22–67% of critical care stays are complicated by AKI.[1-4] Even the mildest
forms of AKI (serum creatinine rise of 27 micromole/L or 50% above baseline) are associated
with substantially higher in-hospital mortality. For the minority of patients with AKI who require
acute dialysis, 60-day mortality is in excess of 50%.[5] These dismal outcomes are further punctu-
ated by the absence of any definitive therapies to prevent AKI, and, once established, there is no
established therapeutic manoeuvre that accelerates kidney recovery or modifies survival.

Comparatively little is known about the outcomes of AKI survivors. It was previously felt that,
following recovery from an acute illness complicated by AKI, kidney function would generally
recover to the level of function that existed prior to the acute illness. However, recent research has
uncovered a compelling relationship between AKI and both *de novo* CKD and the progression
of pre-existing CKD. In addition, survivors of AKI have a high rate of cardiovascular events and
mortality. Whether these epidemiologic findings are indicative of a causal link between AKI and
clinical outcomes remains unclear.

Scientific rationale for the adverse clinical impact of AKI

Animal studies have provided important mechanistic insights on the long-term implications of
AKI. Basile and colleagues induced AKI in rats through bilateral renal artery clamping, with a
comparator group of rats that received a sham procedure.[6] There was a marked initial rise in serum
creatinine among the rats that underwent renal artery clamping, but, by the end of the first week,
serum creatinine levels returned to baseline and approximated those in the sham-operated rats.
Despite the apparent recovery of kidney function, post-AKI rats developed significant proteinuria,
compared to sham-treated animals, at 16 weeks following the initial insult. At 40 weeks following
renal artery clamping, microvascular density was diminished and tubulointerstitial fibrosis was
heightened in rats subjected to experimental AKI. Subsequent work suggested a prominent role
for the profibrotic cytokine transforming growth factor-β (TGF-β) in mediating this process.[7]

A further body of research suggests that an episode of AKI imparts long-term cardiovascular dysfunction. Kelly et al. demonstrated that apoptosis and echocardiographically proven
cardiac dysfunction developed in rats exposed to transient renal ischaemia-reperfusion (I/R).[8]
Furthermore, rats that recovered kidney function after an episode of I/R injury had evidence of
endothelial dysfunction and salt-sensitive hypertension several weeks after the initial insult.[9,10]

In summary, studies in animal models provide a compelling rationale for why AKI may have implications months to years after recovery from the acute illness despite the apparent recovery of kidney function.

The epidemiology of the long-term outcomes of AKI

AKI and progressive CKD

Early studies examining kidney function among AKI survivors were hampered by relatively small sample sizes and often the lack of a comparator cohort comprising non-AKI patients.[11] Moreover, the definition of post-AKI survival and the duration of follow-up were quite variable. Access to administrative datasets encompassing entire populations made it feasible to study large cohorts that were hospitalized with AKI; linkages to laboratory and end-stage renal disease (ESRD) registries permitted the ascertainment of important kidney outcomes over an extended time period following the initial insult.

Using data from the Cooperative Cardiovascular Project, a quality improvement initiative directed at patients hospitalized with myocardial infarction in 1994–1995, Newsome et al. followed the post-discharge course of nearly 90 000 individuals.[12] Over a maximum follow-up of 10 years (median 4.1 years), 1.6% of patients developed ESRD. After adjustment for key clinical and demographic variables, the risk of ESRD was increased 3-fold (adjusted hazard ratio (HR) 3.26 (95% CI 2.73–3.71)) among individuals with the highest quartile of serum creatinine rise (i.e. 0.6–3.0 mg/dL) during the index hospitalization.

Subsequent studies evaluated the link between AKI and progressive CKD in a broader cohort of hospitalized patients. Using American Medicare data from the year 2000, Ishani et al. showed that survivors of hospitalizations complicated by AKI had an ESRD incidence of 5.3 per 1000 person-years.[13] After adjustment for a limited set of covariates, AKI survivors without pre-existing CKD had a 13-fold risk of ESRD (HR 13.0, 95% CI 10.6–16.0), as compared to controls with neither AKI nor CKD. Among AKI survivors and pre-existing CKD, the risk of ESRD was further accentuated (HR 41.2, 95% CI 34.6–49.1).

Two cohort studies, utilizing databases from Kaiser Permanente of Northern California, highlighted the impact of dialysis-requiring AKI on long-term kidney function. In both studies, AKI survivors comprised patients who survived to 30 days following discharge without the development of ESRD. Hospitalized patients with underlying CKD (pre-hospitalization estimated glomerular filtration rate (eGFR) <45 mL/min/1.73m^2) and an episode of AKI requiring dialysis were at significantly higher risk of ESRD (adjusted HR 1.30, 95% CI 1.04–1.64), as compared to those without AKI.[14] A parallel study focused on patients with dialysis-requiring AKI who had relatively preserved kidney function (eGFR >45 mL/min/1.73 m^2) at baseline.[15] After an episode of dialysis-requiring AKI, the risk of CKD stage 4 or worse (i.e. eGFR <30 mL/min/1.73m^2) was increased 28-fold (adjusted HR 28.1, 95% CI 21.1–37.6), as compared to the absence of AKI.

A study using administrative data from across Ontario, Canada, further established the link between dialysis-requiring AKI, defined by diagnosis and billing codes, and subsequent ESRD.[16] The presence of a government-funded, single-payer health care system assured the capture of all events from across the province. Patients suffering an episode of dialysis-requiring AKI between 1996 and 2006 who survived free of dialysis and re-hospitalization for at least 30 days after discharge were identified. A comparator group, hospitalized during a contemporaneous period with neither AKI nor dialysis, was identified by matching patients using a propensity score for the risk of AKI-requiring dialysis. The incidence rate of ESRD (defined as the need for chronic dialysis for ≥90 days) among survivors of dialysis-requiring AKI was 2.63 per 100 person-years, and such individuals had a threefold higher risk (adjusted HR 3.23, 95% CI 2.70–3.86) of ESRD over a median follow-up of 3 years, as compared to controls. In a much larger cohort of patients hospitalized with AKI but who did not require acute dialysis (n = 41 327), the incidence of ESRD among AKI survivors was substantially lower at 1.78 per 100 person-years. However, when compared to a propensity score-matched cohort of individuals with hospitalizations uncomplicated by AKI, the relative risk of developing ESRD was similar to that observed with dialysis-requiring AKI (adjusted HR 2.70, 95% CI 2.42–3.00).[17]

Using a province-wide dataset from Alberta, Canada that enabled linkages to laboratory data, James et al. accurately characterized pre-AKI kidney function by considering the eGFR and the magnitude of proteinuria.[18] While an episode of AKI was independently associated with the progression of kidney disease, as defined by a doubling in serum creatinine or the initiation of chronic dialysis over a median follow-up of 35 months, the magnitude of this association was substantially diminished among individuals with lower premorbid eGFR or high-grade proteinuria. These findings suggest that, in the presence of significant underlying kidney disease, renal prognosis is largely driven by the presence of CKD, as opposed to the episode of AKI. The actual impact of an AKI episode is significantly more pronounced in the setting of preserved premorbid kidney function.

AKI and long-term mortality

Several of the studies cited in the previous paragraphs showed a consistent link between AKI and a heightened risk of long-term mortality. An episode of AKI was associated with an adjusted risk of mortality that was increased twofold among Medicare recipients.[13] In the Kaiser Northern California cohorts, dialysis-requiring AKI, whether occurring on the background of preserved or impaired kidney function, was associated with a higher risk of death among individuals who survived for 30 days, following discharge.[14,15]

The impact of an episode of non-dialysis-requiring AKI on long-term survival was further evaluated in a large cohort of over 800 000 American veterans who survived for 90 days, following hospitalization.[19] Over a mean follow-up of 2.3 years, AKI survivors had a crude mortality of 30%, as compared to 16% among individuals without AKI. Following adjustment for an extensive array of covariates, including post-discharge residual kidney function, AKI was associated with a 40% higher risk of mortality (adjusted HR 1.41, 95% CI 1.39–1.43). Importantly, AKI severity during the index hospitalization was associated with a graded rise in the risk of long-term mortality.

High long-term mortality was also observed among AKI survivors in Ontario, Canada, who survived to 30 days following discharge.[16,17] Crude mortality in the years following an episode of dialysis-requiring AKI and non-dialysis-requiring AKI was 35% and 41%, respectively. However, when compared to propensity-matched cohorts without AKI, dialysis-requiring AKI was not independently associated with death (adjusted HR 0.95, 95% CI 0.89–1.02).[16] The relative risk of death was modestly elevated among survivors of non-dialysis-requiring AKI (adjusted HR 1.10, 95% CI 1.07–1.13).[17]

In summary, while survivors of AKI have a high risk of death in the months and years following their acute illness, the independent impact of AKI is controversial. The divergent effect estimates in studies that utilized different approaches to account for confounding suggest that the relationship between AKI and mortality may not be causal in nature.

The long-term cardiovascular impact of AKI

As described previously, basic scientific investigation suggests that AKI induces cardiovascular toxicity, which may persist well after the initial insult. In a cohort of nearly 2000 patients who experienced an ST-elevation myocardial infarction, individuals with moderate/severe AKI (defined as serum creatinine rise of >0.5 mg/dL on the index hospitalization) that did not completely resolve by the time of discharge from the index hospitalization had a twofold risk of heart failure (HF) after a median follow-up of 36 months.[20] In a secondary analysis of the Survival and Ventricular Enlargement trial that evaluated the role of captopril in patients with a myocardial infarction complicated by severe left ventricular systolic function, an episode of AKI (defined as a serum creatinine of >0.3 mg/dL on the index hospitalization) was associated with a higher risk of the composite endpoint of cardiovascular death, recurrent myocardial infarction, and HF over a 36-month follow-up period (HR 1.32, 95% CI, 1.03–1.70).[21]

Limitations associated with epidemiologic studies of AKI survivors

Although studies rooted in administrative databases provide substantial statistical power and generalizability to large, diverse populations, these studies also have important limitations. Diagnosis codes to identify AKI, especially when dialysis is not administered, have poor sensitivity and may predispose to misclassification of the exposure.[22,23] However, the combination of an AKI diagnosis code and a claim for dialysis is more robust. While 'hard' outcomes, such as ESRD or death, are reliable to discern in administrative datasets, the inability to link to laboratory data in many studies limits the detection of *de novo* CKD or its progression. However, even when linkage to laboratory data is feasible, bloodwork is not always available at consistent time intervals (i.e. every 6 months after discharge). Finally, the mounting epidemiologic data linking AKI and adverse outcomes may be subject to residual confounding due to unavailable or unmeasurable covariates. Most importantly, missing data on premorbid kidney function, as well as the pace of kidney function decline prior to the acute illness on which AKI occurred, make it difficult to establish the actual effect of the AKI event on the long-term trajectory of kidney function[24] (see Figure 15.1). Specifically, are the adverse outcomes attributed to AKI reflective of AKI being a mere surrogate for serious comorbidity or is AKI a direct mediator of progressive kidney disease and death? This issue can only be resolved definitively if future trials for the primary prevention of AKI integrate a long-term follow-up component to establish whether the prevention of AKI confers protection from progressive CKD and death in the ensuing years.

How can we improve the outcomes of AKI survivors?

Prediction of adverse clinical events following an episode of AKI

The accumulating epidemiologic data supporting a link between AKI and subsequent adverse outcomes are tempered by limited data on how to translate this information into clinical practice. Although a significant proportion of AKI survivors will die and a smaller number will experience progressive kidney disease in the 2–5 years following an AKI hospitalization, the majority of AKI survivors will recover kidney function and will not experience an adverse clinical event. Given the high frequency with which AKI complicates an acute hospitalization, the provision of close follow-up or the administration of a putative protective therapy to all AKI survivors may be inefficient. As a result, the early identification of 'high-risk' AKI survivors will help target any potential preventative strategies to individuals who stand to derive the maximum benefit.

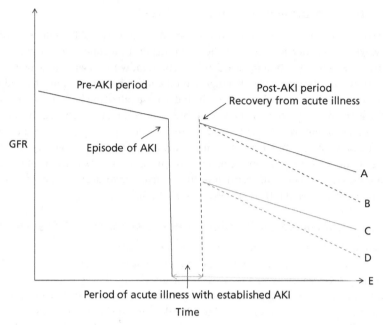

Fig. 15.1 The impact of AKI on long-term kidney function. The figure depicts five hypothetical scenarios after an episode of severe AKI, leading to virtual cessation of endogenous kidney function, as expressed by the GFR (glomerular filtration rate) on the y-axis. During the pre-AKI period, GFR is declining at a stable pace. After a variable period of acute illness, and possibly requirement for RRT, the surviving patient enters a period of recovery that is heralded by the dotted vertical line. In scenarios A and B, kidney function returns to slightly below the GFR that was noted prior to the acute illness. In scenario A, kidney function then declines at the same rate, but in scenario B, the pace of kidney function decline accelerates after the episode of AKI. In scenario A, the episode of AKI did not meaningfully alter the course of kidney function decline, whereas it does in scenario B. In scenarios C and D, kidney function recovers to a level substantially below the level of kidney function present before the episode of AKI. In scenario C, kidney function decline occurs at the same rate as that prior to the acute illness, but, since post-AKI, kidney function was reset at a lower level, the patient depicted in this scenario is more likely to progress to require chronic dialysis. In scenario D, the patient's kidney function returns to a lower level after recovery from the acute illness **and** kidney function declines at an accelerated rate. In scenario E, there is no meaningful recovery of kidney function after the episode of AKI, and the patient remains dependent on RRT. Understanding the true relationship between an episode of AKI and post-AKI kidney function is highly dependent on comprehending the course of kidney function during the pre-AKI period. For example, in scenario A, if one had limited information on the trajectory of kidney function prior to the episode of AKI, one may be tempted to ascribe the lower GFR observed after the acute illness to an 'AKI-induced fall in GFR' when, in fact, the patient's kidney function was on the same trajectory of decline after the episode of AKI as it was prior to the event.

Reproduced from Liu KD, Lo L, Hsu CY, 'Some methodological issues in studying the long-term renal sequelae of acute kidney injury', *Current Opinion in Nephrology and Hypertension*, 18, 3, pp. 241–245, copyright 2009, with permission from Wolters Kluwer.

Chawla and colleagues followed the course of 5351 patients following discharge from a hospitalization complicated by an episode of AKI with the intent of clarifying factors that anticipated progressive CKD.[25] Eligible patients were admitted to a Veterans' Administration hospital between October 1999 and December 2005 and had preserved kidney function (eGFR >60 mL/min/1.73 m^2) prior to the index hospitalization. The primary outcome, persistent stage 4 CKD (eGFR <30 mL/min/1.73 m^2), occurred in 728 (14%) patients. Three separate predictive models were derived in order to maximize clinical applicability, depending on the availability of data. Each model had good discrimination for the development of stage 4 CKD (c-statisitics ranged from 0.77 to 0.82). Older age, mean serum creatinine during the index hospitalization, AKI severity, and the receipt of acute dialysis were all associated with a significantly higher likelihood of CKD progression, whereas serum albumin and African American race were inversely associated with CKD progression.

In a study of 1610 patients with premorbid eGFR >60 mL/min/1.73m^2 who developed AKI during a hospitalization, CKD developed in 841 (52.2%) patients over a median follow-up of 3.3 years. Older age, pre-existing HF and hypertension, lower baseline GFR, higher comorbidity (as quantified by the Charlson Comorbidity Index), and severity of AKI were associated with the development of *de novo* CKD.[26]

A study conducted in Alberta, Canada highlighted the importance of short-term recovery of kidney function after an episode of AKI on long-term outcomes. Among 3231 patients with AKI who survived to 90 days after an episode of AKI, 70% experienced early recovery of kidney function, defined as a return to within 25% of premorbid serum creatinine within 30–150 days of the AKI episode. Mortality over a median follow-up period of 2.8 years was significantly higher for patients who did not recover (HR 1.26, 95% CI 1.10–1.43). Non-recovery of kidney function was also associated with a 4-fold increase in the risk of developing a sustained doubling of serum creatinine or the need for chronic RRT (HR 4.13, 95% CI 3.38–5.04).[27]

Although these findings require validation in different populations before becoming widely applicable, these studies provide preliminary insights into the risk stratification of AKI survivors and suggest subsets of patients that may benefit from more rigorous post-discharge follow-up (see Table 15.1).

Strategies to reduce adverse outcomes following an episode of AKI

Although the causal relationship between AKI and adverse clinical events has not been definitively established, it is unquestionable that an episode of AKI foreshadows a more ominous prognosis with respect to CKD progression and overall survival. The high rate of adverse events among such individuals suggests a pressing need for novel strategies to modify these outcomes. To date, there

Table 15.1 Risk factors for progressive kidney disease following an episode of AKI

Pre-existing factors	Factors associated with acute episode and its aftermath
Older age	Severity of acute kidney injury
Impaired kidney function	Duration of acute kidney injury
Proteinuria	Receipt of intermittent (vs continuous) forms of renal support
History of heart failure	Extent of kidney recovery following acute illness
History of hypertension	
History of diabetes	

has not been a clinical trial dedicated to testing therapeutic strategies in AKI survivors, and thus high-quality evidence to guide the management of this vulnerable population is lacking.

Observational studies provide some hypothesis-generating data on potentially useful strategies for improving long-term outcomes in AKI survivors. For patients with severe AKI requiring RRT, continuous renal replacement therapy (CRRT) presents the theoretical advantage of slow ultra-filtration and solute removal, thereby minimizing haemodynamic perturbation. Although these putative benefits have not translated into any short-term survival advantage of continuous over intermittent modalities in several randomized trials,[28,29] it is possible that, among survivors of the initial critical illness, the haemodynamic stability conferred by CRRT would minimize iatrogenic ischaemia in the injured kidney and improve the likelihood of kidney function recovery.[30] In a multicentre study from Sweden, Bell et al. demonstrated that patients receiving CRRT for the initial management of AKI were more likely to be dialysis-independent at 90 days after dialysis initiation. Among CRRT recipients, a higher likelihood of freedom from chronic dialysis was maintained over a 10-year follow-up, as compared to patients who received intermittent haemodialysis (IHD).[31]

HMG-CoA reductase inhibitors (statins) have been shown to reduce cardiovascular outcomes in a wide array of settings, possibly as a result of their anti-inflammatory properties. In a cohort study of 434 patients undergoing percutaneous coronary intervention at a single centre in Italy, patients who were receiving statins prior to their procedure had a lower risk of post-procedure contrast-induced AKI (3% vs 27% in non-statin users).[32] All patients received statins at the time of discharge. Over a 4-year follow-up, contrast-induced AKI was a strong predictor of major adverse cardiac events (i.e. composite of cardiac death, myocardial infarction, or repeat coronary revascularization), but the pre-procedure use of statins appeared to confer persistent protection. Among patients who experienced AKI, the early receipt of statins was associated with mitigation of the risk of future cardiovascular events.

Process of care following an episode of AKI

Recent research has clarified the nature of care provided to patients after an episode of AKI.[33] AKI survivors who were alive 30 days following discharge from five Veterans' Administration hospitals between 2003 and 2008 were identified. Eligible patients had evidence of some degree of residu-ally impaired kidney function (eGFR <60 mL/min/1.73 m^2) for whom nephrology consultation or co-management would normally be recommended according to prevailing guidelines. Over the 12-month surveillance period, accounting for the competing risks of death, dialysis initiation, or kidney function improvement, only 8.5% of patients were referred to a nephrologist. Nephrology referral rates did not vary appreciably according to the severity of the initial AKI episode.

Survivors of AKI requiring dialysis are especially susceptible to developing progressive CKD and are at high risk of death. In a cohort of 3877 patients from Ontario, Canada, who survived to 90 days after discharge from a hospitalization that was complicated by dialysis-requiring AKI, Harel et al. showed that 1583 (41%) had an early nephrology visit, defined as a visit with a neph-rologist during the 90-day interval following discharge based on provincial claims data.[34] As com-pared to propensity score-matched AKI survivors with no evidence of an early nephrology visit, those with an early nephrology visit had significantly lower mortality over the ensuing 2 years (incidence 8.4 vs 10.6 per 100 person-years among those without early nephrology visit; adjusted HR 0.76, 95% CI 0.62–0.93). The incidence of ESRD was substantially higher among those with an early nephrology visit (7.0 vs 2.7 per 100 person-years among those with no early nephrology visit; adjusted HR 2.71, 95% CI 1.76–4.19). The datasets used for the study could not evaluate specific interventions offered by nephrologists that could explain the aforementioned relation-ships. Nonetheless, one may speculate that several benefits may be attributed to post-discharge nephrology care which may reduce the risk of death. Nephrologists are well versed in delivering optimal CKD care and are optimally positioned to address an array of CKD-associated complications while facilitating the preparation for chronic dialysis, as appropriate. It has been shown that patients with CKD who consult a nephrologist relatively later or infrequently experience excess mortality after starting maintenance dialysis.[35] Notably, the association between early nephrology visit and the subsequent risk of ESRD suggests that referrals to nephrologists were preferentially made for patients who had less residual kidney function at the conclusion of the index hospitalization, in whom kidney disease progression was felt to be more likely.

Implications for current clinical practice and suggestions for future research

Hospitalized patients who survive an episode of AKI remain at risk for serious adverse outcomes, including ESRD and death. These risks persist for several years after discharge from the hospitalization on which the initial AKI episode occurred. Basic science data, emanating from animals subjected to experimental AKI, demonstrate irreversible renal scarring and vascular abnormalities long after the initial insult despite the ostensible recovery of kidney function. These data provide a plausible mechanism to explain the accumulating epidemiologic data that has linked AKI with progressive kidney disease, cardiovascular events, and mortality. Nonetheless, it remains unclear if AKI is a direct mediator of long-term adverse outcomes or whether the reported relationships are confounded by patient demographics and comorbid conditions, most notably the extent of CKD prior to hospitalization. Ultimately, the true long-term implications of AKI will only be known once patients enrolled in trials of AKI prevention are followed for several years to see whether the initial reduction of AKI risk translates into improved outcomes that are sustained over time.

Irrespective of the true biologic significance of an AKI event, AKI survivors represent a high-risk group for whom no high-quality evidence exists to guide clinical practice. Given the increasing incidence of AKI, ensuring the optimal management of AKI survivors is of great relevance to public health.[36] RCTs testing strategies that are plausibly nephroprotective and/or cardioprotective (e.g. renin-angiotensin system blockade (RAS), blood pressure control, statins, smoking cessation) are urgently needed. Rather than testing a single intervention, a multi-pronged, pragmatic strategy that integrates numerous therapies stands to have the highest likelihood of success. Until the completion of such trials, post-discharge follow-up with a nephrologist should be provided to all patients who experienced dialysis-requiring AKI as well as those individuals with residual CKD (eGFR <60 mL/min/1.73 m^2) following an acute illness. Close monitoring of kidney function and proteinuria, and modulation of blood pressure and cardiovascular risk factors are likely warranted.

References

1 Hoste EA, Clermont G, Kersten A, et al. RIFLE criteria for acute kidney injury are associated with hospital mortality in critically ill patients: a cohort analysis. *Crit Care* 2006;**10**:R73.

2 Thakar CV, Christianson A, Freyberg R, Almenoff P, Render ML. Incidence and outcomes of acute kidney injury in intensive care units: a Veterans Administration study. *Crit Care Med* 2009;**37**:2552–8.

3 Mandelbaum T, Scott DJ, Lee J, et al. Outcome of critically ill patients with acute kidney injury using the Acute Kidney Injury Network criteria. *Crit Care Med* 2011;**39**:2659–64.

4 Nisula S, Kaukonen KM, Vaara ST, et al. Incidence, risk factors and 90-day mortality of patients with acute kidney injury in Finnish intensive care units: the FINNAKI study. *Intensive Care Med* 2013;**39**:420–8.

5 Palevsky PM, Zhang JH, O'Connor TZ, et al. Intensity of renal support in critically ill patients with acute kidney injury. *N Engl J Med* 2008;**359**:7–20.

6 Basile DP, Donohoe D, Roethe K, Osborn JL. Renal ischemic injury results in permanent damage to peritubular capillaries and influences long-term function. *Am J Physiol Renal Physiol* 2001;**281**: F887–99.

7 Spurgeon KR, Donohoe DL, Basile DP. Transforming growth factor-beta in acute renal failure: receptor expression, effects on proliferation, cellularity, and vascularization after recovery from injury. *Am J Physiol Renal Physiol* 2005;**288**:F568–77.

8 Kelly KJ. Distant effects of experimental renal ischemia/reperfusion injury. *J Am Soc Nephrol* 2003;**14**:1549–58.

9 Phillips SA, Pechman KR, Leonard EC, et al. Increased ANG II sensitivity following recovery from acute kidney injury: role of oxidant stress in skeletal muscle resistance arteries. *Am J Physiol Regul Integr Comp Physiol* 2010;**298**:R1682–91.

10 Spurgeon-Pechman KR, Donohoe DL, Mattson DL, Lund H, James L, Basile DP. Recovery from acute renal failure predisposes hypertension and secondary renal disease in response to elevated sodium. *Am J Physiol Renal Physiol* 2007;**293**:F269–78.

11 Coca SG, Yusuf B, Shlipak MG, Garg AX, Parikh CR. Long-term risk of mortality and other adverse outcomes after acute kidney injury: a systematic review and meta-analysis. *Am J Kidney Dis* 2009;**53**:961–73.

12 Newsome BB, Warnock DG, McClellan WM, et al. Long-term risk of mortality and end-stage renal disease among the elderly after small increases in serum creatinine level during hospitalization for acute myocardial infarction. *Arch Intern Med* 2008;**168**:609–16.

13 Ishani A, Xue JL, Himmelfarb J, et al. Acute kidney injury increases risk of ESRD among elderly. *J Am Soc Nephrol* 2009;**20**:223–8.

14 Hsu CY, Chertow GM, McCulloch CE, Fan D, Ordonez JD, Go AS. Nonrecovery of kidney function and death after acute on chronic renal failure. *Clin J Am Soc Nephrol* 2009;**4**:891–8.

15 Lo LJ, Go AS, Chertow GM, et al. Dialysis-requiring acute renal failure increases the risk of progressive chronic kidney disease. *Kidney Int* 2009;**76**:893–9.

16 Wald R, Quinn RR, Luo J, et al. Chronic dialysis and death among survivors of acute kidney injury requiring dialysis. *JAMA* 2009;**302**:1179–85.

17 Wald R, Quinn RR, Adhikari NK, et al. Risk of chronic dialysis and death following acute kidney injury. *Am J Med* 2012;**125**:585–93.

18 James MT, Hemmelgarn BR, Wiebe N, et al. Glomerular filtration rate, proteinuria, and the incidence and consequences of acute kidney injury: a cohort study. *Lancet* 2010;**376**:2096–103.

19 Lafrance JP, Miller DR. Acute kidney injury associates with increased long-term mortality. *J Am Soc Nephrol* 2010;**21**:345–52.

20 Goldberg A, Kogan E, Hammerman H, Markiewicz W, Aronson D. The impact of transient and persistent acute kidney injury on long-term outcomes after acute myocardial infarction. *Kidney Int* 2009;**76**:900–6.

21 Jose P, Skali H, Anavekar N, et al. Increase in creatinine and cardiovascular risk in patients with systolic dysfunction after myocardial infarction. *J Am Soc Nephrol* 2006;**17**:2886–91.

22 Waikar SS, Wald R, Chertow GM, et al. Validity of International Classification of Diseases, Ninth Revision, Clinical Modification Codes for Acute Renal Failure. *J Am Soc Nephrol* 2006;**17**:1688–94.

23 Hwang YJ, Shariff SZ, Gandhi S, et al. Validity of the International Classification of Diseases, Tenth Revision code for acute kidney injury in elderly patients at presentation to the emergency department and at hospital admission. *BMJ Open* 2012;**2**:pii:e001821.

24 Liu KD, Lo L, Hsu CY. Some methodological issues in studying the long-term renal sequelae of acute kidney injury. *Curr Opin Nephrol Hypertens* 2009;**18**:241–5.

25 Chawla LS, Amdur RL, Amodeo S, Kimmel PL, Palant CE. The severity of acute kidney injury predicts progression to chronic kidney disease. *Kidney Int* 2011;**79**:1361–9.

26 Bucaloiu ID, Kirchner HL, Norfolk ER, Hartle JE, 2nd, Perkins RM. Increased risk of death and *de novo* chronic kidney disease following reversible acute kidney injury. *Kidney Int* 2012;**81**:477–85.

27 Pannu N, James M, Hemmelgarn B, Klarenbach S. Association between AKI, recovery of renal function, and long-term outcomes after hospital discharge. *Clin J Am Soc Nephrol* 2013;**8**:194–202.

28 Vinsonneau C, Camus C, Combes A, et al. Continuous venovenous haemodiafiltration versus intermittent haemodialysis for acute renal failure in patients with multiple-organ dysfunction syndrome: a multicentre randomised trial. *Lancet* 2006;**368**:379–85.

29 Bagshaw SM, Berthiaume LR, Delaney A, Bellomo R. Continuous versus intermittent renal replacement therapy for critically ill patients with acute kidney injury: a meta-analysis. *Crit Care Med* 2008;**36**:610–17.

30 Schneider AG, Bellomo R, Bagshaw SM, et al. Choice of renal replacement therapy modality and dialysis dependence after acute kidney injury: a systematic review and meta-analysis. *Intensive Care Med* 2013;**39**:987–97.

31 Bell M, Granath F, Schon S, Ekbom A, Martling CR. Continuous renal replacement therapy is associated with less chronic renal failure than intermittent haemodialysis after acute renal failure. *Intensive Care Med* 2007;**33**:773–80.

32 Patti G, Nusca A, Chello M, et al. Usefulness of statin pretreatment to prevent contrast-induced nephropathy and to improve long-term outcome in patients undergoing percutaneous coronary intervention. *Am J Cardiol* 2008;**101**:279–85.

33 Siew ED, Peterson JF, Eden SK, et al. Outpatient nephrology referral rates after acute kidney injury. *J Am Soc Nephrol* 2012;**23**:305–12.

34 Harel Z, Wald R, Bargman JM, et al. Nephrologist follow-up improves all-cause mortality of severe acute kidney injury survivors. *Kidney Int* 2013;**83**:901–08.

35 Winkelmayer WC, Owen WF, Jr, Levin R, Avorn J. A propensity analysis of late versus early nephrologist referral and mortality on dialysis. *J Am Soc Nephrol* 2003;**14**:486–92.

36 Hsu CY. Where is the epidemic in kidney disease? *J Am Soc Nephrol* 2010;**21**:1607–11.

Chapter 16

Severe Burn Injuries and Their Long-Term Implications

Eva C. Diaz, Celeste C. Finnerty, and David N. Herndon

Introduction

Burn trauma has a prolonged severity and greater duration when compared to other critical illnesses. Burn injury triggers a dramatic stress response that is characterized by disturbances in the immune and endocrine systems and increased insulin resistance, muscle wasting, and marked hypermetabolism.[1]

Progress in the acute care setting has improved survival of severely burned patients. Forty years ago, the LD50 (lethal dose resulting in a 50% survival rate) approached approximately 40% of total body surface area burned (TBSA-B). Currently, the LD50 approaches 80% of TBSA-B, and, if inhalation injury is absent, children with lesions exceeding 80–90% usually survive.[2] Nevertheless, these survivors face severe disabilities and impairments that represent an increasing challenge in burn patient management.[3] Even though scarring, functional limitations, and psychological problems are the most notorious sequelae, the profound and complex metabolic changes that arise after burn injury may persist for years after the initial event, impacting every system in the body and delaying recovery and rehabilitation.[2,4]

Pharmacological and non-pharmacological interventions have been implemented to attenuate the burn-induced hypermetabolic response and provide metabolic support to burn victims. The goal is to not only ensure that the patient survives, but also to modify the pathophysiologic events associated with the response to burn injury and improve long-term outcomes.[5]

This chapter reviews the long-term metabolic and hormonal changes associated with severe burn injury and their effect on muscle metabolism, growth delay, and bone wasting. It also addresses scarring as an important sequela of burn injury and therapeutic interventions during the recovery phase of the injury.

The post-burn hypermetabolic response

Severe thermal injury, defined as lesions exceeding 40% of the total body surface area, triggers the most aggressive hypermetabolic and hypercatabolic responses seen in the trauma setting.[6,7] Immediately after severe burn injury, oxygen consumption, glucose tolerance, and cardiac output (CO) are low. This so-called 'ebb' phase occurs within the first 3 days after injury. After this, the 'flow' phase ensues, with hyperdynamic circulation, a gradual incremental increase in the metabolic rate, increased lipolysis, glycolysis, proteolysis and body temperature, and futile substrate cycling.[4,7,8]

Contrary to what was previously believed, this phase lasts well beyond wound healing and the acute hospitalization.[9] Hypermetabolic physiology involves dramatic endocrine and immunologic responses that linger years after the initial event and adversely affect long-term outcomes.

Extent of the hypermetabolic response

The intensity of the hypermetabolic response to burn is determined by the TBSA-B and the time elapsed since injury. Accordingly, patients with less than 10% of TBSA-B exhibit insignificant modifications of the resting energy expenditure (REE), whereas patients with more than 40% of TBSA-B may have REEs that exceed twice that of normal, non-burnt patients.[10] After severe burns, the resting metabolic rate at a thermally neutral temperature (33°C) reaches 180% of the basal rate during acute admission, 150% when the burn wound is fully healed, 140% at 6 months post-burn, 120% at 9 months post-burn, and 110% at 12 months post-burn.[9,10]

In a large prospective study,[11] we assessed the pathophysiologic events associated with burn injury during the first 3 years after the initial trauma. Even at 3 years, burn survivors continued to exhibit elevated levels of stress hormones, inflammatory markers, and abnormally elevated REE, indicating long-term persistence of the hypermetabolic response.

Mediators of the hypermetabolic response

Corticosteroids, pro-inflammatory cytokines, and catecholamines orchestrate the cascade of events that follow major thermal injuries and are considered to be the primary mediators of the hypermetabolic state seen after burn trauma.[6]

Plasma levels of catecholamines surge immediately after burn and remain increased for up to 9 months, while urinary norepinephrine (NE) undergoes a 10-fold increase and remains significantly elevated for 18 months. In addition to inducing metabolic disturbances, catecholamines prompt post-burn cardiac stress and subsequent myocardial depression. Therefore, the reported persistence of the sympathetic response may explain the long-term elevations in cardiac parameters, such as CO and cardiac index, for up to 6 months post-injury as well as dramatic tachycardia (120–180% of the predicted heart rate) for at least 36 months post-injury.[11,12]

Similar to catecholamines, urinary and serum cortisol increase immediately after burn and remain significantly elevated 3 years after injury.[8,11,13] Cortisol influences metabolic and immune responses following burn trauma. Specifically, it induces increments in REE, acute phase protein synthesis, proteolysis, lipolysis, and gluconeogenesis and decreases in bone formation.[12]

Tissue damage, inflicted by direct thermal injury and by mediators of I/R injury, precipitates an immediate inflammatory response characterized by a surge in cytokines.[14] Overexpression of several cytokines leads to alterations in the immune system, protein metabolism, insulin sensitivity, and multiple organ systems.[11,15,16] Immediately after burn, IL-6, IL-8, and MCP-1 undergo a striking 2000-fold increase and, together with IL-2, GM-CSF, IFN-γ, and tumour necrosis factor alpha (TNF-α), remain significantly elevated at 3 years post-burn.[8,11]

Long-term insulin resistance

All the aforementioned metabolic alterations cause important modifications in energy substrate metabolism.[17] Catecholamines, cortisol, and glucagon are diabetogenic hormones that stimulate glucose production by the liver, amino acid release from muscle, and free fatty acid and glycerol release from fat.[6,18] All these changes lead to hyperglycaemia and impaired insulin sensitivity related to post-receptor insulin resistance, as demonstrated by elevated levels of insulin and fasting glucose as well as important reductions in glucose clearance.[6]

It is well established that hyperglycaemia and insulin resistance are associated with detrimental outcomes, specifically increased graft loss, impaired wound healing, increased protein catabolism, immunologic compromise, increased risk of infections, and death.[19,20]

Gauglitz et al.[8] reported that blood glucose levels are persistently elevated for 6 months after burn injury in the presence of normal pancreatic β-cell function. Even though euglycaemia is eventually reached, serum levels of insulin and C-peptide remain elevated at 3 years post-burn, indicating that insulin resistance persists for a prolonged time.

Mechanisms of chronic insulin resistance

Molecular mechanisms underlying post-burn insulin resistance are complex. Catecholamines and cytokines, such as IL-6, MCP-1, and TNF, can inhibit insulin action by modifying signalling properties of the insulin receptor substrate 1 (IRS-1) and translocation of the glucose transporter (GLUT)-4.[16,17,21]

Normally, phosphorylation of IRS-1 leads to activation of the phosphatidylinositol-3 kinase (PI3K)/AKT pathway, which plays a major role in stimulating glucose transport within hepatocytes, skeletal muscle, and adipose tissue. The PI3K/AKT pathway is also key in stimulating protein synthesis through activation of the protein kinase mammalian target of rapamycin (mTOR).[17]

Insulin resistance is also attributable to mitochondrial dysfunction. Mitochondrial dysfunction following burn injury attenuates the suppressive actions of insulin on hepatic glucose production and decreases muscle glucose oxidation, contributing to hyperglycaemia and peripheral insulin resistance. Furthermore, a massive loss of muscle mass in the acute and convalescent phase of the disease may also contribute to insulin resistance, since 70–80% of insulin-induced glucose uptake occurs in skeletal muscle.[17,21]

Muscle catabolism and burn injury

Muscle wasting, defined as the unintentional loss of 5–10% of muscle mass, is a hallmark of the post-burn hypermetabolic response. It leads to immunologic compromise, decreased strength, growth delay, failure to undergo full rehabilitation, and decreased QoL.[6,8,22] After burn injury, protein synthesis and protein breakdown are both increased. However, muscle protein is degraded much faster than it is synthesized, leading to a negative net protein balance.[7] Significant wasting of LBM can lead to loss of important structural and functional proteins, resulting in increased morbidity and mortality.[23] For instance, a 10% loss of total body mass is associated with immune system dysfunction. A 20% loss decreases wound healing. A 30% loss increases the risk of pneumonia and pressure sores. Finally, a 40% loss can lead to death.[6]

Burn victims that survive the acute phase of injury are not free from risk of complications. In fact, a major determinant of morbidity is the degree and length of the catabolic state.[24]

Muscle catabolism after major thermal injury

Hart et al.[9] studied the extent of burn-induced muscle catabolism by measuring the cross-leg phenylalanine balance. This study revealed that a negative net balance in protein occurs at 9 months post-injury, and an improved, but not positive, balance occurs at 12 months. This improvement is due solely to a decrease in protein breakdown rate. In the same study, modifications in LBM mirrored changes in protein kinetics, in that build-up of LBM was seen at 12 months after injury. Interestingly, further studies have shown that burnt children do not attain normal LBM values at 2, or even 3, years after injury.[11,24] Similar to critically ill adults, they may regain their weight but not their LBM.

At our centre, we recently found that muscle fractional synthetic rate (FSR) remains elevated for at least 18 months post-injury (unpublished data). This persistent alteration in the kinetics of muscle protein correlates with the long-lasting disturbances in metabolic homeostasis seen after severe burns. Further studies to characterize protein synthesis and protein breakdown balance after the first year post-injury in a larger sample population are warranted.

Biological mechanisms associated with long-term muscle protein wasting

Under physiologic conditions, IGF-1 plays a unique role in skeletal muscle by virtue of its ability to stimulate myoblast proliferation and differentiation.[25] However, immediately after severe burn injuries, serum levels of IGF-1 and its major binding protein IGFBP-3 decrease and remain decreased for at least 3 years.[3,11] Both IGF-1 and insulin are important determinants of muscle mass due to their ability to promote protein translation through activation of mTOR. Severe thermal injuries decrease IGF-1 levels and impair insulin signalling pathways by elevating levels of GCs, TNF-α, and other cytokines. These changes decrease phosphorylation of the FOX-O transcription factors (Forkhead box-containing protein, O-subfamily). This, in turn, increases the expression of ubiquitin proteasome system components (e.g. Atrogin-1 and MuRF1), which mediate protein degradation and muscle atrophy.[22,26]

Growth delay

Linear growth and weight gain are dynamic processes that generally reflect the state of a child's health.[27] They are dependent on many factors: nutritional intake, pituitary and thyroid hormone release, energy expenditure, and psychosocial environment.[28] Severe thermal injury is a catastrophic disease in which prolonged hospitalization, long-term alterations of the GH-hypophysis-IGF-1-IGFBP-3 axes, vast muscle wasting, high nutritional requirements, and hypermetabolism seem to interact and contribute to growth arrest in children.[8,17,29] Rutan and Herndon showed that major thermal injuries reduce weight, height, and growth velocities for up to 3 years. Significant changes in per cent height and weight gain have been reported to begin at 18 months post-burn;[24] however, weight and height remain significantly lower in burnt children than in non-burnt matched controls after 3 years.[11]

The effect of burn injury on growth delay appears to vary with the developmental stage of the child at the time of injury. Previous studies suggest that physiological increments in GH during the juvenile (6–8 years) and adolescent growth spurts (10.5–13 years for girls and 12.5–15 years for boys) can sustain normal growth after severe injury. On the other hand, children injured during non-growth spurt phases undergo obvious growth delays.[30]

rhGH therapy after severe thermal injuries can markedly improve linear growth, weight gain, and body composition.[31] An RCT revealed that paediatric patients receiving rhGH therapy from discharge to 12 months post-injury were able to reach an average height at the 50th percentile at 12 months, and even at 1 year, after discontinuation of treatment. In contrast, children who did not receive rhGH showed growth arrest, with a mean height percentile at 12 and 24 months that did not differ from that seen at discharge.[32]

Even though high doses of rhGH have been associated with increased morbidity and mortality in critically ill, non-burnt adult patients,[33] neither short-term nor long-term administration of rhGH has been associated with these complications in severely burnt children.[32]

Bone wasting

Severe burn injury adversely affects calcium and bone metabolism. In adults, iliac crest bone biopsies have demonstrated that bone formation is reduced at 3 weeks after burn.[13] Adults with less than 50% TBSA-B show uncoupled bone remodelling, i.e. a reduction in bone formation without a concomitant decrease in resorption. However, the long-term effects of bone injury on bone density in the adult population remain unknown.[34] In children, the effects of thermal injury on bone turnover are more severe and long-lasting. Histomorphometric analyses have shown that bone formation is almost absent at 26 ± 10 days post-burn, as seen by an almost non-existent uptake of doxycycline into trabecular bone.[34] In a cross-sectional study, Klein et al.[35] demonstrated that bone mass is decreased 5 years after burn injury in 60% of the subjects. In children, this sustained, pervasive loss of bone leads to an increased annual fracture incidence by twofold in boys and one-third in girls. Axial and appendicular fractures have been reported to occur with age-appropriate physical activity.[13,35]

Biological mechanism in acute and long-term bone wasting

Osteopaenia occurs rapidly following severe burns and is a sustained phenomenon involving multiple interacting mechanisms. First, the pro-inflammatory cytokines IL-1β and IL-6 stimulate osteoblasts to increase production of the ligand of the receptor activator of nuclear transcription factor κB (RANKL), which stimulates osteoclast differentiation to increase bone resorption. Second, cortisol can stimulate osteoblast production of RANKL, producing further bone wasting.[13] Third, immediately after burn injury, parathyroid hormone (PTH) decreases by 8-fold and remains significantly decreased for at least 3 years after injury.[11] Hypoparathyroidism, PTH resistance, hypocalcaemia, and hypercalciuria are characteristic alterations occurring after burn injury. Hypoparathyroidism is exacerbated by upregulation of the calcium-sensing receptor, which reduces the set point for calcium stimulation of PTH secretion.[36] Urinary calcium wasting and decreased osteoblastic activity can potentially interfere with deposition of calcium in the bone.[13]

Another factor that may contribute to bone disease is altered body biomechanics, produced by burn-induced damage to soft tissue.[35] Muscle atrophy and failure to return to pre-burn levels of physical activity also contribute to reduced bone mineralization.[37]

Finally, burn patients may become progressively vitamin D-deficient due to biochemical abnormalities of the skin. Burn scars, and even the adjacent normal skin, have reduced amounts of 7-dehydrocholesterol substrate and therefore diminished capacity to convert this vitamin D precursor to pre-vitamin D3. Supplementation with vitamin D is recommended, since previous studies have demonstrated that a correlation exists between low levels of 25(OH) vitamin D and lumbar spine bone mineral density (BMD).[13,38]

Management

Rehabilitation and limitation of adverse outcomes begin at the time of admission. Bone atrophy cannot be prevented, but it can be lessened by early mobilization. Thus, standing is a priority measure, since weight bearing is the most efficient strategy for stressing the bones of the axial skeleton, pelvis, and lower extremities. In addition, muscle isometric contractions can be used for bone stress and for maintaining muscle tone and bulk.[37]

Anabolic agents, like rhGH and oxandrolone, have been used to modulate the hypermetabolic response and improve outcomes. The effects of rhGH on bone mineral content (BMC) are dose-related. Administration of 0.05 mg/kg/day rhGH from discharge to 12 months after injury significantly improves BMC at 12 months, and even 2 years, after the injury when compared to placebo. However, 0.2 mg/kg/day rhGH is associated with a significant decrease in BMC at 9 and 12 months after injury.

In a controlled, prospective study of severely burnt children, oxandrolone was administered from discharge to 12 months after injury, and patients were monitored for 12 months after discontinuation of oxandrolone. At a dose of 0.1 mg/kg/bd, oxandrolone significantly improved BMC at 12 months but not at 18 or 24 months. On the other hand, improvements in body composition, weight, height, and strength were considerable and sustained.[39]

Reduction in bone wasting after the administration of anabolic agents may be partly and indirectly mediated by increased skeletal loading due to an increase in muscle skeletal mass.[36]

Finally, in severely burnt children, IV administration of a dose of the bisphosphonate pamidronate (1.5 mg/kg/day) within 10 days post-burn and then a second dose 1 week later was found to preserve lumbar spine BMC from admission to discharge. Patients receiving acute treatment with pamidronate had a better lumbar spine BMC than the placebo group at 6 and 24 months after burn injury.[40]

The burn scar

Scar tissue is defined as the fibrous tissue replacing normal tissue destroyed by injury or disease. After injury, if the scar is not managed appropriately, it may become hypertrophic.[41] Hypertrophic scarring is a frequent and severe form of fibrosis of the skin, which limits movement and compromises the cosmetic appearance and function of the skin.[42] It drastically affects the patient's QoL both physically and psychologically, by causing pain, pruritus, and contractures.[43]

Hypertrophic scars occur after deep dermal injury and are characterized by the overproduction of collagen.[44] Factors contributing to the formation of excessive scarring may include wound infection, genetics, immunological factors, repeated harvesting of donor sites, age, chronic inflammatory processes, location of the injury, and tension.[41]

Burn scar contracture is probably the most frequently seen cause of impairment in burn survivors. Contractile forces can result in marked skin shortage, decreasing the arc of motion of not only underlying joints, but also adjacent joints. When the scar contracture is severe, several staged surgical procedures may be needed until functionality and cosmesis are achieved. In addition to producing contractures, scar tissue is fragile and therefore prone to chronic ulceration. Loss of sweat gland function and hair growth, altered pigment formation, cold and heat intolerance, and altered sensation are other abnormalities associated with burn scar that limit restoration of function.[2]

Pathophysiology of the burn scar

Normal wound repair occurs in three different phases: inflammation, proliferation, and remodelling. During the inflammation phase, platelet degranulation is responsible for the release of potent cytokines, such as epidermal growth factor (EGF), IGF-1, platelet-derived growth factor (PDGF), and TGF-β, which serve as chemotactic agents for the recruitment of inflammatory cells. Transition to the second phase occurs within 48–72 hours after the initial event and lasts for up to 3–6 weeks. At this time, fibroblasts synthesize a scaffold of reparative tissue known as extracellular matrix (ECM), which forms a structural repair framework to bridge the wound and allow vascular ingrowth. Transition to the final maturation phase occurs once the wound is closed and may last several months. The abundant ECM is degraded, and the immature type III collagen of the early wound can be modified into mature type I collagen.[45] Alterations in the delicate balance between ECM protein deposition and degradation lead to abnormal scarring. Inflammation and alterations in the phenotype of fibroblasts, which have an increased number of growth factor receptors, produce this aberrant fibrotic response.[43]

Burn scar management

Pressure therapy has been the preferred conservative approach for both the prophylaxis and treatment of hypertrophic scars and keloids in burns.[43] During their early stages of development, burn scar contractures may often be corrected through the use of splints and pressure therapy.[2] Options for pressure therapy include pressure garments, inserts, and conforming orthotics.[41] The mechanism of action of pressure therapy remains poorly understood; however, possible mechanisms are increased apoptosis and decreased collagen synthesis, attributable to limiting the supply of blood, oxygen, and nutrients to the scar tissue.[45]

Pharmacological and non-pharmacological strategies and long-term outcomes after severe burn injury

Scientific evidence that burn injury induces a stress response and profound metabolic, hormonal, and immunologic alterations that persist for at least 3 years after injury augments the need for optimal pharmacological interventions that modulate the hypermetabolic response not only acutely, but also chronically.

Long-term persistence of elevated REE and decreased muscle mass, strength, and growth contribute significantly to delays in recovery and reintegration back into society.[39] This section provides a brief summary of the pharmacologic and non-pharmacologic interventions that have been studied in the acute setting and are intended to enhance recovery and rehabilitation as well as decrease morbidity and mortality associated with the prolonged hypermetabolic and catabolic state seen after major thermal injuries.

Oxandrolone

Oxandrolone, a testosterone analogue with only 5% of the virilizing effects of this steroid hormone, lessens muscle protein wasting by enhancing protein synthesis, reduces weight loss, decreases length of hospital stay, and increases donor site wound healing during the acute admission.[46] Beneficial effects of long-term administration of oxandrolone have also been documented.

In a prospective randomized trial, 61 burnt paediatric patients received either 0.1 mg/kg/day oxandrolone or placebo from discharge to 12 months after injury and were evaluated at discharge as well as at 6, 12, 18, and 24 months after injury. Oxandrolone-treated patients showed improved LBM, BMD, and strength during the treatment period, and significant differences in weight and height were detected between groups after discontinuation of treatment. Interestingly, a significant increment in serum IGF-1 levels was noted in oxandrolone-treated patients at 12 and 18 months. In addition, oxandrolone induced no significant changes in scar assessments or predicted REE.[39]

Oxandrolone in combination with exercise

Synergistic effects of oxandrolone and exercise have been documented. In one trial, 51 severely burnt children were assigned to receive oxandrolone (OX), oxandrolone and exercise (OXEX), placebo and no exercise (PL), or placebo and exercise (PLEX). Oxandrolone was administered from discharge to 12 months post-injury. OXEX was found to improve the per cent change in weight and LBM to a greater extent than the other three treatments. Changes in LBM in the OX and PLEX groups were superior to those seen in the PL group. Muscle strength was significantly better in the OXEX, OX, and PLEX groups than in the PL group. However, OXEX was not superior to OX and PLEX. Interestingly, OX was able to improve muscle strength, an effect that is not seen with rhGH alone (see Figure 16.1).[47]

rhGH

rhGH enhances immune function and wound healing as well as decreases the hypermetabolic response. In addition, rhGH stimulates protein synthesis and attenuates protein catabolism in the acute phase of burn trauma.[3]

A prospective, randomized trial was conducted to evaluate the long-term efficacy of rhGH in 205 paediatric patients with 40% of TBSA-B. Patients received either placebo or long-term rhGH treatment (0.05, 0.1, or 0.2 mg/kg/day) from discharge to 12 months post-injury. Evaluations were made at discharge and at 6, 9, 12, 18, and 24 months post-burn.[31] When compared to placebo, rhGH significantly improved LBM from 6 to 12 months post-burn. The greatest improvement in LBM was seen at a dose of 0.2 mg/kg/day, with this improvement remaining significant for the entire study duration (see Figure 16.2).

CO decreased at 12 and 18 months in the entire rhGH group, whereas REE significantly decreased at all time points, with the exception of 24 months. The largest decrease in REE was seen in the 0.1 mg/kg/day rhGH group. Improvements in cardiac stress and hypermetabolism may be related to decreases in cortisol levels seen after rhGH therapy. rhGH therapy was also associated with improvements in the hormonal panel, as manifested by increased levels of IGF-1/IGFBP-3 and endogenous GH, especially at 0.1 or 0.2 mg/kg/day. No significant alterations in glucose levels were reported in this study. However, improved scar scores (indicating reduced scarring) were noted at 12 months in the 0.1 and 0.2 mg/kg/day rhGH groups.

In summary, long-term administration of rhGH has the following dose-related effects: improvement in growth and LBM, reduction in hypermetabolism, increased IGF-1/IGFBP-3 serum levels, diminished cardiac stress, and attenuation of scarring.

Exercise

Therapeutic exercise is the motion of the body or its parts to relieve symptoms or improve function. The need for therapeutic exercise begins acutely and continues throughout the months of healing from burn injury. The goals of this strategy are to reduce the effect of oedema and immobilization, maintain functional joint motion and muscle strength, stretch the scar tissue, and return the patient to an optimal level of function.[41]

Exercise training is an essential adjunct to any metabolic treatment. Celis et al.[48] showed that incorporation or implementation of a supervised exercise programme at 6 months post-injury decreases the number of functional surgical releases at 9 months post-burn and, even more dramatically, at 24 months post-burn.

The addition of a 12-week resistance and aerobic exercise programme to the standard hospital rehabilitation plan has been shown to improve total LBM, strength, and overall cardiopulmonary capacity.[49] Suman et al. demonstrated that greater than 20-fold difference in the mean rate of increase in total LBM exists between patients undergoing resistance and aerobic exercise and those in the standard of care group. In this study, changes in LBM occurred in parallel to increments in muscle strength, total work, and power.

Patients with severe thermal injuries should participate in a structured exercise programme as soon as possible after hospital discharge. The programme should be individualized and based on progressive resistance. The improvements associated with exercise should increase the patient's capacity to return to normal daily activities and gain more physical independence.[41,49]

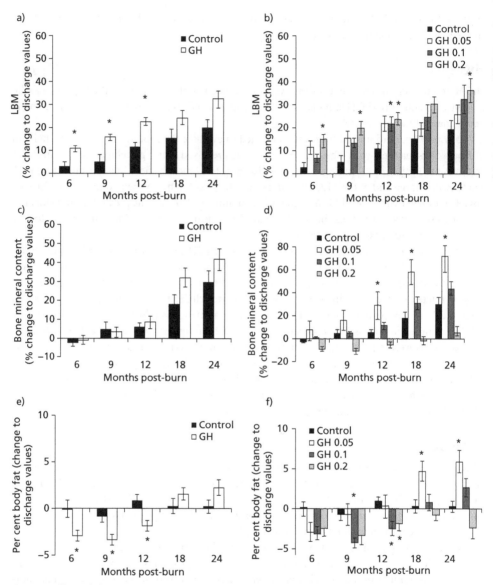

Fig. 16.1 Effect of rhGH therapy on body composition in severely burnt children. The per cent change from hospital discharge to 24 months post-burn is shown for (A, B) LBM, (C, D) bone mineral content, and (E, F) per cent body fat. Data are expressed as mean ± SEM. * *P* <0.05 vs control.

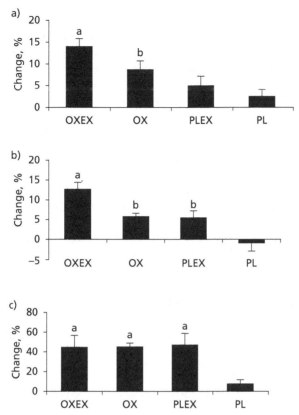

Fig. 16.2 Effect of oxandrolone and a 12-week exercise programme, alone or in combination, on (A) weight, (B) LBM, and (C) muscle strength in severely burnt children. Patients received oxandrolone (OX), oxandrolone + exercise (OXEX), placebo (PL), or placebo + exercise (PLEX). Data are expressed as the per cent change (mean ± SEM) from 6 months to 9 months post-burn, after completion of the exercise programme. For (A) and (B), [a] $P <0.05$ vs OX, PLEX, and PL; [b] $P <0.05$ vs PL. For (C), [a] $P <0.05$ vs PL.

Reproduced with permission from *Pediatrics*, Przkora R, Herndon DN, Suman OE, 'The effects of oxandrolone and exercise on muscle mass and function in children with severe burns', 119, 1, pp. e109–16, Copyright © 2007 by the AAP.

Conclusion

Severe thermal injury is a catastrophic condition associated with profound and long-lasting metabolic and hormonal disturbances that hamper recovery and rehabilitation for years after the initial trauma. Long-term outcomes depend on the unique characteristics of the post-burn stress response. Therefore, modulation of the hypermetabolic response is necessary if structural and functional restoration is to be achieved. Exercise has clear benefits in burn patients. In addition, oxandrolone and rhGH are two therapeutic strategies that have been shown to be effective in abating the hypermetabolic response after discharge and in improving long-term outcomes. Nonetheless, further studies are necessary to determine the optimal pharmacologic regimens for survivors of severe thermal injuries.

References

1 Mann EA, Mora AG, Pidcoke HF, Wolf SE, Wade CE. Glycemic control in the burn intensive care unit: focus on the role of anemia in glucose measurement. *J Diabetes Sci Technol* 2009;3:1319–29.

2 Warden GD, Warner P. Functional sequelae and disability assessment. In: Herndon DN (ed.) *Total burn care*. 2nd ed. London: WB Saunders; 2002. p. xv, p. 817, 4 p. of plates.

3 Jeschke MG, Chinkes DL, Finnerty CC, et al. Pathophysiologic response to severe burn injury. *Ann Surg* 2008;**248**:387–401.

4 Herndon DN, Tompkins RG. Support of the metabolic response to burn injury. *Lancet* 2004;**363**: 1895–902.

5 Desai SV, Law TJ, Needham DM. Long-term complications of critical care. *Crit Care Med* 2011;**39**: 371–9.

6 Williams FN, Jeschke MG, Chinkes DL, Suman OE, Branski LK, Herndon DN. Modulation of the hypermetabolic response to trauma: temperature, nutrition, and drugs. *J Am Coll Surg* 2009;**208**: 489–502.

7 Williams FN, Herndon DN, Jeschke MG. The hypermetabolic response to burn injury and interventions to modify this response. *Clin Plast Surg* 2009;**36**:583–96.

8 Gauglitz GG, Herndon DN, Kulp GA, Meyer WJ 3rd, Jeschke MG. *Abnormal insulin sensitivity persists up to three years in pediatric patients post-burn. J Clin Endocrinol Metab* 2009;**94**:1656–64.

9 Hart DW, Wolf SE, Mlcak R, et al. Persistence of muscle catabolism after severe burn. *Surgery* 2000;**128**:312–19.

10 Pereira CT, Jeschke MG, Herndon DN. Beta-blockade in burns. *Novartis Found Symp* 2007;**280**:238–48; discussion 248–51.

11 Jeschke MG, Gauglitz GG, Kulp GA, et al. Long-term persistance of the pathophysiologic response to severe burn injury. *PLoS One* 2011;**6**:e21245.

12 Jones SB ea. Significance of the adrean and sympathetic response to burn injury. In: Herndon DN (ed.) *Total burn care*. 2nd ed. London: WB Saunders; 2002. p. xv, p. 817, 4 p. of plates.

13 Klein GL. Burn-induced bone loss: importance, mechanisms, and management. *J Burns Wounds* 2006;**5**:e5.

14 Sherwood ER. The systemic inflammatory response syndrome. In: Herndon DN (ed.) *Total burn care*. 2nd ed. London: WB Saunders; 2002. p. xv, p. 817, 4 p. of plates.

15 Finnerty CC, Herndon DN, Przkora R, et al. Cytokine expression profile over time in severely burned pediatric patients. *Shock* 2006;**26**:13–19.

16 Sell H, Dietze-Schroeder D, Kaiser U, Eckel J. Monocyte chemotactic protein-1 is a potential player in the negative cross-talk between adipose tissue and skeletal muscle. *Endocrinology* 2006;**147**:2458–67.

17 Gauglitz GG, Herndon DN, Jeschke MG. Insulin resistance postburn: underlying mechanisms and current therapeutic strategies. *J Burn Care Res* 2008;**29**:683–94.

18 Cochran A, Saffle JR, Caran G. Nutritional support of the burned patient. In: Herndon DN (ed.) *Total burn care*. 2nd ed. London: WB Saunders; 2002. p. xv, p. 817, 4 p. of plates.

19 Gore DC, Chinkes DL, Hart DW, Wolf SE, Herndon DN, Sanford AP. Hyperglycemia exacerbates muscle protein catabolism in burn-injured patients. *Crit Care Med* 2002;**30**:2438–42.

20 Gore DC, Chinkes D, Heggers J, Herndon DN, Wolf SE, Desai M. Association of hyperglycemia with increased mortality after severe burn injury. *J Trauma* 2001;**51**: 540–4.

21 Padfield KE, Astrakas LG, Zhang Q, et al. Burn injury causes mitochondrial dysfunction in skeletal muscle. *Proc Natl Acad Sci USA* 2005;**102**:5368–73.

22 Heszele MF, Price SR. Insulin-like growth factor I: the yin and yang of muscle atrophy. *Endocrinology* 2004;**145**:4803–5.

23 Chang DW, DeSanti L, Demling RH. Anticatabolic and anabolic strategies in critical illness: a review of current treatment modalities. *Shock* 1998;**10**:155–60.

24 Przkora R, Barrow RE, Jeschke MG, et al. Body composition changes with time in pediatric burn patients. *J Trauma* 2006;**60**:968–71; discussion 971.

25 Roberts CT, Rosenfeld RG. The IGF system: molecular biology, physiology, and clinical applications. In: *Contemporary endocrinology*. Totowa, NJ: Humana Press; 1999. p. xii, p. 787.

26 Norbury WB. Modulation of the hypermetabolic response after burn injury. In: Herndon DN (ed.) *Total burn care*. 2nd ed. London: WB Saunders; 2002. p. xv, p. 817, 4 p. of plates.

27 Rogol AD, Clark PA, Roemmich JN. Growth and pubertal development in children and adolescents: effects of diet and physical activity. *Am J Clin Nutr* 2000;72(2 Suppl):521S–8S.

28 Rutan RL, Herndon DN. Growth delay in postburn pediatric patients. *Arch Surg* 1990;**125**:392–5.

29 Suman OE. Mitigation of the burn induced hypermetabolic response during convalescence. In: Herndon DN (ed.) *Total burn care*. 2nd ed. London: WB Saunders; 2002. p. xv, p. 817, 4 p. of plates.

30 Low JF, Herndon DN, Barrow RE. Effect of growth hormone on growth delay in burned children: a 3-year follow-up study. *Lancet* 1999;**354**:1789.

31 Przkora R, Herndon DN, Suman OE, et al. Beneficial effects of extended growth hormone treatment after hospital discharge in pediatric burn patients. *Ann Surg* 2006;**243**:796–801; discussion 801–3.

32 Branski LK, Herndon DN, Barrow RE, et al. Randomized controlled trial to determine the efficacy of long-term growth hormone treatment in severely burned children. *Ann Surg* 2009;**250**:514–23.

33 Takala J, Ruokonen E, Webster NR, et al. Increased mortality associated with growth hormone treatment in critically ill adults. *N Engl J Med* 1999;**341**:785–92.

34 Klein GL, Herndon DN, Goodman WG, et al. Histomorphometric and biochemical characterization of bone following acute severe burns in children. *Bone* 1995;**17**:455–60.

35 Klein GL, Herndon DN, Langman CB, et al. Long-term reduction in bone mass after severe burn injury in children. *J Pediatr* 1995;**126**:252–6.

36 Klein G. Effects of burn injury on bone and mineral metabolism. In: Herndon DN (ed.) *Total burn care*. 2nd ed. London: WB Saunders; 2002. p. xv, p. 817, 4 p. of plates.

37 Evans E. Musculoskeletal changes secondary to thermal burns. In: Herndon DN (ed.) *Total burn care*. 2nd ed. London: WB Saunders; 2002. p. xv, p. 817, 4 p. of plates.

38 Klein GL, Langman CB, Herndon DN. Vitamin D depletion following burn injury in children: a possible factor in post-burn osteopenia. *J Trauma* 2002;**52**:346–50.

39 Przkora R, Jeschke MG, Barrow RE, et al. Metabolic and hormonal changes of severely burned children receiving long-term oxandrolone treatment. *Ann Surg* 2005;**242**:384–9, discussion 390–1.

40 Przkora R, Herndon DN, Sherrard DJ, Chinkes DL, Klein GL. Pamidronate preserves bone mass for at least 2 years following acute administration for pediatric burn injury. *Bone* 2007;**41**:297–302.

41 Serghiou MA. Comprehensive rehabilitation of the burn patient. In: Herndon DN (ed.) *Total burn care*. 2nd ed. London: WB Saunders; 2002. p. xv, p. 817, 4 p. of plates.

42 Tredget EE, Yang L, Delehanty M, Shankowsky H, Scott PG. Polarized Th2 cytokine production in patients with hypertrophic scar following thermal injury. *J Interferon Cytokine Res* 2006;**26**:179–89.

43 Gauglitz GG, Korting HC, Pavicic T, Ruzicka T, Jeschke MG. Hypertrophic scarring and keloids: pathomechanisms and current and emerging treatment strategies. *Mol Med* 2011;**17**:113–25.

44 Oliveira GV, Hawkins HK, Chinkes D, et al. Hypertrophic versus non hypertrophic scars compared by immunohistochemistry and laser confocal microscopy: type I and III collagens. *Int Wound J* 2009;**6**:445–52.

45 Slemp AE, Kirschner RE. Keloids and scars: a review of keloids and scars, their pathogenesis, risk factors, and management. *Curr Opin Pediatr* 2006;**18**:396–402.

46 Jeschke MG, Finnerty CC, Suman OE, Kulp G, Mlcak RP, Herndon DN. The effect of oxandrolone on the endocrinologic, inflammatory, and hypermetabolic responses during the acute phase postburn. *Ann Surg* 2007;**246**:351–60; discussion 360–2.

47 **Przkora R, Herndon DN, Suman OE.** The effects of oxandrolone and exercise on muscle mass and function in children with severe burns. *Pediatrics* 2007;**119**:e109–16.

48 **Celis MM, Suman OE, Huang TT, Yen P, Herndon DN.** Effect of a supervised exercise and physiotherapy program on surgical interventions in children with thermal injury. *J Burn Care Rehabil* 2003;**24**:57–61; discussion 56.

49 **Suman OE, Spies RJ, Celis MM, Mlcak RP, Herndon DN.** Effects of a 12-wk resistance exercise program on skeletal muscle strength in children with burn injuries. *J Appl Physiol* 2001;**91**:1168–75.

Chapter 17

Consequences of Endotracheal Intubation and Tracheostomy

Bernd Schönhofer and Stefan Kluge

Background and history

The incidence of MV is increasing worldwide. Endotracheal intubation and tracheostomy are the main airway access techniques in the ICU. However, these procedures are associated with a spectrum of complications, ranging from injury to the airway to nosocomial lower respiratory infections. In this chapter, we will summarize the acute and late complications directly attributable to endotracheal intubation and tracheostomy in adult patients. Previously, post-intubation lesions were the single most common indication for tracheal resection and reconstruction. Fortunately, with recent improvements in design and management of endotracheal and tracheostomy tubes, the incidence of these injuries has declined.[1]

Historically, the earliest account of tracheostomy can be traced back to 2000 BC in Hindu scripts. In more recent history, there are reports of endotracheal intubation first applied in the 17th century to resuscitate drowning victims. In 1833, Trousseau reported on his experience with 200 cases of respiratory faliure in the treatment of diphtheria.[2] This was followed in 1880 by Macewan's publication of the first academic paper, introducing endotracheal intubation in four patients for up to 35 hours in duration. This early publication also highlighted complications of endotracheal intubation such as cough, discomfort, tracheal mucosal congestion, and thickening of the vocal cords.[3] The more widespread clinical implementation of endotracheal intubation started in Scandinavia; endotracheal intubation was introduced both by Nilsson as an alternative to tracheostomy for patients with respiratory failure caused by barbiturate poisoning and Ibsen for the treatment of respiratory failure caused by polio.[4,5]

Complications of intubation and tracheostomy are often caused by a number of factors such as blind emergency intubations, improper patient positioning, inexperienced operators, and abnormal anatomy. Furthermore, mechanical properties of the tube and/or cuff, including ETT size, shape, pressure, and movement, are factors contributing to pathological changes. Also, the patient's underlying illness, e.g. rheumatoid arthritis with involvement of the cricoarytenoid joint, and the duration of invasive MV increase the propensity for complications.

Many of the long-term complications of endotracheal intubation and tracheostomy are similar and overlapping. Prevention and early evaluation of complications are important to minimize the risk of long-term morbidities.

The laryngotracheal complications of endotracheal intubation and tracheostomy may be divided into early complications, related to the intubation attempt, and those occuring late in the weeks to months following extubation.

Endotracheal intubation

Complications—early after endotracheal intubation, during MV, and shortly after extubation

Complications during placement of the ETT mostly result from suboptimal technique of the inexperienced physician who intubated the patient or by the presence of a difficult airway. More injuries are associated with the establishment of an emergency airway, compared with elective anaesthetic intubation, but the majority of these are transient and completely reversible by a self-healing process.

In a prospective study performed in two teaching hospitals in 1981, Stauffer et al. reported early adverse events of endotracheal intubation in 62% of 226 intubations.[6] In descending order of frequency, the following injuries were found: excessive cuff pressure required to seal the airway, self-extubation, instability to seal the airway, right main bronchus intubation, and aspiration. In a recent series of over 3400 emergent intubations, the following acute complications occurred in 4.2% of patients: aspiration (2.8%), oesophageal intubation (1.3%), dental injury (0.2%), and pneumothorax (0.1%).[7] Independent predictors of complications were: three or more intubation attempts, grade III or IV view, general care floor location, and emergency department location. The incidence of difficult intubation in this series was 10.3%.

Extrapulmonary injuries

Although a broad spectrum of extrapulmonary adverse effects (e.g. haemodynamic instability) may occur during intubation, only some of these are serious and influence life after ICU. An example is oesophageal intubation, with a complication in 1% of intubations in critically ill adults,[6] which may be associated with serious local and systemic complications such as oesophageal perforation and cardiac arrest.[8,9]

Oro-nasal injuries

In the oral area, both during the insertion of the ETT and after successful endotracheal intubation, dental injuries are relatively common. In an analysis of 598 904 patients receiving general anaesthetics, the dental injury rate in those with tracheal intubation was 1 in 2805.[10] Dental injuries during endotracheal intubation are one of the most important reasons for anaesthesia-related malpractice claims. Pressure-induced ulcerations of the lips and oropharyngeal structures are also important sequelae that can be caused by the ETT.

Paranasal sinusitis

In addition to nasotracheal intubation and nasogastric tubes, risk factors for paranasal sinusitis include head trauma, prior steroid exposure, and previous antibiotic therapy.

Nasal tubes have the disadvantage of occluding the ostia of the maxillary sinus which commonly results in the accumulation of fluid in the sinuses and development of sinusitis. In a prospective study of 16 patients, CT imaging performed on the eighth day after nasotracheal intubation showed the following: the maxillary and sphenoid sinuses were each affected in 87% of patients, and this was followed by ethmoid (50%) and frontal (12.5%) sinus involvement, including fluid accumulation, opacification, and mucosal thickening.[11] Furthermore, some studies reported paranasal sinusitis secondary to prolonged nasotracheal intubation as a source of sepsis.[12,13] Holzapfel et al. found that nasotracheal intubation was significantly associated with ventilator-associated pneumonia and increased 2-month mortality.[14] Based on these data, the preferred intubation route for most physicians today is orotracheal.

Pharyngeal and laryngeal injuries

During the ETT placement, pharyngeal injury of the naso-, oro-, and hypopharynx may occur and include lacerations, bleeding (see Figure 17.1), contusions, submucosal haemorrhage, and oedema. Perforations of the posterial pharyngeal wall or hypopharynx and trauma of the cricoarytenoid joint, mainly as subluxation and luxation of the arytenoid cartilage, are rare, but serious, complications.

Laryngeal oedema and mucosal ulcerations occur in almost all patients intubated for 4 or more days.[15] In a recent study, 136 patients, with a median duration of intubation of 3 days, underwent fibreoptic endoscopic examination of the larynx within 6 hours after extubation. Laryngeal injuries occurred in 73% of patients and were associated with the duration of intubation and absence of myorelaxant drug use at intubation.[16] Severe lesions of the larynx were detected in 6% of a series of 1000 patients after anaesthetic intubations.[17]

Laryngeal ulcerations from endotracheal intubation are typically symmetrical and occur in the posterior and medial parts of the vocal cords and arytenoids and posterolateral area of the cricoid cartilages.[18] Laryngeal ulceration from endotracheal intubation may remain clinically silent until extubation. Ulceration of the true vocal cords and arytenoids occur in more than 50% of endotracheal intubations.[6]

Colice et al. prospectively followed 82 patients who underwent endotracheal intubation for more than 4 days.[19] At the time of extubation and again after 2 weeks, direct laryngoscopy was performed in these patients. One typical pattern of laryngeal damage was mucosal ulcerations along the posterior-medial part of the vocal cords, and these resolved in the majority of patients within 4 weeks. The post-intubation laryngeal sequelae were prospectively studied by Thomas et al. in patients requiring MV longer than 24 hours.[20] Immediately after extubation, 87.6% of patients (n = 131) had visible laryngeal pathology and 8.6% of this same study sample had long-term sequelae.

Tracheal injuries

During intubation, tracheal perforation, laceration, and rupture are rare complications and mostly result from forceful intubation, tearing of the posterior membranous trachea, or overinflated cuff. In this context, the rare, but severe, complication of post-intubation tracheobronchial laceration must be mentioned.

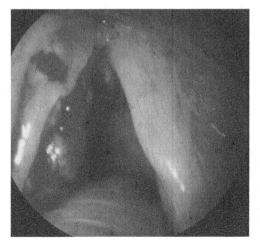

Fig. 17.1 Acute bleeding in the left vocal cord caused by difficult intubation.

Courtesy of Prof Dr H-J Welkoborsky, Klinikum Region Hannover.

Lung injuries

Intubation of a main-stem bronchus occurs usually on the right side. Complications include hyperinflation of the right lung, right pneumothorax, and atelectasis of the non-inflated part of the predominantly left lung.

Pulmonary complications during an attempt to place the ETT include pulmonary aspiration which has been reported in 8–19% of adult non-anaesthetic intubations.[6,21] Furthermore, different types of baro- and volutrauma are known injuries during ETT placement. In the context of this book, residual lung injuries as a long-term consequence of endotracheal intubation and tracheostomy are relatively seldom, since they mostly are reversible.

Swallowing dysfunction

The transient development of post-extubation swallowing dysfunction occurs in approximately every second patient; however, clinically important aspiration is much less common. In a recent study, 41% of trauma patients had swallowing dysfunction after a mean intubation time of 9.2 days. Patients older than 55 years and duration of endotracheal intubation were independent risk factors for post-extubation swallowing dysfunction.[22]

Late complications of endotracheal intubation

Late complications occur weeks to months after extubation. During prolonged endotracheal intubation, tracheal injuries typically occur at the site of the inflated cuff, at the level of the tip of the tracheal tube, or in the area where the tip of the suction catheter damages the mucosa of the tracheal wall. One major pathophysiological mechanism underlying these injuries is high ETT cuff pressure. Elevated cuff pressures exceeding the capillary perfusion pressure of the mucosa are followed by mucosal ischaemia, inflammation, necrosis, and ulceration. Abnormal healing with fibrosis or granuloma formation accounts for the most significant late complications of endotracheal intubation. Serious late complications include the following: tracheal granuloma formation, tracheal stenosis or destruction of the tracheal cartilage, dilation or fistula to adjacent organs such as the oesophagus. Tracheomalacia, another severe complication after endotracheal intubation, is caused by airway ischaemia where the resultant chondritis leads to destruction and necrosis of the tracheobronchial cartilage. Following the introduction of high-volume, low-pressure cuffs, the occurrence of cuff injury has been markedly reduced.

Laryngeal injuries

An important late complication is granuloma formation (see Figure 17.2), primarily affecting the larynx. The rate of granuloma formation varies broadly across studies from 3%[6] to 7%[19] to 27%.[23] Laryngeal stenosis is located in the glottic and subglottic regions, either alone or in combination. Adults tend to have the majority of post-intubation stenosis in the posterior glottis.[6]

Tracheal stenosis

Tracheal stenosis usually presents as inspiratory stridor and shortness of breath. In every patient who has these symptoms after MV, tracheal stenosis needs to be excluded. However, symptoms usually do not occur at rest and only occur when the lumen of the trachea has been reduced by 50–75%. Taking the results of prospective studies together,[6,19,24–26] laryngeal stenosis is found in approximately 3% of patients after extubation. The frequency of injuries also depends on the duration of MV. In a special subgroup of patients with PMV (defined as 11 days or longer), laryngeal

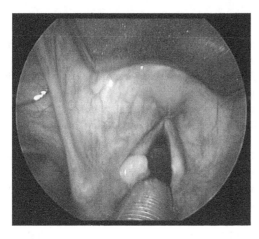

Fig. 17.2 Granuloma in the left vocal cord after 12 days lasting endotracheal intubation.

Courtesy of Prof Dr H-J Welkoborsky, Klinikum Region Hannover.

stenosis was found in 14%.[26] In an evaluation of the long-term adverse effects of endotracheal intubation in patients with ARDS, Elliott et al. noted symptomatic upper airway obstruction from laryngotracheal stenosis in 10% (3/30) of patients at 4 to 12 months after hospital discharge.[27] These patients suffered mainly from symptoms of dyspnoea, and risk factors included difficult intubation and high ETT cuff pressures.

Tracheo-oesophageal fistula

Tracheo-oesophageal fistula is an uncommon, but potentially life-threatening, complication occurring after endotracheal intubation or tracheostomy. With the use of modern tubes with low-pressure cuffs and close monitoring of the cuff pressure, its occurrence has become rare.

Prevention of complications

A registry of the major complications of airway management in the UK identified important gaps in care that included poor identification of at-risk patients, incomplete planning, inadequate provision of skilled staff and equipment to manage these events successfully, delayed recognition of events, and failed rescue due to lack or failure of interpretation of capnography.[28] One important method to prevent many of the above described complications is the implementation of an educational programme and adoption of feasible algorithms about how to perform intubation, with particular emphasis on the management of the difficult airway.

Studies have shown that the implementation of an ICU-based endotracheal intubation care bundle strategy can reduce immediate and severe life-threatening complications associated with intubation of patients.[29] However, it is unclear whether this affects the prevalence of long-term airway complications. The size of the ETT may influence the complication rate, since it has been demonstrated that tubes of size 8 are a significant risk factor for adverse airway sequelae in patients with PMV.[30] Careful monitoring of cuff pressures and tube stability is required. Cuff pressures greater than 20–30 cmH_2O are thought to cause mucosal ischaemia and subsequent larygngeal and tracheal injuries.[31] Compared to low-volume, high-pressure, low-compliance cuffs, fewer injuries are caused by artificial airways using high-volume, low-pressure, and high-compliance cuffs (the so-called 'soft cuffs').[31,32] The best prophylaxis to prevent nasal tube-induced sinusitis is avoiding nasal intubation.

Diagnostic approach

Laryngeal and tracheal injuries incurred during endotracheal intubation mostly remain unknown, since an accurate diagnostic approach is not possible. Sometimes, tracheal injury may be found by fibreoptic bronchoscopy after deflating the cuff and moving the tube upward. This technique is not standardized and therefore cannot be recommended.

Flow-volume curves may demonstrate fixed airway obstruction. Physical examination and lung function are basic tools to diagnose complications of endotracheal intubation and MV. Post-extubation injuries are assessed by indirect and direct laryngoscopy, fibreoptic bronchoscopy, cervical CT, and MRI. Additionally, EMG of the larynx may be important in differentiating arytenoid dislocation from true vocal cord paralysis from nerve damage.

After PMV and difficult weaning, late manifestations of tracheal stenosis may become apparent. Patients with symptoms caused by stenosis usually present when the lumen of airways is reduced by 50–60%, as discussed previously. In light of this, we recommend close follow-up of these patients, e.g. at 4 weeks and 3 months after discharge from hospital. If there remains any clinical suspicion of tracheal stenosis, the above mentioned diagnostic package must be performed. In particular, those patients who successfully underwent thoracic surgery to repair tracheobronchial damage caused by intubation require close follow-up in order to detect tracheal stenosis.

Tracheostomy

Tracheostomy is a frequently performed surgical procedure in the ICU and has undergone a substantial change in the last few decades. The fear of the previously mentioned complications of endotracheal intubation is the leading rationale for performing tracheostomy for long-term airway maintenance. The main indication for tracheostomy is the need for PMV; however, the ideal timing for this is still a subject of debate, as there is no evidence that early tracheostomy improves long-term clinical outcomes.[33] However, since the introduction and widespread acceptance of percutaneous techniques in the ICU setting, the number of critically ill patients undergoing tracheostomy has increased and the procedure is being performed significantly earlier during the intensive care stay. Many studies have highlighted the advantage of improved patient comfort, better oral hygiene, and fewer requirements for sedation. Furthermore, tracheostomy may shorten the duration of MV because of reduced WOB and decreased dead space ventilation. However, tracheostomy may be associated with numerous severe complications. The objective of this chapter is to give an overview of the procedure-related complications, with a special focus on late complications.

Techniques of tracheostomy

Percutaneous tracheostomy has gained widespread acceptance in the ICU setting, and six different percutaneous tracheostomy techniques have been developed over the last several years. Recent literature suggests that percutaneous tracheostomy offers several potential advantages, and many specialists in intensive care view this as the method of choice for critically ill patients who require tracheostomy. A meta-analysis of trials, comparing percutaneous to surgical tracheostomy, revealed significantly fewer complications in the percutaneous group, with respect to wound infection and unfavourable scarring. However, there was a statistically significant and clinically important increased risk for decannulation and tube obstruction in those undergoing percutaneous tracheostomy. The incidence of overall number of complications and mortality, however, was not different between the procedures. Furthermore, percutaneous tracheostomies are more cost-effective and provide greater feasibility in terms of bedside capability and operation.[34] The single-step dilation or modified Ciaglia technique has become the most popular technique for percutaneous tracheostomy and is currently the most reliable for safety and success rate.[35,36] Surgical tracheostomy is usually reserved for patients with contraindications to percutaneous tracheostomy.

Early complications of tracheostomy

In a large case series, the prevalence of early complications (procedural or immediately post-procedure) was 3%.[37] Complications include the following:

- Bleeding is reported to be the most common complication but usually is low-volume and seldom life-threatening or fatal. The percutaneous technique is associated with less perioperative and stomal bleeding, because the tight fit of the stoma effectively tamponades blood vessels.

- Accidental decannulation of an existing tracheostomy or tube obstruction is a major problem of the percutaneous technique. These are frequently occurring airway management problems in the ICU which can lead to morbidity and mortality.[28] The open technique allows the insertion of a tracheostomy tube more easily.

- Subcutaneous emphysema and pneumothorax are relevant, but infrequent, complications of percutaneous tracheostomy, occurring in 1.4% and 0.8% patients, respectively.[37]

- Posterior tracheal wall injury, occurring in fewer than 1% of patients after surgical or percutaneous tracheostomy, can be a severe complication requiring surgical repair.

- Wound infections are frequent after surgical tracheostomy and are less often seen after percutaneous tracheostomy due to the smaller size of the skin incision and the smaller wound.

Some studies have reported the association of a tracheostomy tube left in place after ICU discharge with a higher risk of post-ICU mortality.[37] Recent data show that patients with a tracheostomy tube *in situ* at the time of ICU discharge to a general ward and who also receive follow-up from a dedicated multidisciplinary team(compared with standard care), have reductions in time to decannulation, length of stay, and adverse events.[38]

Late complications of tracheostomy

In comparison to early complications of tracheostomy, late complications are more difficult to quantify, as long-term follow-up of ICU survivors is often challenging and frequently difficult to determine if complications are secondary to tracheostomy or endotracheal intubation or a combination of each procedure. In this section, more current data were emphasized to highlight the change in incidence of tracheostomy complications over the last decades.

Granulation tissue

A frequent phenomenon after tracheostomy is the development of granulation tissue, and many patients have some degree of tracheal narrowing at the site of the tracheostoma. This complication is often subclinical but may result in airway occlusion or tracheal stenosis.[39]

Tracheal stenosis

Tracheal stenosis is the most common, relevant late airway complication after tracheostomy. Associated risk factors for tracheal stenosis include sepsis, stomal infection, mucosal ischaemia from excessive cuff pressure, older age, exposure to systemic corticosteroids, and prolonged tube placement.[39] Higher puncture site with injury of the cricoid is also associated with an increased risk of tracheal stenosis. Due to the introduction of high-volume, low-pressure endotracheal cuffs, the prevalence of severe (>50%) tracheal stenosis has fallen. The incidence of clinically important tracheal stenosis has been reported in more recent studies between 1.7% and 5.9%.[40,41] Obese patients experience more complications after tracheostomy. Halum et al. reviewed the charts of 1175 tracheostomy procedures for tracheostomy complications in the US and found a significant association between the development of airway stenosis and a BMI >30.[40]

The presence of a subclinical tracheal stenosis is frequent in patients who have undergone percutaneous tracheostomy in the ICU setting. However, the stenosis is generally mild. Norwood et al. followed 48 patients for 30 months after percutaneous tracheostomy with tracheal CT and found more than 10% tracheal stenosis in 15 of 48 patients (31%). However, only one of these patients had greater than 50% narrowing of the lumen of the airway. With the exception of one patient, all of the stenoses occurred at the stoma level.[42]

It is often difficult to separate the effect of prior endotracheal intubation from that of tracheostomy, since each can lead to tracheal stenosis. However, tracheal stenosis after tracheostomy differs from tracheal stenosis after endotracheal intubation. Tracheal stenosis following tracheostomy most commonly results from abnormal wound healing, with excess granulation tissue formation around the tracheal stoma site.[43] Excess granulation tissue can also develop over a fractured cartilage, which can occur during the tracheostomy procedure. However, it has been challenged whether tracheal ring fractures truly are associated with the subsequent development of tracheal stenosis. Sixteen patients with tracheal ring fractures were followed up by an experienced ear, nose, and throat consultant and their tracheas examined with nasoendoscopy. There were no reported cases of tracheal stenosis at follow-up in this study.[44]

One widely debated issue is whether the percutaneous technique results more frequently in tracheal stenosis. Current evidence shows that this complication develops with both techniques to an equal extent.[45] Silvester et al. conducted a prospective randomized controlled study, comparing percutaneous tracheostomy (by the Ciaglia technique) and surgical tracheostomy. Follow-up occurred at a median of 20 months in 29 patients in the percutaneous tracheostomy group and 42 patients in the surgical tracheostomy group for assessment of long-term sequelae. No patient from either group demonstrated any evidence of tracheal stenosis.[46]

Scar formation

Procedures like tracheostomy in ICU patients can lead to persistent, and often unsightly, scars. As the incision in percutaneous tracheostomy is small, there is less tissue damage and the production of a more aesthetically acceptable scar. Badia and co-workers examined 189 patients 12 months after ICU discharge to define the skin lesions produced by procedures used in the ICU. A total of 189 patients were interviewed, and 93 patients (49%) reported some skin lesions after 12 months. All patients who had undergone surgical tracheostomy reported the presence of a scar, but 4 of 24 patients who had undergone percutaneous tracheostomy reported no tracheostomy scar.[47] Assessment of the tracheostomy cutaneous scar at a median of 20 months in the study by Sylvester et al. revealed that the scar length was significantly longer in the surgical tracheostomy (ST) group and that there was a trend to be abnormally coloured, puckered, hypertrophied, visible, or unsightly.[46]

Voice changes

In the previously mentioned study by Norwood et al., 100 patients were interviewed after percutaneous tracheostomy. Voice changes were reported in 27% of patients, with 2% of patients noting severe hoarseness.[42] Another study evaluated 66 patients 16 months after decannulation.

Voice changes, mostly minor, were identified in 21% of patients.[48] One year after tracheostomy, Antonelli et al. interviewed and examined 31 patients who had survived hospitalization after long-term ventilation. Five of the 13 patients in the percutaneous tracheostomy group (38%) and six of the 18 from the surgical tracheostomy group (33%) reported subjective phonetic or respiratory problems, described as mild or moderate.[45]

Swallowing dysfunction

It has been demonstrated that the presence of a tracheostomy tube often induces or increases aspiration. Mechanisms that may explain this effect include tethering of the larynx, desensitization of the upper airway, impairment of the vocal cord closure reflex, disuse atrophy of the laryngeal muscles, oesophageal compression by the inflated cuff, and loss of subglottic air pressure during swallowing.[49] Romero et al. examined 40 non-neurologic, critically ill tracheotomized patients with fibreoptic endoscopic evaluation of swallowing at 3–5 days after discontinuation of MV. They found an incidence of 38% of swallowing dysfunction in this group.[50] Of these patients, 73% (11/15) had silent aspiration.[50] Of note, patients with neurologic disorders, a group with known high incidence of swallowing dysfunction, were excluded from this study. The patients with swallowing dysfunction experienced a significant delay in their tracheostomy decannulation process. With regard to these findings, we recommend a routine formal swallowing evaluation before decannulation.

Fistula

Tracheo-oesophageal fistula is a relatively unusual complication, occurring in fewer than 1% of patients, and is usually the result of iatrogenic damage to the posterior tracheal wall.

A rare (incidence <1%), but devastating, complication after any form of tracheostomy is the development of a tracheoarterial fistula with massive haemorrhage. The majority of cases will occur within 3 days to 6 weeks after tracheostomy placement. The risk factors include pressure necrosis from high cuff pressure, mucosal trauma from malpositioned cannula tip, low tracheal incision, and excessive neck movement. This condition is usually fatal, unless treatment is instituted immediately.[51]

Tracheomalacia

Another possible late, but rare, complication is tracheomalacia. It occurs from pressure necrosis, impaired blood flow, and recurrent infections, usually with destruction of the supporting cartilage. This weakness of the airway can cause expiratory airway collapse.[39]

Long-term outcome after tracheostomy

Engoren et al. studied post-hospital survival and functional outcome in a group of 429 patients who received a tracheostomy for respiratory failure between 1998 and 2000 (see Figure 17.3).[52] Hospital mortality was 19%; survivors were younger, more often surgical patients who received more rehabilitation after hospital discharge. Only 57% of survivors were liberated from MV. At 1 year after discharge, 36% of hospital survivors had died. Patients discharged without tracheostomy tubes also had the best 1-year survival (92%); the mortality of ventilator-dependent patients was highest (57%). Sixty-six patients completed the SF-36 for functional status. At follow-up, most responders had good emotional health but remained with major physical limitations. Decannulated patients had better social functioning than patients discharged partially or totally ventilator-dependent.[52]

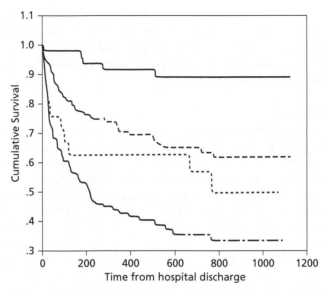

Fig. 17.3 Kaplan–Meier survival of ventilator-dependent patients (dashed and dotted line), partially dependent patients (dotted line), patients liberated from MV but with tracheostomy tube still present (dashed line), and patients liberated and tracheostomy tube removed (straight line).[52]

In a follow-up evaluation by Antonelli et al., over half of the interviewed survivors of each group rated their physical health as moderately or severely compromised and emotional health ratings were even lower. Ratings for patients with open stomas were significantly lower than those for patients whose stomas had been closed. The tracheostomy technique (percutaneous vs surgical) had no significant effect on the outcomes measured.[45]

Prevention of complications

As in any other invasive procedures, the rate of complications depends on the experience of the operator and the anatomical characteristics of the patient.[48,53] Therefore, it is of major relevance that complications can be avoided when contraindications to percutaneous tracheostomy (altered neck anatomy, irreversible coagulopathy, etc.) are noted. However, most contraindications are relative and are dependent on the skill of the operator.

We advocate performing the procedure under videobronchoscopic guidance to enable the operator to view the bronchoscopic procedure which may minimize perioperative complications. This can help to visualize correct placement of the needle, guidewire, dilator, and tracheostomy cannula. Furthermore, it can prevent iatrogenic damage to the posterior tracheal wall. However, disadvantages of bronchoscopy include compromised ventilation, carbon dioxide (CO_2) retention, increased cost, and time. Studies have shown that preoperative ultrasound of the neck can identify aberrant blood vessels and the use of a laryngeal mask airway (LMA) improves visualization of the trachea and larynx during fibreoptically assisted percutaneous tracheostomy. These procedures may all improve safety; however, more research is needed before these approaches can be recommended for routine use. Careful monitoring of cuff pressure to avoid overinflation is recommended to prevent tracheal stenosis. The use of outer flange sutures to anchor the tracheostomy tube seems to reduce complications.[40] In conclusion, it should be emphasized that the implementation of a standardized strategy for the care of tracheostomized patients and the existence of local guidelines can reduce the rate of tracheostomy complications.[54]

Treatment of complications

Laryngeal granulomas may by treated with topical inhalant steroids as first-line treatment[55] before considering surgical or endoscopical interventions. Laryngeal stenosis requires more invasive interventions such as laser therapy, dilation, and/or stenting. Reconstructive surgical procedures are applied to treat complex pathology such as cricoarytenoid joint fibrosis. The treatment strategy for tracheal stenosis depends on symptoms and their degree of severity. Patients with mild stenosis (<25% of airway diameter) and no symptoms may be observed without treatment. Interventions for patients with severe tracheal stenosis include non-surgical and surgical procedures, including balloon dilatation, laser resection, cryotherapy, stent placement, and tracheal resection of the stenotic segment and re-anastomosis/construction. Stenoses in excess of 4 cm in length are traditionally managed with a tracheal sleeve resection. Patients with mild stenosis which progresses slowly often benefit from mechanical dilation with a flexible or rigid bronchoscope, followed by laser intervention and/or stent placement. Rahman evaluated the flexible bronchoscopic management of tracheal stenosis in 76 patients after endotracheal intubation and 30 patients post-tracheostomy.[56] In the majority of patients, the balloon dilation and laser treatment was performed, rather than stent placement and brachytherapy. Even in this elderly population with a significant burden of comorbid disease, there was an almost 90% success rate, following flexible bronchoscopic treatment modalities, at a median follow-up of 51 months. Nouraei evaluated the outcome of endoscopic treatment of post-intubation tracheal stenosis in adults.[57] In total, 53 of 62 patients had a tracheostomy; the length of intubation was 26 ± 28 days, and the latency between intubation and intervention was 29 ± 47 months in this population. In addition to balloon dilation, laser treatment, and stent placement, this group locally instilled mitomycin C or steroids as an anti-inflammatory strategy. Noppen et al. published a series of 15 patients after multiple weaning failures from MV, caused by benign post-intubation airway stenosis.[58] After successful treatment with dilatation procedures and stent insertion, almost all patients (14/15 patients) were successfully extubated/decannulated.

Depending on the extent and location of tracheal lacerations both nonsurgical and surgical strategies are successfully performed.[59,60] Furthermore the tracheal rupture during emergent endotracheal intubation requires surgical repair.[61]

In the management of tracheal stenosis after endotracheal intubation, we prefer to apply rigid bronchoscopy, combined with flexible bronchoscopy, under anaesthesia to perform the above mentioned interventions and stent insertion, in particular (see Figure 17.4).

The success rate of stenting to treat tracheal stenosis depends on a series of co-factors such as location of the lesion, its distance to the glottis, the remaining degree of the stenosis, and the type of stent. An important challenge is the fixation of the stent within the trachea.

If stents are used to stabilize the effect of dilation and laser intervention during the healing period, they may be removed some weeks or months later.

Treatment of tracheomalacia depends on its degree. Mild cases are followed with a conservative strategy. In severe cases, management options include stent placement, tracheal resection with end-to-end anastomosis or tracheoplasty.

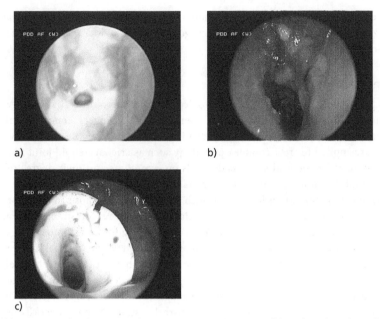

Fig. 17.4 (a) Severe tracheal stenosis after long-term tracheotomy. (b) Widened trachea after laser resection. (c) Stent placement after laser resection.

References

1 Wain JC, Jr Postintubation tracheal stenosis. *Semin Thorac Cardiovasc Surg* 2009;**21**:284–9.

2 Frost EA. Tracing the tracheostomy. *Ann Otol Rhinol Laryngol* 1976;**85**:618–24.

3 Macewen W. Clinical observations on the introduction of tracheal tubes by the mouth, instead of performing tracheotomy or laryngotomy. *Br Med J* 1880;**2**:163–5.

4 Nilsson E. On treatment of barbiturate poisoning; a modified clinical aspect. *Acta Med Scand Suppl* 1951;**253**:1–127.

5 Ibsen B. The anaesthetist's viewpoint on the treatment of respiratory complications in poliomyelitis during the epidemic in Copenhagen, 1952. *Proc R Soc Med* 1954;**47**:72–4.

6 Stauffer JL, Olson DE, Petty TL. Complications and consequences of endotracheal intubation and tracheotomy. A prospective study of 150 critically ill adult patients. *Am J Med* 1981;**70**:65–76.

7 Martin LD, Mhyre JM, Shanks AM, Tremper KK, Kheterpal S. 3,423 emergency tracheal intubations at a university hospital: airway outcomes and complications. *Anesthesiology* 2011;**114**:42–8.

8 Phillips LG, Jr, Cunningham J. Esophageal perforation. *Radiol Clin North Am* 1984;**22**:607–13.

9 Keenan RL, Boyan CP. Cardiac arrest due to anesthesia. A study of incidence and causes. *JAMA* 1985;**253**:2373–7.

10 Warner ME, Benenfeld SM, Warner MA, Schroeder DR, Maxson PM. Perianesthetic dental injuries: frequency, outcomes, and risk factors. *Anesthesiology* 1999;**90**:1302–5.

11 Fassoulaki A, Pamouktsoglou P. Prolonged nasotracheal intubation and its association with inflammation of paranasal sinuses. *Anesth Analg* 1989;**69**:50–2.

12 O'Reilly MJ, Reddick EJ, Black W, et al. Sepsis from sinusitis in nasotracheally intubated patients. A diagnostic dilemma. *Am J Surg* 1984;**147**:601–4.

13 Deutschman CS, Wilton P, Sinow J, Dibbell D, Jr, Konstantinides FN, Cerra FB. Paranasal sinusitis associated with nasotracheal intubation: a frequently unrecognized and treatable source of sepsis. *Crit Care Med* 1986;**14**:111–14.

14 Holzapfel L, Chastang C, Demingeon G, Bohe J, Piralla B, Coupry A. A randomized study assessing the systematic search for maxillary sinusitis in nasotracheally mechanically ventilated patients. Influence of nosocomial maxillary sinusitis on the occurrence of ventilator-associated pneumonia. *Am J Respir Crit Care Med* 1999;**159**:695–701.

15 Wittekamp BH, van Mook WN, Tjan DH, Zwaveling JH, Bergmans DC. Clinical review: post-extubation laryngeal edema and extubation failure in critically ill adult patients. *Crit Care* 2009;**13**:233.

16 Tadie JM, Behm E, Lecuyer L, et al. Post-intubation laryngeal injuries and extubation failure: a fiberoptic endoscopic study. *Intensive Care Med* 2010;**36**:991–8.

17 Kambic V, Radsel Z. Intubation lesions of the larynx. *Br J Anaesth* 1978;**50**:587–90.

18 Burns HP, Dayal VS, Scott A, van Nostrand AW, Bryce DP. Laryngotracheal trauma: observations on its pathogenesis and its prevention following prolonged orotracheal intubation in the adult. *Laryngoscope* 1979;**89**:1316–25.

19 Colice GL, Stukel TA, Dain B. Laryngeal complications of prolonged intubation. *Chest* 1989;**96**:877–84.

20 Thomas R, Kumar EV, Kameswaran M, et al. Post intubation laryngeal sequelae in an intensive care unit. *J Laryngol Otol* 1995;**109**:313–16.

21 Taryle DA, Chandler JE, Good JT, Jr, Potts DE, Sahn SA. Emergency room intubations—complications and survival. *Chest* 1979;**75**:541–3.

22 Bordon A, Bokhari R, Sperry J, Testa D, Feinstein A, Ghaemmaghami V. Swallowing dysfunction after prolonged intubation: analysis of risk factors in trauma patients. *Am J Surg* 2011;**202**:679–82.

23 Santos PM, Afrassiabi A, Weymuller EA, Jr Prospective studies evaluating the standard endotracheal tube and a prototype endotracheal tube. *Ann Otol Rhinol Laryngol* 1989;**98**:935–40.

24 Pecora DV, Seinige U. Prolonged endotracheal intubation. *Chest* 1982;**82**:130.

25 Kastanos N, Estopa MR, Marin PA, Xaubet MA, Agusti-Vidal A. Laryngotracheal injury due to endotracheal intubation: incidence, evolution, and predisposing factors. A prospective long-term study. *Crit Care Med* 1983;**11**:362–7.

26 Whited RE. A prospective study of laryngotracheal sequelae in long-term intubation. *Laryngoscope* 1984;**94**:367–77.

27 Elliott CG, Rasmusson BY, Crapo RO. Upper airway obstruction following adult respiratory distress syndrome. An analysis of 30 survivors. *Chest* 1988;**94**:526–30.

28 Cook TM, Woodall N, Harper J, Benger J. Major complications of airway management in the UK: results of the Fourth National Audit Project of the Royal College of Anaesthetists and the Difficult Airway Society. Part 2: intensive care and emergency departments. *Br J Anaesth* 2011;**106**:632–42.

29 Jaber S, Jung B, Corne P, et al. An intervention to decrease complications related to endotracheal intubation in the intensive care unit: a prospective, multiple-center study. *Intensive Care Med* 2010;**36**: 248–55.

30 Santos PM, Afrassiabi A, Weymuller EA, Jr Risk factors associated with prolonged intubation and laryngeal injury. *Otolaryngol Head Neck Surg* 1994;**111**:453–9.

31 Tu HN, Saidi N, Leiutaud T, Bensaid S, Menival V, Duvaldestin P. Nitrous oxide increases endotracheal cuff pressure and the incidence of tracheal lesions in anesthetized patients. *Anesth Analg* 1999; **89**:187–90.

32 Grillo HC, Cooper JD, Geffin B, Pontoppidan H. A low-pressure cuff for tracheostomy tubes to minimize tracheal injury. A comparative clinical trial. *J Thorac Cardiovasc Surg* 1971;**62**:898–907.

33 Wang F, Wu Y, Bo L, et al. The timing of tracheotomy in critically ill patients undergoing mechanical ventilation: a systematic review and meta-analysis of randomized controlled trials. *Chest* 2011;**140**: 1456–65.

34 **Higgins KM, Punthakee X.** Meta-analysis comparison of open versus percutaneous tracheostomy. *Laryngoscope* 2007;**117**:447–54.

35 **Kluge S, Baumann HJ, Maier C, et al.** Tracheostomy in the intensive care unit: a nationwide survey. *Anesth Analg* 2008;**107**:1639–43.

36 **Cabrini L, Monti G, Landoni G, et al.** Percutaneous tracheostomy, a systematic review. *Acta Anaesthesiol Scand* 2012;**56**:270–81.

37 **Fikkers BG, van Veen JA, Kooloos JG, et al.** Emphysema and pneumothorax after percutaneous tracheostomy: case reports and an anatomic study. *Chest* 2004;**125**:1805–14.

38 **Garrubba M, Turner T, Grieveson C.** Multidisciplinary care for tracheostomy patients: a systematic review. *Crit Care* 2009;**13**:R177.

39 **Epstein SK.** Late complications of tracheostomy. *Respir Care* 2005;**50**:542–9.

40 **Halum SL, Ting JY, Plowman EK, et al.** A multi-institutional analysis of tracheotomy complications. *Laryngoscope* 2012;**122**:38–45.

41 **Fikkers BG, Staatsen M, van den Hoogen FJ, van der Hoeven JG.** Early and late outcome after single step dilatational tracheostomy versus the guide wire dilating forceps technique: a prospective randomized clinical trial. *Intensive Care Med* 2011;**37**:1103–9.

42 **Norwood S, Vallina VL, Short K, Saigusa M, Fernandez LG, McLarty JW.** Incidence of tracheal stenosis and other late complications after percutaneous tracheostomy. *Ann Surg* 2000;**232**:233–41.

43 **Zias N, Chroneou A, Tabba MK, et al.** Post tracheostomy and post intubation tracheal stenosis: report of 31 cases and review of the literature. *BMC Pulm Med* 2008;**8**:18.

44 **Higgins D, Bunker N, Kinnear J.** Follow-up of patients with tracheal ring fractures secondary to antegrade percutaneous dilational tracheostomy. *Eur J Anaesthesiol* 2009;**26**:147–9.

45 **Antonelli M, Michetti V, Di PA, et al.** Percutaneous translaryngeal versus surgical tracheostomy: a randomized trial with 1-yr double-blind follow-up. *Crit Care Med* 2005;**33**:1015–20.

46 **Silvester W, Goldsmith D, Uchino S, et al.** Percutaneous versus surgical tracheostomy: a randomized controlled study with long-term follow-up. *Crit Care Med* 2006;**34**:2145–52.

47 **Badia M, Trujillano J, Servia L, March J, Rodriguez-Pozo A.** Skin lesions after intensive care procedures: results of a prospective study. *J Crit Care* 2008;**23**:525–31.

48 **van Heurn LW, Goei R, de P, I, Ramsay G, Brink PR.** Late complications of percutaneous dilatational tracheotomy. *Chest* 1996;**110**:1572–6.

49 **Prigent H, Lejaille M, Terzi N, et al.** Effect of a tracheostomy speaking valve on breathing-swallowing interaction. *Intensive Care Med* 2012;**38**:85–90.

50 **Romero CM, Marambio A, Larrondo J, et al.** Swallowing dysfunction in nonneurologic critically ill patients who require percutaneous dilatational tracheostomy. *Chest* 2010;**137**:1278–82.

51 **Grant CA, Dempsey G, Harrison J, Jones T.** Tracheo-innominate artery fistula after percutaneous tracheostomy: three case reports and a clinical review. *Br J Anaesth* 2006;**96**:127–31.

52 **Engoren M, Arslanian-Engoren C, Fenn-Buderer N.** Hospital and long-term outcome after tracheostomy for respiratory failure. *Chest* 2004;**125**:220–7.

53 **Diaz-Reganon G, Minambres E, Ruiz A, Gonzalez-Herrera S, Holanda-Pena M, Lopez-Espadas F.** Safety and complications of percutaneous tracheostomy in a cohort of 800 mixed ICU patients. *Anaesthesia* 2008;**63**:1198–203.

54 **Cosgrove JE, Sweenie A, Raftery G, et al.** Locally developed guidelines reduce immediate complications from percutaneous dilatational tracheostomy using the Ciaglia Blue Rhino technique: a report on 200 procedures. *Anaesth Intensive Care* 2006;**34**:782–6.

55 **Roh HJ, Goh EK, Chon KM, Wang SG.** Topical inhalant steroid (budesonide, Pulmicort nasal) therapy in intubation granuloma. *J Laryngol Otol* 1999;**113**:427–32.

56 **Rahman NA, Fruchter O, Shitrit D, Fox BD, Kramer MR.** Flexible bronchoscopic management of benign tracheal stenosis: long term follow-up of 115 patients. *J Cardiothorac Surg* 2010;**5**:2.

57 **Nouraei SA, Ghufoor K, Patel A, Ferguson T, Howard DJ, Sandhu GS.** Outcome of endoscopic treatment of adult postintubation tracheal stenosis. *Laryngoscope* 2007;**117**:1073–9.

58 **Noppen M, Stratakos G, Amjadi K, et al.** Stenting allows weaning and extubation in ventilator- or tracheostomy dependency secondary to benign airway disease. *Respir Med* 2007;**101**:139–45.

59 **Carbognani P, Bobbio A, Cattelani L, Internullo E, Caporale D, Rusca M.** Management of postintubation membranous tracheal rupture. *Ann Thorac Surg* 2004;**77**:406–9.

60 **Massard G, Rouge C, Dabbagh A, et al.** Tracheobronchial lacerations after intubation and tracheostomy. *Ann Thorac Surg* 1996;**61**:1483–7.

61 **Fan CM, Ko PC, Tsai KC, et al.** Tracheal rupture complicating emergent endotracheal intubation. *Am J Emerg Med* 2004;**22**:289–93.

Part 3

Cognitive and Behavioural Disorders Following Critical Illness

Chapter 18

Introduction: Cognitive and Behavioural Disorders Following Critical Illness

E. Wesley Ely

An admission to the ICU is in itself often considered a tragic life occurrence by the lay public and by medical professionals alike. However harrowing the events of the ICU may be, though, we are now aware of the life-changing 'legacy' of brain and behavioural disorders that ICU survivors suffer in the months and years following critical illness. In just the past decade or so, investigators, such as the authors of the four chapters in this section, have published data that clearly illustrate a spectrum of acquired or exacerbated 'neck-up' disorders that often dismantle the lives of our patients and seriously delay or outright prevent their recovery. First and foremost among these disorders is a potentially life-altering, 'dementia-like' long-term cognitive impairment (see Chapter 19) that occurs in 60–80% of ICU survivors and which is most often characterized by memory and executive dysfunction. These problems have real-world, ecologically valid implications, as they assault patients' ability to return to work, find their car in a parking lot, go shopping, balance a cheque book, and, although most people can remember the names of people they know well, they have trouble remembering new events, facts, and their schedule. These extremely troublesome neuropsychological deficits are compounded by mood disorders such as major depression (see Chapter 20) as well as PTSD (see Chapter 21). These two diagnoses (depression and PTSD) are oft missed despite their occurrence in 25–30% and 10–20% of ICU survivors, respectively. As a profession, we are just beginning to address the risk factors for these 'newly acquired' and/or 'accelerated-from-baseline' diseases.

How might we incorporate these issues into our life as a health care professional? It is important, I think, to envision your patient rolling in on a gurney with an dangerous disease, such as pneumonia or cholecystitis, and then remind yourself that, during the ensuing days under your care, this person with a 'lung or gall bladder problem' will literally acquire new 'neck-up' and 'neck-down' (brain/central nervous system plus neuromuscular/neuroskeletal) diseases. These two new or acquired elements of disease burden have to be a major focus of our attention during and following our patients' ICU stays. It is also important to recognize that these two categories of body decay are inextricably connected. As we move to identify means of intervention both to prevent and treat these problems, we would be wise to focus on the following modifiable risk factors during our patients' ICU stay and recovery: total exposure to potent psychoactive medications, duration of delirium, sleep deficits and derangements (see Chapter 27), and periods of immobilization. These and other aspects of care are well addressed within the covers of this book, published at a pivotal time of dramatic change in critical care, both within the walls of the ICU and beyond into the world of cognitive and physical rehabilitation following ICU discharge.

Chapter 19

Cognitive Impairment Following Critical Illness

Ramona O. Hopkins and James C. Jackson

Introduction

Advancement in the treatment of critical illness has resulted in reduced mortality, along with a substantial and growing number of patients who survive a critical illness,[1] many of whom will develop significant physical, cognitive, and psychiatric morbidities. A editorial noted that surviving critical illness is the major challenge of critical care medicine.[2] A stakeholders' conference, sponsored by the SCCM, regarding improving outcomes after ICU discharge identified these constellation of morbidities as 'post-intensive care syndrome (PICS)' which includes physical, cognitive, or psychiatric morbidities, acquired following critical illness.[3] These morbidities adversely impact survivors' functional status, ability to return to work, and QoL and are associated increased health care costs.[2] This chapter will focus on cognitive impairment following critical illness, potential mechanisms and risk factors of the cognitive impairments, and recovery and rehabilitation of post-ICU cognitive impairment.

Cognitive impairment

Investigations to date indicate that survivors of critical illness have substantial cognitive impairments, with a high prevalence rate, which develop during critical illness, are severe in intensity, affect multiple cognitive domains (e.g. memory, executive function, attention, mental processing speed), can last for years, and may be permanent.[4] Studies describe a prevalence range of cognitive impairment of about 9–70% of ICU survivors in the first year after discharge.[5,6] Higher prevalence rates are documented when cognitive impairments are assessed at hospital discharge (78–100%)[7,8] and remain as high as 45% at 2 years after discharge.[7] Cognitive impairments improve during the first 6–12 months post-hospital discharge,[7] at least in some individuals, and this is similar to the recovery observed following other acquired brain injuries such as TBI. The cognitive impairments are often severe in nature, and many patients continue to experience significant chronic cognitive impairments years after ICU discharge. A number of factors, such as age, likely influence the rate of cognitive impairment, as age over 65 years is associated with an increased risk for the development of cognitive impairments. In an older ICU population (mean age 61), Girard and colleagues found 80% of ICU survivors had cognitive impairment at 3 months and 70% had cognitive impairment at 12 months, a rate higher than reported in most previous studies.[6] In patients with CCI, a prospective study of 126 patients with PMV found only 56% of patients survived to 1 year and 65% of these survivors had severe cognitive impairment.[9] Since only severe cognitive impairment was assessed in this study, it is likely that many other survivors had mild to moderate cognitive disability. Of the survivors, 82% had a poor outcome (e.g. complete functional dependency), 26% had a fair outcome (e.g. moderate dependency), and only 9% had a good outcome (e.g. no functional dependency).[9] These data suggest that cognitive impairment following critical illness is not only common but is often severe, affects functional outcomes, and appears to be permanent in nature.

Critical illness-acquired brain injury

Current cognitive and neuroimaging data indicate that critical illness is associated with new non-specific acquired brain injury.[4,10,11] By definition, acquired brain injury has an acute onset, may occur at any age, is due to external environmental or internal insults, remains static or improves over time (not decline), and likely responds to rehabilitation. In the case of critical illness, discrete insults, such as hypoxia, cytokine-activated immune system dysregulation, hypotension, glucose dysregulation, neurotoxic effects of medications (e.g. sedatives), and delirium (see section on biological mechanisms), are implicated in brain injury.

One requirement of an acquired brain injury is an acute onset. Recent investigations suggest that critical illness-acquired brain injury and associated cognitive impairment onset are acute, following critical illness. Three recent population-based studies demonstrate that newly acquired cognitive impairments occur, following an episode of critical illness, sepsis, or hospitalization.[12-14] A longitudinal cohort study of older, cognitively healthy adults, in whom cognitive function was assessed every 2 years, found critical illness was associated with greater cognitive decline, compared to patients who did not experience critical illness.[12] A second longitudinal cohort study of 1194 healthy older adults found that an episode of severe sepsis was associated with the development of new cognitive impairment.[14] Finally, a recent longitudinal, population-based cohort study of 1870 older adults, in whom cognitive function was assessed every 3 years, found the rate of cognitive decline increased 2.4-fold in older adults who were hospitalized (only 3% were ICU hospitalizations), compared to the rate of decline in the first year after hospitalization, controlling for older age, illness severity, and pre-hospital cognitive decline.[13] There was a 3.3-fold decline in memory and 1.7-fold decline in executive function.[13] These data suggest that sepsis, critical illness, and hospitalization, in general, result in new abrupt cognitive impairments in healthy older populations without pre-existing cognitive dysfunction.

Aetiology of cognitive impairments

Another requirement of an acquired brain injury is that it the result of an external environmental or internal insult. Cognitive outcomes have been assessed in a variety of ICU populations, including ARDS, post-MV, sepsis, surgery, and trauma patients without intracranial haemorrhage. Table 19.1 shows the prevalence rate of cognitive impairment by aetiology (see Table 19.1). No studies to date have directly compared the rates of cognitive impairment, using specific aetiologies of critical illness; however, high prevalence rates of cognitive impairments are consistently found across the various ICU populations,[15] including medical,[16] surgery,[17] ARDS,[7] and sepsis.[14] Approximately one-third of general medical ICU patients have cognitive impairment at 6 months.[18] In older medical ICU survivors, 70% have cognitive impairments at 12 months, one of the highest rates reported, suggesting that not only aetiology, but population characteristics, such as older age, may influence outcomes.[6] Among the sickest of these populations, in individuals with ARDS, the prevalence of long-term cognitive impairment is particularly high: 74% at hospital discharge and approximately 46% at 1 and 2 years.[7] A recent multicentre study that assessed cognitive outcomes in ARDS patients found 55% of patients had cognitive impairments and 13%

Table 19.1 Cognitive impairments by aetiology of critical illness

Population	Study	Design	Prevalence of cognitive impairment
ARDS	Kapfhammer et al. (2004)[5]	Retrospective cohort	9%
	Hopkins et al. (2005)[7]	Prospective cohort	78% hospital discharge 45% at 1 and 2 years
	Mikkelsen et al. (2009)[65]	Cross-sectional cohort	56%
	Rothenhausler et al. (2001)[66]	Retrospective cohort	24%
	Mikkelsen et al. (2012)[19]	Prospective multicentre cohort study of survivors of ARDSNet Fluid and Catheter Treatment Trial	55% cognitive impairment 13% impaired memory 16% impaired verbal fluency 49% executive dysfunction
Chronically critically ill	Unroe et al. (2010)[9]	Prospective cohort	65%
Medical	Jackson et al. (2003)[18]	Prospective cohort	32%
	Girard et al. (2010)[6]	Prospective cohort	80% impaired at 3 months 70% impaired at 12 months
	Jones et al. (2006)[8]	Prospective cohort	100% hospital discharge 31% impaired memory at 2 months 50% impaired executive function at 2 months
	Sukantarat et al. (2005)[16]	Prospective cohort	55%
Sepsis	Iwashyna et al. (2010)[14]	Prospective cross-sectional cohort	Cognitive impairment increased from 6.1% before to 16.7% after severe sepsis 59.3% had worsening cognitive or physical function after severe sepsis
Surgical	Torgersen et al. (2011)[67]	Prospective cohort	64% at ICU discharge 11% at 3 months
	Duning et al. (2010)[17]	Prospective cohort	Impaired attention, executive function, visuospatial skills, and memory (percentage not reported)
Trauma	Jackson et al. (2007)[20]	Prospective cohort	43%
	Jackson et al. (2011)[21]	Prospective cohort	55%

had impaired memory, 16% had impaired verbal fluency, and 49% had impaired executive function.[19] Not surprisingly, trauma populations appear to have poor cognitive outcome, as 57% of critically ill trauma patients (without intracranial haemorrhage) have moderate to severe cognitive impairments, and the likelihood of cognitive impairment doubled in patients with a skull fracture or concussion.[20] A second prospective study in trauma ICU survivors (without intracranial haemorrhage) found 55% of patients had moderate to severe cognitive impairments and the proportion with cognitive impairments did not differ for patients with moderate injury (injury severity score >15 and <25), compared to patients with severe injury (injury severity score >25).[21] As already noted, approximately 65% of survivors of CCI have cognitive impairments.[9] These data suggest that the aetiology of the critical illness appears to be less crucial to the development of cognitive impairment than having a critical illness event or its associated treatment. The lack of discrimination, based on aetiology, may be due to common insults, and, therefore, common mechanisms are likely responsible for the observed cognitive impairments.

Biological mechanisms

The mechanisms of cognitive impairments in critically ill patients are multifactorial and are undoubtedly interrelated. Research regarding the mechanisms of critical illness-acquired cognitive impairment is limited but increasing. Current data suggest that pathophysiologic mechanisms of unfavourable cognitive sequelae include hypoxaemia,[7] hypotension,[22] glucose dysregulation,[23] and inflammation and cytokine-activated immune system dysregulation.[24]

Hypoxaemia

Hypoxia has been associated with cognitive impairments in a variety of populations, including patients with cardiac and pulmonary disorders. The relationship between the duration and severity of hypoxaemia and cognitive outcome was evaluated in a prospective cohort of mechanically ventilated ARDS survivors and demonstrated that the duration of hypoxaemia was significantly associated with cognitive sequelae.[7] Consistent with previous work, a recent adjunct study to the Acute Respiratory Distress Syndrome Clinical Trials Network Fluid and Catheter Treatment Trial (FACTT) the Adult Respiratory Distress Syndrome Cognitive Outcomes Study (ACOS) found hypoxaemia was a potential risk factor for the development of long-term cognitive impairment.[19] Hypoxaemia during the trial, enrolment in the conservative fluid management strategy, and lower central venous pressure during FACTT were each associated with worse executive function. After controlling for covariates, hypoxaemia and enrolment in the conservative fluid management strategy were independently associated with cognitive impairment at 12 months' follow-up.[19]

Hypoxia injures the brain via a biochemical cascade, including: (1) decreased adenosine triphosphate (ATP) production,[25] (2) lactic acidosis,[26] (3) excitotoxicity due to excessive release of excitatory neurotransmitters (e.g. glutamate),[27] (4) increased calcium influx and intracellular calcium accumulation due to ionic pump failure,[28] (5) reperfusion injury,[29] (6) necrosis,[29] and apoptosis.[30] For a review of mechanisms of hypoxia-induced brain injury, see reference 31.[31]

Hypotension

Limited data suggest that hypotension is associated with cognitive impairments. A study in ARDS patents found the duration of hypotension was associated with impaired memory at hospital discharge but not at 1 or 2 years.[7] As noted previously, outcomes of the ACOS study found lower central venous pressure during FACTT was associated with worse executive function and cognitive impairment.[19] However, there was no indirect evidence for hypotension, such as reduced cerebral perfusion, low cardiac index, or low systolic pressure, in this study. Additional research is needed to determine if hypotension in critically ill populations is a risk factor for development of cognitive impairment.

Glucose dysregulation

Blood glucose dysregulation is associated with cognitive impairments in ARDS patients at 1-year follow-up.[23] Blood glucose values greater than 153 mg/dL (moderate hyperglycaemia) predicted adverse cognitive sequelae, but the effect did not worsen as blood glucose values increased. In addition, blood glucose variability (blood glucose SD >15.9) increased the risk of cognitive sequelae.[23] A second study evaluated surgical critically ill patients with at least one episode of hypoglycaemia who were matched to critically ill patients without hypoglycaemia.[17] Patients in each group had cognitive impairments in the domains of attention, executive function, working memory, memory, and visual-spatial skills. Critical illness-induced cognitive impairments were worsened by hypoglycaemia, but the effect of blood glucose dysregulation, including hyperglycaemia and blood glucose variability, also contributed to adverse cognitive sequelae.[17] A recent post-mortem study of patients who died in the ICU assessed neuropathologic changes associated with normoglycaemia, moderate hyperglycaemia, or hyperglycaemia.[32] Patients with hyperglycaemia had increased microglial activation, reduced astrocyte number and activation, increased neuronal apoptosis, and increased neuronal damage in the hippocampus and frontal cortex. Normoglycaemia prevented injury, and moderate hyperglycaemia attenuated the neuropathologic changes.[32]

Hyperglycaemia decreases cerebral blood flow (CBF),[33] damages the vascular endothelium,[34] increases blood-brain barrier (BBB) permeability,[35] and increases the release of excitatory neurotransmitters, with subsequent neuronal death.[36] Pathologic mechanisms of hyperglycaemia-induced brain injury include increased lactic acidosis and impaired phosphorus metabolism,[37] increased calcium release and influx, increased catecholamine release,[38] and neuronal necrosis.[39] Hyperglycaemia also results in the formation of oxygen radicals, cytolytic proteases, and release of pro-inflammatory cytokines, resulting in neuronal injury.[40]

Risk factors for cognitive impairment

Delirium

Up to 80% of mechanically ventilated ICU patients develop delirium that is associated with longer hospital stays and increased mortality.[41] Delirium is a nearly ubiquitous acute neurologic dysfunction that is associated with adverse cognitive outcomes in critically ill patients. Studies of older hospitalized patients found delirium to be an independent risk factor for the development of cognitive impairment,but the relationship between delirium and cognitive impairment remains poorly understood.[42] Delirium may be a risk factor for neurologic injury and cognitive impairment in survivors of critical illness. A study that assessed the relationship between delirium and cognitive outcomes in critically ill patients found the mean delirium duration was 2 days and the prevalence of cognitive impairments at 3 and 12 months was ~70%.[6] Delirium duration independently predicted 3 and 12 month cognitive impairment in survivors of critical illness.[6] A prospective cohort study, using diffusion tensor imaging (DTI), assessed the relationships among delirium, white matter integrity, and cognitive impairments in survivors of critical illness.[43] Greater duration of delirium was associated with white matter disruption in the corpus callosum and anterior limb of the internal capsule, and white matter disruption was associated with cognitive impairment at 3 and 12 months.[43] A magnetic resonance imaging (MRI) study found septic patients with delirium had lesions in the centrum semiovale, including small multiple focal diffuse lesions.[44]

The pathophysiologic mechanisms of delirium are complex and thought to be related to imbalances in synthesis, release, and inactivation of neurotransmitters, including dopamine excess or acetylcholine depletion,[45] serotonin imbalance and increased noradrenergic activity are also associated with delirium.[46] Other mechanisms of delirium include inflammation due to endotoxin and cytokine release,[47] insufficient cerebral perfusion,[48] metabolic derangements,[49] and activation of the hypothalamic-pituitary axis.[50]

Sedatives or analgesics

Not surprisingly, medications routinely administered in the ICU have effects on neurotransmitters (e.g. acetylcholine, dopamine, serotonin, gamma-aminobutyric acid (GABA), glutamate, and NE). For example, tricyclic antidepressants, H2 blockers, opiates, furosemide, and benzodiazepines have central anticholinergic effects.[51] Excess dopamine is a risk factor for the development of delirium,[52] and GABA abnormalities contribute to delirium.[53] Medications, such as sedatives, narcotics, and paralytics, play a role in the development of delirium,[54] but less is known regarding their effects on cognitive function. A recent study assessed cognitive outcomes in patients who received SBTs and a wake up-and-breathe protocol that interrupts and reduces sedative exposure, compared to SBTs alone.[55] Cognitive impairment was common, affecting 79% of patients at 3 months and 71% at 12 months. Cognitive impairments were less common in patients who had reduced sedative exposure at 3 months, but not at 12 months, suggesting the effect of sedatives may only affect short-term outcomes.[55]

Recovery and rehabilitation

Recovery

As numerous studies have demonstrated, there is a natural recovery curve that often occurs among critically ill survivors, although the recovery they experience is generally partial and very rarely complete.[6,7] The temporal course of spontaneous recovery is months to years, and the recovery rate likely varies from patient to patient and over time. It is simplistic to think that all patients recover. Survivors of critical illness likely have variable outcome trajectories. Such trajectories include individuals who recover to their pre-illness baseline function, individuals whose cognitive function declines, and individuals with no change in cognitive function or who remain stable over time. For the group that remains stable over time, there are two subgroups, those who have normal pre-critical illness cognitive function and remain normal post-critical illness and individuals who have cognitive impairments at ICU discharge and remain impaired (no recovery) over time. Figure 19.1 shows hypothetical trajectories of cognitive function after critical illness, superimposed on age-related cognitive changes. Hypothetical outcomes after the onset of critical illness include new cognitive impairments which can recover over time to the individual's prior level of cognitive function (spontaneous recovery), decline and partial recovery to a new cognitive level of performance, decline to a new cognitive baseline with no recovery, or decline after critical illness and continued decline with ageing. There are other possible outcome trajectories such as improvement followed by decline. Spontaneous recovery via neuroplasticity appears to occur for at least some patients. However, spontaneous recovery does not include the benefits of cognitive

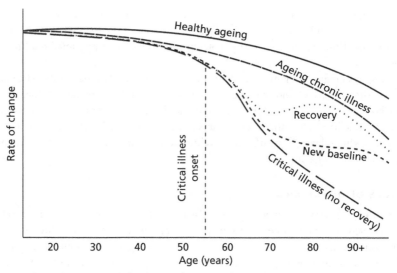

Fig. 19.1 Hypothetical trajectories of cognitive function after critical illness superimposed on age-related cognitive changes.

The timing of critical illness could occur at any time point, but age 55 was selected, as it is nearing the time that normal age-related cognitive decline may occur in some individuals and helps to illustrate possible cognitive outcome trajectories in the context of ageing. The solid line shows a hypothetical rate of cognitive decline in cognitive function in healthy ageing, reflecting a gradual, but relatively modest, change. The close dashed line shows a hypothetical rate of cognitive decline in individuals with chronic disease and ageing. The dotted line shows hypothetical cognitive function before and after critical illness, showing some decline, then recovery of function. The small dashed line shows hypothetical cognitive function before and after critical illness, showing cognitive impairment, little or no recovery, and then a new baseline of cognitive function. The large dashed line shows hypothetical cognitive function before and after critical illness, showing cognitive impairment, then continued decline in cognitive function with ageing.

rehabilitation, as such a one-size-fits-all approach to recovery and rehabilitation will likely not be effective in promoting optimal outcomes after critical illness.

Rehabilitation

As we have previously observed, there are numerous risk factors implicated in the development of cognitive impairment after intensive care, some of which are clearly not modifiable, whereas other risk factors are potentially modifiable. Until such a time as these risk factors can be reduced or eliminated, an important pathway to improved cognitive functioning for ICU survivors may be through cognitive rehabilitation. Cognitive rehabilitation is widely employed in diverse populations, including individuals with various kinds of acquired brain injuries.[56] While a common approach in the management of individuals treated in the trauma or neurological ICUs, cognitive rehabilitation is rarely used with general medical or general surgical ICU survivors,[57] perhaps because the insults they sustain do not fit the commonly understood paradigms for brain injuries, lack of funding, and regulatory requirements for acute inpatient rehabilitation that require at least 60% of patients having a diagnosis from a list of approved diagnoses.[3] Nonetheless, cognitive rehabilitation may be appropriate and effective for individuals following intensive care.

Cognitive rehabilitation has been defined in various ways, though Cicerone and colleagues[58] have developed a widely utilized definition which posits that it is 'the systematic, functionally oriented service of therapeutic activities that is based on assessment and understanding of the patient's brain-behavior deficits.' Cognitive rehabilitation is based on two fundamental principles: (1) the brain has the capacity to recover from insult or injury (to a greater or lesser degree) and (2) individuals have the potential to adjust and adapt to the effects of brain damage, resulting in more effective coping.[59] While the 'promise' of plasticity and spontaneous recovery may provide reason for optimism for some brain-injured individuals, it clearly applies more to some circumstances than others and depends on a number of factors such as the age of the individual and the timing of rehabilitation.[60] Brain plasticity is strongly influenced by age, as reflected in numerous rodent studies which demonstrate that younger animals have substantial neuronal changes in response to behavioural stresses, in contrast to older animals whose brains remain essentially unchanged.[61] Similarly, plasticity is time-dependent, as relatively large changes occur in the first weeks and months following brain injury, but they gradually dissipate over time.[60] On the basis of these facts, individuals with the greatest recovery potential after intensive care are likely younger and include those individuals who engage in cognitive rehabilitation shortly after their brain injury.

While cognitive functioning can improve via cognitive rehabilitation, it is also the case that brain-injured individuals (including ICU survivors) can become more functional, even in the absence of fundamental neuroplasticity, through the use of robust compensatory strategies.[62] Compensatory strategies, in theory, can be employed at virtually any time after brain injury and are not dependent on the time-dependent factors that influence plasticity. Compensatory strategies refer to approaches by which individuals leverage existing skills and abilities or develop new ones to 'offset' the impact of the cognitive impairment following brain injury. For example, these may include the use of a memory book, daily planner, or smart phone (schedule and alarms) to compensate for impaired memory. Alternatively, compensation can involve an adjustment of goals or desires so that they are more compatible with post-injury abilities.[63] For a young brain-injured ICU survivor, it may be that the rigorous mechanical engineering programme he was pursuing at a large elite university is no longer a viable choice in view of his difficulties with executive dysfunction, which contribute to poor decision making and planning. Compensatory strategies, for him, might involve harnessing his considerable interpersonal skills which have been relatively less affected and using these to successfully engage in the study of sales and marketing in a smaller and less demanding college where he can find relatively more social support. Of course, such a change is often not accomplished easily and frequently requires significant mental health treatment, as people often experience important depression and anxiety in such circumstances and grieve their lost abilities. Indeed, a central goal of rehabilitation may be helping these individuals grieve and develop a new post-injury identity that corresponds more accurately to their post-injury abilities.[64]

The impact of early cognitive rehabilitation for ICU patients is not well studied but, if positive, holds promise of improving cognitive outcomes. To date, a single investigation—the RETURN Trial—focused specifically on the efficacy of the rehabilitation of executive dysfunction. This randomized trial by Jackson et al. focused on general medical and surgical ICU patients and employed a protocolized approach to rehabilitation called goal management training.[57] Baseline (pre-intervention) neuropsychological testing results were well matched. At 3-month follow-up, however, intervention group patients demonstrated significantly improved executive functioning on the study's primary outcome measure the Tower Test ($P < 0.01$). While the RETURN Trial was a small pilot investigation with clear limitations, it has demonstrated, in an admittedly preliminary way, that rehabilitation of executive functioning in ICU survivors may be accomplished—but will the effect persist over time? Future studies should engage this question more fully and with larger populations to definitively determine whether executive impairments can be improved and sustained.

Conclusion

Cognitive impairment in ICU survivors has been the subject of increased investigation in the last decade and a half. Significant knowledge has been generated, as evidence increasingly shows ICU survivors display marked cognitive deficits following critical illness. Nearly 20 studies report, with striking unanimity, that cognitive problems occur in more than two out of three individuals after hospital discharge and persist for years, often in the absence of premorbid cognitive difficulties. However, many key questions remain, including the trajectories of change over time, whether ICU survivors experience continued cognitive decline, and how cognitive impairments pertain to the so-called 'real-world' outcomes (ecological validity). With respect to trajectories of change over time, these have been widely investigated in other populations but rarely, if ever, explored following intensive care due to limited duration of follow-up that has been employed (typically followed at one time point only). As such, much remains unknown about the long-term natural history and recovery of ICU-acquired cognitive impairments. Importantly, studies need to more fully assess the degree to which persistent cognitive decline occurs after, or is accelerated by, critical illness, particularly in older populations, and whether differential risk factors contribute to distinct patterns of outcomes. It may be that the increasing rates of Alzheimer's disease could be driven, in part, by the effects of critical illness and its treatment,[4,10,11] although this is speculative and remains to be proven.

Key questions remain regarding the functional or real-world effects of the cognitive impairments that are common in ICU survivors. Unfortunately, little attention has been paid to this. These outcomes, increasingly explored in other cognitively impaired populations, include activities like driving, managing medications, financial abilities (e.g. balancing a cheque book), shopping for groceries, and map reading. Functional outcomes are not easy to measure, and they often require specialized facilities and extensive training. Furthermore, normative data for tasks of ecological validity, such as managing medications, either do not exist or are limited. These barriers should not dim the enthusiasm for determining the impact of cognitive deficits on real-world activities, since these studies will allow us to more fully understand the functional consequences of post-ICU cognitive impairments.

Cognitive impairment in ICU survivors remains a public health problem. In recent years, more attention has been paid to this phenomenon, both in clinical and research settings and in the popular media. Current efforts to improve post-ICU morbidities are promising, and studies of the effects of rehabilitation after intensive care is a particularly exciting area of investigation. Still, there is much to learn. Future efforts should reflect the increasing sophistication and granularity in the assessment of cognitive outcomes and should address the vital questions elucidated in this chapter. In time, these efforts will contribute directly to the QoL and well-being of ICU survivors and will ultimately enhance public health.

References

1 Adhikari NK, Fowler RA, Bhagwanjee S, Rubenfeld GD. Critical care and the global burden of critical illness in adults. *Lancet* 2010;**376**:1339–46.

2 Iwashyna TJ. Survivorship will be the defining challenge of critical care in the 21st century. *Ann Intern Med* 2010;**153**:204–5.

3 Needham DM, Davidson J, Cohen H, et al. Improving long-term outcomes after discharge from intensive care unit: report from a stakeholders' conference. *Crit Care Med* 2012;**40**:502–9.

4 Hopkins RO, Jackson JC. Long-term neurocognitive function after critical illness. *Chest* 2006;**130**: 869–78.

5 Kapfhammer HP, Rothenhausler HB, Krauseneck T, Stoll C, Schelling G. Posttraumatic stress disorder and health-related quality of life in long-term survivors of acute respiratory distress syndrome. *Am J Psychiatry* 2004;**161**:45–52.

6 Girard TD, Jackson JC, Pandharipande PP, et al. Delirium as a predictor of long-term cognitive impairment in survivors of critical illness. *Crit Care Med* 2010;**38**:1513–20.

7 Hopkins RO, Weaver LK, Collingridge D, Parkinson RB, Chan KJ, Orme JF, Jr. Two-year cognitive, emotional, and quality-of-life outcomes in acute respiratory distress syndrome. *Am J Respir Crit Care Med* 2005;**171**:340–7.

8 Jones C, Griffiths RD, Slater T, Benjamin KS, Wilson S. Significant cognitive dysfunction in non-delirious patients identified during and persisting following critical illness. *Intensive Care Med* 2006;**32**:923–6.

9 Unroe M, Kahn JM, Carson SS, et al. One-year trajectories of care and resource utilization for recipients of prolonged mechanical ventilation: a cohort study. *Ann Intern Med* 2010;**153**: 167–75.

10 Hopkins RO, Gale SD, Weaver LK. Brain atrophy and cognitive impairment in survivors of acute respiratory distress syndrome. Brain Inj 2006;**20**:263–71.

11 Suchyta MR, Jephson A, Hopkins RO. Neurologic changes during critical illness: brain imaging findings and neurobehavioral outcomes. *Brain Imaging Behav* 2010;**4**:22–34.

12 Ehlenbach WJ, Hough CL, Crane PK, et al. Association between acute care and critical illness hospitalization and cognitive function in older adults. *JAMA* 2010;**303**:763–70.

13 Wilson RS, Hebert LE, Scherr PA, Dong X, Leurgens SE, Evans DA. Cognitive decline after hospitalization in a community population of older persons. *Neurology* 2012;**78**:950–6.

14 Iwashyna TJ, Ely EW, Smith DM, Langa KM. Long-term cognitive impairment and functional disability among survivors of severe sepsis. *JAMA* 2010;**304**:1787–94.

15 Hopkins RO, Jackson JC. Short- and long-term cognitive outcomes in intensive care unit survivors. *Clin Chest Med* 2009;**30**:143–53.

16 Sukantarat KT, Burgess PW, Williamson RC, Brett SJ. Prolonged cognitive dysfunction in survivors of critical illness. *Anaesthesia* 2005;**60**:847–53.

17 Duning T, van den Heuvel I, Dickmann A, et al. Hypoglycemia aggravates critical illness-induced neurocognitive dysfunction. *Diabetes Care* 2010;**33**:639–44.

18 Jackson JC, Hart RP, Gordon SM, et al. Six-month neuropsychological outcome of medical intensive care unit patients. *Crit Care Med* 2003;**31**:1226–34.

19 Mikkelsen ME, Christie JD, Lanken PN, et al. The adult respiratory distress syndrome cognitive outcomes study: Long-term neuropsychological function in survivors of acute lung injury. *Am J Respir Crit Care Med* 2012;**185**:1307–15.

20 Jackson JC, Obremskey W, Bauer R, et al. Long-term cognitive, emotional, and functional outcomes in trauma intensive care unit survivors without intracranial hemorrhage. *J Trauma* 2007;**62**:80–8.

21 Jackson JC, Archer KR, Bauer R, et al. A prospective investigation of long-term cognitive impairment and psychological distress in moderately versus severely injured trauma intensive care unit survivors without intracranial hemorrhage. *J Trauma* 2011;**71**:860–6.

22 Hopkins RO, Weaver LK, Chan KJ, Orme JF, Jr. Quality of life, emotional, and cognitive function following acute respiratory distress syndrome. *J Int Neuropsychol Soc* 2004;**10**:1005–17.

23 Hopkins RO, Suchyta MR, Snow GL, Jephson A, Weaver LK, Orme JF. Blood glucose dysregulation and cognitive outcome in ards survivors. *Brain Inj* 2010;**24**:1478–84.

24 Elenkov IJ, Iezzoni DG, Daly A, Harris AG, Chrousos GP. Cytokine dysregulation, inflammation and well-being. *Neuroimmunomodulation* 2005;**12**:255–69.

25 Lutz PL, Nilsson GE. *The brain without oxygen: causes of failure—physiological and molecular mechanisms for survival.* Austin, TX: RG Landes Co; 1994.

26 Michenfelder JD, Sundt TM, Jr. Cerebral ATP and lactate levels in the squirrel monkey following occlusion of the middle cerebral artery. *Stroke* 1971;**2**:319–26.

27 Siesjo BK, Bengtsson F, Grampp W, Theander S. Calcium, excitotoxins, and neuronal death in the brain. *Ann N Y Acad Sci* 1989;**568**:234–51.

28 Schurr A, Lipton P, West CA, Rigor BM. The role of energy in metabolism and divalent cations in the neurotoxicity of excitatory amino acids in vitro. In: Krieglstein J (ed.) *Pharmacology of cerebral ischemia.* Boca Raton, FL: CRC Press LLC; 1990. pp. 217–26.

29 Biagas K. Hypoxic-ischemic brain injury: advancements in the understanding of mechanisms and potential avenues for therapy. *Curr Opin Pediatr* 1999;**11**:223–8.

30 Floyd RA. Role of oxygen free radicals in carcinogenesis and brain ischemia. *FASEB J* 1990;**4**:2587–97.

31 Johnston MV, Nakajima W, Hagberg H. Mechanisms of hypoxic neurodegeneration in the developing brain. *Neuroscientist* 2002;**8**:212–20.

32 Sonneville R, den Hertog HM, Guiza F, et al. Impact of hyperglycemia on neuropathological alterations during critical illness. *J Clin Endocrinol Metab* 2012;**97**:2113–23.

33 Katsura K, Kristian T, Smith ML, Siesjo BK. Acidosis induced by hypercapnia exaggerates ischemic brain damage. *J Cereb Blood Flow Metab* 1994;**14**:243–50.

34 Nabeshima T, Katoh A, Ishimaru H, et al. Carbon monoxide induced delayed amnesia, delayed neuronal death and change in acetylcholine concentration in mice. *J Pharmacol Exp Ther* 1991;**256**:378–84.

35 Dietrich WD, Alonso O, Busto R. Moderate hyperglycemia worsens acute blood-brain barrier injury after forebrain ischemia in rats. *Stroke* 1993;**24**:111–16.

36 McCall AL. The impact of diabetes on the CNS. *Diabetes* 1992;**41**:557–70.

37 Levine SR, Welch KM, Helpern JA, et al. Prolonged deterioration of ischemic brain energy metabolism and acidosis associated with hyperglycemia: human cerebral infarction studied by serial 31p NMR spectroscopy. Ann *Neurol* 1988;**23**:416–18.

38 Rosner MJ, Newsome HH, Becker DP. Mechanical brain injury: the sympathoadrenal response. *J Neurosurg* 1984;**61**:76–86.

39 Siesjo BK, Siesjo P. Mechanisms of secondary brain injury. *Eur J Anaesthesiol* 1996;**13**:247–68.

40 Feuerstein GZ, Liu T, Barone FC. Cytokines, inflammation, and brain injury: Role of tumor necrosis factor-alpha. *Cerebrovasc Brain Metab Rev* 1994;**6**:341–60.

41 Ely EW, Shintani A, Truman B, et al. Delirium as a predictor of mortality in mechanically ventilated patients in the intensive care unit. *JAMA* 2004;**291**:1753–62.

42 Jackson JC, Gordon SM, Hart RP, Hopkins RO, Ely EW. The association between delirium and cognitive decline: A review of the empirical literature. *Neuropsychol Rev* 2004;**14**:87–98.

43 Morandi A, Rogers BP, Gunther ML, et al. The relationship between delirium duration, white matter integrity, and cognitive impairment in intensive care unit survivors as determined by diffusion tensor imaging: The visions prospective cohort magnetic resonance imaging study. *Crit Care Med* 2012;**40**:2182–9.

44 Sharshar T, Carlier R, Bernard F, et al. Brain lesions in septic shock: a magnetic resonance imaging study. *Intensive Care Med* 2007;**33**:798–806.

45 Trzepacz PT. Is there a final common neural pathway in delirium? Focus on acetylcholine and dopamine. *Semin Clin Neuropsychiatry* 2000;**5**:132–48.

46 Meagher DJ, Trzepacz PT. Motoric subtypes of delirium. *Semin Clin Neuropsychiatry* 2000;**5**:75–85.

47 Arvin B, Neville LF, Barone FC, Feuerstein GZ. Brain injury and inflammation. A putative role of TNF alpha. *Ann N Y Acad Sci* 1995;**765**:62–71; discussion 98–9.

48 Bellingan GJ. The pulmonary physician in critical care: the pathogenesis of ALI/ARDS. *Thorax* 2002;**57**:540–6.

49 Francis J, Martin D, Kapoor WN. A prospective study of delirium in hospitalized elderly. *JAMA* 1990;**263**:1097–101.

50 De Kloet ER, Vreugdenhil E, Oitzl MS, Joels M. Brain corticosteroid receptor balance in health and disease. *Endocr Rev* 1998;**19**:269–301.

51 Milbrandt EB, Angus DC. Potential mechanisms and markers of critical illness-associated cognitive dysfunction. *Curr Opin Crit Care* 2005;**11**:355–9.

52 Sommer BR, Wise LC, Kraemer HC. Is dopamine administration possibly a risk factor for delirium? *Crit Care Med* 2002;**30**:1508–11.

53 Fischer JE, Rosen HM, Ebeid AM, James JH, Keane JM, Soeters PB. The effect of normalization of plasma amino acids on hepatic encephalopathy in man. *Surgery* 1976;**80**:77–91.

54 Morrison RS, Magaziner J, Gilbert M, et al. Relationship between pain and opioid analgesics on the development of delirium following hip fracture. *J Gerontol* 2003;**58**:76–81.

55 Jackson JC, Girard TD, Gordon SM, et al. Long-term cognitive and psychological outcomes in the awakening and breathing controlled trial. *Am J Respir Crit Care Med* 2010;**182**:183–91.

56 Stuss DT, Winocur G, Robertson IH (eds.). *Cognitive neurorehabilitation: evidence and applications.* 2nd ed. Cambridge: Cambridge University Press; 2010.

57 Jackson JC, Ely EW, Morey MC, et al. Cognitive and physical rehabilitation of intensive care unit survivors: results of the return randomized controlled pilot investigation. *Crit Care Med* 2012;**40**:1088–97.

58 Cicerone KD, Dahlberg C, Kalmar K, et al. Evidence-based cognitive rehabilitation: recommendations for clinical practice. *Arch Phys Med Rehabil* 2000;**81**:1596–615.

59 Winocur G. Introduction to principles of cognitive rehabilitation. In: Stuss DT, Winocur G, Robertson IH (eds.) *Cognitive neurorehabilitation: evidence and application.* 2nd ed. Cambridge: Cambridge University Press; 2010. pp. 3–5.

60 Kleim JA, Jones TA. Principles of experience-dependent neural plasticity: Implications for rehabilitation after brain damage. *J Speech Lang Hear Res* 2008;**51**:S225–39.

61 Bloss EB, Janssen WG, Ohm DT, et al. Evidence for reduced experience-dependent dendritic spine plasticity in the aging prefrontal cortex. *J Neurosci* 2011;**31**:7831–9.

62 Dixon RA, Garrett DD, Blackman L. Principles of compensation in cognitive neuroscience and neurorehabilitation. In: Stuss DT, Winocur G, Robertson IH (eds.) *Cognitive neurorehabilitation: evidence and application.* 2nd ed. Cambridge: Cambridge University Press; 2010. pp. 22–38.

63 Backman L, Dixon RA. Psychological compensation: a theoretical framework. *Psychol Bull* 1992;**112**:259–83.

64 Gracey F, Evans JJ, Malley D. Capturing process and outcome in complex rehabilitation interventions: a 'y-shaped' model. *Neuropsychol Rehabil* 2009;**19**:867–90.

65 Mikkelsen ME, Shull WH, Biester RC, et al. Cognitive, mood and quality of life impairments in a select population of ards survivors. *Respirology* 2009;**14**:76–82.

66 Rothenhausler HB, Ehrentraut S, Stoll C, Schelling G, Kapfhammer HP. The relationship between cognitive performance and employment and health status in long-term survivors of the acute respiratory distress syndrome: results of an exploratory study. *Gen Hosp Psychiatry* 2001;**23**:90–6.

67 Torgersen J, Hole JF, Kvale R, Wentzel-Larsen T, Flaatten H. Cognitive impairments after critical illness. *Acta Anaesthesiol Scand* 2011;**55**:1044–51.

Chapter 20

Depressive Mood States Following Critical Illness

O. Joseph Bienvenu

Introduction

Patients with critical illnesses treated in ICUs face a number of severe physical and psychic stresses due to their illnesses, associated physiologic disturbances, and life-saving procedures. Specifically, critically ill patients frequently experience respiratory insufficiency, discomfort with ETT suctioning and invasive procedures, activation of the inflammatory cascade, strain on the hypothalamic-pituitary-adrenal axis, high levels of endogenous and exogenous catecholamines, and delirium with associated psychotic experiences, all in the context of a limited ability to communicate and reduced autonomy. In addition, many survivors have residual cognitive impairments and muscle weakness,[1–3] as well as financial burdens, the need for re-hospitalization, and other stresses.[4,5] These stresses likely increase the risk of mood disturbances substantially.

Importantly, depressive symptoms and syndromes may well impede general recovery in critical illness survivors.[6] First, depressive symptoms may decrease motivation for, and reward from, physical activities.[7] This is consistent with clinical experience that depressed patients are more difficult to engage in PT, which is often crucial for the recovery of physical functioning.[8] Second, depressive symptoms can amplify symptoms of general medical illnesses,[9] and an increased physical symptom load could negatively affect function. Third, depressive symptoms can affect adherence to medication regimens,[10] which could worsen the course of general medical illnesses. Fourth, depressive symptoms could affect functioning through direct neurobiologic pathways, including neuroendocrine and inflammatory mechanisms.[11] Importantly, treatment of depressive states has been shown to improve physical functioning in elderly depressed persons.[12,13] In this chapter, I will review what is known about depressive mood states in ICU survivors, point out gaps in our knowledge base, and discuss a future research agenda.

Definitions and considerations

Readers may wonder why I chose the term 'depressive mood states' in the title of this chapter. The main reason is that depressive mood states are typically what has been measured in critical illness/ ICU long-term outcome studies, as opposed to psychiatric diagnoses like major depressive disorder, dysthymic disorder, bipolar disorder with recent depressed episode, adjustment disorder with depressed mood, depressive disorder not otherwise specified, substance-induced mood disorder, or mood disorder due to a general medical condition.

One might assume that, as a psychiatrist, I would find psychiatric diagnoses valuable and information on symptoms of little worth, but this is not the case, for two reasons. First, though psychiatric diagnoses may be made relatively reliably, depending on context, it is unlikely that diagnoses like major depressive disorder correspond to a unitary and specific disease process across individuals.[14,15] That is, major depressive disorder appears to be a relatively heterogeneous condition, sometimes appearing more 'primary' or 'disease-like' (i.e. involving a truly 'disordered' mood) and sometimes more like a reaction to circumstances in persons with varying levels of vulnerability.[16–18] Second, there is growing recognition within the field that many psychiatric diagnoses, including major depression, may reflect the severity of phenomena more than their essence. For example, people experiencing loss or disappointed ambitions can have varying levels of psychic pain and dysfunction, sometimes mild and sometimes severe, without a clear threshold demarcating 'caseness'.[19] In my opinion, data from self-report questionnaires do have intrinsic value, and these data complement those obtained using clinical interviews.

Prevalence and natural history

Prior systematic reviews

A few years ago, our group systematically reviewed the critical care outcomes literature for infor-mation on depressive symptoms and syndromes in survivors of ALI/ARDS.[20] We found that, in 277 patients, the prevalence of substantial depressive symptoms, ascertained using ques-tionnaires, ranged from 17% to 43% (study median 28%) over the first 2 years[21–24] after ALI/ARDS. Questionnaire measures included the Beck Depression Inventory (BDI),[21,23,25] the CES-D scale,[22,26] and the Zung Depression Rating Scale (ZDRS).[24,27] One of the studies examined wheth-er patients evaluated more recently after ALI had more depressive symptoms, and this was indeed the case.[22] One of the studies employed clinicians (specifically, psychiatrists) who administered the Structured Clinical Interview for DSM-IV (SCID) to 46 patients.[28,29] In that study, only 4% of ARDS survivors met criteria for major depressive disorder, but these patients were interviewed a median of 8 years after their critical illness.[29] Notably, this study excluded patients with prior psychiatric illness,[29] and another excluded patients with prior psychotic disorder.[21,23] Thus, the prevalence of substantial depressive symptoms in ALI/ARDS survivors generally is likely in the higher end of the range we reported.

In a separate systematic review of depressive symptoms and syndromes in general ICU survi-vors, we found that, in 1213 patients, the prevalence of substantial depressive symptoms, ascer-tained using questionnaires, ranged from 8% to 61% (study median 28%) over the first year after critical illness.[30] The point prevalence of clinician-diagnosed depressive disorders was also high (33% of 134 patients interviewed with the SCID), though the prevalence of major depression was lower (13% had major depressive disorder or bipolar depression). The most common measure of depressive symptoms (8/14 studies) was the HADS depression subscale;[31–39] all, except two, of the studies[32,35] used the ≥8 threshold to define substantial depressive symptoms (two studies used the more stringent ≥11 threshold). Four studies employed the CES-D scale,[40–43] one employed the Geriatric Depression Rating Scale-Short Form,[44,45] and one employed the BDI-II.[46,47] Five of the 14 reviewed studies excluded patients with known psychiatric illness (i.e. major or unspeci-fied psychiatric illness, psychotic illness, or admission after a suicide attempt).[32,33,35,36,45] Thus, the prevalence of substantial depressive symptoms in critical illness survivors generally may be in the higher end of the range we reported. Also, five of the studies explicitly examined for a change in depressive symptoms over time. In three of these studies, there were significant decreases in depressive symptoms over the first 2–12 months after critical illness.

More recent studies

Tables 20.1 and 20.2 show characteristics of 18 more recent studies (13 unique cohorts, total n = 1652) reporting on depressive symptoms and syndromes in critical illness/ICU survivors;[6,48–64]

Table 20.1 Study cohort characteristics

Study first author	Study design	Inclusion (I) and exclusion (E) criteria	Mean (SD or 95% CI) or median (interquartile range) [absolute range]					
			% male	Age (y)	d in hosp	d in ICU	d of MV	APACHE II score
Jubran (2010)[48]	Prospective cohort	I: referral to long-term acute care hospital with tracheotomy	51	71	–	–	–	16
Treggiari (2009)[49]	Prospective f/u open-label RCT	I: adult, requiring intubation and MV ≥12 h; E: neuro condition w/expected d/c, GCS ≤8, NMD requiring vent support, renal failure, allergy to benzodiazepine or morphine, h/o epilepsy, adm DX of drug overdose, liver failure, pregnancy, mental disability, inability to cooperate, receipt of HIV protease inhibitor or erythromycin	77	61	–	–	–	III: 60 (27)
Cox (2012)[50]	Cross-sectional	I: adult, MV ≥96 h; E: lack of informal caregiver, baseline dementia, brain injury, or acute stroke, language barrier, expected survival <3 m	43	56 (47–74)	28 (18–50)	19 (10–25)	10 (6–21)	25 (18–31)
Rattray (2010)[51]	Prospective cohort	I: adult, ICU stay ≥24 h, MV; E: head injury, neurosurgery, unable to give informed consent	64	60 [17–64]	13 [0–368]	7 [0–63]		19 [6–34]
McKinley (2012)[52]	Prospective f/u MC RCT	I: adult, ICU stay ≥48 h, MV >24 h; E: discharged to a rehabilitation facility	61	57 (16)	18 (12–29)	6 (4–11)	4 (2–8)	18 (7)
Myhren (2009, 2010)[53–55]	Prospective cohort	I: adult ≤75 y old, ICU stay ≥24 h; E: language difficulties, psychosis, severe head injury or cognitive failure	63	48 (16)	–	12 (10–14)	11 (9–13)	–
Dowdy (2008, 2009)[56,57] Bienvenu (2012)[6]	Prospective multisite cohort	I: adult, ALI in non-neuro ICU; E: life expectancy <6 m, cognitive impairment or language barrier, transfer with pre-existing ALI >24 h, >5 d of MV before ALI, no fixed address, request for no escalation of care	56	48 (14)	–	18 (12)	–	24 (6)
Schandl (2011)[58]	Prospective cohort	I: discharge from general ICU; E: ICU stay <4 d	64	53 (18)	–	7 [4–37]	–	21 (9)

Table 20.1 (continued) Study cohort characteristics

Study first author	Study design	Inclusion (I) and exclusion (E) criteria	% male	Age (y)	d in hosp	d in ICU	d of MV	APACHE II score
				Mean (SD or 95% CI) or median (*interquartile range*) [*absolute range*]				
Jackson (2010)[59]	Prospective f/u RCT	I: adult, MV >12 h; E: adm after CP arrest, continuous MV >2 w before enrolment, moribund state and/or withdrawal of life support, profound neuro deficits that prevented independence, enrolment in another clinical trial, cardiac surgery, or neurosurgery or stroke	50	66	–	–	–	28
Cuthbertson (2009)[60]	Prospective f/u NB RCT	I: ICU care, survival to hospital d/c; E: <18 y of age, survival not expected, not able to complete questionnaires or attend clinics	60	60	–	–	–	19 (15–24)
Mikkelsen (2012)[61]	Prospective f/u MC RCT	I: adult, MV, ALI, enrolled in Acute Respiratory Distress Syndrome Clinical Trials Network Fluid and Catheter Treatment Trial and Economic Analysis of the Pulmonary-Artery Catheter study	43	49 (40–58)				III: 85 (63–102)
Strøm (2011)[62]	Prospective f/u SB RCT	I: adult, needing MV >24 h; E: pregnancy, increased IC pressure, or sedative need (e.g. for seizures or therapeutic hypothermia)	66	67	–	–	–	22
Adhikari (2009, 2011)[63,64]	Prospective cohort	I: ARDS at ≥16 y old; E: immobile prior to ICU adm, h/o lung resection, documented neurological disease or psychiatric disorder	54	42 (35–56)		27 (16–51)		23 (15–27)

adm, admission; ALI, acute lung injury; Ap III, Apache III; CP, cardiopulmonary; d, days; d/c, discharge; DX, diagnosis; f/u, follow-up; GCS, Glasgow Coma Scale; h, hours; h/o, history of; hosp, hospital; HIV, human immunodeficiency virus; IC, intracranial; ICU, intensive care unit; m, months; MC, multicentre; MV, mechanical ventilation; neuro, neurologic; NB, non-blinded; NMD, neuromuscular disease; RCT, randomized controlled trial; SB, single-blinded; w, weeks; vent, ventilatory; w/, with; y, years.

Table 20.2 Measurements of depressive symptoms, roughly ordered by follow-up time

Study first author	Instrument (potential range)	Follow-up in months	n	Mean (SD) or *median* (*IQR*) score	Cut-off score	Point prevalence
Jubran (2010)[48]	Clinical interview by psychologist	0	336	n/a	n/a	42%*
Treggiari (2009)[49]	HADSd (0–21)	0	109	5.9	≥11	12%
		1	102	3.2	≥8, ≥11	15%, 6%
Cox (2012)[50]	HADSd (0–21)	1.5	21	–	≥7	58%
Rattray (2010)[51]	HADSd (0–21)	0	43	6.7	≥11	18%
		2	43	7.2		
		6	43	6.9		
McKinley (2012)[52]	DASS-21d (0–42)	0.25	186	*8 (2–12)*	≥14, ≥21	27%, 14%
		2	175	*4 (0–10)*	≥14, ≥21	16%, 9%
		6	164	*4 (0.5–10)*	≥14, ≥21	21%, 9%
Myhren (2009, 2010, 2010)[53–55]	HADSd (0–21)	1–1.5	255	4.8	≥11	12%
		12	192	4.7	≥8, ≥11	27%, 12%
Dowdy (2008, 2009)[56,57]	HADSd (0–21)	3	135	5.5	≥8, ≥11	28%, 11%
		6	184	5.2 (4.2)	≥8, ≥11	26%, 11%
Bienvenu (2012)[6]		12	142	–	≥8	24%
		14	136		≥8	32%
Schandl (2011)[58]	HADSd (0–21)	3	30	5.2 (4.2)	–	–
		6	30	4.5 (4.1)		
		12	30	4.9 (4.0)		
Jackson (2010)[59]	BDI-II (0–63)	3	79	~12	≥11	62%
		12	60	~13	≥11	60%
Cuthbertson (2009)[60]	HADSd (0–21)	6	220	5.3	–	–
Mikkelsen (2012)[61]	ZDRS (20–80)	12	102	–	≥60	36%
Strøm (2011)[62]	BDI-II (0–63)	23	26	3	≥11	19%
Adhikari (2009, 2011)[63,64]	BDI-II (0–63)	22	61	*12 (5–25)*	≥20	41%
		62	43	*10 (3–18)*	≥20	19%

BDI-II, Beck Depression Inventory II; DASS-21d, Depression, Anxiety, and Stress Scales 21 depression subscale; HADSd, Hospital Anxiety and Depression Scale depression subscale; n, number of survivors assessed; n/a, not applicable; ZDRS, Zung Depression Rating Scale.

* Of the 142 patients with DSM-IV depressive disorders, 12% had major depression, 4% dysthymic disorder, and 84% depressive disorder not otherwise specified.

studies reporting on the same patient cohorts are grouped together. Most of these studies had prospective cohort designs, and six involved controlled trials.[49,52,59–62]

Instruments

As in our prior systematic review of depressive symptoms in general ICU survivors,[30] the most common measure of depressive symptoms was the HADS depression subscale (11/17 studies employing questionnaire measures).[6,49–51,53–58,60] In calculating point prevalences of substantial depressive symptoms, investigators varied with regard to HADS depression subscale thresholds, one report using a relatively low threshold (≥7),[50] one report using only the ≥8 threshold,[6] two reports using only the ≥11 threshold,[51,53] and four reports using both the ≥8 and the ≥11 thresholds.[49,54,56,57] The second most common instrument was the BDI-II, used in four studies.[59,62–64] Investigators varied with regard to BDI-II threshold choices, two reports using the ≥11 threshold[59,62] and two reports using the ≥20 threshold.[63,64] Investigators employed the ZDRS in one study,[61] and investigators employed the Depression Anxiety Stress Scales (DASS-21) depression scale in another study.[52]

Results

Similar to our prior systematic reviews,[20,30] the point prevalence of substantial depressive symptoms, ascertained using questionnaires, ranged from 15%[49] to 61%[59] in the first 5 years after critical illness (see Table 20.2), and the median prevalence across studies was 27% (total n = 1316). Notably, investigators excluded patients with known prior psychiatric illness in only three[49,53–55,63,64] of the 12 studies/groups of studies, and, in two of these studies, investigators only excluded patients admitted with drug overdose[49] or prior psychosis.[53–55] The point prevalence of any DSM-IV depressive disorder in tracheostomized patients in an LTAC facility was 42% (n = 336), though only 16% of these were diagnosed with major depression or dysthymia—the majority of patients had depressive disorders not otherwise specified.[48] Evidence for a decrease in depressive symptoms over time was more mixed than in our prior systematic reviews.[20,30] That is, in the first 1–2 years after critical illness, point prevalences and/or symptom levels appeared relatively constant in five[6,51,53–59] studies/groups of studies assessing the same patients over time, while point prevalences and/or symptom levels appeared to decrease over time in only two studies.[49,52] Nevertheless, there was a clear decrease in the prevalence of substantial depressive symptoms between 2 and 5 years after ARDS.[63,64]

Conclusions

Depressive mood states are extremely common in survivors of critical illnesses, with a median point prevalence of approximately 28% across studies (with most studies focusing on the first year after critical illness). Some studies suggest persistence of depressed mood, though not all, at least during the first year or so after critical illness. Depressive disorder diagnoses appear as common as clinically significant depressive symptoms in critical illness survivors; however, severe depressive states (e.g. major depressive episodes), while common, are less common than more minor depressive states. Thus, critical care physicians should be aware that a quarter to a third of their patients who survive may have substantial depressive symptoms during recovery, and survivors should be monitored and treated for this common adverse outcome.

Risk factors and correlates

Prior systematic reviews

ALI/ARDS survivors

Unfortunately, as of the time of our prior systematic review,[20] few researchers had examined the risk factors for depressive symptoms in survivors of ALI/ARDS. One group of investigators found that days of sedation, days of MV, and days in ICU were positively correlated with the severity of depressive symptoms at follow-up.[65]

General ICU survivors

Clinical researchers following general ICU survivors had examined more risk factors for critical illness survivors at the time of our prior systematic review.[30] I summarize results in terms of pre-ICU (baseline) risk factors, critical illness/ICU risk factors/correlates, and post-ICU risk factors/correlates.

Pre-ICU risk factors

In three studies examining demographic risk factors, female sex was associated with more depressive symptoms in one study, but age was not associated with depressive symptoms in any of the three studies.[34,38,42] One study examined prior depression and physical functioning as a predictor of post-ICU depression; the authors found that poor pre-ICU physical functioning and proxy-reported depression in the month before ICU predicted post-ICU depressive symptoms, but not antidepressant prescription in the 6 months before ICU.[42]

Critical illness/ICU risk factors

In one study, investigators examined ICU admission diagnosis as a potential risk factor for post-ICU depressive symptoms, but no association was evident.[33] Three studies examined the relationship between ICU length of stay and post-ICU depressive symptoms, but none found a relationship.[33,34,37] Similarly, APACHE II scores at ICU admission did not predict later depressive symptoms in any of these three studies.[33,34,37] Also, in-ICU duration of sedation[33] and daily interruption of continuous sedation[47] were not associated with post-ICU depressive symptoms.

Critical illness/ICU correlates

Poor recall of the ICU at hospital discharge, but not memories of frightening experiences, predicted depressive symptoms at 6-month follow-up in one study.[34] However, in another study, memories of extremely stressful in-ICU nightmares or fearfulness 5 days post-ICU predicted depressive symptoms 2 months post-ICU.[32] Finally, memories of in-ICU psychotic/nightmare experiences were cross-sectionally associated with more depressive symptoms 14 days after ICU discharge in a third study.[33]

Post-ICU risk factors/correlates

Neuropsychiatric symptoms at hospital discharge and afterward were prospective predictors or cross-sectional correlates of post-ICU depressive symptoms in all of five studies.[32,34,37,42,45] Specifically, depressive symptoms at hospital discharge were a strong predictor of depressive symptoms at 6- and 12-month follow-ups in one study,[34] and depressive symptoms at 2-month follow-up were a strong predictor of depressive symptoms at 6-month follow-up in another study.[42] Post-ICU symptoms of PTSD were strongly correlated cross-sectionally with post-ICU depressive symptoms in the two studies that examined this issue.[32,37] Similarly, post-ICU non-specific anxiety symptoms were strongly correlated with post-ICU depressive symptoms in the one study that examined the issue.[42] Finally, cognitive impairment at 6-month follow-up was cross-sectionally associated with depressive symptoms in the one study that examined this issue.[45]

Two studies examined the relationship between post-ICU physical functioning and depressive symptoms.[37,42] In the first, improvement in physical functioning was associated with a concomitant improvement in depressive symptoms between 2- and 6-month follow-up but not between hospital discharge and 2-month follow-up.[42] In the second study, an increased burden of physical symptoms was cross-sectionally associated with depressive symptoms at both 3- and 9-month follow-ups.[37]

More recent studies

Table 20.3 shows the risk factor and correlate information garnered from more recent studies of depressive symptoms and syndromes in critical illness/ICU survivors. Again, I summarize results in terms of pre-ICU (baseline) risk factors, critical illness/ICU risk factors/correlates, and post-ICU risk factors/correlates.

Pre-ICU risk factors

Demographic risk factors for depressive symptoms included female sex in two studies,[52,66] younger age in one study,[66] less education in two independent cohorts,[6,53,57] and baseline unemployment/disability in two studies.[6,53] Baseline general medical morbidity was a risk factor for depressive disorders/symptoms in two studies.[6,48] Baseline functional dependency was associated with later depressive disorders/symptoms in one study[48] but not another.[57] Baseline morbid obesity was a risk factor for depressive symptoms in one group of studies.[56,57] Dispositional pessimism, measured at 4- to 6-week follow-up, was associated with depressive symptoms in one set of studies.[53,54] Pre-ICU depression/anxiety, assessed retrospectively before hospital discharge, was associated with later depressive symptoms in one set of studies.[56,57] Prior psychiatric history was associated with depressive disorders in one study in which both factors were measured concurrently.[48] Finally, prior alcohol dependence was associated with later depressive symptoms in one study.[66]

Critical illness/ICU risk factors

Surgery or surgical ICU admission were associated with depressive symptoms in two studies.[54,57] In-ICU hypoglycaemia/low blood glucose was a risk factor for early depressive symptoms in one set of studies.[6,56,57] Maximum organ failure or slower organ recovery were associated with later depressive symptoms in two studies of ALI/ARDS survivors.[57,64] Finally, longer durations of MV and ICU stay were associated with more depressive symptoms in one study of ARDS survivors.[64]

Critical illness/ICU correlates

Patients who received high doses of benzodiazepines in the ICU had more depressive symptoms in one set of studies.[56,57] Patients who had less recall of the ICU, remembered more frightening experiences, and expressed less satisfaction with care had more depressive symptoms cross-sectionally at hospital discharge in one study.[51] Also, patients who recalled not being able to express their needs in the ICU had more depressive symptoms cross-sectionally in one study.[53] Patients who used adaptive coping measures infrequently had more depressive symptoms in one study. Interestingly, patients with depressive disorders in an LTAC hospital had longer durations of MV, a higher rate of weaning failure, and higher mortality.[48]

Post-ICU risk factors/correlates

Having earlier post-ICU depressive symptoms was a potent risk factor for later depressive symptoms in two studies.[64,66] Depressive symptoms were associated with not returning to work in two studies,[55,63] with worse sleep in one study[52] and with worse memory function in one set of studies.[63,64] Cognitive sequelae 1 year after ARDS was associated with depressive symptoms cross-sectionally and at later follow-up in one study.[66] Finally, depression at last follow-up was associated with later incidence of impaired physical functioning (decrements in IADL) in one study.[6]

Table 20.3 Identified risk factors for depressive symptoms/syndromes, with correlates/outcomes

Study first author	Identified risk factors	What was measured and when	Correlates
Jubran (2010)[48]	– More baseline functional dependency – More baseline medical morbidity – Previous psychiatric history	DSM-IV depressive disorders in patients being weaned from prolonged MV	– Higher rate of weaning failure – Longer duration of ventilation – Higher mortality
Rattray (2010)[51]		HADSd score at hospital d/c (continuous)	– More frightening experiences, less recall, and less satisfaction with care at hospital discharge
Cox (2012)[50]		HADSd score 6 w post-d/c (continuous)	– Infrequent use of adaptive coping
McKinley (2012)[52]	– Female sex	DASS-21d score in the 6 m after ICU (continuous)	– Worse sleep
Myhren (2009)[53]	– Less education – Baseline unemployment/disability – Dispositional pessimism – Inability to express needs in ICU	HADSd score at 4–6 w post-ICU (continuous)	
Myhren (2010)[54,55]	– Dispositional pessimism – Surgery	HADSd score at 12 m post-ICU (score ≥11)	– Not returning to work
Dowdy (2008)[56]	– Baseline BMI > 40 kg/m² – Pre-admission depression/anxiety – Hypoglycaemia in ICU – High-dose benzodiazepines in ICU	HADSd score 3 m post-ALI (continuous and/or score ≥8)	
Dowdy (2009)[57]	– ≤12 years of education – Baseline BMI > 40 kg/m² – Pre-admission depression/anxiety – Surgical ICU admission – Maximum daily SOFA score in ICU – High-dose benzodiazepines in ICU	HADSd score 6 m post-ALI (continuous and/or score ≥8)	
Bienvenu (2012)[6]	– ≤12 years of education – Baseline disability/unemployment – More baseline medical morbidity – Lower blood glucose in the ICU	HADSd score ≥8 3–24 m post-ALI in patients w/o baseline depression – Depression at last follow-up	– Later incident impaired physical functioning

Table 20.3 (continued) Identified risk factors for depressive symptoms/syndromes, with correlates/outcomes

Study first author	Identified risk factors	What was measured and when	Correlates
Hopkins (2010)[66]	– History of alcohol dependence – Female sex, younger age – BDI score ≥17 12 m post-d/c – Cognitive sequelae 12 m post-d/c	BDI score ≥17 12 m post-d/c; BDI score ≥17 24 m post-d/c	Cognitive sequelae 12 m post-d/c
Adhikari (2009)[63]		BDI-II score ≥20 ~22 m post-ALI	– Worse memory function – Not returning to work
Adhikari (2011)[64]	– Higher earlier BDI-II score (~22 m) – Slower organ function recovery in ICU – Longer duration of MV, ICU stay	BDI-II score at 60 m post-ARDS (continuous and/or score ≥20)	– Worse memory function

ALI, acute lung injury; BDI-II, Beck Depression Inventory II; DASS-21d, Depression, Anxiety, and Stress Scales 21 depression subscale; HADSd, Hospital Anxiety and Depression Scale depression subscale; h/o, history of; ICU, intensive care unit; m, months; MV, mechanical ventilation; QOL, quality of life; SOFA, sequential organ failure assessment; w, weeks; w/o, without.

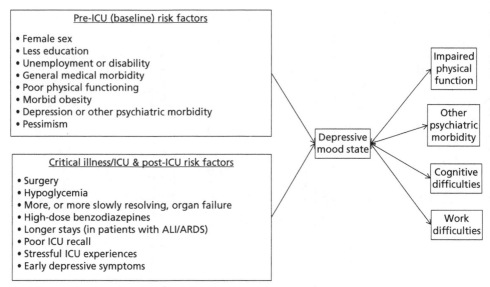

Fig. 20.1 Theoretical model of the aetiology and potential consequences of depressive mood states in critical illness survivors.

Conclusions

Figure 20.1 illustrates a theoretical model of the aetiology and consequences of depressive mood states in critical illness survivors. One-sided arrows indicate possible causal directionality, while two-sided arrows indicate more unclear causal directionality (i.e. correlates). Note that many potential risk factors for depressive symptoms and syndromes have apparently not been measured in studies of critical illness survivors, e.g. family/genetic risk for anxiety/depression, childhood family environmental disturbance, childhood sexual abuse, childhood parental loss, the broad personality trait neuroticism (proneness to negative emotions), low self-esteem, early anxiety or conduct disorder, lifetime traumas, poor social support, marital problems, and other stressful life events.[67–69]

Given this information, clinicians and researchers can attempt to reduce the suffering in their patients via prevention and early intervention. Both non-modifiable and modifiable risk factors are relevant. Specifically, the presence of non-modifiable risk factors like prior psychiatric illness should alert clinicians to provide ongoing monitoring and early psychiatric referral, as needed. Also, minimizing delirium and associated frightening experiences via more judicious use of sedative medications in the ICU may have a preventative effect. Finally, it is crucial that clinicians note early distress and refer, as needed, as early symptoms are strong predictors of prolonged suffering.

Association with quality of life

Depressive symptoms appear to have a substantial negative effect on HRQoL. In ALI/ARDS survivors, one group found that depressive symptoms, as measured with the BDI, were negatively correlated with both mental health and physical domains of the Medical Outcomes Study SF-36 instrument,[70] especially the mental health domains. Specifically, the correlations were: physical functioning = –0.29, role physical = –0.46, bodily pain = –0.56, general health = –0.59, vitality = –0.57, social functioning = –0.56, role emotional = –0.65, and mental health = –0.76.[21] Another group found a particularly strong correlation between CES-D depression symptoms and the SF-36 MCS score (r = –0.94); in that study, depressive symptoms were not significantly correlated with the SF-36 PCS score (r = –0.17).[22]

In general ICU survivors, one group found that incident depressive disorders (major depressive disorder or depressive disorder not otherwise specified) were associated with a lower SF-36 physical functioning domain score (T-score = 14 vs T-score = 43 in those without incident depressive disorder).[42] Another group found that the HADS depression subscale was negatively correlated with the EuroQoL Visual Analogue Scale[71] at 3 months (r = –0.63) and 9 months (r = –0.67); similarly, the HADS depression subscale was negatively correlated with SF-36 PCS and MCS scores (r = –0.44 and r = –0.48 at 3 months, and r = –0.44 and r = –0.62 at 9 months, respectively).[37] Finally, in a recent study, BDI-II depressive symptoms were negatively correlated with SF-36 mental health domains (Spearman coefficients between –0.50 and –0.82).[64]

Prevention and treatment

Though there are little hard data to guide prevention and treatment of depressive states after critical illness, there is a wealth of information regarding the treatment of depressive states generally,[72] and there is little reason, at present, to predict that this information would not generalize well to the treatment of critical illness survivors. However, it is worth reviewing some broad interventions that have been tried to improve recovery after critical illness.

An in-ICU psychological intervention

In a recent study of major trauma patients,[73] Peris and colleagues examined outcomes of patients treated before and after the institution of an in-ICU psychological intervention. The authors used the HADS to measure depressive symptoms 12 months after ICU discharge. They found a lower prevalence (threshold > 11 on the depression subscale) in the intervention cohort (6.5%) than in the pre-intervention cohort (13%), though the difference did not reach statistical significance. Interestingly, at 12-month follow-up, patients in the intervention cohort had a substantially lower point prevalence of psychiatric medication use than those in the pre-intervention cohort (8.1% vs 42%, respectively, P <0.0001).

ICU sedation strategies

Four randomized studies have examined the long-term psychological effects of alternate sedation strategies for critically ill patients. One motivation for these studies was to ensure that reducing benzodiazepines and other sedatives did not worsen psychiatric outcomes. First, as noted previously, Kress and colleagues[47] found that DIS was not associated with depressive symptoms at ≥6-month follow-up. Second, Treggiari and colleagues[49] found that patients randomized to light sedation had no more depressive symptoms at 4-week follow-up than patients randomized to deep sedation. Third, Jackson and colleagues[59] found that patients randomized to spontaneous awakening trials had no more depressive symptoms than those in the control group at 3- and 12-month follow-ups. Finally, Strøm and colleagues[62] found that patients treated with morphine-only sedation had no more depressive symptoms than those treated with propofol/midazolam infusions at 2-year follow-up.

Rehabilitation strategies

Jones and colleagues randomized critical illness survivors to receive or not receive a 6-week self-help rehabilitation manual, designed to aid physical and psychological recovery.[35] The authors found that patients in the intervention group tended to have a lower prevalence of HADS depression scores ≥11 (12%) at 8-week follow-up, compared to those in the control group (25%). Antidepressant medications appeared to boost the effect of the intervention.

Elliott and colleagues randomized critical illness survivors to an 8-week, home-based, individually tailored physical rehabilitation programme vs usual care,[74] hypothesizing that the intervention would affect both physical and psychological recovery. Unfortunately, there were no differences in depressive symptoms in the intervention and control groups.[52]

Nurse-led intensive care follow-up programmes

Cuthbertson and colleagues randomized critical illness survivors to a nurse-led intensive follow-up programme vs usual care.[60] Patients in the intervention group were introduced to a manual-based, self-directed, physical rehabilitation programme developed by physiotherapists that began in the hospital and continued for 3 months after discharge. These patients monitored their own adherence and progress with the manual-based treatments and were assessed at nurse-led clinics 3 and 9 months after discharge. If nurses were concerned about psychiatric problems or physical weakness, they referred patients to a mental health professional or physiotherapist, offered a visit to the ICU, if appropriate, and referred patients for review of their current drug treatment. The nurses also sent letters to each patient's GP regarding the patient's progress. Unfortunately, there were no differences in depressive symptoms in the intervention and control groups at 1-year follow-up.

Conclusion

Thus far, the most promising interventions for the prevention of, or early intervention in, depressive mood states are an in-ICU psychological intervention and a self-help rehabilitation manual, focused on both physical and psychological recovery. Though earlier studies showed that in-ICU high-dose benzodiazepines were associated with later depressive mood states, recent randomized trials have not shown a benefit of reduced benzodiazepine doses. As noted, however, this is a young field, with great opportunity for major advances.

Utilizing risk factor information could greatly enhance the benefit of interventions, targeting those patients at greatest risk for long-term depressive symptoms. Targeting patients with prior anxiety and depressive disorders, and those with early post-ICU distress, should maximize the benefit of early post-ICU antidepressant and psychotherapeutic interventions.

References

1 Herridge MS, Cheung AM, Tansey CM, et al. One-year outcomes in survivors of the acute respiratory distress syndrome. *N Engl J Med* 2003;**348**:683–93.

2 Herridge MS, Tansey CM, Matté A, et al. Functional disability 5 years after acute respiratory distress syndrome. *N Engl J Med* 2011;**364**:1293–304.

3 Needham DM, Davidson J, Cohen H, et al. Improving long-term outcomes after discharge from intensive care unit: report from a stakeholders' conference. *Crit Care Med* 2012;**40**:502–9.

4 Cheung AM, Tansey CM, Tomlinson G, et al. Two-year outcomes, health care use, and costs of survivors of acute respiratory distress syndrome. *Am J Respir Crit Care Med* 2006;**174**:538–44.

5 Unroe M, Kahn JM, Carson SS, et al. One-year trajectories of care and resource utilization for recipients of prolonged mechanical ventilation: a cohort study. *Ann Intern Med* 2010;**153**:167–75.

6 Bienvenu OJ, Colantuoni E, Mendez-Tellez PA, et al. Depressive symptoms and impaired physical function after acute lung injury: a 2-year longitudinal study. *Am J Respir Crit Care Med* 2012;**185**: 517–24.

7 Roshanaei-Moghaddam B, Katon WJ, Russo J. The longitudinal effects of depression on physical activity. *Gen Hosp Psychiatry* 2009;**31**:306–15.

8 Desai SD, Law TJ, Needham DM. Long-term complications of critical care. *Crit Care Med* 2011;**39**:371–9.

9 Katon W, Lin EHB, Kroenke K. The association of depression and anxiety with medical symptom burden in patients with chronic medical illness. *Gen Hosp Psychiatry* 2007;**29**:147–55.

10 DiMatteo MR, Lepper HS, Croghan TW. Depression is a risk factor for noncompliance with medical treatment: meta-analysis of the effects of anxiety and depression on patient adherence. *Arch Intern Med* 2000;**160**:2101–7.

11 Tsigos C, Chrousos GP. Hypothalamic-pituitary-adrenal axis, neuroendocrine factors and stress. *J Psychosom Res* 2002;**53**:865–71.

12 Oslin DW, Streim J, Katz IR, Edell WS, TenHave T. Change in disability follows inpatient treatment for late life depression. *J Am Geriatr Soc* 2000;**48**:357–62.

13 Callahan CM, Kroenke K, Counsell SR, et al. Treatment of depression improves physical functioning in older adults. *J Am Geriatr Soc* 2005;**53**:367–73.

14 Shorter E. *Before Prozac: the troubled history of mood disorders in psychiatry.* New York, NY: Oxford University Press; 2009.

15 Roth M. Unitary or binary nature of classification of depressive illness and its implications for the scope of manic depressive disorder. *J Affect Disord* 2001;**64**:1–18.

16 McHugh PR, Slavney PR. *The perspectives of psychiatry.* 2nd ed. Baltimore, MD: Johns Hopkins University Press; 1998.

17 McHugh PR. Striving for coherence: psychiatry's efforts over classification. *JAMA* 2005;**293**:2526–8.

18 Bienvenu OJ, Davydow DS, Kendler KS. Psychiatric 'diseases' versus behavioral disorders and degree of genetic influence. *Psychol Med* 2010;**41**:33–40.

19 Andrews G, Brugha T, Thase ME, Duffy FF, Rucci P, Slade T. Dimensionality and the category of major depressive episode. *Int J Methods Psychiatr Res* 2007;**16**(Suppl 1):541–51.

20 Davydow DS, Desai SV, Needham DM, Bienvenu OJ. Psychiatric morbidity in survivors of the acute respiratory distress syndrome: a systematic review. *Psychosom Med* 2008;**70**:512–19.

21 Hopkins RO, Weaver LK, Chan KJ, Orme JF, Jr. Quality of life, emotional, and cognitive function following acute respiratory distress syndrome. *J Int Neuropsychol Soc* 2004;**10**:1005–17.

22 Weinert CR, Gross CR, Kangas JR, Bury CL, Marinelli WA. Health-related quality of life after acute lung injury. *Am J Respir Crit Care Med* 1997;**156**:1120–8.

23 Hopkins RO, Weaver LK, Collingridge D, Parkinson RB, Chan KJ, Orme JF, Jr. Two-year cognitive, emotional, and quality-of-life outcomes in acute respiratory distress syndrome. *Am J Respir Crit Care Med* 2005;**171**:340–7.

24 Christie JD, Biester RC, Taichman DB, et al. Formation and validation of a telephone battery to assess cognitive function in acute respiratory distress syndrome survivors. *J Crit Care* 2006;**21**:125–32.

25 Beck AT. *Beck Depression Inventory: manual.* San Antonio, TX: Psychology Corporation; 1987.

26 Radloff LS. The CES-D scale: a self-report depression scale for research in the general population. *Appl Psychol Meas* 1977;**1**:385–401.

27 Zung WWK. A self-rating depression scale. *Arch Gen Psychiatry* 1965;**12**:63–70.

28 First MB, Spitzer RL, Gibbon M, Williams JBW. *Structured clinical interview for DSM-IV axis I disorders, clinician version (SCID-CV).* Washington, DC: American Psychiatric Press, Inc; 1996.

29 Kapfhammer HP, Rothenhausler HB, Krauseneck T, Stoll C, Schelling G. Posttraumatic stress disorder and health-related quality of life in long-term survivors of acute respiratory distress syndrome. *Am J Psychiatry* 2004;**161**:45–52.

30 Davydow DS, Gifford JM, Desai SV, Bienvenu OJ, Needham DM. Depression in general intensive care unit survivors: a systematic review. *Intensive Care Med* 2009;**35**:796–809.

31 Zigmond AS, Snaith RP. The Hospital Anxiety and Depression Scale. *Acta Psychiatr Scand* 1983;**67**:361–70.

32 Samuelson KAM, Lundberg D, Fridlund B. Stressful memories and psychological distress in adult mechanically ventilated intensive care patients: a 2-month follow-up study. *Acta Anaesthesiol Scand* 2007;**51**:671–8.

33 Jones C, Griffiths RD, Humphris G, Skirrow PM. Memory, delusions, and the development of acute posttraumatic stress disorder-related symptoms after intensive care. *Crit Care Med* 2001;**29**:573–80.

34 Rattray JE, Johnston M, Wildsmith JA. Predictors of emotional outcomes of intensive care. *Anaesthesia* 2005;**60**:1085–92.

35 Jones C, Skirrow P, Griffiths RD, et al. Rehabilitation after critical illness: a randomized, controlled trial. *Crit Care Med* 2003;**31**:2456–61.

36 Young E, Eddleston J, Ingleby S, et al. Returning home after intensive care: a comparison of symptoms of anxiety and depression in ICU and elective cardiac surgery patients and their relatives. *Intensive Care Med* 2005;**31**:86–91.

37 Sukantarat K, Greer S, Brett S, Williamson R. Physical and psychological sequelae of critical illness. *Br J Health Psychol* 2007;**12**:65–74.

38 Eddleston JM, White P, Guthrie E. Survival, morbidity, and quality of life after discharge from intensive care. *Crit Care Med* 2000;**28**:2293–9.

39 Scragg P, Jones A, Fauvel N. Psychological problems following ICU treatment. *Anaesthesia* 2001;**56**:9–14.

40 Boyle M, Murgo M, Adamson H, Gill J, Elliott D, Crawford M. The effect of chronic pain on health related quality of life amongst intensive care survivors. *Aust Crit Care* 2004;**17**:108–13.

41 Guentner K, Hoffman LA, Happ MB, et al. Preferences for mechanical ventilation among survivors of prolonged mechanical ventilation and tracheostomy. *Am J Crit Care* 2006;**15**:65–77.

42 Weinert C, Meller W. Epidemiology of depression and antidepressant therapy after acute respiratory failure. *Psychosomatics* 2006;**47**:399–407.

43 Chelluri L, Im KA, Belle SH, et al. Long-term mortality and quality of life after prolonged mechanical ventilation. *Crit Care Med* 2004;**32**:61–9.

44 Sheikh JL, Yesavage JA. Geriatric Depression Scale (GDS): Recent evidence and development of a shorter version. *Clin Gerontol* 1986;**5**:165–73.

45 Jackson JC, Hart RP, Gordon SM, et al. Six-month neuropsychological outcome of medical intensive care unit patients. *Crit Care Med* 2003;**31**:1226–34.

46 Beck AT, Steer RA, Brown GK. *Beck Depression Inventory: second edition manual.* San Antonio, TX: Psychological Corporation, Harcourt, Brace; 1980.

47 Kress JP, Gehlbach B, Lacy M, Pliskin N, Pohlman AS, Hall JB. The long-term psychological effects of daily sedative interruption on critically ill patients. *Am J Respir Crit Care Med* 2003;**168**:1457–61.

48 Jubran A, Lawm G, Kelly J, et al. Depressive disorders during weaning from prolonged mechanical ventilation. *Intensive Care Med* 2010;**36**:828–35.

49 Treggiari MM, Romand JA, Yanez ND, et al. Randomized trial of light versus deep sedation on mental health after critical illness. *Crit Care Med* 2009;**37**:2527–34.

50 Cox CE, Porter LS, Hough CL, et al. Development and preliminary evaluation of a telephone-based coping skills training intervention for survivors of acute lung injury and their informal caregivers. *Intensive Care Med* 2012;**38**:1289–97.

51 Rattray J, Crocker C, Jones M, Connaghan J. Patients' perceptions of and emotional outcome after intensive care: results from a multicentre study. *Nurs Crit Care* 2010;**15**:86–93.

52 McKinley S, Aitken LM, Alison JA, et al. Sleep and other factors associated with mental health and psychological distress after intensive care for critical illness. *Intensive Care Med* 2012;**38**:627–33.

53 Myhren H, Tøien K, Ekeberg O, Karlsson S, Sandvik L, Stokland O. Patients' memory and psychological distress after ICU stay compared with expectations of the relatives. *Intensive Care Med* 2009;**35**:2078–86.

54 Myhren H, Ekeberg O, Tøien K, Karlsson S, Stokland O. Posttraumatic stress, anxiety and depression symptoms in patients during the first year post intensive care unit discharge. *Crit Care* 2010;**14**:R14.

55 Myhren H, Ekeberg Ø, Stokland O. Health-related quality of life and return to work after critical illness in general intensive care unit patients: a 1-year follow-up study. *Crit Care Med* 2010;**38**:1554–61.

56 Dowdy DW, Dinglas V, Mendez-Tellez PA, et al. Intensive care unit hypoglycemia predicts depression during early recovery from acute lung injury. *Crit Care Med* 2008;**36**:2726–33.

57 Dowdy DW, Bienvenu OJ, Dinglas VD, et al. Are intensive care factors associated with depressive symptoms 6 months after acute lung injury? *Crit Care Med* 2009;**37**:1702–7.

58 Schandl AR, Brattström OR, Svensson-Raskh A, Hellgren EM, Falkenhav MD, Sackey PV. Screening and treatment of problems after intensive care: a descriptive study of multidisciplinary follow-up. *Intensive Crit Care Nurs* 2011;**27**:94–101.

59 Jackson JC, Girard TD, Gordon SM, et al. Long-term cognitive and psychological outcomes in the awakening and breathing controlled trial. *Am J Respir Crit Care Med* 2010;**182**:183–91.

60 Cuthbertson BH, Rattray J, Campbell MK, et al. The PRaCTICaL study of nurse led, intensive care follow-up programmes for improving long term outcomes from critical illness: a pragmatic randomised controlled trial. *BMJ* 2009;**339**:b3723.

61 Mikkelsen ME, Christie JD, Lanken PN, et al. The adult respiratory distress syndrome cognitive outcomes study: long-term neuropsychological function in survivors of acute lung injury. *Am J Respir Crit Care Med* 2012;**185**:1307–15.

62 Strøm T, Stylsvig M, Toft P. Long term psychological effects of a no sedation protocol in critically ill patients. *Crit Care* 2011;**15**:R293.

63 Adhikari NK, McAndrews MP, Tansey CM, et al. Self-reported symptoms of depression and memory dysfunction in survivors of ARDS. *Chest* 2009;**135**:678–87.

64 Adhikari NK, Tansey CM, McAndrews MP, et al. Self-reported depressive symptoms and memory complaints in survivors five years after ARDS. *Chest* 2011;**140**:1484–93.

65 Nelson BJ, Weinert CR, Bury CL, Marinelli WA, Gross CR. Intensive care unit drug use and subsequent quality of life in acute lung injury patients. *Crit Care Med* 2000;**28**:3626–30.

66 Hopkins RO, Key CW, Suchyta MR, Weaver LK, Orme JF, Jr. Risk factors for depression and anxiety in survivors of acute respiratory distress syndrome. *Gen Hosp Psychiatry* 2010;**32**:147–55.

67 Kendler KS, Gardner CO, Prescott CA. Toward a comprehensive developmental model for major depression in women. *Am J Psychiatry* 2002;**159**:1133–45.

68 Kendler KS, Gardner CO, Prescott CA. Toward a comprehensive developmental model for major depression in men. *Am J Psychiatry* 2006;**163**:115–24.

69 Kendler KS, Gardner CO. A longitudinal etiologic model for symptoms of anxiety and depression in women. *Psychol Med* 2011;**41**:2035–45.

70 Ware JE. *SF-36 health survey manual and interpretation guide*. Boston, MA: The Health Institute, New England Medical Center; 1993.

71 Nord E. EuroQol: health-related quality of life measurement. Valuations of health states by the general public in Norway. *Health Policy* 1991;**18**:25–36.

72 American Psychiatric Association. Practice guideline for the treatment of patients with major depressive disorder (revision). *Am J Psychiatry* 2000;**157**(4 Suppl):1–45.

73 Peris A, Bonizzoli M, Iozzelli D, et al. Early intra-intensive care unit psychological intervention promotes recovery from post traumatic stress disorders, anxiety and depression symptoms in critically ill patients. *Crit Care* 2011;**15**:R41.

74 Elliott D, McKinley S, Alison JA, Aitken LM, King MT. Study protocol: home-based physical rehabilitation for survivors of a critical illness. *Crit Care* 2006;**10**:R90.

Chapter 21

Post-Traumatic Stress Disorder Following Critical Illness

Christina Jones and Richard D. Griffiths

Introduction

What is post-traumatic stress disorder?

PTSD is classed as an anxiety disorder and can develop after a very frightening event, such as rape, warfare, or natural disasters such as earthquakes. The symptoms fall into three groups:

1 Avoidance—where the individual tries to avoid reminders of the traumatic event.

2 Re-experiencing—the individual re-experiences aspects of the traumatic event; this may be through recurrent nightmares or flashback where it feels as if the event is happening again.

3 Arousal—e.g. difficulties concentrating, exaggerated startle reflex, sleeplessness.

For acute PTSD, the symptoms have to have been present for 1 month following the traumatic event, and, for chronic PTSD, it is 3 months or more.[1] The final diagnostic category is that the symptoms should affect the individual's ability to function in some aspect of their everyday life. PTSD is a major challenge, as it is a key factor that compromises the ability of our patients to recover their well-being and return their lives to normal. The symptoms and the patients' reaction to them can affect every part of their lives and leave them isolated in their own homes; in addition, in an effort to cope with their distress, individuals can turn to self-medication in the form of alcohol and drugs.

There are a number of models to explain the development of PTSD, but all of them have at their core the assumption that PTSD symptoms are mainly caused by the unique characteristics of trauma memories and the difficulty of integrating them into other autographical memories. It has been suggested that the helplessness experienced during the traumatic event can lead to the changes seen in PTSD.[2] Ehlers and Clark's PTSD model[3] hypothesizes that it is the individuals' ability to cognitively process during the traumatic event that is involved in the development of chronic PTSD. Those who feel confused and overwhelmed during the traumatic situation are more likely to develop chronic PTSD. Key to understanding how PTSD develops in ICU is the appreciation that ICU patients' ability to process information may be disturbed by acute brain dysfunction as a consequence of the critical illness (with delirium and amnesia as a manifestation of this) and sleep deprivation, sedation, and opiates additionally contributing. The implication is that, due to acute brain dysfunction, ICU patients are unable to correctly process the meaning of the events happening to them.

PTSD following critical illness

It was not appreciated until fairly recently that patients who had suffered a critical illness necessitating a stay in an ICU could develop PTSD. In fact, one of the aims of sedation in critical illness

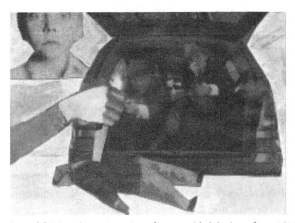

Fig. 21.1 Representation of frightening memories of paranoid delusions from ICU.[41]

Reproduced from *British Medical Journal*, Griffiths RD, Jones C, 'ABC of intensive care: Recovery from intensive care', 319, pp. 427–429, copyright 1999, with permission from BMJ Publishing Group Ltd.

was to ensure that patients would be amnesic for the experience and so, it was thought, not have frightening memories. This model of patient care was taken from the experience of surgical patients where being awake during surgery is a powerful precipitant of PTSD.[4] This, however, was not achieved with critically ill patients, as real memories for the illness were frequently replaced by very frightening and realistic delusional memories,[5] such as hallucinations, nightmares, and paranoid delusions of, for example, staff trying to kill them or being abducted by aliens[6] (see Figure 21.1). This was contrary to the established belief that it was the real, factual experiences of intensive care that were traumatic and why we observed that patients who sustain distressing delusional experience without any factual, real experience were at increased risk of developing acute stress reactions that can go onto develop PTSD. The key to this was realizing that the delusional experiences appear very real and frightening, while the absence of real experiences denies them the protective reassurance and feeling of safety provided by a contact with a health care professional. Procedures that we may think unpleasant and distressing may not be recalled or their impact may not be considered distressing, because they are associated with human contact, support, or comfort (e.g. endotracheal suctioning). It is important not to underestimate the feeling of safety a patient has to see a health care professional around them frequently. It is important to stress that particular delusional beliefs by patients that something happened may be very strongly held, even if they can be shown to be completely fictitious. In addition, many so-called real experiences can be misinterpreted. The experience of a psychotic episode in psychiatric illness, such as schizophrenia, can be a trigger for PTSD, especially when the individuals experienced a sense of helplessness and uncontrollability at the time or had frightening content of persecutory delusions.[7]

The lack of factual memories for the period of critical illness, including their admission to hospital prior to ICU admission, has a direct effect on the way patients think about the physical after-effects of their illness. As they have no real experience of their illness, they do not understand why they feel so weak and have pains on their joints.[8] In addition, the recall of delusional memories from the ICU period during convalescence can adversely affect the patients' QoL,[9,10] result in unexplained feelings of panic,[11] and be a powerful trigger for the development of PTSD.[3,12,13] Factors found to influence the recall of delusional memories fall into two categories:

first, patient factors such as a previous history of psychological problems;[9] and, second, care factors in the ICU such as depth of sedation,[9] with deeper, prolonged sedation increasing the risk of having such memories. A number of predictors of the development of PTSD have been shown, and a systematic review of general ICU studies found a number of consistent predictors, including a prior history of psychological problems, high doses of benzodiazepines during the ICU stay, and memories for frightening or psychotic experiences during the period of critical illness.[14] A separate review of studies with ARDS patients found that the consistent predictors for PTSD in this patient group were longer periods of MV, longer ICU stays, and sedation.[15] One of the earliest ARDS studies showed an association between the number of adverse memories, such as nightmares, anxiety, breathlessness, and pain recalled by patients after their ICU stay, and the development of PTSD.[16]

The incidence of PTSD following critical illness varies considerably among different studies, with reports varying between 8 and 51%[17] (see Table 21.1). This has been attributed to a number of possible factors; first, a significant number of the studies rely on the use of a screening tool for assessing PTSD-related symptoms and use a cut-off score to diagnose PTSD, which can overestimate the incidence; second, the case-mix or sedation practices of the study ICU may influence the

Table 21.1 Summary of PTSD studies in critical care patients

Study	Subgroup	n	PTSD
Schelling et al. (1998)[42]	ARDS	80	27.5%
Schelling et al. (1999)[43]	Septic shock	54	38%
Stoll et al. (1999)[44]	ARDS	52	25%
Nelson et al. (2000)[28,45]	ARDS	24	25%
Eddleston et al. (2000)[46]	–	227	36%
Shaw et al. (2001)[47]	ARDS	20	35%
Schnyder et al. (2001)[48]	Trauma	106	14%
Scragg et al. (2001)[49]	–	80	15%
Jones et al. (2001)[6]	–	126	51%
Kress et al. (2003)[50]	Sedation break	32	54% controls
Cuthbertson et al. (2004)[51]	–	78	5–15%
Kapfhammer et al. (2004)[52]	ARDS	80	43%
Capuzzo et al. (2005)[53]	-	84	5%
Rattray et al. (2005)[54]	–	109	20%
Deja et al. (2006)[55]	ARDS	129	29%
Jones et al. (2007)[13]	–	231	3–15%
Girard et al. (2007)[56]	–	43	14%
Davydow et al. (2009)[57]	Trauma	1906	25%
Myhren et al. (2010)[58]	–	194	27%
Jackson et al. (2011)[59]	Trauma	108	26%
Jones et al. (2012)[32]	–	352	13% controls

incidence;[9] and, finally, most studies do not examine when the traumatic memories precipitating the PTSD occurred. This may mean that patients with undiagnosed pre-existing psychiatric problems are included in the figures, and this may inflate the incidence by as much as 5%.[9] This can be quite easily ascertained by asking the patient how long they have had their PTSD symptoms or using a diagnostic tool such as the Post-traumatic Diagnostic Scale (PDS),[18] which makes an assessment of previous traumatic events and allows the recognition of pre-existing PTSD. The gold standard for making the diagnosis is a clinical interview using the DSM-IV criteria;[1] however, this requires funding for a clinical psychologist, and, in the clinical setting, this is not always feasible. The use of a screening tool, such as the PTSS-14,[19] to recognize the level of PTSD-related symptoms, coupled with a key question about how the symptoms are affecting the patients' everyday life and how long they have been present, gives enough information for an appropriate referral for therapy. Another alternative is the IES-R.[20] The original IES, developed by Horowitz et al. in 1979,[21] is the most widely used of all the PTSD measures and had good psychometric properties. It has been used with ICU patients.[6] The revision was to take account of symptoms of hyperarousal, and more information is still needed on its reliability and validity. However, the tool has the advantage of being short and easily understood by patients. This makes it an excellent screening tool as an adjunct to a more detailed diagnostic interview.[22]

Relatives of ICU patients can also develop PTSD, and this may mean that family therapy is necessary.[23,24] Patients and their relatives can both suffer from PTSD at the same time,[13] and this can mean that they are not able to support each other and can lead to family and marital breakdown.[25] Where the patients' delusional memories revolve around a member of their family being harmed in some way, then this can similarly precipitate relationship problems. One of our patients remembered seeing during her critical illness her teenage daughter being sexually abused, and, in her delusion, the ICU staff had stopped her from intervening by giving her sedation. This was remembered as such a real experience that she became panic-stricken on the general ward afterwards and could not sleep. It took some time for her to trust one of the authors (CJ) enough to be able to tell her what she remembered. She required therapy for PTSD, and, for some time, her relationship with her daughter was affected as she tried to stop her from leaving her side once she was discharged home. Factors shown to be associated with high levels of PTSD-related symptoms in relatives are patients admitted following trauma, high levels of anxiety during the ICU stay, where insurance is the mode of payment for the illness period,[26] and in family members who felt information given in ICU was incomplete, who shared in decision making, and where the patient died in ICU, those who shared in end-of-life decisions.[24] An association has also been shown between high levels of PTSD-related symptoms in the patient and high scores in their relatives.[23]

Long-term impact of PTSD

Long-term follow-up studies of other patient groups, such as traffic accident victims, have shown that PTSD is associated with problems returning to work and impairments in social interaction and leisure activities.[27] In addition, PTSD has been shown to be associated with elevated rates of medically unexplained physical symptoms and high levels of health care use, with significant implications for health care cost in women.[28] A recent very large study of returning military personnel who have sustained mild TBI highlights that danger of attributing disturbed health and functional problems to purely the organic injury.[29] While the TBI appeared to predict the wide range of health problems, it was no longer a significant factor once PTSD and depression were considered. Indeed, associated PTSD was the primary cause of their myriad of neurological and physical health problems. It is an important lesson not

Box 21.1 Case study

A clinical example of established PTSD in a post-ICU patient who was referred to one of the authors (CJ) for therapy to allow him to have surgery on his knee. He was too frightened to go into hospital to have the surgery. He had been admitted to a neighbouring ICU 12 years previously, following a road traffic accident, and had developed a fat embolus, resulting in prolonged ventilation. During those 12 years, he had not worked (he had been a trained engineer), could not allow his wife to work, as this would require him being left at home on his own, and he was fearful of being taken ill while he was alone. He had also developed chronic pain and was abusing alcohol and cocaine. After 18 months of weekly PTSD therapy, he had stopped drinking and taking drugs and retrained as an alcohol worker, successfully getting a job doing this. His wife had been able to train as a teaching assistant and also was in work. They paid off the debts they had built up over 12 years of being on social security benefits and were able to take their first family holiday since he had been ill. He felt that he had finally got his life back and decided to postpone his knee surgery until he physically could not cope any more. Four years after his therapy finished, he is still working and does not feel that his surgery is needed yet.

to attribute physical disease to acute brain injury without regard to the coexisting functional psychological processes.

Patients need information about the possibility of developing PTSD and other psychological problems. Recently, one of the authors was contacted by e-mail from a patient based in the US who had been in ICU with bronchiolitis obliterans organizing pneumonia and ARDS. After some years of not understanding why she was suffering from recurrent nightmares, anxiety, and panic attacks, she had found a presentation on the internet, given by one of the authors, about delusional memories in ICU, physical restraint, and PTSD and felt it put into words just how she felt. Since this, she has seen a psychologist and started on treatment as well as contributing to the ARDS forum to help other patients early in their recovery to come to terms with their illness experience.

PTSD has a massive effect on the patients' and their relatives' lives and can result in financial hardship, relationship breakdown, alcohol and drug abuse,[30] chronic pain, unexplained medical problems, poor HRQoL,[14] and premature death[19] Rehabilitation from critical illness requires the patient to be able to engage in exercise and eat well to rebuild muscle; the presence of PTSD endangers this recovery and therefore needs to be addressed as a priority early in their recovery. Once established, chronic PTSD is more resistant to treatment and may require different treatment modalities and psychosocial rehabilitation.[31] It is therefore important to prevent this complication of a critical illness (see Box 21.1 for patient case study).

Preventing the development of PTSD and treatment

The patient story (see Box 21.1) about the impact of chronic PTSD shows that reducing the risk of patients developing this debilitating syndrome and offering early therapy where acute symptoms are not settling is very important to allow patients to return to as normal a life as possible after critical illness. Simple changes in care while the patient is in ICU may have a significant impact on their experience, e.g. changes in sedation practice to keep the patient more awake, but still comfortable, or the recognition and treatment of any periods of delirium may impact on what the patient remembers afterwards, and so reduce their risk of developing PTSD.[32] After the patient is discharged to the general ward, they should be given information about how common delusional memories are and their ICU experience normalized. Keeping an ICU diary that gives a daily account in everyday language, also coupled with photographs, can give them information about what happened while they were in ICU. The family are invited to contribute to these diaries and not only write about what is happening in the hospital, but also how they feel and what is happening at home, which the patient will also not know. A recent study has looked at the impact of such ICU diaries on the incidence of new-onset PTSD following critical illness. This study showed that the rate of PTSD could be more than halved by the simple provision of a diary, from 13% in the controls to 5% in the intervention patients.[33] In addition, a proportion of the families were asked to take part in this study, and the results suggested that, where the patient received a diary, the family members' symptoms of PTSD were also reduced.[34] A recently published study supports both these findings in patients and their families.[35] In addition to the impact on PTSD, the provision of an ICU diary has also been shown to reduce the patients' anxiety and depression.[36]

Early psychological distress in the first month following critical illness may resolve spontaneously without any therapy. But very high early levels of anxiety, depression, or PTSD symptoms may require some help to resolve. The key to appropriate intervention is being able to recognize those patients and/or families who are not coping with their symptoms and then offering them help without interfering unnecessarily.[37] Counselling services following critical illness can be needed for severe anxiety, depression, and PTSD and has been shown to be effective in helping both patients and their relatives to get back to their normal functioning.[38] Specific therapies, such as cognitive behavioural therapy (CBT) and eye movement desensitization and reprocessing (EMDR), have been demonstrated to be effective. CBT uses a goal-oriented, systematic procedure which is designed to change the individuals' feelings and thoughts about their present psychological problems.[39] EMDR was developed initially to reduce the distress individuals feel, following events such as rape.[40] When a traumatic experience occurs, the individuals' normal coping mechanisms may be overwhelmed and the memories of the experience are inadequately processed. EMDR has, as its goal, the processing of these distressing memories, allowing individuals to develop more adaptive coping mechanisms. For ICU patients, EMDR can be used to help them process their delusional memories and so reduce the intensity of distress that they feel when these memories are re-experienced through recurrent nightmares or flashback. Reducing the patients' distress at these memories allows them to reduce their avoidance behaviours, such as not attending outpatient appointments or not talking about their experiences, which they use to avoid being triggered into flashbacks. It is the avoidance behaviours which can make PTSD difficult to recognize, particularly when it is chronic, as patients will say they are fine, rather than becoming triggered by revealing their frightening experiences. This may explain why some ICU clinicians are convinced that their patients do not suffer from PTSD!

Conclusion

PTSD is a debilitating and severe disorder, the incidence of which can be reduced in both ICU patients and their families with appropriate measures. Where it does develop, despite our best efforts, there are now good and effective therapies that can help them to recover and return to a normal life. As clinicians, we have a responsibility to our patients to ensure that this happens, because we have the information about their experience that no one else has and the care we provide can both cause the problem and aid its recovery.

References

1 **American Psychiatric Association.** *The diagnostic and statistical manual of mental disorders.* 4th ed. Arlington, VA: American Psychiatric Publishing; 2000.

2 **Van der Volk B, Greenberg M, Boyd J, Krystal J.** Inescapable shock, neurotransmitters and addiction to trauma: towards a psychobiology of post traumatic stress. *Biol Psychiatry* 1985;**20**:314–25.

3 **Ehlers A, Clark DM.** A cognitive model of posttraumatic stress disorder. *Behav Res Ther* 2000;**38**: 319–45.

4 **Osterman JE, Hopper J, Heran WJ, van der Volk BA.** Awareness under anaesthesia and the development of posttraumatic stress disorder *Gen Hosp Psychiatry* 2001;**23**:198–204.

5 **Skirrow P.** Delusional memories of ITU. In: Griffiths RD, Jones C (eds.) *Intensive care aftercare.* Oxford: Butterworth-Heinemann; 2002. pp. 28–35.

6 **Jones C, Griffiths RD, Humphris GH, Skirrow PM.** Memory, delusions, and the development of acute posttraumatic stress disorder-related symptoms after intensive care. *Crit Care Med* 2001;**29**:573–80.

7 **Chisholm B, Freeman D, Cooke A.** Identifying potential predictors of traumatic reactions to psychotic episodes. *Br J Clin Psychol* 2006;**45**:545–59.

8 **Griffiths RD, Jones C, Macmillan RR.** Where is the harm in not knowing? Care after intensive care. *Clin Intensive Care* 1996;**7**:144–5.

9 **Granja C, Lopes A, Moreira S, et al.** Patients' recollections of experiences in the intensive care unit may affect their quality of life. *Crit Care* 2005;**9**:R96–109.

10 **Ringdal M, Plos K, Örtenwall P, Bergbom I.** Memories and health-related quality of life after intensive care: a follow-up study. *Crit Care Med* 2010;**38**:38–44.

11 **Ringdal M, Johansson L, Lundberg D, Bergbom I.** Delusional memories from the intensive care unit— experienced by patients with physical trauma. *Intensive Crit Care Nurs* 2006;**22**:346–54.

12 **Jones C, Skirrow P, Griffiths RD, et al.** Rehabilitation after critical illness: a randomized, controlled trial. *Crit Care Med* 2003;**31**:2456–61.

13 **Jones C, Backman C, Capuzzo M, Flaatten H, Rylander C, Griffiths RD.** Precipitants of post-traumatic stress disorder following intensive care: a hypothesis generating study of diversity in care. *Intensive Care Med* 2007;**33**:978–85.

14 **Davydow DS, Gifford JM, Desai SV, Needham DM, Bienvenu OJ.** Posttraumatic stress disorder in general intensive care unit survivors: a systematic review. *Gen Hosp Psychiatry* 2008;**30**:421–34.

15 **Davydow DS, Desai SV, Needham DM, Bienvenu OJ.** Psychiatric morbidity in survivors of the acute respiratory distress syndrome: a systematic review *Psychosom Med* 2008;**70**:512–19.

16 **Schelling G, Stoll C, Meier M, et al.** Health-related quality of life and posttraumatic stress disorder in survivors of adult respiratory distress syndrome. *Crit Care Med* 1998;**26**:651–9.

17 **Jubran A, Lawm G, Duffner LA, et al.** Post traumatic stress disorder after weaning from prolonged mechanical ventilation. *Intensive Care Med* 2010;**36**:2030–7.

18 **Foa EB, Cashman L, Jaycox L, Perry K.** The validation of a self-reported measure of posttraumatic stress disorder: the Posttraumatic Diagnostic Scale. *Psychological Assessment* 1997;**9**:445–51.

19 **Twigg E, Jones C, McDougall M, Griffiths RD, Humphris GH.** Use of a screening questionnaire for post-traumatic stress disorder (PTSD) on a sample of UK ICU patients. *Acta Anaesthesiol Scand* 2008;**52**:202–8.

20 **Weis DS, Marmar CR.** The impact of event scale—revised. In: Wilson JP, Keane TM (eds.). *Assessing psychological trauma and PTSD.* New York: Guildford Press; 1997. pp. 399–428.

21 **Horowitz M, Wilner N, Alvarez W.** Impact of events scale: a measure of subjective stress. *Psychosom Med* 1979;**41**:209–18.

22 **Keane TM, Weathers FW, Foa EB.** Diagnosis and assessment. In: Foa EB, Keane TM, Friedman MJ (eds.) *Effective treatments for PTSD. Practice guidelines from the International Society for Traumatic Stress.* London: The Guildford Press; 2000. pp. 18–36.

23 Jones C, Skirrow P, Griffiths RD, et al. Post traumatic stress disorder-related symptoms in relatives of patients following intensive care. *Intensive Care Med* 2004;**30**:456–60

24 Azoulay E, Pouchard F, Kentish-Barnes N, et al. Risk of post traumatic stress symptoms in family members of intensive care unit patients' families. *Am J Respir Crit Care Med* 2005;**163**:135–9.

25 Neis LA, Erbes CR, Polusny MA, Compton JS. Intimate relationships among returning soldiers: the mediating and moderating roles of negative emotionality, PTSD symptoms, and alcohol problems. *J Trauma Stress* 2010;**23**:564–72.

26 Pillai L, Aigalikar S, Vishwasrao SM, Husainy SM. Can we predict intensive care relatives at risk for posttraumatic stress disorder? *Indian J Crit Care Med* 2010;**14**:83–7.

27 Barth J, Kopfmann S, Nyberg E, Angenendt J, Frommberger U. Posttraumatic stress disorders and extent of psychosocial impairments five years after a traffic accident. *Psychosoc Med* 2005;**2**:Doc09.

28 Walker EA, Katon W, Russo J, Ciechanowski P, Newman E, Wagner AW. Health care costs associated with posttraumatic stress disorder symptoms in women. *Arch Gen Psychiatry* 2003;**60**:369–74.

29 Hoge CW, McGurk D, Thomas JL, et al. Mild traumatic brain injury in US soldiers returning from Iraq. *N Engl J Med* 2008;**358**:453–63.

30 Foa EB, Keane TM, Friedman MJ (eds.) Introduction. In: *Effective treatments for PTSD*. New York: The Guilford Press; 2000. p. 8.

31 Foa EB, Keane TM, Friedman MJ (eds.) *Effective treatments for PTSD*. New York: The Guilford Press; 2000. p. 5.

32 Kress JP, Gehlbach B, Lacy M, Pliskin N, Pohlman AS, Hall JB. The long-term psychological effects of daily sedative interruption on critically ill patients *Am J Respir Crit Care Med* 2003;**168**:1457–61.

33 Jones C, Bäckman C, Capuzzo M, et al.; RACHEL group. Intensive care diaries reduce new onset PTSD following critical illness: a randomised, controlled trial. *Crit Care* 2012;**14**:R168.

34 Jones C, Bäckman C, Griffiths RD. Intensive care diaries reduce PTSD-related symptom levels in relatives following critical illness: a pilot study *Am J Crit Care* 2012;**21**:172–6.

35 Garrouste-Orgeas M, Coquet I, Perier A, et al. Impact of an intensive care unit diary on psychological distress in patients and relatives *Crit Care Med* 2012;**40**:2033–40.

36 Knowles RE, Tarrier N. Evaluation of the effect of prospective patient diaries on emotional well-being in intensive care unit survivors: a randomized controlled trial *Crit Care Med* 2009;**37**:184–91.

37 Jones C, Griffiths RD. Patient and caregiver counselling after the intensive care unit: what are the needs and how should they be met? *Curr Opin Crit Care* 2007;**13**:503–7.

38 Jones C, Hall S, Jackson S. Benchmarking a nurse-led ICU counselling initiative. *Nurs Times* 2008;**104**:32–4.

39 Foa E, Rothbaum, B, Furr J. Augmenting exposure therapy with other CBT procedures. *Psychiatric Ann* 2011;**33**:47–56.

40 Shapiro F. *EMDR as an integrative psychotherapy approach: experts of diverse orientations explore the paradigm prism*. Washington, DC: American Psychological Association; 2002.

41 Griffiths RD, Jones C. ABC of intensive care: recovery from intensive care. *BMJ* 1999;**319**:427–9.

42 Schelling G, Stoll C, Haller M, et al. Health-related quality of life and post-traumatic stress disorder in survivors of adult respiratory distress syndrome. *Crit Care Med* 1998;**25**:651–9.

43 Schelling G, Stoll C, Kapfhammer HP, et al. The effect of stress doses of hydrocortisone during septic shock on posttraumatic stress disorder and health-related quality of life in survivors. *Crit Care Med* 1999;**27**:2678–83.

44 Stoll C, Kapfhammer HP, Rothenhäusler HB, et al. Sensitivity and specificity of a screening test to document traumatic experiences and to diagnose post-traumatic stress disorder in ARDS patients after intensive care treatment. *Intensive Care Med* 1999;**25**:697–704.

45 Nelson BJ, Weinert CR, Bury CL, Marinelli WA, Gross CR. Intensive care unit drug use and subsequent quality of life in acute lung injury patients. *Crit Care Med* 2000;**28**:3626–30.

46 **Eddleston JM, White P, Guthrie E.** Survival, morbidity, and quality of life after discharge from intensive care. *Crit Care Med* 2002;**28**:2293–9.

47 **Shaw RS, Harvey JE, Nelson KL, Gunary R, Kruk H, Steiner H.** Linguistic analysis to assess medically related posttraumatic stress symptoms. *Psychosomatics* 2001;**41**:35–40.

48 **Schnyder U, Moergeli H, Klaghofer R, Buddeberg C.** Incidence and prediction of posttraumatic stress disorder symptoms in severely injured accident victims incidence and prediction of posttraumatic stress disorder symptoms in severely injured accident victims. *Am J Psychiatry* 2001;**158**:594–9.

49 **Scragg P, Jones A, Fauvel N.** Psychological problems following ICU treatment. *Anaesthesia* 2001;**56**:9–14.

50 **Kress JP, Gehlbach B, Lacy M, Pliskin N, Pohlman AS, Hall JB.** The long-term psychological effects of daily sedative interruption on critically ill patients. *Am J Respir Crit Care Med* 2003;**168**:1457–61.

51 **Cuthbertson BH, Hull A, Strachan M, Scott J.** Post-traumatic stress disorder after critical illness requiring general intensive care. *Intensive Care Med* 2004;**30**:450–5.

52 **Kapfhammer HP, Rothenhäusler HB, Krauseneck T, Stoll C, Schelling G.** Posttraumatic stress disorder and health-related quality of life in long-term survivors of acute respiratory distress syndrome. *Am J Psychiatry* 2004;**161**:45–52.

53 **Capuzzo M, Valpondi V, Cingolani E, et al.** Post-traumatic stress disorder-related symptoms after intensive care. *Minerva Anestesiol* 2005;**71**:167–79.

54 **Rattray JE, Johnston M, Wildsmith JA.** Predictors of emotional outcomes of intensive care. *Anaesthesia* 2005;**60**:1085–92.

55 **Deja M, Denke C, Weber-Carstens S, et al.** Social support during intensive care unit stay might reduce the risk for the development of posttraumatic stress disorder and consequently improve health related quality of life in survivors of acute respiratory distress syndrome. *Crit Care* 2006;**10**:R157.

56 **Girard TD, Shintani AK, Jackson JC, et al.** Risk factors for post-traumatic stress disorder symptoms following critical illness requiring mechanical ventilation: a prospective cohort study. *Crit Care* 2007;**11**:R28.

57 **Davydow DS, Zatzick DF, Rivara FP, et al.** Predictors of posttraumatic stress disorder and return to usual major activity in traumatically injured intensive care survivors. *Gen Hosp Psychiatry* 2009;**31**:428–35.

58 **Myhren H, Ekeberg O, Tøien K, Karlsson S, Stokland O.** Post-traumatic stress, anxiety and depression symptoms in patients and relatives during the first year post intensive care discharge. *Crit Care* 2010;**14**:R14.

59 **Jackson JC, Archer KR, Bauer R, et al.** A prospective investigation of long-term cognitive impairment and psychological distress in moderately versus severely injured trauma intensive care unit survivors without intracranial hemorrhage. *J Trauma* 2011;**71**:860–6.

Chapter 22

Sleep Disorders and Recovery from Critical Illness

Scott Hoff and Nancy A. Collop

Introduction

The ICU is a chaotic environment, with limited opportunities for high-quality sleep. Relatively little is known about how components of the ICU environment, or critical illness, affect sleep or recovery from critical illness. The complexities involved in objectively assessing sleep in the ICU result from the layers of electrical, physiologic, and biochemical signals surrounding the critically ill and complicate the study of the relationships between sleep and aspects of critical illness. This chapter will attempt to describe some of what is known about the interactions between sleep and critical illness.

Sleep physiology

Sleep is a complex, dynamic, but organized, collection of cognitive and behavioural states that results in multifaceted restoration of body and mind (see Figure 22.1). Sleep is categorized into N sleep (non-rapid eye movement (NREM)) and R sleep (REM). More recent nomenclature subdivides N sleep into N1, N2, and N3. Stage N3 sleep was historically known as stage 3 and stage 4 sleep, delta sleep, or slow-wave sleep (SWS) and is thought to be the restorative stage of sleep. Stage R sleep is most commonly associated with story-plot dreaming and a highly active cognitive state. Respiratory and cardiovascular instability commonly characterizes R sleep, likely through centrally generated autonomic activity.

A sleep cycle comprises a stereotypic progression through the sleep stages. In adults, N1 sleep is generally a transition stage and normally occupies the smallest percentage of total sleep. Stage N2 usually occupies the greatest percentage of total sleep and is distinguished by characteristic architectural findings, namely K-complexes and sleep spindles. Stage N3 occupies a progressively smaller percentage of total sleep, as a person ages, and predominates in the first half of the sleep period. The electroencephalogram (EEG) of N3 sleep is characterized by 75 microvolt waves in the delta frequency (0.5–2 Hz). Stage R sleep follows a circadian pattern, with increasing duration of R stage, occurring as the sleep period proceeds, correlating with the normal decline in body temperature toward its nadir. Twenty per cent of the total sleep time (TST) is usually R sleep. An abrupt change in EEG pattern lasting for at least 3 seconds, termed an arousal, often interrupts the continuity of the EEG and can be a cause of excessive daytime sleepiness when it occurs with sufficient frequency. A sleep cycle typically evolves over approximately 90–110 minutes.

The wake-sleep cycle is normally regulated by a complex interaction between the endogenous **circadian rhythm** and a **homeostatic drive**. The circadian rhythm of the body is orchestrated

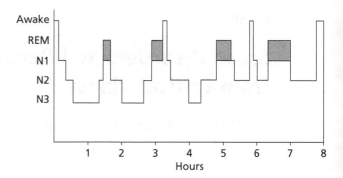

Fig. 22.1 The normal sleep hypnogram demonstrating the progression of sleep through different stages as the sleep period unfolds.

by the suprachiasmatic nucleus (SCN) found in the anterior hypothalamus. This regulatory clock has an intrinsic cycle of slightly greater than 24 hours. Direct input from the retina via the retinohypothalamic tract allows light to assume the predominant synchronizing role between the SCN and the external environment. The homeostatic drive for sleep is determined by an accumulation of adenosine and perhaps other substances during periods of progressive wakefulness.

There are several prominent physiologic systems that demonstrate circadian rhythms, and loss of those rhythms may have significant consequences on the recovery from illness. Prominent among these is the hypothalamic-pituitary-adrenal axis. The circadian pattern of cortisol secretion has been well documented. Melatonin, which is synthesized and secreted by the pineal gland, also follows a circadian pattern and has immunomodulatory properties.

Sleep in the ICU

Sleep in the ICU is a challenging process to objectively measure. Obtaining polysomnographic recordings in the ICU is hampered by the electrical signal interference generated by numerous other electronic devices in the environment such as mechanical ventilators, IV delivery pumps, and video monitors. Nurses have been noted to be inaccurate appraisers of a patient's sleep and provided overestimates of TST when their assessments were compared to polygraphic measures in post-operative ICU patients.[1]

There are conflicting data with regards to the total quantity of sleep patients attain in the ICU and the relative quality of that sleep. The sleep EEG in critically ill patients can demonstrate a wide variety of patterns, ranging from one with usual architectural features to one blending features of wakefulness and sleep, rendering the classification impossible by conventional definitions.[2] Non-septic patients may demonstrate a predominance of stage 1 sleep with decreased amounts of stage 2, stage 3, and REM sleep, whereas septic patients can demonstrate EEG features of encephalopathy without distinguishable sleep and wake periods.[3] Post-operative patients in the ICU were found to be sleep-deprived, with reduced SWS and REM sleep.[1] TST over a 24-hour period may be as long as 8.3 hours but occurs in periods as short as 15 minutes and with up to 54% of sleep occurring during the day.[3–7] It is not known whether these abnormal patterns of sleep described in critically ill patients fulfil the same functions as the usual nocturnal, consolidated pattern of sleep in normal subjects.

Effects of the ICU environment on sleep

See Box 22.1.

Box 22.1 Factors that might lead to improved sleep in the ICU

- Maximize patient-ventilator synchrony for intubated patients
- Minimize sedation
- Reduce noise
- Adjust lighting to match circadian rhythm
- Reduce nocturnal disruptions from patient care activities
- Heightened awareness of potential withdrawal from outpatient medications

---

Noise

The ICU is an environment with ubiquitous noise generated by a variety of sources. The Environmental Protection Agency published recommendations in 1974, specifying that noise levels in hospitals should not exceed 45 dB during the day and 35 dB at night. Studies that continuously monitored ICU noise demonstrated peak noise levels, ranging from 66 to 86 dB, with 150–200 sound peaks in excess of 80 dB occurring between the hours of midnight and 6 a.m. Peak noise levels and sound peak frequency were both found to decrease during night-time hours, compared with daytime levels.[3,5,8,9] The magnitude of the noise levels in the ICU may not be appreciated until one realizes that the decibel scale is a logarithmic one; hence, a perceived doubling of loudness represents a change of approximately 10 dB.

The relationship between noise and sleep disruption appears to be more complex than simply noise peaks triggering arousals and awakenings. Studies evaluating the association between arousals and awakenings and noise demonstrate that only 11–12% of abrupt increases in noise triggered arousals.[3,5] There may be a threshold change in sound level above the baseline that is required to elicit an arousal or awakening, such that a given sound peak may not result in an arousal, despite a high absolute decibel level, if it originates from a high baseline decibel level. Adding white noise to the ambient ICU noise diminishes the frequency of arousals elicited by the same frequency and intensity of noise peaks.[10] Also, patients may accommodate to noise so that greater changes in sound may become necessary to elicit arousals or awakenings.

Despite the intensity of ambient noise and the frequency and magnitude of noise peaks, noise does not seem to be a significant cause of sleep disruption perceived by patients. Measurements of vital signs and phlebotomy were reported by patients as the most disruptive factors to sleep, and noise was as disruptive as the mean of other factors surveyed. Of different categories of noise, staff conversations and telemetry alarms were perceived by patients as the most disruptive environmental noises.[5,11]

Patient-care activities

Patient-care activities, including administration of medications, ventilator changes, bathing, and hygiene activities, often occur during the night. Interruptions by ICU staff can occur more frequently than once per hour, preventing opportunity for consolidated sleep.[8] Despite the frequency of occurrences, these interruptions were not perceived as significant contributors to sleep disruption by ICU patients.[11]

Light

Light is essential in modulating circadian rhythms. Therefore, light in the ICU may be expected to play a role in sleep disruption. Exposure to light of even normal indoor intensity, approximately 180 lx, can significantly advance the endogenous component of the core body temperature cycle.[12] Furthermore, light as dim as 100–500 lx has been shown to reduce the secretion of melatonin and delay its onset.[12] Light intensities in various ICUs continue to demonstrate day-to-night variations, with increased mean maximal intensities during the day (2229–5090 lx) and lower intensities at night (190–1445 lx).[8] Consequently, sleep disruption may occur as a result of circadian alterations and suppression of melatonin secretion due to light exposure.

Effects of critical illness on sleep

Critical illnesses exert diverse effects on sleep. Consistent changes in sleep architecture, resulting from critical illness, consist of an increase in N sleep and a decrease in R sleep. These changes can be seen in healthy human volunteers inoculated with rhinovirus or low doses of endotoxin, or in patients in the early stages of HIV infection. The cytokines TNF-α and IL-1β increase as part of the acute phase response and possess both pyogenic and somnogenic properties. Disruptions of systems with a strong circadian component, including the body temperature cycle and the hypothalamic-pituitary-adrenal axis, may lead to disruption of sleep.

Effects on melatonin

Melatonin is a hormone produced by the pineal gland. The secretion of melatonin typically follows a circadian pattern of release, with peaks between 1 and 3 a.m. Melatonin has potential effects on sleep latency as well as on circadian periods. Recently, melatonin has been found to have immunomodulatory effects. Critical illness affects the secretion pattern and peak levels of melatonin, potentially disrupting maintenance of the circadian pattern of sleep. Septic patients lost the circadian pattern of 6-sulfatoxymelatonin excretion (a melatonin metabolite), had lower peak values relative to mean levels, and had a later peak when compared to non-septic patients and healthy controls. These abnormalities improved but persisted for several weeks after recovery from sepsis.[13] A study, using actigraphy to assess sleep, demonstrated that conscious patients in the ICU lost the nocturnal rise of 6-sulfatoxymelatonin excretion and had lower average peak levels of excretion, compared with patients from general medical wards.[6]

Melatonin, administered as a therapeutic agent to improve sleep in the ICU, potentially has beneficial effects. In a small trial of non-sedated patients on MV, melatonin (10 mg), given at 9 p.m., did not result in a statistically significant improvement in nocturnal sleep quantity, as measured using the bispectral index (BIS) sleep efficiency index, but did show a statistically significant lower bispectral index area under the curve, suggesting improved sleep quality.[14] In a small trial of patients with respiratory failure in a pulmonary ICU, the administration of melatonin (3 mg) led to increased TST and sleep consolidation when compared to stable patients with COPD on a general medical ward. The data for the patients receiving placebo were not presented.[15] Septic newborns treated with two doses of melatonin (10 mg), given 1 hour apart, demonstrated statistically significant improvements in white blood cell counts, absolute neutrophil counts, and markers of lipid peroxidation 24 hours after receiving melatonin when compared with controls.[16]

EEG changes

The spectrum of EEG findings in critically ill patients varies from discrete disturbances of sleep to patterns lacking any defining features of typical wake-sleep states. In 20 patients with technically interpretable EEGs, 12 patients did not manifest sleep, as conventionally defined,[2] whereas five of 22 patients in another study demonstrated EEGs which lacked features defining sleep.[3] Hardin et al. demonstrated an increase in delta sleep of nearly threefold in ICU patients randomized to either intermittent sedation, continuous sedation, or continuous sedation with neuromuscular blockade, but without a statistically significant difference between the groups. Although the doses of benzodiazepines and opiates were significantly lower in the intermittent sedation group, the small sample size may have precluded finding a correlation between drug dosage and the amount of time in any stage of sleep.[7] A minority of patients with sepsis who were not continuously sedated developed an EEG pattern, characterized by low-amplitude waves of varying frequency with interspersed bursts of theta and delta waves, a so-called 'septic encephalopathy'. This pattern often precedes the appearance of clinical manifestations of sepsis by up to 8 hours and occurs with the patient's eyes open or closed, rendering the wake-sleep state's discriminatory ability of the EEG lacking.[3] In 12 of 20 patients studied by Cooper et al., there was no sleep, according to conventional definitions, and there was no correlation between the presence of sepsis and the demonstration of the atypical EEG patterns. Many patients demonstrated a pattern the authors called pathologic wakefulness, in which manifestations of wakefulness, such as saccadic eye movements with increased EMG activity, were noted in the presence of delta frequency EEG activity.[2]

There does not appear to be a correlation between the severity of illness and sleep disruption that can be discerned, independent of the effects of sedation. In one study, TST or time spent in any particular stage of sleep, was not correlated with severity of illness scores in patients with EEGs scorable for sleep by conventional definitions.[3] In another study, the group demonstrating conventional hallmarks of sleep architecture had lower acute physiology scores and higher Glasgow Coma Scores (GCSs) than the combined groups lacking conventional architectural features of sleep. The combined atypical EEG and coma group received higher doses of benzodiazepines and opiates. The authors speculated that the EEG changes between groups may be drug-induced.[2] A third study demonstrated no correlation between TST, or time in any particular sleep stage, and APACHE II scores.[7] No correlation was noted between nocturnal sleep quantity, using BIS measures, and APACHE II scores in non-sedated and mechanically ventilated patients; however, the CI was wide.[14]

Effects of therapeutic interventions on sleep

Different therapeutic interventions can have a disruptive effect on sleep. These include sedatives, analgesics, vasopressors, and MV. Abrupt withdrawal of chronically prescribed medications can have dramatic effects on sleep, as can withdrawal from recreational drugs. In addition, changes in volume of distribution and hepatic or renal metabolism altering clearance of medications can lead to modulation of sleep. Multiple classes of agents, including opiates, selective serotonin reuptake inhibitors, vasopressors, benzodiazepines, and antipsychotics, have been demonstrated to affect sleep architecture, specifically to decrease the amount of R sleep. Also, abrupt discontinuation of these classes of agents can lead to rebound of R stage sleep, which can have significant cardiovascular, respiratory, and neurologic effects, especially in critically ill patients. This has not been well studied in critically ill patients but should be considered in the long list of potential 'sleep disruptors' when a patient enters the ICU. Other contributors to sleep disruption in the ICU include the pattern of sleep that the patient may have experienced prior to the ICU admission and the presence of sleep disorders in the premorbid condition.

Sedatives

Sedation is a vital component of many aspects of patient care in the ICU. The use of sedatives may facilitate initiation and subsequent tolerability of intubation and MV and invasive procedures, such as central line placement, and enhance patient comfort while relieving anxiety. A spectrum of sedatives may be employed in the ICU, with various effects on sleep. An unresolved issue is how the physiologic effects of sedation compare with those of naturally occurring sleep.

Benzodiazepines are commonly used agents in ICU practice. Benzodiazepines work via the GABA-type A receptors. Benzodiazepines tend to shorten sleep onset latency, increase TST, and increase spindle density (N2 sleep) while reducing N3 and R stages of sleep. At higher doses, they can cause diffuse slowing of the EEG, eventually leading to global cerebral dysfunction and death. Sedation with midazolam for MV led to overall slowing of the EEG, manifested by progressive loss of power in the beta frequency range (12.5–30 Hz), median frequency, and spectral edge (95th percentile of the total power spectrum), all of which correlated with increasing levels of sedation. Delta power (1–3.5 Hz) occupied the largest proportion of total power at all levels of sedation, indicating the central nervous system (CNS) slowing, even with mild sedation.[17] A population of mainly post-surgical patients sedated with isofluorane demonstrated a statistically significant higher percentage of time at the desired sedation levels and lower catecholamine levels during the 24-hour study period than those sedated with midazolam.[18]

One of the most significant potential consequences of benzodiazepine use is the increased risk of the development of delirium. Lorazepam, in daily doses greater than 1.8 mg, conferred an OR of over 3 of developing delirium in a univariate analysis.[19] In one study, 34% of patients who developed delirium in the ICU died during the 6-month follow-up, compared with 15% of those who did not develop delirium, and the overall length of hospital stay was a median of 10 days longer.[20] An increasing number of days with delirium progressively increased the HRs for 30-day all-cause mortality, duration of intubation, and length of ICU stay.[21]

Propofol is another commonly used ICU sedative and anaesthetic that acts as a type A GABA receptor agonist but likely acts at a different binding site than do the benzodiazepines. Propofol has been demonstrated in human studies to reduce N3 sleep but does not appear to affect R sleep or lead to an overall state of sleep deprivation.[22] There is evidence from studies in rats suggesting that sedation with propofol does not interfere with the restorative properties of sleep, and a study in human volunteers found that sleep latency increased after receiving a 1-hour continuous infusion of propofol 8 hours prior to habitual bedtime.[23]

In a study performed comparing the two classes of GABA-type A receptors agonists, midazolam and propofol produced similar levels of anxiety and depression in non-intubated, nocturnally sedated patients, and no statistically significant difference in patient-rated quality of sleep. Of note, 25% of the patients randomized to midazolam were excluded because of confusion, dysphoria, and restlessness experienced after receiving the medication.[24]

Dexmedetomidine is an α2-agonist with mixed anaesthetic and analgesic properties, the latter by virtue of receptors in the dorsal horn of the spinal cord. The analgesic properties, without significant respiratory depression, theoretically make this agent potentially valuable for use in critically ill patients. In contrast to benzodiazepines, dexmedetomidine increases N3 sleep and reduces NE release from the locus coeruleus.[23]

Sedation with dexmedetomidine produces similar mean spindle densities, amplitudes, and frequencies as physiologic sleep does, although spindle durations may be longer with dexmedetomidine.[25] Mechanically ventilated patients sedated with dexmedetomidine had an increased number of days free from delirium or coma when compared with those sedated with continuously infused lorazepam, and they spent increased time at the target level of sedation.[26] Another study demonstrated that patients randomized to dexmedetomidine spent statistically similar time at the target level of sedation as patients sedated with midazolam but were extubated in 3.7 days, compared with 5.6 days, and had a prevalence of delirium of 54%, compared with 77%, respectively.[27] A study in cardiac surgery patients demonstrated a reduced incidence of delirum when dexmedetomidine was used, compared with propofol or midazolam.[28] Despite the potential advantages, dexmedetomidine did not lead to patient-perceived improvement in communication, analgesia, anxiolysis, or sleeping and resting when compared with propofol.[29]

Sedation may be important for critically ill patients' comfort and safety, especially those requiring MV, but there can be unintended consequences. Continuous IV sedation is associated with longer durations of MV, longer ICU stays, and longer hospital stays.[30,31] The increased incidence of delirium, with its attendant morbidity and mortality, should be considered when one chooses a sedative class in the ICU.

Analgesics

Opiates exhibit several sleep architecture-changing properties. Opiates can precipitate central apnoeas, leading to fragmented sleep. A single, oral dose of morphine or methadone increased stage 2 sleep and decreased stages 3 and 4 sleep by 30–50% in healthy volunteers.[32] A very small study of surgical patients compared epidurally administered fentanyl with bupivacaine and demonstrated significant sleep disruption in both groups, with decreased slow-wave and REM sleep in the post-operative period. Between-groups comparison revealed a statistically significant decrease in the amount of SWS in patients receiving epidurally administered fentanyl, but not in REM sleep, despite equivalent pain scores.[33] There was suppression of R stage sleep for the 2–3 days following abdominal surgery, followed by a progressive increase in the amount of R stage sleep over post-operative days 4 and 5 to levels that exceeded those preoperatively. The amount of R stage sleep was found to be linearly and inversely related to the post-operative opiate dose. Associated with this rebound of R stage sleep are vivid and distressing dreams.[34] Given the previously mentioned increased cardiovascular instability during R stage sleep, one might wonder how an increased quantity of R stage sleep post-operatively might contribute to post-operative cardiac complications.

Vasopressors

NE is a neurotransmitter with high signalling activity in the locus coeruleus and is thought to act in a wake-promoting or activating fashion. Its role as a vasopressor and one of the main constituents of the adrenergic nervous system likely contributes to sleep disruption in critically ill patients.

MV

Many features associated with receiving MV might be expected to contribute to sleep disruption. Of the many discomforts reported by patients receiving MV, anxiety and fear were reported by 47%, not being able to talk by 46%, difficulties sleeping by 35%, and nightmares by 26%.[35] Sleep while receiving MV is highly fragmented, with a combined arousal and awakening index ranging from 22 to 79 events per hour and a sleep efficiency as low as 43%.[2,5,36,37] Choosing an adequate control group, with whom the effects of MV on sleep can be compared, is challenging, as there are many factors related to MV use that might confound the comparison such as sedation and the presence of an ETT.[38]

The effects of different modes of MV on sleep have received modest interest. PSV has a propensity to induce more sleep fragmentation related to central apnoeas than does assist control ventilation (ACV). The propensity for central apnoea is large when parameters are set during wakefulness to deliver the same tidal volume as ACV (8 mL/kg), especially in patients with HF.[36] However, when PSV is set to a lower tidal volume (6–8 mL/kg) and to limit excessive respiratory rates (<35), no apparent differences in sleep fragmentation occur.[37] A case report has described sleep fragmentation resulting from sudden changes in pressure support while using volume-assured PSV.[39] The range of respiratory frequencies to which an individual can entrain may be less during N sleep than wakefulness.[23] Setting excessive respiratory rates or tidal volumes may contribute to excessive ventilation and consequent central apnoea and sleep fragmentation.

Some of the contribution of MV to sleep disruption may be related to mismatching ventilator settings with patient mechanics, leading to decreased patient-ventilator synchrony. When PSV and proportional assist ventilation (PAV) parameters were set, based on measurements of individual patients' inspiratory efforts, there was no significant difference in TST but sleep quality was improved on PAV, as reflected by a lower arousal and awakening index and greater amounts of N3 and R sleep. Patient-ventilator asynchronies significantly correlated with the arousal index and inversely with the amount of R sleep. Therefore, synchrony between ventilator timing and breathing pattern, as well as balance between ventilator-delivered pressure and patient-generated pressure, affects sleep quality.[40,41] This evidence suggests that the mode of ventilation may be less important than efforts to maximize patient-ventilator synchrony.

Physiological effects of sleep deprivation

The effects of sleep deprivation on recovery from critical illness are not known. The literature is replete with studies investigating the effects of sleep deprivation on healthy volunteers, but data on patients with critical illness are lacking. In addition, there are at least three models of sleep deprivation, including total sleep deprivation (in which the subject has no sleep during the test period), partial sleep deprivation (in which the TST per night over consecutive nights is curtailed), and sleep stage deprivation (in which the subject has restriction of particular stages of sleep). Whether the effects of a particular model of sleep deprivation used in the methodology of a study are generalizable remains to be proven.

The validity of extrapolating physiologic observations from sleep-deprived, healthy volunteers to the critically ill has never been established. Changes in secretory patterns of endocrine organs in sleep-deprived healthy subjects are often opposite to what has been observed in the critically ill or reflect the loss of characteristic circadian patterns, especially with glucose metabolism and catecholamine release. Sleep deprivation does not appear to affect chemoreceptor responsiveness but may lead to reduced respiratory muscle endurance, spirometric indices, and upper airway tone; however, it is not known what effect these may have on liberation from MV. Modulation of various components of the immune system has been described to occur with sleep deprivation, but it is not clear what these alterations may mean for response to, and recovery from, critical illness. Healthy subjects with sleep deprivation frequently demonstrate symptoms shared by patients diagnosed with delirium and neurocognitive deficits.

Conclusion

There is consensus that critically ill patients in the ICU have a high likelihood of experiencing disturbances in sleep architecture, even if their TST is normal. Some of these changes are related to illness factors, while others are related to the ICU environment or associated treatments. While there are data on the physiologic effects of sleep deprivation in healthy subjects, it is not known how these data apply to critically ill patients. Until better methods are available to measure sleep in an environment burdened with electromagnetic signals and to control for the interacting biologic complexities inherent in the critically ill, it will remain difficult to characterize sleep in critically ill patients and to know what role sleep disruption may be playing in the severity of illness or from its recovery.

Many aspects of ICU care must evolve in order to improve sleep and its study in critically ill patients. The ICU culture must shift to emphasize opportunities for consolidated sleep and circadian rhythm preservation, rather than the work shift assignments of the ICU staff. Further investigation into the potential effects of pharmacologic agents, such as melatonin, on enhancing and regulating sleep and circadian rhythm in the ICU and modulating the underlying illness may augment the therapeutic arsenal. In addition, more firmly describing both the beneficial and deleterious profiles of commonly used pharmacologic agents, such as the different sedative classes, may clarify best practice options and drive further drug development. Developing methodologies to accurately define and monitor sleep in critically ill patients is essential in overcoming limitations from population heterogeneities and technological deficiencies. Further investigation of the roles that different modes of MV have on sleep disruption may lead to strategies that limit agitation and delirium and decrease the time a patient spends on the ventilator and in the ICU. As we gain further insight into the multifaceted interactions between sleep and critical illness, the concepts of sleep preservation and avoidance of sleep disruption may emerge as essential elements of ICU care.

References

1 Aurell J, Elmqvist D. Sleep in the surgical intensive care unit: continuous polygraphic recording of sleep in nine patients receiving postoperative care. *Br Med J* 1985;**290**:1029–32.

2 Cooper AB. Sleep in critically ill patients requiring mechanical ventilation. *Chest* 2000;**117**:809–18.

3 Freedman NS, Gazendam J, Levan L, Pack AI, Schwab RJ. Abnormal sleep/wake cycles and the effect of environmental noise on sleep disruption in the intensive care unit. *Am J Respir Crit Care Med* 2001;**163**:451–7.

4 Friese RS, Diaz-Arrastia R, McBride D, Frankel H, Gentilello LM. Quantity and quality of sleep in the surgical intensive care unit: are our patients sleeping? *J Trauma* 2007;**63**:1210–14.

5 Gabor JY, Cooper AB, Crombach SA, et al. Contribution of the intensive care unit environment to sleep disruption in mechanically ventilated patients and healthy subjects. *Am J Respir Crit Care Med* 2003;**167**:708–15.

6 Shilo L, Dagan Y, Smorjik Y, et al. Patients in the intensive care unit suffer from severe lack of sleep associated with loss of normal melatonin secretion pattern. *Am J Med Sci* 1999;**317**:278–81.

7 Hardin KA, Seyal M, Stewart T, Bonekat HW. Sleep in critically ill chemically paralyzed patients requiring mechanical ventilation. *Chest* 2006;**129**:1468–77.

8 Meyer TJ, Eveloff SE, Bauer MS, Schwartz WA, Hill NS, Millman RP. Adverse environmental conditions in the respiratory and medical ICU settings. *Chest* 1994;**105**:1211–16.

9 Aaron JN, Carlisle CC, Carskadon MA, Meyer TJ, Hill NS, Millman RP. Environmental noise as a cause of sleep disruption in an intermediate respiratory care unit. *Sleep* 1996;**19**:707–10.

10 Stanchina ML, Abu-Hijleh M, Chaudhry BK, Carlisle CC, Millman RP. The influence of white noise on sleep in subjects exposed to ICU noise. *Sleep Med* 2005;**6**:423–8.

11 Freedman NS, Kotzer N, Schwab RJ. Patient perception of sleep quality and etiology of sleep disruption in the intensive care unit. *Am J Respir Crit Care Med* 1999;**159**:1155–62.

12 Boivin DB, Duffy JF, Kronauer RE, Czeisler CA. Dose-response relationships for resetting of human circadian clock by light. *Nature* 1996;**379**:540–2.

13 Mundigler G, Delle-Karth G, Koreny M, et al. Impaired circadian rhythm of melatonin secretion in sedated critically ill patients with severe sepsis. *Crit Care Med* 2002;**30**:536–40.

14 Bourne RS, Mills GH, Minelli C. Melatonin therapy to improve nocturnal sleep in critically ill patients: encouraging results from a small randomised controlled trial. *Crit Care* 2008;**12**:R52.

15 Shilo L, Dagan Y, Smorjik Y, et al. Effect of melatonin on sleep quality of COPD intensive care patients: a pilot study. *Chronobiol Int* 2000;**17**:71–6.

16 Gitto E, Karbownik M, Reiter RJ, et al. Effects of melatonin treatment in septic newborns. *Pediatr Res* 2001;**50**:756–60.

17 Veselis RA, Reinsel R, Marino P, Sommer S, Carlon GC. The effects of midazolam on the EEG during sedation of critically ill patients. *Anaesthesia* 1993;**48**:463–70.

18 Kong KL, Willatts SM, Prys-Roberts C, Harvey JT, Gorman S. Plasma catecholamine concentration during sedation in ventilated patients requiring intensive therapy. *Intensive Care Med* 1990;**16**:171–4.

19 Dubois MJ, Bergeron N, Dumont M, Dial S, Skrobik Y. Delirium in an intensive care unit: a study of risk factors. *Intensive Care Med* 2001;**27**:1297–304.

20 Ely EW, Shintani A, Truman B, et al. Delirium as a predictor of mortality in mechanically ventilated patients in the intensive care unit. *JAMA* 2004;**291**:1753–62.

21 Shehabi Y, Riker RR, Bokesch PM, et al. Delirium duration and mortality in lightly sedated, mechanically ventilated intensive care patients. *Crit Care Med* 2010;**38**:2311–18.

22 Weinhouse GL, Watson PL. Sedation and sleep disturbances in the ICU. *Anesthesiol Clin* 2011;**29**:675–85.

23 Weinhouse GL, Schwab RJ. Sleep in the critically ill patient. *Sleep* 2006;**29**:707–16.

24 Treggiari-Venzi, Borgeat A, Fuchs-Buder T, Gachoud JP, Suter PM. Overnight sedation with midazolam or propofol in the ICU: effects on sleep quality, anxiety and depression. *Intensive Care Med* 1996;**22**;1186–90.

25 Huupponen E, Maksimow A, Lapinlampi P, et al. Electroencephalogram spindle activity during dexmedetomidine sedation and physiological sleep. *Acta Anaesthesiol Scand* 2008;**52**:289–94.

26 Pandharipande PP, Pun BT, Herr DL, et al., Effect of sedation with dexmedetomidine vs lorazepam on acute brain dysfunction in mechanically ventilated patients: the MENDS randomized controlled trial. *JAMA* 2007;**298**:2644–53.

27 Riker RR, Shenabi Y, Bokesch PM, et al. Dexmedetomidine vs midazolam for sedation of critically ill patients: a randomized trial. *JAMA* 2009;**301**:489–99.

28 Maldonado JR, Wysong A, van der Starre PJ, Block T, Miller C, Reitz BA. Dexmedetomidine and the reduction of postoperative delirium after cardiac surgery. *Psychosomatics* 2009;**50**:206–17.

29 Corbett SM, Rebuck JA, Greene CM, et al. Dexmedetomidine does not improve patient satisfaction when compared with propofol during mechanical ventilation*. *Crit Care Med* 2005;**33**:940–5.

30 Kollef MH, Levy NT, Ahrens TS, Schaiff R, Prentice D, Sherman G. The use of continuous IV sedation is associated with prolongation of mechanical ventilation. *Chest* 1998;**114**:541–8.

31 Kress JP, Pohlman AS, O'Connor MF, Hall JB. Daily interruption of sedative infusions in critically ill patients undergoing mechanical ventilation. *N Engl J Med* 2000;**342**:1471–7.

32 Dimsdale JE, Norman D, DeJardin D, Wallace MS. The effect of opioids on sleep architecture. *J Clin Sleep Med* 2007;**3**:33–6.

33 Cronin AJ, Keifer JC, Davies MF, King TS, Bixler EO. Postoperative sleep disturbance: influences of opioids and pain in humans. *Sleep* 2001;**24**:39–44.

34 **Knill RL, Moote CA, Skinner MI, Rose EA.** Anesthesia with abdominal surgery leads to intense REM sleep during the first postoperative week. *Anesthesiology* 1990;**73**:52–61.

35 **Bergbom-Engberg I, Haljamae H.** Assessment of patients' experience of discomforts during respirator therapy. *Crit Care Med* 1989;**17**:1068–72.

36 **Parthasarathy S, Tobin MJ.** Effect of ventilator mode on sleep quality in critically ill patients. *Am J Respir Crit Care Med* 2002;**166**:1423–9.

37 **Cabello B, Thille AW, Drouot X, et al.** Sleep quality in mechanically ventilated patients: comparison of three ventilatory modes. *Crit Care Med* 2008;**36**:1749–55.

38 **Parthasarathy S, Tobin MJ.** Sleep in the intensive care unit. *Intensive Care Med* 2004;**30**:197–206.

39 **Carlucci A, Fanfulla F, Mancini M, Nava S.** Volume assured pressure support ventilation—induced arousals. *Sleep Med* 2012;**13**:767–8.

40 **Bosma K, Ferreyra G, Ambrogio C, et al.** Patient-ventilator interaction and sleep in mechanically ventilated patients: pressure support versus proportional assist ventilation. *Crit Care Med* 2007;**35**:1048–54.

41 **Fanfulla F, Delmastro M, Berardinelli A, Lupo ND, Nava S.** Effects of different ventilator settings on sleep and inspiratory effort in patients with neuromuscular disease. *Am J Respir Crit Care Med* 2005;**172**:619–24.

Part 4

Neuromuscular and Musculoskeletal Disorders Following Critical Illness

Chapter 23

Introduction: Neuromuscular and Musculoskeletal Disorders Following Critical Illness

Naeem A. Ali

It is estimated that 13–20 million people annually require life support in ICUs worldwide.[1] In the US alone, more than 750 000 people receive MV,[2,3] with some estimates suggesting that almost 300 000 require prolonged support annually.[4–6] The intensity of this experience has been shown to have measurable impact on those involved. ICU patients, families, and providers all appear to be affected by the experience.[7–9] For ICU survivors specifically, multiple studies have demonstrated that this care and the diseases that necessitate life support have long-lasting effects on various aspects of their recovery. Depressive and other psychiatric symptoms,[7,10,11] cognitive impairment,[12–14] and decrements in physical function[15–17] have all been observed and may ultimately influence morbidity and mortality.[18] Recent stakeholder discussions have recommended that this array of problems for both patients and their caregivers should be characterized as the post-ICU syndrome (PICS).[19]

While PICS includes concerns with cognitive, mental, and physical recovery, effects on the physical function of recovering patients appears to be particularly prevalent.[17,20–22] In studies using QoL surveys, deficits in reported physical domains appear to be more dramatically and persistently affected.[16,23] The reasons for this perception of physical deficit is unclear, but, in several surveys of survivors of acute illness, pain was a dominant symptom.[24,25] Pain could be the result of joint, muscle, or nerve injury during critical illness[15] and potentially lead to physical disability due to inhibited effort. Additionally, pain from physical wounds can also contribute to immobilization-induced muscle atrophy and further functional limitation. Despite the potential that physical deficits may be more pronounced, there is no doubt that there is a high burden of physical, cognitive, and emotional effects in survivors of the ICU. Given the wide range of physical deficits observed in ICU patients and how early in recovery they manifest,[26] physical deficits have the potential to impact clinical decision making for those providing care to these patients from the first days of MV.

Early clinical care ascertainment of physical debility can be difficult. Physical manifestations can be masked by treatments like sedatives or cognitive dysfunction associated with a patient's primary illness. However quickly after the presence of physical disability can impact clinical decisions. Ventilator liberation is known to take longer in patients with acquired weakness,[20,27,28] which could then influence decisions regarding how life support should be valued or administered. It is still unknown whether the duration of time on MV causes the weakness or weakness itself leads to slower liberation. Because the presence of peripheral muscle weakness is a clear marker of respiratory muscle weakness,[29] the likelihood that patients will exhibit rapid shallow breathing is clearly increased. Most studies define an increase in duration of MV of around 3–12 days after awakening[17,20,28] for patients with severe diffuse weakness. For this delay to be a **result** of the initial weakness, muscle strength recovery should occur during this time frame, which is inconsistent with most observations of ICUAW. However, accelerated recovery still remains a possibility, because we still have a significant amount to learn about the natural history of critical illness-associated weakness. In this way, it may be more satisfying to perceive that the duration of ventilation is a marker of the duration of immobilization and therefore muscle injury; however, this issue has not been clearly settled.

Unfortunately, after ventilator liberation, patients with acquired weakness have additional risks for morbidity. When patients with significant weakness are discharged from the ICU, there appears to be an increased risk of the need for ICU readmission, often for the use of recurrent MV.[20] The reasons for this are unclear, but weakness and aspiration could be a link. At least one report suggests that patients with ICUAW have an increase in the risk for nosocomial pneumonia.[30] Whether this need for ICU readmission is entirely driven by 'late' extubation failure or a new infection or respiratory problem is unknown, but awareness of these problems could feasibly inform treatment plans or the attendance of respiratory therapists.

Finally, for those patients ready to leave the hospital, the ability to perform ADLs at all or with sufficient endurance to remain independent must be recognized. While increasing attention has been paid to reasons for hospital readmission,[31] there is little known about the causes in patients recovering from critical illness. This is despite the fact that health care utilization and costs of care are clearly increased.[22] Physical disability could contribute to increased morbidity after hospitalization through an inability to deliver self-care or attend appointments, or through further disuse atrophy. Accordingly, the recognition of the problem of newly acquired physical disability is important at all phases of the recovery of critically ill patients.

While the need to recognize this illness is evident, many factors have made this difficult. First, the spectrum of physical disability after ICU care is broad. In fact, there is such a range of physical disability that no single term appears to encompass this spectrum.[19,32] Mild deconditioning, local peripheral neuropathies, or diffuse polyneuromyopathy can all occur, depending on the circumstances, and each can impact the nature of a patient's recovery. Perhaps the strongest evidence of the range and persistence of these physical abnormalities is the finding that survivors of ARDS, most of whom did not have clear ICUAW,[15] uniformly have lower physical function and 6-minute walk distances for at least 5 years after their illness.[16] It stands to reason that these symptoms would be even worse in those who incur physical deficits that are severe.

When these deficits manifest as profound weakness,[32] they certainly worsen the near-term patient outcome.[20] Multiple series estimate that approximately 25% of patients who require PMV develop global, profound, and persistent weakness.[17,20] In the US alone, more than 750 000 people receive MV,[2,3] with almost 300 000 requiring prolonged support.[4–6] Thus, more than 75 000 patients in the US, and almost one million worldwide, may develop the clinical syndrome of profound, global weakness acquired during critical illness, termed ICUAW.[17,32] While no definitive treatments have been tested to reverse this syndrome, many preventive approaches show promise.[33–37] Importantly, there are established patterns for the use of physical rehabilitation in the functional recovery of patients with physical diseases like acute cerebrovascular accidents[38,39] that could be applied to this vulnerable population. Before critical care practitioners can apply these interventions and take ownership of the long-term outcomes of our critically ill charges, a better understanding of the true scope of this problem, the assessments needed to determine the need for interventions, and the type of interventions needed is required. In subsequent chapters, we intend to outline these clinical problems to advance our understanding of this 'silent' clinical disorder.

References

1 Adhikari NK, Fowler RA, Bhagwanjee S, Rubenfeld GD. Critical care and the global burden of critical illness in adults. *Lancet* 2010;**376**:1339–46.

2 Kahn JM, Goss CH, Heagerty PJ, Kramer AA, O'Brien CR, Rubenfeld GD. Hospital volume and the outcomes of mechanical ventilation. *N Engl J Med* 2006;**355**:41–50.

3 Zilberberg MD, Luippold RS, Sulsky S, Shorr AF. Prolonged acute mechanical ventilation, hospital resource utilization, and mortality in the United States. *Crit Care Med* 2008;**36**:724–30.

4 Cox CE, Martinu T, Sathy SJ, et al. Expectations and outcomes of prolonged mechanical ventilation. *Crit Care Med* 2009;**37**:2888–94.

5 MacIntyre NR, Epstein SK, Carson S, Scheinhorn D, Christopher K, Muldoon S. Management of patients requiring prolonged mechanical ventilation: report of a NAMDRC consensus conference. *Chest* 2005;**128**:3937–54.

6 Frutos-Vivar F, Esteban A, Apezteguia C, et al. Outcome of mechanically ventilated patients who require a tracheostomy. *Crit Care Med* 2005;**33**:290–8.

7 Adhikari NK, Tansey CM, McAndrews MP, et al. Self-reported depressive symptoms and memory complaints in survivors five years after ARDS. *Chest* 2011;**140**:1484–93.

8 Azoulay E, Pochard F, Kentish-Barnes N, et al. Risk of post-traumatic stress symptoms in family members of intensive care unit patients. *Am J Respir Crit Care Med* 2005;**171**:987–94.

9 Ali NA, Hammersley J, Hoffmann SP, et al. Continuity of care in intensive care units: a cluster-randomized trial of intensivist staffing. *Am J Respir Crit Care Med* 2011;**184**:803–8.

10 Davydow DS, Desai SV, Needham DM, Bienvenu OJ. Psychiatric morbidity in survivors of the acute respiratory distress syndrome: a systematic review. *Psychosom Med* 2008;**70**:512–19.

11 Bienvenu OJ, Colantuoni E, Mendez-Tellez PA, et al. Depressive symptoms and impaired physical function after acute lung injury: a 2-year longitudinal study. *Am J Respir Crit Care Med* 2011;**185**: 517–24.

12 Jackson JC, Obremskey W, Bauer R, et al. Long-term cognitive, emotional, and functional outcomes in trauma intensive care unit survivors without intracranial hemorrhage. *J Trauma* 2007;**62**:80–8.

13 Jackson JC, Girard TD, Gordon SM, et al. Long-term cognitive and psychological outcomes in the awakening and breathing controlled trial. *Am J Respir Crit Care Med* 2010;**182**:183–91.

14 Iwashyna TJ, Ely EW, Smith DM, Langa KM. Long-term cognitive impairment and functional disability among survivors of severe sepsis. *JAMA* 2010;**304**:1787–94.

15 Angel MJ, Bril V, Shannon P, Herridge MS. Neuromuscular function in survivors of the acute respiratory distress syndrome. *Can J Neurol Sci* 2007;**34**:427–32.

16 Herridge MS, CM Tansey, A Matte, et al. Functional disability 5 years after acute respiratory distress syndrome. *N Engl J Med* 2011;**364**:1293–304.

17 De Jonghe B, Sharshar T, Lefaucheur JP, et al. Paresis acquired in the intensive care unit: a prospective multicenter study. *JAMA* 2002;**288**:2859–67.

18 Wunsch H, Guerra C, Barnato AE, Angus DC, Li G, Linde-Zwirble WT. Three-year outcomes for Medicare beneficiaries who survive intensive care. *JAMA* 2010;**303**:849–56.

19 Needham DM, Davidson J, Cohen H, et al. Improving long-term outcomes after discharge from intensive care unit: report from a stakeholders' conference. *Crit Care Med* 2011;**40**:502–9.

20 Ali NA, J O'Brien, SP Hoffmann, et al. Acquired weakness, handgrip strength and mortality in critically ill patients. *Am J Respir Crit Care Med* 2008;**178**:261–8.

21 Herridge MS, Cheung AM, Tansey CM, et al. One-year outcomes in survivors of the acute respiratory distress syndrome. *N Engl J Med* 2003;**348**:683–93.

22 Cheung AM, Tansey CM, Tomlinson G, et al., and for the Canadian Critical Care Trials Group. Two-year outcomes, health care use, and costs of survivors of acute respiratory distress syndrome. *Am J Respir Crit Care Med* 2006;**174**: 538–44.

23 Orwelius L, Nordlund A, Nordlund P, et al. Pre-existing disease: the most important factor for health related quality of life long-term after critical illness: a prospective, longitudinal, multicentre trial. *Crit Care* 2010;**14**:R67.

24 Desbiens NA, Mueller-Rizner N, Connors AF, Jr, Wenger NS, Lynn J. The symptom burden of seriously ill hospitalized patients. SUPPORT Investigators. Study to Understand Prognoses and Preferences for Outcome and Risks of Treatment. *J Pain Symptom Manage* 1999;**17**:248–55.

25 Johansen KL, Smith MW, Unruh ML, Siroka AM, O'Connor TZ, Palevsky PM. Predictors of health utility among 60-day survivors of acute kidney injury in the Veterans Affairs/National Institutes of Health Acute Renal Failure Trial Network Study. *Clin J Am Soc Nephrol* 2010;**5**:1366–72.

26 Khan J, Harrison TB, Rich MM, Moss M. Early development of critical illness myopathy and neuropathy in patients with severe sepsis. *Neurology* 2006;**67**:1421–5.

27 De Jonghe B, Bastuji-Garin S, Sharshar T, Outin H, Brochard L. DoesICU-acquired paresis lengthen weaning from mechanical ventilation? *Intensive Care Med* 2004;**30**:1117–21.

28 Garnacho-Montero J, Amaya-Villar R, Garcia-Garmendia JL, Madrazo-Osuna J, Ortiz-Leyba C. Effect of critical illness polyneuropathy on the withdrawal from mechanical ventilation and the length of stay in septic patients. *Crit Care Med* 2005;**33**:349–54.

29 De Jonghe B, Bastuji-Garin S, Durand M, et al. Respiratory weakness is associated with limb weakness and delayed weaning in critical illness. *Crit Care Med* 2007;**35**:2007–15.

30 Garnacho-Montero J, Madrazo-Osuna J, Garcia-Garmendia JL, et al. Critical illness polyneuropathy: risk factors and clinical consequences. A cohort study in septic patients. *Intensive Care Med* 2001;**27**:1288–96.

31 Epstein AM, AK Jha, EJ Orav.The relationship between hospital admission rates and rehospitalizations. *N Engl J Med* 2011;**365**:2287–95.

32 Stevens RD, Marshall SA, Cornblath DR, et al. A framework for diagnosing and classifying intensive care unit-acquired weakness. *Crit Care Med* 2009;**37**:S299–308.

33 Van den Berghe G, Schoonheydt K, Becx P, Bruyninckx F, Wouters PJ. Insulin therapy protects the central and peripheral nervous system of intensive care patients. *Neurology* 2005;**64**:1348–53.

34 Burtin C, Clerckx B, Robbeets C, et al. Early exercise in critically ill patients enhances short-term functional recovery. *Crit Care Med* 2009;**37**:2499–505.

35 Hermans G, A Wilmer, W Meersseman, et al. Impact of intensive insulin therapy on neuromuscular complications and ventilator dependency in the medical intensive care unit. *Am J Respir Crit Care Med* 2007;**175**:480–9.

36 Schweickert WD, Pohlman MC, Pohlman AS, et al. Early physical and occupational therapy in mechanically ventilated, critically ill patients: a randomised controlled trial. *Lancet* 2009;**373**:1874–82.

37 Routsi C, Gerovasili V, Vasileiadis I, et al. Electrical muscle stimulation prevents critical illness polyneuromyopathy: a randomized parallel intervention trial. *Crit Care* 2010;**14**:R74.

38 Khadilkar A, Phillips K, Jean N, Lamothe C, Milne S, Sarnecka J. Ottawa panel evidence-based clinical practice guidelines for post-stroke rehabilitation. *Top Stroke Rehabil* 2006;**13**:1–269.

39 Gordon NF, Gulanick M, Costa F, et al. Physical activity and exercise recommendations for stroke survivors: an American Heart Association scientific statement from the Council on Clinical Cardiology, Subcommittee on Exercise, Cardiac Rehabilitation, and Prevention; the Council on Cardiovascular Nursing; the Council on Nutrition, Physical Activity, and Metabolism; and the Stroke Council. *Circulation* 2004;**109**:2031–41.

Chapter 24

Long-Term Implications of ICU-Acquired Muscle Weakness

Nicola Latronico, Simone Piva, and Victoria McCredie

Introduction

Muscle wasting, the 'rapid loss of flesh' first described by Osler,[1] is a common observation in acutely ill patients. With the advent of intensive care medicine and the improvement in the standard of care and survival of critically ill patients around the world, muscle weakness and wasting are increasingly recognized as common and severe complications arising during the ICU stay.

This chapter will describe the incidence, risk factors, pathology, mechanisms, clinical presentation, and impact on long-term outcome of ICUAW.[2,3] Acute muscle weakness can be caused by pre-existing CNS or neuromuscular disorders. These conditions will not be discussed in this chapter, but differential diagnosis can be difficult in previously undiagnosed conditions causing acute respiratory failure and ICU admission.[4]

Definition

ICUAW is a generalized, diffuse muscle weakness that complicates the clinical course of patients who are in a critical condition. These patients are usually seen in the ICU where they have been admitted because of a variety of acute diseases. The term ICUAW refers to the presence and severity of muscle weakness and is a clinical diagnosis. Terms, such as CIP, CIM, combined neuropathy and myopathy, disuse or cachectic myopathy, refer to underlying pathology and need electrophysiological and muscle biopsy study to be defined.[5] Not all patients with ICUAW have CIP or CIM; conversely, not all patients with an electrophysiological diagnosis of neuropathy or a myopathy have ICUAW, although they are at increasing risk of developing it.[6]

Incidence and risk factors

The frequency of ICUAW is influenced by diagnostic criteria used, timing of evaluation, and mostly by the different patient populations considered. Estimates are difficult to generalize, because ICU admission and discharge policies vary greatly.[7] If manual muscle strength testing[2] or handgrip dynamometry[8] is used, a quarter of critically ill patients with PMV (>5–7 days) are diagnosed with ICUAW. Frequency is higher, 50[9]–100%, when the diagnosis is based on electrophysiological criteria or muscle biopsy findings, and selected populations of patients with sepsis, MOF, or protracted MV are considered.[9,10]

To better appreciate the impact of the patient population considered on ICUAW frequency, it would be instructive to look at the data from the University of Pittsburgh Medical Center; here, the frequency of ICU-acquired neuromuscular complications was 0.09% when the authors considered all admissions to the six ICUs of the University of Pittsburgh Medical Center over a 5-year period (39 patients with CIM out of 44 000 patients admitted),[11] and 7% when the patient population was limited to 100 critically ill patients undergoing liver transplantation in the same institution.[12] In a well-designed single-centre prospective study, 1.7% of critically ill paediatric patients developed generalized muscle weakness.[13]

Risk of ICUAW is increased among the most severely ill ICU patients[14,15] and in those with SIRS, sepsis, MOF, or PMV.[2,10,16–19] Risk is also increased in female sex.[2] Several drugs, including NMBAs, corticosteroids, catecholamines, and propofol, may injure the muscle and have been investigated as possible causes of ICUAW;[20] however, their pathogenetic role is difficult to separate from that of the ongoing critical illness, which may act as a priming factor (see Figure 24.1).[21] As a general rule, it should not be forgotten that the patients are critically ill, with catastrophic events on admission and multiple organ dysfunctions during the clinical course, rather than simply patients receiving drugs.[22]

Prolonged block of the neuromuscular transmission can be observed after protracted infusion of non-depolarizing NMBAs in patients with hepatic or renal insufficiency.[23] Muscle weakness commonly lasts few hours.[24] Cases of several days' duration are probably the consequence of CIP and CIM,[25] because many patients receiving an NMBA infusion have ongoing ARDS, SIRS, or MOF (see Figure 24.1).[21] In ARDS, high-dose 48-hour cisatracurium besylate, an NMBA, decreases mortality and increases ventilator-free and organ failure-free days, with apparently no increase in ICUAW.[26]

Chronic steroid administration has been long recognized as a cause of myopathy.[27] Acute myopathy after high-dose steroids is a rare event,[28] although it is well demonstrated in experimental rat models of high-dose steroids and muscle denervation. The direct evidence of an acute steroid myopathy in critically ill patients is lacking. As for NMBAs, critically ill patients receiving steroids also have infection, SIRS, or MOF, and it is therefore difficult to separate the relative contribution of concurrent events.[29] Endogenous corticosteroids, together with catecholamines, represent the primary end-product of the stress response, which characterizes the critical illness (see Figure 24.1).[21] Short-term treatment with high-dose steroids conveys no benefit and may prove harmful. Megadose methylprednisolone in spinal cord injury has uncertain benefit that does not outweigh the risks to the patient and the cost of the additional resources required to treat the complications.[30] High-dose corticosteroids in patients with septic shock are associated with a greater risk of secondary infections and renal and hepatic dysfunction and mortality.[31] Low-dose steroids have marginal benefit, if any, in septic shock patients[32] and are only recommended if blood pressure is poorly responsive to fluid resuscitation and vasopressor therapy.[33] Consensus exists for steroid treatment in patients previously receiving steroids for different medical disorders who develop septic shock. Steroids are not recommended to prevent or treat early ALI although may offer some benefits in within the first two weeks terms of gas exchange and haemodynamic stability in the treatment of established ALI.[34] Steroids, in conjunction with intensive insulin treatment and strict blood glucose control, might exert a protective effect on muscle, possibly because its beneficial anti-inflammatory effect is not counteracted by hyperglycaemia and insulin resistance.[35] In longitudinal studies in ARDS patients, steroids were the main determinant of impaired ability to exercise at 3 months, but their effect was lost at 6 months.[36] In summary, there is no firm evidence that steroids contribute significantly to acute myopathy and ICUAW during critical illness. In deciding whether or not to use steroids during the ICU stay, a balanced analysis of risks and benefits should be done.

Hyperglycaemia has been recognized as a risk factor for CIP since long term,[17] with an important potential impact in terms of prevention and treatment.

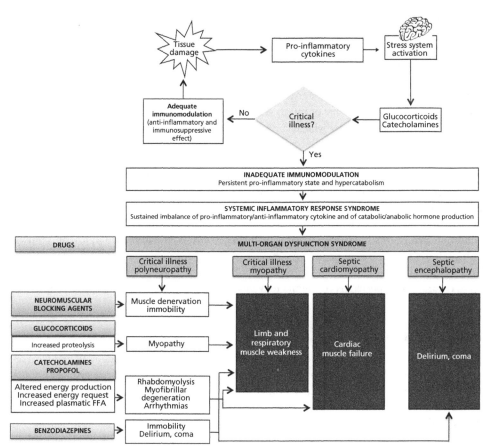

Fig. 24.1 Interplay between critical illness, the priming factor, and drugs, the triggering factors, in causing ICUAW. Pro-inflammatory cytokines produced at the site of tissue damage activate the stress system, causing glucocorticoid and catecholamine secretion. Stress response usually has an anti-inflammatory and immunosuppressive effect. If this is inadequate, the susceptibility to inflammatory diseases is enhanced. The persistent pro-inflammatory state with hypercatabolism causes progressive organ dysfunction, including cardiac and skeletal muscle dysfunction.

Reproduced from: Vasile B, Rasulo F, Candiani A, Latronico N., 'The pathophysiology of propofol infusion syndrome: a simple name for a complex syndrome', *Intensive Care Medicine*, 29, 9, 2003, pp. 1417–1425. With kind permission from Springer Science and Business Media and European Society of Intensive Care Medicine.

Benzodiazepines and narcotics are given to ensure comfort and to minimize pain and distress, but oversedation causes immobility and is associated with PMV and increased ICU length of stay.[37] Risk of ICU-acquired delirium can be increased with the use of benzodiazepines and with immobility (see Figure 24.1).[37]

Immobility is a powerful contributor to reduced muscle mass and strength in healthy people.[38] During critical illness, patients may lose half their muscle mass, resulting in severe physical disability.[39,40] The diaphragm is not spared from such process. The duration of MV, a proxy of diaphragm immobility, is associated with ICUAW;[2] moreover, impaired diaphragmatic function and increased fibre atrophy and injury occur within hours of the onset of controlled MV.[41]

Pathology

CIP and CIM alone, or in combination, are the major causes of ICUAW.[5] Immobilization and muscle wasting are also key events.

CIP is a distal axonal polyneuropathy, affecting both sensory and motor nerves. NCS show reduced amplitude of compound muscle action potentials (CMAPs) and sensory nerve action potentials (SNAPs), with normal or mildly reduced nerve conduction velocity.

CIM is a primary myopathy whose clinical features are the same as for CIP, with difficulty in weaning from the ventilator, flaccid limbs, and reduced deep tendon reflexes but, if testable, normal sensation. Major electrophysiological features are reduced CMAP amplitude with increased duration, normal SNAPs, reduced muscle excitability on direct stimulation, and myopathic motor unit potentials on needle EMG. On muscle biopsy, selective loss of myosin filaments, varying degrees of muscle fibre necrosis, and atrophy are common findings. Rhabdomyolysis is the rapid disintegration of skeletal muscle and may be caused by any condition that results in muscle damage. In rhabdomyolysis, electrophysiological and muscle biopsy findings are normal or near normal, consistent with a rapid and complete recovery.[5] In the ICU patient, rhabdomyolysis associated with cardiac failure, severe metabolic acidosis, renal failure, and hypertriglyceridaemia may be caused by prolonged IV infusion of high-dose propofol.[21]

Pathophysiology

The pathophysiology of ICUAW is complex and still incompletely understood. CIP and CIM are not isolated events but rather represent the failure of the neuromuscular system in the context of MOF, which is caused by inflammatory mediators that are produced during sepsis and SIRS.

Altered microcirculation is a key factor leading to ischaemic hypoxia of muscle, with a striking, though heterogeneous, reduction of perfused capillaries of striated muscles.[5] Calpain and ubiquitin proteasome-mediated myofibrillar protein breakdown is another key event, particularly during sepsis, leading to loss of myosin filaments, disorganization of sarcomeres, and muscle atrophy. This increased muscle protein breakdown (MPB) is potentiated by immobility. Immobility, as occurs in all patients with critical illness, alters skeletal muscle morphology, the proportion of slow- and fast-twitch muscle fibres, contractility, aerobic capacity, and muscle protein synthesis (MPS). All of these factors contribute, in turn, to decreased muscle strength, power, and fatigue resistance. Muscle mitochondrial function is also altered; this condition of cytopathic hypoxia leads to ATP and intracellular antioxidant depletion and increased nitric oxide production. Finally, muscle can be electrically inexcitable as a consequence of denervation and steroid administration. Some of these effects might be mediated by a myotoxic serum factor.[42]

Nerve microcirculation is probably impaired as a consequence of enhanced expression of E-selectin in the vascular endothelium of the peripheral nerves, with a consequent activation of leucocytes within the endoneurial space.[43] This then leads to local cytokine production with increased microvascular permeability, with the formation of endoneurial oedema. Hyperglycaemia and hypoalbuminaemia also impair the microcirculation and supply of nutrients to the peripheral nerves, leading to ischaemic hypoxia, energy depletion, and axonal degeneration. Nerve membrane depolarization, associated with endoneurial hyperkalaemia, hypoxia, or both, has been demonstrated in critically ill patients,[44] but it is unknown if it is secondary to nerve hypoxia or cytopathic hypoxia. In rats, a shift in the voltage dependence of sodium channel fast inactivation towards more negative potentials or a reduced density of functional sodium channels is the key mechanism, leading to nerve inexcitability.[45]

Clinical presentation and diagnosis

Metabolic and electrolyte disorders, including hyponatraemia, hypokalaemia, hypo- and hyper-magnesaemia, hypercalcaemia, and hypophosphataemia, may cause profound muscle weakness and paralysis and should be systematically investigated before CIP and CIM are considered. Likewise, the function of the cardiovascular, respiratory, hepatic, gastrointestinal, haematological, and renal systems, and nutritional status should be assessed before attention is directed to the consideration of neuromuscular problems.

In the acute stage, the typical presentation of ICUAW is that of generalized, symmetric, flaccid muscle weakness that affects the limb and respiratory muscles but spares the facial muscles.[5] Limb muscle weakness is diffuse, affecting both proximal and distal muscles, and can be associated with prominent muscle wasting. In patients with altered consciousness, painful stimulation to gauge the level of consciousness causes facial grimacing but reduced or absent movement of limbs.[5,10] Deep tendon reflexes are usually reduced or absent. Difficult weaning from the ventilator is a cardinal sign of ICUAW and is often the first sign noted;[5,16,46] indeed, ICUAW is an independent predictor of difficult weaning and PMV.[35,47,48]

In alert patients, limb muscle strength can be tested, using the MRC scale or dominant-hand dynamometry.[2,8] An MRC sum score, combining the individual scores of 12 muscle groups, yields an overall estimation of limb motor function. An MRC score of less than 48 or handgrip strength below sex-specific thresholds (males, <11 kg-force; females, <7 kg-force) are associated with prolongation of MV and length ICU stay, increased mortality, and reduced QoL in survivors of critical illness. Milder degrees of muscle weakness are probably overlooked.

Respiratory muscle strength can be tested by measurement of the maximal inspiratory and expiratory pressures and vital capacity. Low scores on these measures are correlated with limb muscle weakness[5] and are associated with delayed extubation, prolonged ventilation, and unplanned readmission to the ICU.[49] These scores depend much on the patient's alertness and cooperation, which can be compromised by concurred delirium, sedation, coma, or injury.[50]

Electrophysiological investigations of peripheral nerves, neuromuscular transmission and muscle, as well as muscle biopsy can usefully contribute to the diagnosis. Several algorithms for an ordered approach to bedside muscle strength testing, electrophysiological, and muscle biopsy investigations are available.[3,5,51]

Outcome

Physical impairments impeding ADLs are extremely common in the early post-ICU period and are only partly explained by reduced muscle strength. If patients are assessed in the first week after ICU discharge, the vast majority, particularly those with prolonged ICU stay, are dependent on others in basic life activities, cannot walk without assistance, and have reduced handgrip muscle strength but only mildly reduced limb muscle strength measured with the MRC scale.[52] Functional independence is improved by early ICU rehabilitation and OT, but still one-third of patients do not reach functional independence despite treatment.[53] MRC examination and handgrip strength are not significantly modified by early rehabilitation.[53] Poor swallowing control and impaired cough increase the risk of pulmonary aspiration of airway secretions, pulmonary atelectasis, and pneumonia that may cause acute respiratory failure and ICU readmission.[54]

Rebuilding muscle mass losses and regaining muscle strength and functional independence can take weeks, months, or years after discharge from the acute-care hospital.[55,56] One-third of patients may not recover to their condition before critical illness.[56] Physical impairments are an important contributor to PICS, which is defined as new or worsening impairments in physical, cognitive, or mental health status arising after critical illness and persisting beyond acute care hospitalization.[57] Functional independence in daily life activities at 1 month after ICU discharge remains an unmet target in a substantial proportion of ARDS survivors[58] who may also fail to return to their baseline health status at 1 year.[58] At this stage, muscle wasting and weakness are prominent features.[39] More than half of survivors of critical illness still complain of restricted walking activity, i.e. walking slowly or having problems with walking stairs, hills, and distances.[59] Improvement is commonly observed over time. In ARDS survivors, muscle wasting and weakness are no longer detected after 5 years.[36] Despite this, patients have persisting reduced ability to walk and exercise and a reduced physical QoL.[36] Younger patients may recover faster and better than older patients, but both may fail to return to normal predicted levels of physical function at 5 years.[36]

Peripheral nerve, muscle, joint, and bone alterations concur, often inextricably, to physical disability. CIP and CIM are relevant causes of prolonged disability in survivors of critical illness.[56] Mild physical disturbances include unsteady gait, reduced or absent deep tendon reflexes, stocking-and-glove sensory loss, muscle atrophy, painful hyperaesthesia, and foot drop. The latter is usually bilateral, as opposed to unilateral, foot drop, caused by peroneal nerve entrapment; however, persisting unilateral foot drop is also reported as a consequence of CIP.[56] In the most severe cases, the patient can be bedridden, with persistent tetraparesis or tetraplegia and ventilator dependency.[56] Neuropathic pain, possibly caused by small-fibre neuropathy,[60] can be disabling.[61]

Other musculoskeletal sequelae reported among ICU survivors include ulnar and peroneal nerve entrapment neuropathy, joint contractures, heterotopic ossification (HO), frozen shoulder, limb amputation, and increased risk of limb fractures in women.[36,39,62] These factors concur to reduced mobility and are an obstacle to effective rehabilitation.

Weakness is remarkably persistent,[63,64] even though the muscle strength and mass have returned to baseline.[36] Weakness can be psychogenic in nature or may overlap with fatigue.[65] Fatigue is described as an overwhelming sense of tiredness, lack of energy, and feeling of exhaustion and is associated with anxiety and depression, which are components of PICS. It is important to distinguish muscle weakness from fatigue, as the latter may recognize distinctive pathogenetic mechanisms and potential treatments.[66]

Variability of the rate of recovery in survivors of critical illness is a poorly defined issue. Patient characteristics, disease-specific patterns, underlying neuromuscular pathology, the presence of structured rehabilitation programmes, and methodological aspects of published research are possible explanations. Faster resolution of lung injury and organ dysfunction, younger age, and the absence of coexisting illness are associated with greater recovery of physical function in ARDS survivors.[36] However, patterns of recovery can be different in patients with other types of acute illnesses such as coma,[10] major trauma,[67] or cardiac surgery.[68]

The underlying pathology can be an important explanatory variable in patients with ICUAW: CIM has a better prognosis than CIP;[69] electrical muscle inexcitability and selective loss of myosin filaments have a better prognosis than muscle fibre necrosis.[5,45]

Early rehabilitation and OT started in the first ICU days[53] have only recently been investigated, and no evidence of long-term benefit exists as yet; however, coordinated rehabilitation applied to ICU patients after discharge from the acute care hospital may influence rates of recovery and long-term outcome.[70,71] The available evidence stems from studies of variable methodological quality, including small-sized retrospective cohort studies, cross-sectional studies, and case series, using different outcome measurement tools. The outcome itself is variously defined, encompassing muscle weakness, fatigue, and (dis)ability to perform specific physical tasks.

Treatment

Intensive insulin treatment is the only therapeutic strategy that has been demonstrated to reduce the incidence and duration of electrophysiologycally proven CIP.[72] Unfortunately, the optimum blood glucose target remains undetermined, because IIT, aiming at maintaining normoglycaemia, also increases mortality.[73,74] Supportive treatment with rehabilitation started in the early ICU days improves functional exercise capacity, quadriceps muscle force, perceived functional status[75] as well as short-term functional independence of patients; however, long-term effects are not established. EMS during ICU stay and rehabilitation after ICU discharge are promising, but yet unproved, methods to improve ICUAW.

Conclusion

Weakness of limb and respiratory muscles is a common complication in critically ill patients during their ICU stay. Bedside diagnosis can be achieved at an early stage in alert collaborative patients, while specific pathological diagnosis can be established, based on electrophysiological and muscle biopsy investigations whenever needed.

Control of ongoing risk factors and early rehabilitation are effective measures to improve patient functional independence at discharge from the acute care hospital, but long-term effects need to be evaluated.

Recovery of muscle strength and functional independence may take days, weeks, months, or even years after discharge from the acute care hospital for several, yet incompletely understood, reasons.

Recovery of muscle strength and functional independence can have different determinants, as some patients may achieve functional independence, in spite of persisting muscle weakness, indicating that patients learn how to adapt to persisting handicap. Finally, weakness, as it is perceived and suffered by patients, can differ from objective muscle weakness and can be associated with anxiety and depression, which are important components of PICS.

Prospective cohort studies of representative populations of critically ill patients, with comprehensive physical, cognitive, and mental assessment, during long-term follow-up are needed to clarify prognosis and to define relevant outcome measures.

The definition of proper outcomes in future studies should consider incorporating the patient perspective, because outcomes that are important for patients may be ignored by clinicians and researchers. The lesson comes from researchers assessing treatments for rheumatoid arthritis who showed that, for most patients, the dominant symptom of concern was fatigue; it was not pain, as researchers had assumed.[76]

References

1 **Osler W.** *The principles and practice of medicine.* New York: D Appleton; 1892.

2 **De Jonghe B, Sharshar T, Lefaucheur JP, et al.** Paresis acquired in the intensive care unit: a prospective multicenter study. *JAMA* 2002;**288**:2859–67.

3 **Stevens RD, Marshall SA, Cornblath DR, et al.** A framework for diagnosing and classifying intensive care unit-acquired weakness. *Crit Care Med* 2009;**37**(Suppl):299–308.

4 **Cabrera Serrano M, Rabinstein AA.** Causes and outcomes of acute neuromuscular respiratory failure. *Arch Neurol* 2010;**67**:1089–94.

5 **Latronico N, Bolton CF.** Critical illness polyneuropathy and myopathy: a major cause of muscle weakness and paralysis. *Lancet Neurol* 2011;**10**:931–41.

6 Latronico N, Shehu I, Guarneri B. Use of electrophysiologic testing. *Crit Care Med* 2009;**37**:S316–20.

7 Latronico N, Rasulo FA. Presentation and management of ICU myopathy and neuropathy. *Curr Opin Crit Care* 2010;**16**:123–7.

8 Ali NA, O'Brien JM, Jr, Hoffmann SP, et al. Acquired weakness, handgrip strength, and mortality in critically ill patients. *Am J Respir Crit Care Med* 2008;**178**:261–8.

9 Stevens RD, Dowdy DW, Michaels RK, Mendez-Tellez PA, Pronovost PJ, Needham DM. Neuromuscular dysfunction acquired in critical illness: a systematic review. *Intensive Care Med* 2007;**33**:1876–91.

10 Latronico N, Fenzi F, Recupero D, et al. Critical illness myopathy and neuropathy. *Lancet* 1996; **347**:1579–82.

11 Lacomis D, Petrella JT, Giuliani MJ. Causes of neuromuscular weakness in the intensive care unit: a study of ninety-two patients. *Muscle Nerve* 1998;**21**:610–17.

12 Campellone JV, Lacomis D, Kramer DJ, Van Cott AC, Giuliani MJ. Acute myopathy after liver transplantation. *Neurology* 1998;**50**:46–53.

13 Banwell BL, Mildner RJ, Hassall AC, Becker LE, Vajsar J, Shemie SD. Muscle weakness in critically ill children. *Neurology* 2003;**61**:1779–82.

14 de Letter MA, Schmitz PI, Visser LH, et al. Risk factors for the development of polyneuropathy and myopathy in critically ill patients. *Crit Care Med* 2001;**29**:2281–6.

15 Nanas S, Kritikos K, Angelopoulos E, et al. Predisposing factors for critical illness polyneuromyopathy in a multidisciplinary intensive care unit. *Acta Neurol Scand* 2008;**118**:175–81.

16 Zochodne DW, Bolton CF, Wells GA, et al. Critical illness polyneuropathy. A complication of sepsis and multiple organ failure. *Brain* 1987;**110**:819–41.

17 Witt NJ, Zochodne DW, Bolton CF, et al. Peripheral nerve function in sepsis and multiple organ failure. *Chest* 1991;**99**:176–84.

18 Bednarik J, Vondracek P, Dusek L, Moravcova E, Cundrle I. Risk factors for critical illness polyneuromyopathy. *J Neurol* 2005;**252**:343–51.

19 Latronico N, Bertolini G, Guarneri B, et al. Simplified electrophysiological evaluation of peripheral nerves in critically ill patients: the Italian multi-centre CRIMYNE study. *Crit Care* 2007;**11**:R11.

20 Hermans G, De Jonghe B, Bruyninckx F, Van den Berghe G. Clinical review: critical illness polyneuropathy and myopathy. *Crit Care* 2008;**12**:238.

21 Vasile B, Rasulo F, Candiani A, Latronico N. The pathophysiology of propofol infusion syndrome: a simple name for a complex syndrome. *Intensive Care Med* 2003;**29**:1417–25.

22 Latronico N. Acute myopathy of intensive care. *Ann Neurol* 1997;**42**:131–2.

23 Segredo V, Caldwell JE, Matthay MA, Sharma ML, Gruenke LD, Miller RD. Persistent paralysis in critically ill patients after long-term administration of vecuronium. *N Engl J Med* 1992;**327**:524–8.

24 Gorson KC. Approach to neuromuscular disorders in the intensive care unit. *Neurocrit Care* 2005; **3**:195–212.

25 Zohar M, Latronico N. Neuromuscular complications in intensive care patients. In: Biller J, Ferro JM (eds.) *Handbook of clinical neurology, Volume 121 (3rd series). Neurological aspects of systemic disease Part III.* Edinburgh: Elsevier; 2014. pp. 1–13.

26 Papazian L, Forel JM, Gacouin A, et al. Neuromuscular blockers in early acute respiratory distress syndrome. *N Engl J Med* 2010;**363**:1107–16.

27 Dubois EL. Triamcinolone in the treatment of systemic lupus erythematosus. *JAMA* 1958;**167**:1590–9.

28 Khan MA, Larson E. Acute myopathy secondary to oral steroid therapy in a 49-year-old man: a case report. *J Med Case Reports* 2011;**5**:82.

29 MacFarlane IA, Rosenthal FD. Severe myopathy after status asthmaticus. *Lancet* 1977;**2**:615.

30 Miller SM. Methylprednisolone in acute spinal cord injury: a tarnished standard. *J Neurosurg Anesthesiol* 2008;**20**:140–2.

31 Cronin L, Cook DJ, Carlet J, et al. Corticosteroid treatment for sepsis: a critical appraisal and meta-analysis of the literature. *Crit Care Med* 1995;**23**:1430–9.

32 Sprung CL, Annane D, Keh D, et al. Hydrocortisone therapy for patients with septic shock. *N Engl J Med* 2008;**358**:111–24.

33 Dellinger RP, Levy MM, Carlet JM, et al. Surviving Sepsis Campaign: international guidelines for management of severe sepsis and septic shock: 2008. *Intensive Care Med* 2008;**34**:17–60.

34 Steinberg KP, Hudson LD, Goodman RB, et al. Efficacy and safety of corticosteroids for persistent acute respiratory distress syndrome. *N Engl J Med* 2006;**354**:1671–84.

35 Hermans G, Wilmer A, Meersseman W, et al. Impact of intensive insulin therapy on neuromuscular complications and ventilator dependency in the medical intensive care unit. *Am J Respir Crit Care Med* 2007;**175**:480–9.

36 Herridge MS, Tansey CM, Matte A, et al. Functional disability 5 years after acute respiratory distress syndrome. *N Engl J Med* 2011;**364**:1293–304.

37 Vasilevskis EE, Ely EW, Speroff T, Pun BT, Boehm L, Dittus RS. Reducing iatrogenic risks: ICU-acquired delirium and weakness—crossing the quality chasm. *Chest* 2010;**138**:1224–33.

38 Kortebein P, Ferrando A, Lombeida J, Wolfe R, Evans WJ. Effect of 10 days of bed rest on skeletal muscle in healthy older adults. *JAMA* 2007;**297**:1772–4.

39 Herridge MS, Cheung AM, Tansey CM, et al. One-year outcomes in survivors of the acute respiratory distress syndrome. *N Engl J Med* 2003;**348**:683–93.

40 Lightfoot A, McArdle A, Griffiths RD. Muscle in defense. *Crit Care Med* 2009;**37**:S384–90.

41 Jaber S, Petrof BJ, Jung B, et al. Rapidly progressive diaphragmatic weakness and injury during mechanical ventilation in humans. *Am J Respir Crit Care Med* 2011;**183**:364–71.

42 Friedrich O, Hund E, Weber C, Hacke W, Fink RH. Critical illness myopathy serum fractions affect membrane excitability and intracellular calcium release in mammalian skeletal muscle. *J Neurol* 2004;**251**:53–65.

43 Fenzi F, Latronico N, Boniotti C, et al. Critical illness polyneuropathy: nerve findings in 12 patients. *Clin Neuropathol* 1994;**13**:150–1.

44 Z'Graggen WJ, Lin CS, Howard RS, Beale RJ, Bostock H. Nerve excitability changes in critical illness polyneuropathy. *Brain* 2006;**129**:2461–70.

45 Novak KR, Nardelli P, Cope TC, et al. Inactivation of sodium channels underlies reversible neuropathy during critical illness in rats. *J Clin Invest* 2009;**119**:1150–8.

46 Bolton CF, Gilbert JJ, Hahn AF, Sibbald WJ. Polyneuropathy in critically ill patients. *J Neurol Neurosurg Psychiatry* 1984;**47**:1223–31.

47 De Jonghe B, Bastuji-Garin S, Sharshar T, Outin H, Brochard L. Does ICU-acquired paresis lengthen weaning from mechanical ventilation? *Intensive Care Med* 2004;**30**:1117–21.

48 Garnacho-Montero J, Amaya-Villar R, Garcia-Garmendia JL, Madrazo-Osuna J, Ortiz-Leyba C. Effect of critical illness polyneuropathy on the withdrawal from mechanical ventilation and the length of stay in septic patients. *Crit Care Med* 2005;**33**:349–54.

49 De Jonghe B, Bastuji-Garin S, Durand MC, et al. Respiratory weakness is associated with limb weakness and delayed weaning in critical illness. *Crit Care Med* 2007;**35**:2007–15.

50 Hough CL, Lieu BK, Caldwell ES. Manual muscle strength testing of critically ill patients: feasibility and interobserver agreement. *Crit Care* 2011;**15**:R43.

51 Schweickert WD, Hall J. ICU-acquired weakness. *Chest* 2007;**131**:1541–9.

52 van der Schaaf M, Dettling DS, Beelen A, Lucas C, Dongelmans DA, Nollet F. Poor functional status immediately after discharge from an intensive care unit. *Disabil Rehabil* 2008;**30**:1812–18.

53 Schweickert WD, Pohlman MC, Pohlman AS, et al. Early physical and occupational therapy in mechanically ventilated, critically ill patients: a randomised controlled trial. *Lancet* 2009;**373**:1874–82.

54 Latronico N, Guarneri B, Alongi S, Bussi G, Candiani A. Acute neuromuscular respiratory failure after ICU discharge. Report of five patients. *Intensive Care Med* 1999;**25**:1302–6.

55 Fletcher SN, Kennedy DD, Ghosh IR, et al. Persistent neuromuscular and neurophysiologic abnormalities in long-term survivors of prolonged critical illness. *Crit Care Med* 2003;**31**:1012–16.

56 Latronico N, Shehu I, Seghelini E. Neuromuscular sequelae of critical illness. *Curr Opin Crit Care* 2005; **11**:381–90.

57 Needham DM, Davidson J, Cohen H, et al. Improving long-term outcomes after discharge from intensive care unit: report from a stakeholders' conference. *Crit Care Med* 2011;**40**:502–9.

58 Angus DC, Clermont G, Linde-Zwirble WT, et al. Healthcare costs and long-term outcomes after acute respiratory distress syndrome: a phase III trial of inhaled nitric oxide. *Crit Care Med* 2006;**34**:2883–90.

59 van der Schaaf M, Beelen A, Dongelmans DA, Vroom MB, Nollet F. Functional status after intensive care: a challenge for rehabilitation professionals to improve outcome. *J Rehabil Med* 2009;**41**:360–6.

60 Angel MJ, Bril V, Shannon P, Herridge MS. Neuromuscular function in survivors of the acute respiratory distress syndrome. *Can J Neurol Sci* 2007;**34**:427–32.

61 Latronico N, Filosto M, Fagoni N, et al. Small nerve fiber pathology in critical illness. *PLoS ONE* 2013;**8**(9):e75696.

62 Orford NR, Saunders K, Merriman E, et al. Skeletal morbidity among survivors of critical illness. *Crit Care Med* 2011;**39**:1295–300.

63 Iwashyna TJ. Survivorship will be the defining challenge of critical care in the 21st century. *Ann Intern Med* 2010;**153**:204–5.

64 van der Schaaf M, Beelen A, Dongelmans DA, Vroom MB, Nollet F. Poor functional recovery after a critical illness: a longitudinal study. *J Rehabil Med* 2009;**41**:1041–8.

65 Latronico N. Muscle weakness during critical illness. *Eur Crit Care Emerg Med* 2010;**2**:61–4.

66 Hagell P, Brundin L. Towards an understanding of fatigue in Parkinson disease. *J Neurol Neurosurg Psychiatry* 2009;**80**:489–92.

67 Livingston DH, Tripp T, Biggs C, Lavery RF. A fate worse than death? Long-term outcome of trauma patients admitted to the surgical intensive care unit. *J Trauma* 2009;**67**:341–8; discussion 8–9.

68 Skinner EH, Warrillow S, Denehy L. Health-related quality of life in Australian survivors of critical illness. *Crit Care Med* 2011;**39**:1896–905.

69 Guarneri B, Bertolini G, Latronico N. Long-term outcome in patients with critical illness myopathy or neuropathy: the Italian multicentre CRIMYNE study. *J Neurol Neurosurg Psychiatry* 2008;**79**:838–41.

70 Dennis DM, Hebden-Todd TK, Marsh LJ, Cipriano LJ, Parsons RW. How do Australian ICU survivors fare functionally 6 months after admission? *Crit Care Resusc* 2011;**13**:9–16.

71 Intiso D, Amoruso L, Zarrelli M, et al. Long-term functional outcome and health status of patients with critical illness polyneuromyopathy. *Acta Neurol Scand* 2011;**123**:211–19.

72 Van den Berghe G, Schoonheydt K, Becx P, Bruyninckx F, Wouters PJ. Insulin therapy protects the central and peripheral nervous system of intensive care patients. *Neurology* 2005;**64**:1348–53.

73 Finfer S, Chittock DR, Su SY, et al. Intensive versus conventional glucose control in critically ill patients. *N Engl J Med* 2009;**360**:1283–97.

74 Qaseem A, Humphrey LL, Chou R, Snow V, Shekelle P. Use of intensive insulin therapy for the management of glycemic control in hospitalized patients: a clinical practice guideline from the American College of Physicians. *Ann Intern Med* 2011;**154**:260–7.

75 Burtin C, Clerckx B, Robbeets C, et al. Early exercise in critically ill patients enhances short-term functional recovery. *Crit Care Med* 2009;**37**:2499–505.

76 Kirwan JR, Hewlett SE, Heiberg T, et al. Incorporating the patient perspective into outcome assessment in rheumatoid arthritis—progress at OMERACT 7. *J Rheumatol* 2005;**32**:2250–6.

Chapter 25

Bone and Joint Disease Following Critical Illness

Amelia Barry and Guy Trudel

Introduction

Bone and joint diseases can cause significant impairment to critical care patients. During the acute phase, the focus is on survival. Bone and joint processes take second stage to acute medical interventions and pulmonary therapy. However, in the long term, the patient's return to pre-admission function is often limited by acquired bone and joint complications. This chapter will examine common bone and joint pathologies affecting patients after intensive care treatment of their critical illness. Mandatory physical examination and early mobilization of patients are fundamental to prevent joint contractures, hypercalcaemia, and HO.

Joint contractures

Definition

A joint contracture is defined as a fixed limitation in passive range of motion of a joint. This occurs as a result of changes to periarticular structures, including bone, muscle, soft tissues, and skin[1,2,3] (see Table 25.1).

Joint contractures can complicate patient recovery after ICU, causing more disability, resource utilization, and long-term limitations. Clavet et al. studied 150 patients in ICU for 2 weeks or longer. At discharge home, more patients with joint contractures had a lower ambulation level, compared to the patients without joint contractures.[4] They received more physiatry consultation, had a longer length of stay in hospital after transfer out of intensive care (38 days vs 23 days), cost more to treat, and were transferred to a rehabilitation centre more often.[4] At follow-up, an average of 3 years after their ICU stay, a larger proportion of patients with contractures had died and a larger proportion of patients with contractures still reported limitations in their mobility, compared to patients with no contractures in ICU (personal communication).

Risk factors

A significant risk factor for the development of contractures is immobility.[5-10] Patients in the intensive care setting are immobile, predisposing them to alterations in joint structures. Time in ICU was found to be a significant risk factor for developing joint contracture, and patients admitted for >8 weeks in intensive care were seven times more likely to develop joint contracture relative to the patients admitted for 2–3 weeks.[11]

Other risk factors in critical care patients include neurologic injury, oedema, contusions, fractures,[12-14] and limb amputation.[15] Intensive care patients with central and peripheral neurologic

Table 25.1 Classification of joint contractures

Type	Example
Arthrogenic	
Bony	Intra-articular fracture
Cartilage	Osteochondritis dissecans
Synovium	Synovial chondromatosis
Capsular	Secondary to immobility, adhesive capsulitis, arthrofibrosis
Other	Meniscal tear, labrum tear
Myogenic	
Muscle	Muscle fibrosis, changes due to altered neurologic supply (i.e. spasticity)
Fascia	Eosinophilic fasciitis
Tendinous	Tendon transposition, shortening
Cutaneous	Burn, scleroderma
Mixed (any combination)	Burn and adhesive capsulitis

This table was published in *Essentials of Physical Medicine and Rehabilitation*, Second Edition, Frontera WR et al., pp. 651–655, Copyright Elsevier 2008.

conditions, such as brain injury, spinal cord injury, and stroke, in addition to patients with critical illness myopathy and neuropathy (CRIMYE), are predisposed to developing contractures.[16–18] These patients are often immobilized, and spasticity and paralysis may disrupt the balance between agonist/antagonist transarticular muscles, with resulting loss of range of the joint.[2,19–20] Other risk factors for joint contractures include burns, rheumatologic conditions, age, and haemophilia.[21–24]

Epidemiology

A cohort of patients of all aetiologies who stay more than 2 weeks in ICU demonstrated evidence of at least one joint contracture in 39% of cases. Contractures were graded as functionally significant in 34% of patients.[11] Contractures were present in the elbow in approximately one-third of cases, followed, in declining frequency, by the ankle, the knee, the hip, and the shoulder.[11]

In brain-injured patients, one study found incidence of joint contracture of 84% of all joints combined. Other studies demonstrated slightly lower rates for ankle (16%) and shoulder (52%) contractures.[18,25,26] Greater than half of stroke patients demonstrated contractures, occurring as early as 2 months post-stroke.[17] On admission to a rehabilitation unit, approximately 15% of spinal cord patients had functionally significant contractures.[27] In patients with spinal cord injury over age 20, the incidence of contractures climbs to 30%.[24,28] Elbow contractures were more common in tetraplegic than in paraplegic joints, with an incidence of 50% in tetraplegia.[28,29,30]

Twelve per cent of elbow fractures are associated with contractures.[14] Burn patients are a specific population at high risk of developing joint contractures, with incidence ranging from 50 to 95%, based on the joints affected and management.[22]

Pathological changes

Changes occur in the soft tissues of immobile joints, leading to contracture. When immobilized, there is an absence of mechanical tensile forces on the joints. There is shortening of the capsule and decreased proportion of proliferating synoviocytes in animal studies of contractures. Further evidence shows increased type 1 collagen and less type 3 collagen in the capsule, consistent with a fibrotic picture.[31] These changes lead to capsular stiffness. These changes in the soft tissue are dependent on their location in the joint and occur only on the side not subjected to tensile forces.[32] Animal work suggests there may be a genetic susceptibility to joint contractures secondary to immobility.[3] If the immobility is long-standing, chondrocytes not stimulated by mechanical forces can die, causing destruction of the ECM and joint degeneration.[33] Joint ankylosis is the final stage.

Symptoms and signs

Joint contractures are pain-free and often asymptomatic. The critical care team should be vigilant, especially in sedated patients. Patients may report stiffness in the affected joint, and pain and limitation at the end of the affected joint range of motion.[27,34] Pain and stiffness may also disrupt sleep patterns.[34] Functionally significant contractures impair a patient's ability to perform specific tasks. Patients or caregivers may report difficulty with ADLs such as transfers, ambulation, or self-care.[35,36] Contractures may also pose difficulty for positioning patients, including for seating.[36]

Assessment of contractures involves completing a musculoskeletal physical examination. This is often neglected in the ICU assessment but should be carried out in all patients. There may be deformity of the joint on inspection. Oedema and skin breakdown over the joint should be noted, as pressure ulcers can be found in conjunction with contracture.[19] Range of motion of the joint should be examined, both actively and passively and bilaterally, with a goniometer. Special tests exist to assess specific joints (e.g. Thomas test for hip flexion contracture).[1] Neurologic exam often allows the clinician to diagnose conditions predisposing to the contracture, e.g brain injury, spinal cord injury, stroke, or neuromuscular condition such as CRIMYNE. Weakness, absent or enhanced reflexes, or the presence of tone and spasticity will reveal these diagnoses.[19]

Investigation

Joint contractures are diagnosed, based on clinical presentation and physical examination. The differential diagnosis includes bony pathology such as fractures, HO, arthritis; soft tissue pathology, such as ligamentous or meniscal damage; and neurologic abnormalities such as spasticity (see Figure 25.1). Radiological imaging may help to rule out these differential diagnoses.

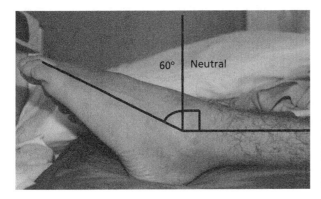

Fig. 25.1 Plantarflexion contracture of 60° after prolonged immobilization.

Reproduced with kind permission from Dr Sreenivasan.

Management

Early mobilization

Early mobilization of patients, when possible, is important for prevention of contractures. Mobilization protocols vary across ICUs, and positive outcomes have been associated with early mobilization.[37] Early mobilization led to a higher percentage of functionally independent patients at discharge.[38] Involvement of a multidisciplinary team led to earlier mobilization of critically ill patients[39] and reduced intensive care length of stay by 3 days.[40]

Stretching

Stretching is the primary means used to prevent and treat joint contractures and includes passive stretch, positioning, static and dynamic splinting, and casting. Despite its ubiquitous recommendation, evidence regarding the benefit of stretching in both prevention and treatment is mixed. Animal studies demonstrate that 30 minutes of daily stretch will prevent the loss of sarcomeres in an immobilized limb.[41] A 2010 systematic review of the available literature failed to demonstrate a significant benefit for stretching on range of motion, pain, spasticity, activity limitation, participation restriction, or QoL in mixed treatment and prevention studies.[42] This review included all aetiologies of contractures, both neurologic and non-neurologic, and all interventions, including sustained passive stretching, positioning, splinting, and serial casting.[42] Despite this, stretching continues to be current practice in most facilities for the prevention and treatment of joint contractures. However, the time of onset, specific dosage, modality of delivery, frequency, and intensity have yet to be clearly defined for clinical subgroups and individual joints.[7,16,43]

Passive stretch

One clinical study reported that physiotherapists provided routine passive range of motion to only 14% of ICU patients; however, rates were higher in high-risk patients.[44] Current recommendation is for passive stretch daily for 30 minutes. This is despite studies in spinal cord patients by one group of investigators showing no benefit to 30 minutes of daily passive stretching of the hamstrings or at the ankle for 4 weeks, compared to controls receiving usual care.[16,45,46] Although research is necessary to delineate which patient population would most benefit from joint stretching, this is considered standard practice and should be incorporated into ICU management, along with positioning.

Positioning/orthoses

Prolonged stretching can be administered through positioning, static orthoses, serial casting, and dynamic orthoses.[7,16] A longer stretch is applied using these devices than would be achieved by therapists alone. Static orthoses may be applied to joints at risk for contracture. For treatment with serial interventions, the joint is stretched to its endpoint, then the cast or static orthoses is applied. It is maintained for 2–3 days, then it is removed. The joint is stretched again to its new maximal range with reapplication of the device. Benefits of dynamic orthoses for stretching are the need for only one device and the easy adjustment to various angles. Disadvantages are the higher cost of the device.

Critical care patients may benefit from static orthoses to prevent contracture development on joints at risk such as the ankle.[2] This is routinely done at many centres; however, no evidence supports its use in the ICU population.[44] Similarly, positioning is important for prevention of joint contractures, though no published evidence could be retrieved for the ICU population.[44] Examples include positioning the patient prone to stretch the hip joint in extension or maintaining shoulders in external rotation or abduction by arm boards attached to the bed.[47] An ICU survey showed that 44% of staff considered varying the position of joints as a means of contracture prevention, and joint repositioning is one of the most frequent ICU interventions performed by physiotherapists.[44,48]

In **stroke** patients, night splints 7 days per week or use of a tilt table for 30 minutes five times per week have both prevented ankle contracture.[49] Conversely, in the upper limb, similar hand splinting failed to reduce contracture rate in two RCTs.[50-52] However, another prospective RCT of stroke patients demonstrated that 30 minutes of daily shoulder positioning started an average of 14 days after hemiparesis reduced contracture formation.[53]

In **brain-injured** patients, wearing ankle foot orthoses for 23 hours per day for a total of 2 weeks or serial casting for 1–4 days improved dorsiflexion in patients with plantar flexion contracture.[25,54-6] Conversely, neither hand splints nor serial casting of the upper limb showed long-term gains in range of motion.[51,57,58]

In **spinal cord-injured patients**, static orthoses demonstrated no significant prevention of thumb contractures.[59] For non-ambulatory patients, standing on a tilt table for 30 minutes, three times per week for 3 months, achieved a 4° improvement in ankle range.[60] Harvey et al. suggested that stretching likely needs to be applied for longer than 30 minutes per day and for more than 3 months, assisted by orthoses.[16]

Continuous passive movement

Continuous passive movement (CPM) has mainly been used to assist orthopaedic patients after total knee arthroplasty (TKA), ligament repair, and fractures.[20] It could potentially be used in ICU. For patients post-TKA, it is applied for 8–12 hours per day, for up to 5 days after surgery.[20] Unfortunately, its benefit in increasing knee flexion is small, approximately 2° in passive range of motion and 3° in active range of motion, in TKA patients.[61]

Surgery

Surgery can correct severe or disabling joint contractures. Tendon lengthening, tenotomy, capsular release, joint reconstruction, or replacement may be used. Tendon lengthening is predicted to improve joint range of motion at the expense of muscle strength.[62]

Spasticity management

In neurologic conditions, spasticity plays an important role in managing joint mobility. This includes removal of noxious stimuli that could exacerbate spasticity. The treatment of spasticity with agents, such as baclofen, dantrolene, tizanidine, the use of botulinum toxin or phenol injected at neuromuscular junction, and, in severe cases, intrathecal baclofen pumps can facilitate the mobility of joints.

Medication

No medication has been found effective in preventing joint contractures or treating established contractures. In animal models, corticosteroids and ketotifen have shown positive results, but they have restricting side effect profiles or are yet to be tested in humans.[63] Interestingly, patients who received steroids during their ICU stay had decreased odds of developing joint contracture.[11]

In summary, alternating limb positioning and joint stretching by the critical care team is important to prevent contractures in immobile critical care and neurologically impaired patients. In addition, static and dynamic orthoses are commonly applied at the ankle to prevent plantarflexion contracture (see Figure 25.1), although other joints may be braced in an effort to prevent contractures while the patient is sedated. As soon as feasible, early mobilization should be added to this regimen.

Heterotopic ossification

Definition

HO is defined as the formation of calcified lamellar bone in soft tissue or muscle.[64–67] HO can functionally impair patients long after ICU discharge. It is therefore important for the intensive care team to detect HO.

Risk factors

HO may develop in multiple populations (see Table 25.2). Neurologic or traumatic insults (or both) are major risk factors. In brain injury, spasticity, immobilization, and duration of coma may contribute to the development of HO.[65,66] In spinal cord injury, spasticity, pressure ulcers, and time of injury are independent risk factors for the development of HO.[68] However, HO can be found in the critical care population in the absence of an identifiable neurologic or traumatic lesion. These patients are typically immobilized, mechanically ventilated, with or without neuromuscular blockade.[69–72]

Pathophysiology

In the initial phase of heterotopic bone formation, there is an inflammatory response in the affected soft tissue region with increased blood flow.[73] This leads to mesenchymal stem cell (MSC) proliferation; however, their origin is unknown and may either be from local or distant sites. Some of these MSC will differentiate into osteoblasts. Osteoblasts lay down cartilaginous osseous matrix that will mineralize, thus forming ectopic bone. Multiple factors, including local, neuroimmunological, and humoral, have been identified that modulate the process.[67,73]

Symptoms and signs

HO presents most commonly with decreased joint range of motion.[64] Patients may complain of joint pain or localized soft tissue pain, and there is often associated tenderness on physical exam.

Table 25.2 Classification and epidemiology of heterotopic ossification

Type	Aetiology	Incidence	References
Neurologic	Spinal cord injury	10–78%	65, 66, 73, 77
	TBI	11–77%	65, 66, 147, 148
	Neuromuscular blockade	Case reports	70
	Polio	Case reports	149
	Acute inflammatory demyelinating polyneuropathy	Case reports	150
Traumatic	Acetabular fractures	26%	151
	Hip arthroplasty	5–90%, mean 50%	152, 153
	Burns	1–3%	75
Non-neurologic, non-traumatic	Critical care population (MV, neuromuscular blockade, idiopathic)	5%	71

Other findings that may lead to diagnosing HO in a sedated population in ICU include swelling, erythema, and warmth at the joint or over the HO site.[69,70,72,74]

HO primarily targets large joints. Joints most commonly affected in non-traumatic, non-neurologic critical care populations include hips, shoulders, and knees.[69,70,72,74] Burn patients develop HO in elbow joints, followed less frequently by hips, knees, hands, and shoulders.[75,76]

The mean time of diagnosis of HO is 2 months, but it varies, based on aetiology.[64] Neurogenic HO in TBI patients usually appears 2–3 weeks post-injury; however, diagnosis can be made between 1 and 7 months post-injury.[65,66] In spinal cord patients, HO has been identified on screening bone scan at 1 month post-event and typically becomes clinically overt within the initial 2 months post-injury.[77,78] HO has been identified in the critical care population at a mean of 48 days post-neuromuscular blockade and 32 days post-MV without neuromuscular blockade.[70,79]

Investigations

Serum markers

Serum alkaline phosphatase (alkP) rose in HO at 2 weeks post-injury and peaked at 10 weeks in heterogeneous populations, including neurologic, traumatic, and critical care patients.[70,80,81] However, one study in spinal cord patients has shown no correlation between alkP levels and HO.[82] Serum creatine kinase (CK) is often elevated in spinal cord patients with HO and may also be associated with increased severity of disease.[82,83] Non-specific inflammatory markers, including ESR and CRP, are elevated at the time of diagnosis. CRP demonstrated greater specificity than ESR in following disease resolution.[84]

Imaging

When investigating clinical findings of HO, initial X-rays are often negative, because ossification has not yet occurred. Triple phase bone scan with technetium-99m (^{99m}Tc) tagged diphosphate demonstrates HO earlier than plane films. Triple phase scans will detect radioisotope uptake in the first and second phases, respectively, corresponding to increased vascularity and blood pooling.[67,81] The third phase will detect bony radioisotope uptake after mineralization of HO occurs.[73] Bone scans are positive 4–6 weeks sooner than the detection of HO on X-ray.[80] Bone scan phases 1 and 2 will become negative after 6–18 months.[81] Since bone scan has greater sensitivity than plane films, other causes of increased radionuclide uptake, such as musculoskeletal tumour and soft tissue infection, should be ruled out.[85] MRI in a small heterogeneous critical care population demonstrated HO, on average, at day 20 post-admission in contrast to day 40 on plane films.[86] The differential diagnoses of HO include thrombophlebitis, septic arthritis, and deep vein thrombosis.

Management

Prevention

NSAIDs

Non-steroidal anti-inflammatory drugs (NSAIDs) are thought to prevent heterotopic bone formation by inhibiting the early stages of bone formation.[87] Anti-inflammatories decrease the inflammatory response by inhibition of the prostaglandin-H synthase (PGHS). NSAIDs are also believed to hinder differentiation and migration of precursor cells.[88] NSAIDs post-total hip arthroplasty reduced the risk by one-half to two-thirds of heterotopic bone formation on radiographic follow-up.[89] In acetabular fractures, reviews of the literature recommended indomethacin 25 mg orally three times daily over 6 weeks for prophylaxis, based on 12-month and 14-month radiographic follow-up.[90–92] Similarly, in patients with spinal cord injury treated with indomethacin 75 mg daily for 3 weeks, there was a lower incidence of HO diagnosed on triple phase bone scan (both early and up to 12 months) and lower clinical symptoms, compared to placebo.[78] Rofecoxib, a PGHS-2 selective inhibitor, administered 25 mg daily for 4 weeks, prevented HO formation clinically and on bone scan at an unspecified follow-up period.[78,88,93] No trials have proven the efficacy of NSAIDs to prevent HO in other neurologic populations, including brain injury patients, burn patients, or critical care patients.[70,75]

Bisphosphonates

Bisphosphonates are chemically related to inorganic pyrophosphates and have been used to prevent ectopic bone formation. This is thought to occur by preventing bone mineralization by inhibiting the replacement of amorphous calcium phosphate by hydroxyapatite crystals.[87] Some bisphosphonates also decrease the number of osteoblasts as another mechanism of preventing ectopic bone formation.[73] Etidronate disodium, given within 1 week of head injury and continued for a total of 6 months, decreased the incidence of HO.[94] Patients with a spinal cord injury and negative X-rays, treated with etidronate for 8–12 weeks, had reduced incidence of HO at 12 weeks but a similar prevalence of HO at 1 year. This may be because, when bisphosphonate therapy is stopped, mineralization of the bone is allowed to proceed.[91] In this study, early administration (within 44 days) was more beneficial than late treatment, and the duration of treatment did not affect outcomes.[95,96] One retrospective study in a burn population found an increased incidence of HO in the etidronate-treated patients.[97] After total hip arthroplasty, mixed results and lack of long-term follow-up prevented recommending the routine use of bisphosphonate prophylaxis.[91]

Radiation therapy

Radiation stops the development of HO by inhibiting the differentiation of mesenchymal cells into osteoblasts.[98] Single-dose, 800 cGy external beam radiation has prevented heterotopic bone formation in selected populations. Singl-dose radiation following total hip arthroplasty and following open repair of hip fractures at 800 cGy was effective in preventing HO, although a meta-analysis failed to find a significant difference between radiation and NSAID use in both of these surgical groups.[99] For acetabular fractures, local radiation at 800 cGy was equally effective as indomethacin in preventing HO on radiographs at 12- and 14-month follow-up.[90,92] However, one systematic review favours radiation over indomethacin, because indomethacin was associated with non-union of long bone fractures.[100,101] But choosing the therapeutic approach of choice has been further complicated by one randomized trial suggesting that radiation therapy itself increased the rate of non-union post-surgical repair of elbow fracture.[102] Radiation over a non-fracture site may be safe. No studies have been done using radiation therapy in primary prophylaxis of neurogenic HO.

Medical treatment

After the diagnosis of heterotopic bone has been established, some of the same agents used in prophylaxis have been administered to limit its extent.

NSAIDs

Two ICU case reports mentioned improved function after treatment of HO with indomethacin and physiotherapy in patients with neuromuscular blockade.[69,70]

Bisphosphonates

IV etidronate, followed by oral etidronate, decreased the swelling related to established HO in spinal cord patients.[103] Three studies showed evidence that etidronate limited the progression of established HO.[65,66,77,104,105] One case series failed to show such benefit.[65,66] Various case reports of HO in ICU patients with neuromuscular blockade confirmed etidronate and physiotherapy to decrease warmth or oedema and improve range of motion.[69,70] In patients with burns, two studies using bisphosphonate for established HO showed mixed results, and this constitutes insufficient evidence to guide management.[106,107]

Radiation therapy

Radiation therapy administered in ranges of 2–10 Gy, in either single dose or multiple fractions, to established HO limited the progression of the disease in spinal cord-injured patients.[108–110]

Surgical management

Surgical excision is a treatment option for HO of all patient groups (see Figure 25.2).

In neurogenic HO, surgical excision of heterotopic bone improved transfers, gait, pain levels, and range of motion of joints in patients with a TBI.[111–119] Surgical excision of HO over large joints in patients with a spinal cord injury also improved range of motion.[120,121]

The excision of heterotopic bone in traumatic and non-traumatic, non-neurologic causes, including fractures, burn patients, and medical ICU patients have all shown benefit of improved range of motion, sitting ability, and ambulation.[75,122–125]

Optimal time for excision is controversial because of possibilities of recurrence.[75,93,123,124] Proponents of late excision (at 12–18 months) suggest that mature bone on bone scan and stable alkP levels will prevent recurrence. But some evidence does indicate that early excision may be warranted, as bone scan and alkP levels may not reliably predict the likelihood of recurrence.[126]

Recurrence rates of HO after surgical excision are higher for neurogenic HO than post-trauma,[122] and higher in brain-injured than in spinal cord-injured patients.[93,116,119,120,127] Recurrence rates in brain injury were linked to the severity of injury more than the timing of excision.[128] Case reports of mechanically ventilated patients treated with surgical resection, with and without indomethacin and etidronate prophylactically post-resection, showed no recurrence.[70,72,74,124]

Management summary

Prophylactic treatment to prevent HO is not routinely practised in ICU. Management of established HO should move from least invasive to most invasive. NSAIDs and radiation can be used

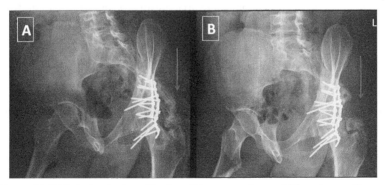

Fig. 25.2 X-ray of left hip heterotopic ossification, (A) preoperative and (B) post-operative resection.

in selected cases as the initial choice. In cases where significant functional gains can be made (e.g seating, mobility, ADLs) or QoL improved (e.g. improved pain), then surgical options should be considered. Physicians should weigh the surgical risk and timing of surgery with the degree of impairment and disability caused to the patient by the HO.

Altered bone metabolism: bone hyperresorption and osteoporosis

The critical care population is at increased risk of abnormal bone metabolism. Alterations in bone turnover are related to the critical illness and to the immobility and predispose to acute hypercalcaemia, osteoporosis, and fragility fractures. In 1998, Nierman et al. found that 92% of mechanically ventilated critically ill patients had increased bone resorption markers when transferred to a step-down unit.[129] Follow-up of 748 patients 3.7 years after ICU discharge demonstrated increased risk of fracture among females >60 years old, with an HR of 1.65, in comparison to age-matched controls in the general population.[130]

Hypercalcaemia

Definition

Hypercalcaemia is defined as serum calcium level >2.6 mmol/L, corrected for albumin level, or an ionized calcium level of >1.4 mmol/L. The corrected calcium (mmol/L) level is equal to measured calcium (mmol/L) + ([40 – albumin (g/L)] × 0.02).[131]

Aetiology

In the critical care patient, immobilization and paralysis may cause hypercalcaemia in spinal cord injury patients. Other causes of elevated calcium in ICU include malignancy-associated (either paraneoplastic or due to bone resorption) or endocrine causes (such as hyperparathyroidism, hyperthyroidism, adrenal insufficiency, or acromegaly), and medications, including thiazide diuretics, lithium, vitamin A, and vitamin D toxicity. Differential diagnoses also include milk alkali syndrome, Paget's disease, sarcoidosis, granulomatous diseases, and renal failure.[132,133]

Clinical presentation

Symptoms and signs of hypercalcaemia include diffuse musculoskeletal pain, lethargy, fatigue, nausea, vomiting, abdominal discomfort, polyuria, polydipsia, and constipation. Patients may also show confusion or psychiatric changes.

Patients with hypercalcaemia demonstrate shortening of the QT interval on ECG and then, in more severe cases, wide T wave and ventricular tachyarrhythmia.[132]

Management

Primary treatment is with IV hydration to increase urinary calcium excretion, typically with normal saline at 200–300 cc/hour, unless contraindicated. Further treatment includes loop diuretics, specifically furosemide. Bisphosphonates are commonly used to stabilize hypercalcaemia secondary to bone destruction in metastatic malignancy. Other alternatives include calcitonin or GCs.[133]

The acute calcium losses and bony matrix deficit can lead to osteoporosis.

Osteoporosis

Definition and classification

Osteoporosis is defined as BMD 2.5 SDs below peak adult bone mass, whether or not a fragility fracture has occurred.[134] BMD screening is performed by dual-energy X-ray absorptiometry (DEXA) scan.[135] Canadian guidelines recommend routine screening for patients >65 or patients >50 presenting with other risk factors. Osteoporosis is classified into primary and secondary forms. Primary osteoporosis occurs in post-menopausal females in type 1, and in both genders after the age of 75 in type 2.[136–138] Secondary osteoporosis results from endocrine or metabolic causes, genetic collagen abnormalities, nutritional problems, systemic illness, hypo- or immobility, and medications such as those in critical care patients.[137,138] (see Table 25.3).

Pathophysiology

In the critical care population, abnormal bone metabolism is multifactorial and summarized in Table 25.3. In addition to the risk factors associated with the general population, including fragility fracture before age 40, parental hip fracture, vertebral fracture, use of steroids or other medication, smoking, alcohol intake, low body weight or major weight loss, rheumatoid arthritis, some risk factors are specific to intensive care patients.[135]

Management

Patients post-ICU with low BMD on DEXA will require specific management.

Vitamin D

In critical care patients, supplementation with 200 IU and 500 IU was insufficient to normalize vitamin D levels.[139] The goal is a level of 25-hydroxyvitamin D >80 nmol/L (32 ng/mL).[140] Current recommendations are to supplement patients with prolonged ventilation and CCI with 2000 IU daily of ergocalciferol (vitamin D2), unless they present with frank hypercalcaemia or hypercalciuria.[141] The activated form of vitamin D (calcitriol 0.25 micrograms daily) may be required in patients with kidney dysfunction that inhibits the enzyme 1α hydroxylase from converting ergocalciferol to the active form calcitriol.[140]

Bisphosphonates

Bisphosphonates are used in critically ill patients to slow bone hyperresorption; however, they are not indicated in patients with adynamic bone disease. Adynamic bone disease is defined by low turnover of bone: fewer osteoblasts and osteoclasts, and less bone formation, however, normal bone mineralization process.[142,143] Investigations reveal low PTH, osteocalcin, and NTX (indicating decreased osteoblast and osteoclast activity, respectively).[143] It occurs most commonly in patients with CKD and on haemodialysis. Should osteocalcin and NTX be elevated, adynamic bone diseases are less probable.[141]

Patients whose increased serum levels of CTX indicated bone resorption were treated with single dose of ibandronate 3 mg IV, ergocalciferol 2000 IU, calcium carbonate 1250 mg, and calcitriol 0.25 micrograms. This treatment blunted bone resorption and osteoclast activity and lowered levels of CTX for 6 days.[144] Critically ill patients demonstrating bone hyperresorption (elevated urine NTX levels) also responded to IV pamidronate 90 mg and calcitriol by decreasing bone resorption markers for 18 days. This was in contrast to treatment with calcitriol alone

Table 25.3 Causes and mechanisms of abnormal bone metabolism in ICU[129,136,140,141,145,146]

Risk factor	Mechanism	Markers	Significance
Immobility	Bone hyperresorption → hypercalcaemia and hypercalcuria→ prevents PTH and vitamin D production[136,140,146,154,155]	Serum calcium (Ca)	Elevated
		Urine Ca	Elevated
		PTH	Low: suppressed by increased calcium during immobilization[140]
		Vitamin D	Low: low PTH leads to suppression of 1,25-vitamin D synthesis[145]
Vitamin D deficiency	Bone hyperresorption leads to increased Ca levels→ low PTH→ downregulation of 1α hydroxylase enzyme that is responsible for low vitamin D production[139,146] **AND/OR** Poor intake/absorption/ hepatic or renal metabolism of vitamin D Thus, failure to mineralize new bone	Vitamin D	Low: poor absorption, intake, decreased renal or hepatic formation
		PTH	Elevated: vitamin D deficiency increases PTH levels
Hormonal abnormalities	Acutely: amplified pituitary stress response → increased ACTH → increased cortisol[146] → persistent stimulation of adrenal gland	ACTH	Elevated
		Cortisol	Elevated
	Subacutely: pituitary blunted → decreased GH, IGF-1 hinder osteoblast activity, and decreased TSH, T4 → osteoclast bone resorption[140]	TSH	Low
		Thyroxine (T4)	Low
Inflammatory cytokines	Elevated cytokines (TNF-α, IL-6, and IL-1) in critical illness→ osteoclast production and activation → bone resorption and inhibit osteoblast formation of new bone[140,146]	Urinary N-telopeptides of type 1 collagen (NTX)*	Specific marker of bone breakdown; elevated in bone hyperresorption[145]
		Serum C- telopeptide of type 1 collagen (CTX)*	Elevated in bone hyperresorption[140]
Medications	Corticosteroids: inhibit osteoblast proliferation[156]		
	Loop diuretics: increase renal Ca excretion[157]	Urine Ca	Elevated

* NTX and CTX are present in all causes of bone hyperresorption when osteoclast function is enhanced.

that did not alter bone resorption markers.[145] Adverse effects of IV bisphosphonates include hypocalcaemia, which may precipitate paraesthesiae, tetany, seizure, cardiac arrhythmia, and death, and usually occurs in the context of hypovitaminosis D. Hypocalcaemia can be prevented by 25-hydroxyvitamin D supplementation.[146] Patients on biphosphonates should be monitored for nephrotoxicity and dosage adjusted as necessary. Ibandronate demonstrated a better renal profile than other bisphosphonates.[144] Other side effects of bisphosphonates include fever or flu-like symptoms, and rarely development of atrial fibrillation, osteonecrosis of the jaw, and skeletal fragility.[146]

Conclusion

Joint contractures, HO, and altered bone metabolism are common bone and joint complications in ICU patients and important to identify. Bone and joint pathology can significantly impair the ICU survivors long after their discharge from the hospital. Early recognition and treatment can improve long-term outcomes.

For the ICU team, the following recommendations may ameliorate bone and joint outcomes after critical illness:

+ Perform **musculoskeletal assessments** on all ICU patients

+ **Early mobilization** of patients is important for prevention of contractures, hypercalcaemia, and HO

+ Maintain a high index of suspicion for **joint contractures**, as they are often asymptomatic but the source of enduring disability once the critical illness had receded. More research is needed to document the effectiveness of alternate positioning, stretching, and bracing as the current standard practice for prevention of contractures

+ **HO** has many common mimickers and should be considered in the context of a swollen, warm, painful musculoskeletal site. Early detection requires triple phase bone scan. In some cases, prophylaxis with NSAIDs or radiation is warranted. When functional impairment is severe, the decision to proceed and timing of surgical resection requires coordinated consideration by the medical and surgical teams

+ **Bone hyperresorption** in ICU patients can be caused by immobility, hormonal changes, heightened inflammatory status, medication, and vitamin D deficiency. Laboratory biomarkers can guide treatment. Hypercalcaemia is managed with rehydration and diuresis; however, severe cases will respond to vitamin D and/or bisphosphonates. This may prevent long-term osteoporosis and fragility fractures.

References

1 **Braddom RL, Chan L, Harrast M.** Spinal cord injury. In: Braddom RL, Chan L, Harrast M, et al. (eds.) *Physical medicine and rehabilitation.* 4th ed. Philadelphia, PA: Saunders/Elsevier; 2011. pp. 1293–346.

2 **Dittmer DK, Teasell R.** Complications of immobilization and bed rest. **Part 1**: Musculoskeletal and cardiovascular complications. *Can Fam Physician* 1993;**39**:1428–32, 1435–7.

3 **Laneuville O, Zhou J, Uhthoff HK, Trudel G.** Genetic influences on joint contractures secondary to immobilization. *Clin Orthop Relat Res* 2007;**456**:36–41.

4 **Clavet H, Hebert PC, Fergusson D, Doucette S, Trudel G.** Joint Contractures in the Intensive Care Unit: Association with Resource Utilization and Ambulatory Status at Discharge. *Disabil Rehabil* 2011;**33**:105–12.

5 **Akeson WH, Ameil D, Woo S.** Immobility effects on synovial joints: The pathomechanics of joint contracture. *Biorheology* 1980;**17**:95–110.

6 **Akeson WH, Ameil D, Abel MF, Garfin SR, Woo SL-Y.** EO Effects of Immobilisation on Joints. *Clin Orthop Relat Res* 1987;**219**:28–37.

7 **Farmer SE, James M.** Contractures in orthopaedic and neurological conditions: a review of causes and treatment. *Disabil Rehabil* 2001;**23**:549–58.

8 **Trudel G, Uhthoff HK, Brown M.** Extent and direction of joint motion limitation after prolonged immobility: an experimental study in the rat. *Arch Phys Med Rehabil* 1999;**80**:1542–47.

9 **Trudel G, Seki M, Uhthoff HK.** Synovial adhesions are more important than pannus proliferation in the pathogenesis of knee joint contracture following immobilization: an experimental investigation in the rat. *J Rheumatol* 2000;**27**:351–7.

10 **Woo SL, Matthews JV, Akeson WH, Amiel D, Convery FR.** Connective tissue response to immobility. Correlative study of biomechanical and biochemical measurements of normal and immobilized rabbit knees. *Arthritis Rheum* 1975;**18**:257–64.

11 **Clavet H, Hébert PC, Fergusson D, Doucette S, Trudel G.** Joint contracture following prolonged stay in the intensive care unit. *CMAJ* 2008;**178**:691–7.

12 **Cohen MS.** Hastings 1H. Post-traumatic contracture of the elbow. *J Bone Joint Surg Br* 1998;**80**–B:805–12.

13 **Hildebrand KA, Sutherland C, Zhang Z.** Rabbit knee model of posttraumatic joint contractures: the long-term natural history of motion loss and myofibroblasts. *J Orthop Res* 2004;**22**:313–20.

14 **Myden C, Hildebrand K.** Elbow joint contracture after traumatic injury. *J Shoulder Elbow Surg* 2011;**20**:39–44

15 **Esquenazi A, Meier RH 3rd.** Rehabilitation in limb deficiency 4. Limb amputation. *Arch Phys Med Rehabil* 1996;**77**(3 Suppl):S18–28.

16 **Harvey LA, Glinsky JA, Katalinic OM, Ben M.** Contracture management for people with spinal cord injuries. *NeuroRehabilitation* 2011;**28**:17–20.

17 **O'Dwyer NJ, Ada L, Neilson PD.** Spasticity and muscle contracture following stroke. *Brain* 1996;**119**:1737–49

18 **Yarkony GM, Sahgal V.** Contractures:a major complication of craniocerebral trauma. *Clin Orthop Relat Res* 1987;**219**:93–6.

19 **Dalyan M, Sherman A and Cardenas DD.** Factors associated with contractures in acute spinal cord injury. *Spinal Cord* 1998;**36**:405–8.

20 **Frontera W.** Joint contractures. In: Delisa's *Physical medicine and rehabilitation: principles and practice.* 5th ed. Philadelphia, PA: Wolters Kluwer/Lippincott Williams & Wilkins; 2010. pp. 1255–61.

21 **Atkins RM, Henderson NJ, Duthie RB.** Joint contractures in hemophilias. *Clin Orthop Relat Res* 1987;**219**:97–1066.

22 **Huang T, Blackwell SJ, Lewis SR.** Ten years of experience in managing patients with burn contractures of axilla, elbow, wrist and knee joints. *Plast Reconstr Surg* 1978;**61**:70–6.

23 **Karten I, Koatz AO, McEwen C.** Treatment of contractures of the knee in rheumatoid arthritis. *Bull N Y Acad Med* 1968;**44**:763–73.

24 **Krause JS.** Aging after spinal cord injury: an exploratory study. *Spinal Cord* 2000;**38**:77–83.

25 **Pohl M, Ruckriem S, Mehrholz J, Ritschel C, Strik H, Pause MR.** Effectiveness of serial casting in patients with severe cerebral spasticity: a comparison study. *Arch Phys Med Rehabil* 2002;**83**:784–90.

26 **Singer BJ, Jegasothy GM, Singer KP, Allison GT.** Incidence of ankle contracture after moderate to severe acquired brain injury. *Arch Phys Med Rehabil* 2004;**85**:1465–9.

27 **Yarkony GM, Bass LM, Keenan V and Meyer PR.** Contractures complicating spinal cord injury: incidence and comparison between spinal cord centre and general hospital acute care. *Paraplegia* 1985;**23**:265–71.

28 **Fergusson D, Hutton B, Drodge A.** The epidemiology of major joint contractures: a systematic review of the literature. *Clin Orthop Relat Res* 2007;**456**:22–9.

29 **Bryden AM, Kilgore KL, Lind BB, Yu DT.** Triceps denervation as a predictor of elbow flexion contractures in C5 and C6 tetraplegia. *Arch Phys Med Rehabil* 2004;**85**:1880–5.

30 **Vogel LC, Krajci JA, Anderson CJ.** Adults with pediatric-onset spinal cord injury: Part 2: musculoskeletal and neurological complications. *J Spinal Cord Med* 2002;**25**:117–23.

31 **Matsumoto F, Trudel G, Uhthoff H.** High collagen type I and low collagen type III levels in knee joint contracture: an immunohistochemical study with histological correlate. *Acta Orthop Scand* 2002;**73**:335–43.

32 **Trudel G, Jabi M, Uhthoff H.** Localized and adaptive synoviocyte proliferation characteristics in rat knee joint contractures secondary to immobility. *Arch Phys Med Rehabil* 2003;**84**:1350–6.

33 **Trudel G, Recklies A, Laneuville O.** Increased Expression of Chitinase 3-like Protein 1 Secondary to Joint Immobility. *Clin Orthop Relat Res* 2007;**456**:92–7.

34 **Scott JA, Donovan WH.** The prevention of shoulder pain and contracture in the acute tetraplegia patient. *Paraplegia* 1981;**19**:313–19.

35 **Grover J, Gellman H, Waters RL.** The effect of a flexion contracture of the elbow on the ability to transfer in patients who have quadriplegia at the sixth cervical level. *J Bone Joint Surg* 1996;**78A**:1397–400.

36 **Harvey LA, Herbert RD.** Muscle stretching for treatment and prevention of contracture in people with spinal cord injury. *Spinal Cord* 2002;**40**:1–9.

37 **Morris PE, Goad A, Thompson C, et al:** Early intensive care unit mobility therapy in the treatment of acute respiratory failure. *Crit Care Med* 2008;**36**:2238–43.

38 **Schweickert WD, Pohlman MC, Pohlman AS, et al.** Early physical and occupational therapy in mechanically ventilated, critically ill patients: a randomized controlled trial. *Lancet* 2009;**373**:1874–82.

39 **Garzon-Serrano J, Ryan C, Waak K, et al.** Early mobilization in critically ill patients: patients' mobilization level depends on health care provider's profession. *PM R* 2011;**3**:307–13.

40 **Hopkins RO, Spuhler VJ, Thomsen GE.** Transforming ICU culture to facilitate early mobility. *Crit Care Clin* 2007;**23**:81–96.

41 **Williams PE.** Use of intermittent stretch in the prevention of serial sarcomere loss in immobilised muscle. *Ann Rheum Dis* 1990;**49**:316–17.

42 **Katalinic OM, Harvey LA, Herbert RD.** Effectiveness of stretch for the treatment and prevention of contractures in people with neurological conditions: a systematic review. *Phys Ther* 2011;**91**:11–24.

43 **Stockley RC, Hughes J, Morrison J, Rooney J.** An investigation of the use of passive movements in intensive care by UK physiotherapists. *Physiotherapy* 2010;**96**:228–33.

44 **Wiles L, Stiller K.** Passive limb movements for patients in an intensive care unit: a survey of physiotherapy practice in Australia. *J Crit Care* 2010;**25**:501–8.

45 **Harvey LA, Byak AJ, Ostrovskaya M, Glinsky J, Katte L, Herbert RD.** Randomised trial of the effects of four weeks of daily stretch on extensibility of hamstring muscles in people with spinal cord injuries. *Aust J Physiother* 2003;**49**:176–81.

46 **Harvey, LA, Batty J, Crosbie J, Poulter S, Herbert RD.** A randomized trial assessing the effects of 4 weeks of daily stretching on ankle mobility in patients with spinal cord injuries. *Arch Phys Med Rehabil* 2000;**81**:1340–7.

47 **Dudek N, Trudel G.** Joint contractures. In: Frontera WR, Silver JK, Rizzo TD (eds.) *Essentials of physical medicine and rehabilitation*. 2nd ed. Philadelphia: Saunders, Elsevier; 2008. pp. 651–5.

48 **Thomas PJ, Paratz JD, Stanton WR, Deans R, Lipman J.** Positioning practices for ventilated intensive care patients: current practice, indications and contraindications. *Aust Crit Care* 2006;**19**:122–6, 128, 130–2.

49 **Robinson W, Smith R, Aung O, Ada L.** No difference between wearing a night splint and standing on a tilt table in preventing ankle contracture early after stroke: a randomised trial. *Aust J Physiother* 2008;**54**:33–8.

50 Foley N, Teasell R, et al. *Upper extremity interventions. Evidence based review of stroke rehabilitation.* Available at: http://www.ebrsr.com/uploads/Module-10_upper-extremity_001.pdf (accessed 21 November 2011).

51 Lannin NA, Horsley SA, Herbert R, McCluskey A, Cusick A. Splinting the hand in the functional position after brain impairment: a randomized, controlled trial. *Arch Phys Med Rehabil* 2003;**84**: 297–302.

52 Lannin NA, Cusick A, McCluskey A, Herbert RD. Effects of Splinting on Wrist Contracture After Stroke: A Randomized Controlled Trial. *Stroke* 2007;**38**:111–16.

53 Ada L, Goddard E, McCully J, Stavrinos T, Bampton J. Thirty minutes of positioning reduces the development of shoulder external rotation contracture after stroke: a randomized controlled trial. *Arch Phys Med Rehabil* 2005;**86**:230–4.

54 Grissom SP, Blanton S. Treatment of upper motoneuron plantarflexion contractures by using an adjustable ankle-foot orthosis. *ArchPhys Med Rehabil* 2001;**82**:270–3.

55 Moseley AM. The effect of casting combined with stretching on passive ankle dorsiflexion in adults with traumatic head injuries. *PhysTher* 1997;**77**:240–7.

56 Verplancke D, Snape S, Salisbury CF, Jones PW, Ward AB. A randomized controlled trial of botulinum toxin on lower limb spasticity following acute acquired severe brain injury. *Clin Rehabil,* 2005;**19**;117–25.

57 Marshall S, Aubut J, Willems G, Teasell R, Lippert C. *Motor & sensory impairment remediation post acquired brain injury. Evidence based review of moderate to severe acquired brain injury.* Available at: http://www.abiebr.com/module/4-motor-sensory-impairment-remediation-post-acquired-brain-injury (accessed 21 November 2011).

58 Moseley AM, Hassett LM, Leung J, Clare JS, Herbert RD, Harvey LA. Serial casting versus positioning for the treatment of elbow contractures in adults with traumatic brain injury: a randomized controlled trial. *Clin Rehabil* 2008;**22**:406–17.

59 Harvey L, de Jong I, Goehl G, Marwedel S. Twelve weeks of nightly stretch does not reduce thumb web-space contractures in people with a neurological condition: a randomized controlled trial. *Aust J Physiother* 2006;**52**:251–8.

60 Ben M, Harvey L, Denis S, et al. Does 12 weeks of regular standing prevent loss of ankle mobility and bone mineral density in people with recent spinal cord injuries? *Aust J Physiother* 2005;**51**:251–6.

61 Harvey LA, Brosseau L, Herbert RD. Continuous passive motion following total knee arthroplasty in people with arthritis. *Cochrane Database Syst Rev* 2010;3:CD004260.

62 Delp SL, Statler K, Carroll NC. Preserving plantar flexion strength after surgical treatment for contracture of the triceps surae: a computer simulation study. *J Orthop Res* 1995;**13**:96–104.

63 Monument MJ, Hart DA, Befus AD, Salo PT, Zhang M, Hildebrand KA. The mast cell stabilizer ketotifen fumarate lessens contracture severity and myofibroblast hyperplasia: a study of a rabbit model of posttraumatic joint contractures. *J Bone Joint Surg Am* 2010;**92**:1468–77.

64 Garland DE. A clinical perspective on common forms of acquired heterotopic ossification. *Clin Orthop* 1991;**263**:13–29.

65 Teasell R, Aubut J, Marshall S, Cullen N. *Heterotopic ossification and venous thromboembolism. Evidence based review of moderate to severe acquire brain injury.* Available at: http://www.abiebr.com/module/11-heterotopic-ossification-venous-thromboembolism (accessed 21 November 2011).

66 Teasell R, Mehta S, Aubut J, et al. *Heterotopic ossification. Spinal cord injury rehabilitation evidence.* Available at: http://www.scireproject.com/rehabilitation-evidence/heterotopic-ossification. (accessed 21 November 2011).

67 Vanden Bossche L, Vanderstraeten G. Heterotopic ossification: a review. *J Rehabil Med* 2005;**37**: 129–36.

68 Coelho CV, Beraldo PS. Risk factors of heterotopic ossification in traumatic spinal cord injury. *Arq Neuropsiquiatr* 2009;**67**:382–7.

69 Clements NC, Camili AE. Heterotopic ossification complicating critical illness. *Chest* 1993;**104**: 1526–8.

70 Goodman TA, Merkel PA, Perlmutter G, Doyle MK, Krane SM, Polisson RP. Heterotopic ossification in the setting of neuromuscular blockade. *Arthritis Rheum* 1997;**40**:1619–27.

71 Herridge MS, Cheung AM, Tansey CM, et al. One-year outcomes in survivors of the acute respiratory distress syndrome. *N Engl J Med* 2003;**348**:683–93.

72 Jacobs JW, De Sonnaville PB, Hulsmans HM, van Rinsum AC, Bijlsma JW. Polyarticular heterotopic ossification complicating critical illness. *Rheumatology (Oxford)* 1999;**38**:1145–9.

73 van Kuijk AA, Geurts AC, van Kuppevelt HJ. Neurogenic ossification in spinal cord injury. *Spinal Cord* 2002;**40**:313–26.

74 Sugita A, Hashimoto J, Maeda A, et al. Heterotopic ossification in bilateral knee and hip joints after long-term sedation. *J Bone Miner Metab* 2005;**23**:329–32.

75 Chen HC, Yang JY, Chuang SS, Huang CY, Yang SY. Heterotopic ossification in burns: our experience and literature reviews. *Burns* 2009;**35**:857–62.

76 Peterson SL, Mani MM, Crawford CM, et al. Postburn heterotopic ossification: insights for management decision making. *J Trauma* 1989;**29**:365–9

77 Banovac K, Gonzalez F. Evaluation and management of heterotopic ossification in patients with spinal cord injury. *Spinal Cord* 1997;**35**:158–62.

78 Banovac K, Williams JM, Patrick LD, Haniff YM. Prevention of heterotopic ossification after spinal cord injury with indomethacin. *Spinal Cord* 2001;**39**:370–4.

79 Dellestable F, Voltz C, Mariot J, Perrier JF, Gaucher A. Heterotopic ossification complicating long-term sedation. *Br J Rheumatol* 1996;**35**:700–1.

80 Freed JH, Hahn H, Menter R, Dillon T. The use of the three-phase bone scan in the early diagnosis of heterotopic ossification (HO) and in the evaluation of didronel therapy. *Paraplegia* 1982;**20**:208–16.

81 Orzel JA, Rudd TG. Heterotopic bone formation: clinical, laboratory, and imaging correlation. *J Nucl Med* 1985;**26**:125–32.

82 Singh RS, Craig MC, Katholi CR, Jackson AB, Mountz JM. The predictive value of creatine phosphokinase and alkaline phosphatase in identification of heterotopic ossification in patients after spinal cord injury. *Arch Phys Med Rehabil* 2003;**84**:1584–8.

83 Sherman AL, Williams J, Patrick L, Banovac K. The value of serum creatine kinase in early diagnosis of heterotopic ossification. *J Spinal Cord Med* 2003;**26**:227–30.

84 Estrores IM, Harrington A, Banovac K. C-reactive protein and erythrocyte sedimentation rate in patients with heterotopic ossification after spinal cord injury. *J Spinal Cord Med* 2004;**27**:434–7.

85 Parikh J, Hyare H, Saifuddin A. The imaging features of post-traumatic myositis ossificans, with emphasis on MRI. *Clin Radiol* 2002;**57**:1058–66.

86 Argyropoulou MI, Kostandi E, Kosta P, et al. Heterotopic ossification of the knee joint in intensive care unit patients: early diagnosis with magnetic resonance imaging. *Crit Care* 2006;**10**:R152.

87 Cullen N, Perera J. Heterotopic ossification: pharmacologic options. *J Head Trauma Rehabil* 2009;**24**: 69–71.

88 Banovac K, Williams JM, Patrick LD, Levi A. Prevention of heterotopic ossification after spinal cord injury with COX-2 selective inhibitor (rofecoxib). *Spinal Cord* 2004;**42**:707–10.

89 Fransen M, Neal B. Non-steroidal anti-inflammatory drugs for preventing heterotopic bone formation after hip arthroplasty. *Cochrane Database Syst Rev* 2004;**3**:CD001160.

90 Burd TA, Lowry KJ, Anglen JO. Indomethacin compared with localized irradiation for the prevention of heterotopic ossification following surgical treatment of acetabular fractures. *J Bone Joint Surg Am* 2001;**83A**:1783–8.

91 Macfarlane RJ, Ng BH, Gamie Z, et al. Pharmacological treatment of heterotopic ossification following hip and acetabular surgery. *Expert Opin Pharmacother* 2008;**9**:767–86.

92 **Moore KD, Goss K, Anglen JO.** Indomethacin versus radiation therapy for prophylaxis against heterotopic ossification in acetabular fractures: a randomised, prospective study. *J Bone Joint Surg Br* 1998;**80**:259–63.

93 **Aubut JA, Mehta S, Cullen N, Teasell RW;** ERABI Group; Scire Research Team. A comparison of heterotopic ossification treatment within the traumatic brain and spinal cord injured population: An evidence based systematic review. *NeuroRehabilitation* 2011;**28**:151–60.

94 **Spielman G, Gennarelli T, Rogers CR.** Disodium etidronate: its role in preventing heterotopic ossification in severe head injury. *Arch Phys Med Rehabil* 1983;**64**:539–42.

95 **Stover S.** Disodium etidronate in the prevention of heterotopic ossification following spinal cord injury. *Paraplegia* 1976;**4**:146–56.

96 **Stover SL.** Didronel in the prevention of heterotopic ossification following spinal cord injury: Determination of an optimal treatment schedule. *Rehabil R D Prog Rep* 1987;**25**:110–11.

97 **Shafer DM, Bay C, Caruso DM, Foster KN.** The use of eidronate disodium in the prevention of heterotopic ossification in burn patients. *Burns* 2008;**34**:355–60.

98 **Ayers DC, Pelligrini VD, Evarts CM.** Prevention of heterotopic ossification in high-risk patients by radiation therapy. *Clin Orthop* 1991;**263**:87–93.

99 **Vavken P, Castellani L, Sculco TP.** Prophylaxis of heterotopic ossification of the hip: systematic review and meta-analysis. *Clin Orthop Relat Res* 2009;**467**:3283–9.

100 **Blokhuis TJ, Frolke JP.** Is radiation superior to indomethacin to prevent heterotopic ossification in acetabular fractures?: a systematic review. *Clin Orthop Relat Res* 2009;**467**:526–30.

101 **Burd TA, Hughes MS, Anglen JO.** Heterotopic ossification prophylaxis with indomethacin increases the risk of long-bone nonunion. *J Bone Joint Surg Br* 2003;**85**:700–5.

102 **Hamid N.** Radiation therapy for heterotopic ossification prophylaxis acutely after elbow trauma: a prospective randomized study. *J Bone Joint Surg Am* 2010; **92**:2032–8.

103 **Banovac K, Gonzalez F, Wade N, Bowker JJ.** Intravenous disodium etidronate therapy in spinal cord injury patients with heterotopic ossification. *Paraplegia* 1993;**31**:660–6.

104 **Banovac K.** The effect of etidronate on late development of heterotopic ossification after spinal cord injury. *J Spinal Cord Med* 2000;**23**:40–4.

105 **Garland DE.** Diphosphonate treatment for heterotopic ossification in spinal cord injury patients. *Clin Orthop Relat Res* 1983;**176**:197–200.

106 **Lippin Y, Shvoron A, Faibel M, Tsur H.** Vocal cords dysfunction resulting from heterotopic ossification in a patient with burns. *J Burn Care Rehabil* 1994;**15**:169–73.

107 **Tepperman PS, Hilbert L, Peters WJ, et al.** Heterotopic ossification in burns. *J Burn Care Rehabil* 1984;**5**:283–7.

108 **Sautter-Bihl ML, Liebermeister E, Nanassy A.** Radiotherapy as a local treatment option for heterotopic ossifications in patients with spinal cord injury. *Spinal Cord* 2000;**38**:33–6.

109 **Sautter-Bihl ML, Hultenschmidt B, Liebermeister E, Nanassy A.** Fractionated and single-dose radiotherapy for heterotopic bone formation in patients with spinal cord injury. A phase-I/II study. *Strahlenther Onkol* 2001;**177**:200–5.

110 **Citak M, Backhaus M, Kalicke T, et al.** Treatment of heterotopic ossification after spinal cord injury—clinical outcome after single-dose radiation therapy. *Z Orthop Unfall* 2011;**149**:90–3.

111 **Charnley G, Judet T, Garreau DL, Mollaret O.** Excision of heterotopic ossification around the knee following brain injury. *Injury* 1996;**27**:125–8.

112 **de Palma L, Rapali S, Paladini P, Ventura A.** Elbow heterotopic ossification in head-trauma patients: diagnosis and treatment. *Orthopedics* 2002;**25**:665–8.

113 **Ippolito E, Formisano R, Caterini R, Farsetti P, Penta F.** Operative treatment of heterotopic hip ossification in patients with coma after brain injury. *Clin Orthop Relat Res* 1999;**365**:130–8.

114 **Ippolito E, Formisano R, Caterini R, Farsetti P, Penta F.** Resection of elbow ossification and continuous passive motion in postcomatose patients. *J Hand Surg Am* 1999;**24**:546–53.

115 **Fuller DA, Mark A, Keenan MA.** Excision of heterotopic ossification from the knee: a functional outcome study. *Clin Orthop Relat Res* 2005;**438**:197–203.

116 **Kolessar DJ, Katz SD, Keenan MA.** Functional outcome following surgical resection of heterotopic ossification in patients with brain injury. *J Head Trauma Rehabil* 1996;**11**:78–87.

117 **Lazarus MD, Guttmann D, Rich CE, Keenan MAE.** Heterotopic ossification resection about the elbow. *NeuroRehabilitation* 1999;**12**:145–53.

118 **Melamed E, Robinson D, Halperin N, Wallach N, Keren O, Groswasser Z.** Brain injury-related heterotopic bone formation: treatment strategy and results. *Am.J Phys. Med Rehabil* 2002;**81**:670–4.

119 **Moore TJ.** Functional outcome following surgical excision of heterotopic ossification in patients with traumatic brain injury. *J Orthop Trauma* 1993;**7**:11–14.

120 **Garland DE, Orwin JF.** Resection of heterotopic ossification in patients with spinal cord injuries. *Clin Orthop Relat Res* 1989;**242**:169–276.

121 **Meiners T, Abel R, Bohm V, Gerner HJ.** Resection of heterotopic ossification of the hip in spinal cord injured patients. *Spinal Cord* 1997;**35**:443–5.

122 **Baldwin K, Hosalkar HS, Donegan DJ, Rendon N, Ramsey M, Keenan MA.** Surgical resection of heterotopic bone about the elbow: an institutional experience with traumatic and neurologic etiologies. *J Hand Surg Am* 2011;**36**:798–803.

123 **Maender C, Sahajpal D, Wright TW.** Treatment of heterotopic ossification of the elbow following burn injury: recommendations for surgical excision and perioperative prophylaxis using radiation therapy. *J Shoulder Elbow Surg* 2010;**19**:1269–75.

124 **Mitsionis GI, Lykissas MG, Kalos N, et al.** Functional outcome after excision of heterotopic ossification about the knee in ICU patients. *Int Orthop* 2009;**33**:1619–25.

125 **Tsionos I, Leclercq C, Rochet JM.** Heterotopic ossification of the elbow in patients with burns: results after early excision. *J Bone J Surg Br* 2004;**86B**:396–403.*il Med* 2005;**37**:129–36.

126 **Freebourn TM.** The treatment of immature heterotopic ossification in spinal cord injury with combination surgery, radiation therapy and NSAID. *Spinal Cord* 1999;**37**:50–3.

127 **Ippolito E, Formisano R, Farsetti P, Caterini R, Penta F.** Excision for the treatment of periarticular ossification of the knee in patients who have a traumatic brain injury. *J Bone Joint Surg Am* 1999;**81**:783–9.

128 **Chalidis B.** Early excision and late excision of heterotopic ossification after traumatic brain injury are equivalent: a systematic review of the literature. *J Neurotrauma* 2007;**24**:1675–86.

129 **Nierman DM, Mechanick JI.** Bone hyperresorption is prevalent in chronically critically ill patients. *Chest* 1998;**114**:1122–8.

130 **Orford NR, Saunders K, Merriman E, et al.** Skeletal morbidity among survivors of critical illness. *Crit Care Med* 2011;**39**:1295–300.

131 **Seccaricia D.** Cancer related hypercalcemia. *Can Fam Physician* 2010;**56**:244–6.

132 **Agus ZS.** Disorders of calcium and magnesium homeostasis. *Am J Med* 1982;**72**:473–88.

133 **Kraft MD, Btaiche IF, Sacks GS, Kudsk KA.** Treatment of electrolyte disorders in adult patients in the intensive care unit. *Am J Health Syst Pharm* 2005;**62**:1663–82.

134 **Woolf AD, Pfleger B.** Burden of major musculoskeletal conditions. *Bull World Health Organ* 2003;**81**:646–56.

135 **Pappaioannou A, Morin S, Cheung AM, et al.** 2010 clinical practice guidelines for the diagnosis and management of osteoporosis in Canada: summary. *CMAJ* 2010;**182**:1864–73.

136 **Griffith D.** Bone loss during critical illness: a skeleton in the closet for the intensive care unit survivor? *Crit Care Med* 2011;**39**:1554–5.

137 **South Paul J.** Osteoporosis: Part 1. *Am Fam Physician* 2001;**63**:897–904, 908.

138 **Templeton K.** Secondary osteoporosis. *J Am Acad Orthop Surg* 2005;**13**:475–86.

139 **Van den Berghe G, Van Roosbroeck, Wouters PJ, et al.** Bone turnover in prolonged critical illness: effect of vitamin D. *J Clin Endocrinol Metab* 2003;**88**:4623–32.

140 Via MA, Gallagher EJ, Mechanick JI. Bone physiology and therapeutics in chronic critical illness. *Ann N Y Acad Sci* 2010;**1211**:85–94.

141 Hollander JM, Mechanick JI. Nutrition support and the chronic critical illness syndrome. *Nutr Clin Pract* 2006;**21**:587–604.

142 Frazao J. Adynamic bone disease: clinical and therapeutic implications. *Curr Opin Nephrol Hypertens* 2009;**18**:303–7.

143 National Kidney Foundation. K/DOQI clinical practice guidelines for bone metabolism and disease in chronic kidney disease. *Am J Kidney Dis* 2003;42(4 Suppl 3):S1–201.

144 Via MA. Intravenous ibandronate acutely reduces bone hyperresorption in chronic critical illness. *J Intensive Care Med* 2012;**27**:312–18.

145 Nierman DM, Mechanick JI. Biochemical response to treatment of bone hyperresorption in chronically critically ill patients. *Chest* 2000;**118**:761–6.

146 Hollander JM, Mechanick J. Bisphosphonates and metabolic bone disease in the ICU. *Curr Opin Clin Nutr Metab Care* 2009;**12**:190–5.

147 Garland DE, Blum CE, Waters RL. Periarticular heterotopic ossification in head-injured adults. Incidence and location. *J Bone Joint Surg. Am* 1980;**62**:1143–6.

148 Simonsen LL, Sonne-Holm S, Krasheninnikoff M, Engberg AW. Symptomatic heterotopic ossification after very severe traumatic brain injury in 114 patients: incidence and risk factors. *Injury* 2007;**38**:1146–50.

149 Larsen L, Wright HH. Para-articular ossification, a complication of anterior poliomyelitis; a case report. *Radiology* 1957;**69**:103–5.

150 Ohnmar H, Roohi SA, Naicker AS. Massive heterotopic ossification in Guillain-Barré syndrome: a rare case report. *Clin Ter* 2010;**161**:529–32.

151 Giannoudis PV, Grotz MR, Papakostidis C, Dinopoulos H. Operative treatment of displaced fractures of the acetabulum: a meta-analysis. *J Bone Joint Surg Br* 2005;**87**:2–9.

152 Brooker AF, Bowerman JW, Robinson RA, Riley RH Jr. Ectopic ossification following total hip replacement. Incidence and method of classification. *J Bone Joint Surg Am* 1973;**55**:1629–32.

153 Kocic M, Lazovic M, Mitkovic M, Djokic B. Clinical significance of the heterotopic ossification after total hip arthroplasty. *Orthopedics* 2010;**33**:16.

154 Sambrook PN, Chen CJ, March L, et al. High bone turnover is an independent predictor of mortality in the frail elderly. *J Bone Miner Res* 2006;**21**:549–55.

155 Ruml LA, Dubois SK, Roberts ML, Pak CY. Prevention of hypercalciuria and stone-forming propensity during prolonged bedrest by alendronate. *J Bone Miner Res* 1995;**10**:655–62.

156 Tsunashima Y. Hydrocortisone inhibits cellular proliferation by downregulating hepatocyte growth factor synthesis in human osteoblasts. *Biol Pharm Bull* 2011;**34**:700–3.

157 Rejnmark L. Loop diuretics increase bone turnover and decrease BMD in osteopenic postmenopausal women: results from a randomized controlled study with bumetanide. *J Bone Miner Res* 2006;**21**:163–70.

Part 5

Biological Mechanisms of Injury and Repair

Chapter 26

Introduction: Biological Mechanisms of Injury and Repair

Robert D. Stevens

This section is devoted to biological mechanisms underpinning organ dysfunction and repair in critical illness. Decades of research in intensive care have centred on the characterization and modulation of physiological perturbations; an emphasis on biological mechanisms is a welcome, albeit much more recent, development. Basic and translational research has generated fundamental insights into the biology of conditions, such as sepsis and ARDS, and has suggested important new therapeutic paradigms. Notwithstanding this progress, effective and safe therapies targeting specific cellular or molecular processes do not exist for the majority of patients suffering from such life-threatening conditions.[1]

The translation of mechanistic hypotheses from the experimental setting into clinically effective interventions poses many challenges. Recent analyses indicate that assumptions of generalizability in well-established animal models of severe illness may be invalid.[2,3,4] This translational gap can only be closed via a thorough reappraisal of disease models and experimental paradigms. The understanding of how tissues and organs undergo repair or remodelling during disease and following severe injury, a central theme of this book, is likely to generate many new insights into the post-critical illness recovery process. The pathophysiologic continuum which extends from acute illness to recovery is heavily determined by premorbid factors, such as genetic susceptibility (Chapter 27), and the degree of cognitive (Chapter 29) or physiological reserve, or deficiency thereof, as discussed in the chapter on frailty (Chapter 28). In addition, recent work has highlighted extremely dynamic cellular systems capable of regenerating and reorganizing tissues after ARDS, AKI (Chapter 30), myocardial ischaemia (Chapter 31), and critical illness muscle wasting (Chapter 35). Collectively, this research has opened a new window on reparative mechanisms which, together with the burgeoning science of regenerative biology and medicine, is likely to effect a major transformation in our approach to the treatment of critically ill patients.

The long-term burdens of critical illness are largely a consequence of neurologic or musculoskeletal injuries incurred in the setting of acute illness.[5,6] The mechanisms underlying these injuries are being progressively unravelled, as detailed in the chapters treating on sepsis-associated encephalopathy (SAE) (Chapter 32), CIP (Chapter 33), and structural muscle alterations in critical illness (Chapter 34). Inferences from this research have already suggested important new treatment possibilities, as discussed in Chapters 37 and 46 of this book.

References

1 **Dyson A, Singer M.** Animal models of sepsis: why does preclinical efficacy fail to translate to the clinical setting? *Crit Care Med* 2009;**37**:S30–7.
2 **Seok J, Warren HS, Cuenca AG, et al.** Genomic responses in mouse models poorly mimic human inflammatory diseases. *Proc Natl Acad Sci USA* 2013;**110**:3507–12.

3 **Perel P, Roberts I, Sena E, et al.** Comparison of treatment effects between animal experiments and clinical trials: systematic review. *BMJ* 2007;**334**:197.

4 **Fisher M, Feuerstein G, Howells DW, et al.** Update of the stroke therapy academic industry roundtable preclinical recommendations. *Stroke* 2009;**40**:2244–50.

5 **Herridge MS, Tansey CM, Matte A, et al., and Canadian Critical Care Trials.** Functional disability 5 years after acute respiratory distress syndrome. *N Engl J Med* 2011;**364**:1293–304.

6 **Iwashyna TJ, Ely EW, Smith DM, Langa KM.** Long-term cognitive impairment and functional disability among survivors of severe sepsis. *JAMA* 2010;**304**:1787–94.

Chapter 27

Genetic Determinants of Sepsis Outcomes

Sachin Yende and Derek C. Angus

Introduction

Infection and severe sepsis are a leading cause of hospital admission and admission to non-coronary ICUs.[1] Although genetics may modify long-term outcomes of several critical illnesses, we will focus on understanding the role of genetics in infection and severe sepsis. This chapter will also review common long-term sequelae of sepsis and potential biological mechanisms and provide a broad outline of commonly used terminology and study designs to ascertain the role of genetic variation in critical care. Genetics may provide insights into biological mechanisms and allow more precise use of interventions. Using targeted therapy (pharmacogenetics or pharmacogenomics), based on an individual's genetic make-up, rather than using it on all patients, is an appealing strategy. We will also examine the role of epigenetics, because several studies suggest that epigenetic changes may occur in severe sepsis due to exposure of cells to the inflammatory environment.[2] The role of epigenetic changes in several conditions that impair recovery after sepsis, such as atherosclerosis[3] and cancer,[4] and other chronic inflammatory conditions, such as rheumatoid arthritis,[5] has been well described. It is therefore rational to consider epigenetics plays an important role in the sequelae of critical illness.

Common sequelae of infection and severe sepsis

Mortality

Although estimates vary, the 1-year mortality after pneumonia varies between 23 and 35%.[6-9] The high mortality persists, even after 1 year, and may remain elevated up to 7 years after the initial hospitalization.[10] In contrast to high long-term mortality, short-term mortality at 28 or 90 days or hospital mortality after pneumonia is less than 10%. Understanding the mechanisms underlying increased long-term mortality are therefore important.

Whether high mortality is due to the acute illness or poor chronic health status before pneumonia and sepsis is difficult to tease out. It is unclear which patients should be included in a control group to compare long-term mortality of sepsis survivors. Furthermore, cross-sectional studies have little information regarding prior events, which may influence long-term trajectories.

Several lines of evidence suggest that sepsis may increase long-term mortality. Individuals hospitalized for pneumonia have 1- and 5-year mortality similar to those hospitalized for chronic diseases, such as CHF, or acute conditions with long-term sequelae such as cerebrovascular accident and hip fracture.[8] The high mortality among pneumonia survivors persists when adjusted for health behaviours, chronic disease burden, and nutritional markers.[6,8,11] Thus, although pneumonia and sepsis are often conceptualized as an acute illness, survivors of the initial hospitalization experience high long-term mortality, compared to individuals with similar chronic health profile.

Understanding the causes of high long-term mortality among survivors of pneumonia and sepsis, especially after hospital discharge, is difficult. Causes of death listed in death certificates are often unreliable, and causes of death for subjects who die at home or in long-term care settings are difficult to ascertain. An alternative approach is to examine the causes of subsequent hospitalizations among survivors of sepsis hospitalization. Cardiovascular disease, including ischaemic heart disease, CHF, and stroke, exacerbation of chronic respiratory disease, repeat infections, and cancer are leading causes of death and repeat hospitalization. These results suggest that sepsis survivors incur high mortality, but causes of death are similar to the general population.

Morbidity

A large body of literature has reported and investigated the non-mortal sequelae after critical illness, sepsis, or ARDS. Morbid sequelae include worsening of kidney disease, cardiovascular disease, physical dysfunction, cognitive impairment, depression, and reduced QoL.

Mechanisms of long-term sequelae

Mechanisms underlying long-term sequelae remain poorly understood. In general, mechanisms that may play a role in long-term sequelae include those underlying chronic disease and ageing that are activated prior to the acute illness, those that are activated during the acute infection, effects of therapies, and pathways that may fail to resolve after infection (see Figure 27.1). Certain

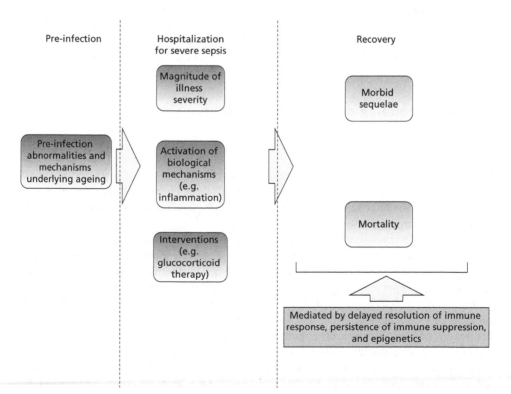

Fig. 27.1 Mechanisms of long-term sequelae of sepsis.

mechanisms may disproportionately influence some sequelae. For example, levels of circulating inflammatory markers may be increased in older adults and in those who are at higher risk of developing an infection. Levels of inflammatory markers are logfold higher during the acute infection, and these levels may be modified by therapeutic interventions, such as GC therapy, and may not resolve in a subset during recovery. Higher levels of these markers may cause instability of the atherosclerotic plaque and increase risk of acute cardiovascular events and may possibly worsen muscle weakness.

Ageing and senescence

Several pathways implicated in ageing and senescence could play an important role in long-term sequelae of critical illness. Several lines of evidence suggest that oxidative stress may play a role in ageing, severe sepsis, and several long-term sequelae of sepsis such as cardiovascular disease. For example, overexpression of p66, silencing of silent information regulator (Sir) proteins (whose mammalian homologue is Sirtuin), and impaired functioning of hormonal pathways (e.g. insulin-like growth factor)[12,13] have been hypothesized to play an important role in lifespan regulation. A mutation in the gene encoding p66 extends the lifespans of mice by about 30%.[14] In line with the free radical theory of ageing, several animal models of lifespan regulation (*C. elegans*, *Drosophila*, and mice) suggest that increased oxidative damage accelerates ageing and increased resistance to oxidative damage can extend lifespan.[13] Cells from p66 mutants are resistant to oxidative stress, while increased p66shc expression within cells may worsen the detrimental effects of reactive oxygen species (ROS).[15]

Oxidative stress is increased in severe sepsis and associated with organ dysfunction.[16] Furthermore, reactive oxygen and nitrogen species may play a role in cardiovascular disease due to their effects on the atherosclerotic plaque and endothelium. For instance, oxidation of low-density lipoprotein (LDL) is essential for uptake by macrophages and for foam cell formation, a key step in plaque formation. Nitric oxide (NO) interacts with superoxide to form peroxynitrate, which can lead to lipid peroxidation and the formation of several NO-derived species, which worsen endothelial function and increase the risk of plaque rupture.[16,17] p66 also accelerates vascular ageing.

Animal studies have shown that p66 plays an important role in age-dependent endothelial dysfunction and p66shc knockout mice have reduced atherosclerosis.[15,18] Thus, mechanisms underlying ageing may be accelerated during severe sepsis and worsen long-term outcomes of critically ill patients.

Immune suppression and resolution

Many patients who develop severe sepsis die due to health care-acquired infections. Furthermore, a common cause of re-hospitalization and death among older adults hospitalized for pneumonia is repeat infections. Thus, alterations in immune response to infection have been hypothesized to play a role in the sequelae of severe sepsis. Several terms are used to describe this phenomenon, including immunoparalysis, lipopolysaccharide (LPS) tolerance, immune remodelling, leucocyte deactivation, and sepsis-inducted immune suppression. A recent study measured several immune suppression markers and the ability to express pro-inflammatory cytokines from spleen and lung antigen-presenting cells in ICU patients who died due to severe sepsis.[19] Results of this study were similar to prior observational studies where immune suppression measures were examined in peripheral blood and showed that many of these patients had severe immune suppression, which may place them at higher risk of subsequent infections. Whether immune suppression occurs when patients recover from critical illness and are discharged from the hospital is not known.

Several preclinical studies also suggest that the resolution of the immune response following an infection is an active and coordinated process.[20,21] Abnormalities in the resolution of inflammation may lead to persistent unresolved inflammation and worsen long-term outcomes. For example, lipoxins, an important mediator of the oxidative stress pathway, have been suggested to play an important role in the resolution of infection.[20,22]

Role of genetics in long-term sequelae

Genetic studies could be used to understand the mechanisms of long-term sequelae. For example, TNF hypersecretor genotypes may be associated with persistently elevated pro-inflammatory levels during recovery. Similarly, PAI-1 hypersecretor genotypes are associated with high risk of pneumonia; PAI-1 levels are increased during sepsis, and hypersecretor genotypes are associated with high risk of cardiovascular disease. Understanding the relationship between PAI-1 genotypes and late outcomes may improve the understanding of the potential role of PAI-1 in long-term sequelae.

Pharmacogenetic studies may help to establish the risk-benefit profile for sepsis therapies. For instance, GC therapy may be more beneficial in individuals who have genetic variants associated with GC resistance such genetic variants within the GC receptor. GC therapy have short- and long-term adverse effects such as secondary infection and reduced long-term physical function. GC therapy could be customized to those who are most likely to benefit from GC therapy, based on an individual's genetic profile.

Finally, measuring genome-wide markers, described later, and determining their association with long-term morbid sequelae could be used to identify novel pathways that mediate long-term sequelae of critical illness.

Mendelian traits or diseases, such as sickle cell disease or cystic fibrosis, are influenced by a single gene. In contrast, most critical illnesses are multifactorial diseases and called 'complex traits' in genetic parlance. Severe sepsis, and its long-term sequelae, is an example of complex traits. For example, physical dysfunction following sepsis may be mediated by pre-illness muscle strength, genetic variations within inflammatory mediators, such as TNFs, and medications, such as GC therapy and neuromuscular blockers received during the acute illness. The relative contribution of host genetic factors in complex traits, such as severe sepsis, is probably modest.

Focusing only on the contribution of genetic variation to disease, the exact pattern of genetic variation influencing complex traits is still unclear, and several theories have been proposed.[23] One model, termed the common disease-rare variant model, suggests that phenotypic variation in complex traits is due to numerous rare genetic variants at multiple loci, with each variant single-handedly causing disease. Although the frequency of each rare variant is low, populations may have several such variants.

In contrast, the common disease-common variant model suggests that common variants underlie complex traits and may be more common in critical care. Such variants may be maintained through generations due to some form of balancing selection where the same genetic variant may be protective for certain diseases and harmful in others. This model may be particularly important in critical illnesses, which often occur due to differences in expression of inflammatory mediators. A robust pro-inflammatory response with TNF and IL-6 release may increase the risk of complications like severe sepsis or ARDS; yet that same response may be critical for an adequate host response to infection. Therefore, genetic variants associated with a pro-inflammatory response could be protective and detrimental under different conditions. An example of balancing selection is the guanine to adenine transition at the +250 site within the lymphotoxin alpha gene, which is associated with increased TNF expression, and also associated with higher risk of severe sepsis but lower risk of PMV after coronary artery bypass graft surgery.[24,25] Complex traits may also occur due to a combination of rare and common variants. Finally, interactions may occur among genes (epistasis) and with environmental factors (gene-environment interactions) to influence the phenotype.

Genetic nomenclature

Polymorphism, mutation, and SNPs

Nucleotides are the building blocks of deoxyribonucleic acid (DNA) and contain one of the following four bases: adenine (A), thymine (T), guanine (G), and cytosine (C). Substitution of one of the four base pairs by another base pair is called single nucleotide polymorphism (SNP or mutation). For example, an SNP may change the DNA sequence from GATAA to GGTAA. Polymorphism and mutations are heritable changes in the DNA sequence. Typically, the frequency of mutations is low (<1%), whereas polymorphisms occur more frequently. Variable number of tandem repeats (VNTR) is also a type of polymorphism where a particular repetitive sequence is present in different numbers in different individuals. An example of a tandem repeat is the tetra-nucleotide $(CATT)_n$ repeat within the promoter region of the macrophage inhibitory factor (MIF) gene where subjects can have five, six, seven, or eight repeats.[26]

The genes in the human genome account for a very small fraction of the total DNA, and more than 90% of the sequences between genes do not encode for any particular protein.[27] Variations within DNA are common, and SNPs occur every 1000 base pairs in the human genome, and most SNPs do not lead to changes in protein structure or secretion. When SNPs lead to changes in amino acids, they are called non-synonymous, or missense, SNPs. Some of the non-synonymous SNPs in the coding region may affect protein structure and lead to alterations in phenotype. An example is the G to A coding polymorphism at the +1691 site in the factor V gene of the coagulation cascade.[28] This polymorphism leads to the substitution of an arginine to a glutamine at amino acid position 506, which is one of the cleavage sites for activated protein C. Factor V inactivation is delayed, because the cleavage site is not present, and leads to a hypercoagulable state.

SNPs in the promoter region do not affect protein structure, but they may affect binding of transcription factors and alter expression of the protein in response to an appropriate stimulus. For example, an insertion/deletion polymorphism, termed 4G/5G, is found 675 base pairs upstream of the transcriptional initiation site in the PAI-1 gene.[29,30] Although both alleles bind a transcriptional activator, the 5G allele reduces transcription by binding a repressor protein and is associated with lower circulating PAI-1 concentrations.[31,32]

Most SNPs have no effect on the phenotype, because they are either in non-coding regions or they are synonymous SNPs. Of the SNPs in the non-coding region, those in the 5' or 3' untranslated region (UTR) are probably more important than those in introns, which is a non-coding sequence of DNA that is initially copied into the ribonucleic acid (RNA) but is cut out of the final RNA transcript. They may play critical roles in the post-transcriptional regulation of gene expression, including modulation of the transport of messenger RNAs (mRNAs) out of the nucleus and stabilization of protein.[33] It is important to understand these distinctions when choosing SNPs during candidate gene analysis for causal variants. In general, the promoter region and non-synonymous SNPs are likely to be more important than those in the non-coding region.

Linkage disequilibrium and haplotype blocks

Knowing the causal SNP may often be difficult. Many of the SNPs 'associated' with a specific phenotype are simply a 'marker', rather than the causal variant. These markers are co-inherited, along with the causal variant, because they tend to be on the same piece of DNA. This phenomenon where two genetic variants are inherited together through generations is called linkage disequilibrium (LD). Several methods can be used to measure LD. Two most commonly used are Lewontin D' and R^2. Both are measures of correlation and expressed on a scale of 0 to 1, with a higher number indicating greater LD or these SNPs are more likely to be inherited together. These measures of LD are statistical measurements in population genetics and do not necessarily imply distance between the two sites. LD maps for SNPs within a single gene are available publicly and provide important insights into choosing marker SNPs for candidate gene analysis. During meiosis, pieces of maternal and paternal DNA are exchanged via recombination. However, markers in LD remain tightly linked and are transmitted through generations as regions of DNA called haplotype blocks. Once an association is determined between a marker and disease, one could focus on the 'block' of DNA to identify the causal polymorphism. These 'blocks' can be identified, or tagged, by one or more polymorphisms on the block. Depending on the size of the gene, often the entire gene or all variants within the haplotype block can be sequenced to identify coding variants.

Study design for genetic studies

Two broad approaches are used to assess the role of genetic variants in disease: linkage analysis and association studies. **Linkage** analysis follows meiotic events through families for co-segregation of disease and genetic variant. In contrast to chronic illnesses, such as diabetes, obtaining an accurate family history about critical illnesses in the past, such as whether a family member developed ARDS after pneumonia, is difficult. Therefore, this approach is less useful in acute illnesses and has not been used widely in the critically ill. In contrast to linkage analysis, **association** studies detect the association between genetic variants and disease across individuals in large populations. Most association studies are population-based, but family-based studies, using parents-affected child trios (transmission disequilibrium test, TDT), can also be conducted. This design tests for an association between a specific allele and disease in the child by testing whether heterozygous parents transmit this allele to affected children more frequently than expected.[34]

Genome-wide association studies

Regardless of the overall study design, one also needs to decide the methodology to examine genetic variation. There are two general approaches: genome wide association studies (GWAS) and candidate gene association studies. GWAS are philosophically similar to whole genome linkage analyses where the investigator does not have an a priori idea of the susceptibility locus but is trying to locate a chromosomal region that is associated with the 'disease' of interest.[35] This approach is hypothesis-generating, and results should be validated. GWAS can be used to identify new pathways or proteins that may play a role in outcomes of a disease. Although GWAS are expensive to conduct, advances in technology are rapidly reducing costs. Current GWAS chips include between 700 000 and 5 million SNPs. Using LD, additional genotypes can be imputed. For instance, a chip that has 700 000 SNPs can be imputed up to 2 million SNPs, using either Hapmap data or data from the 1000 Genome Project. Whole genome sequencing is also increasingly available, and future studies may routinely include this technology. Customized chips with only coding SNPs, which have higher likelihood of being functional, are also available.

Candidate gene approach

The candidate gene approach examines the role of genetic variation in one or more genes most likely to be involved in the biological pathway. This approach requires an understanding of the biological mechanisms to identify candidate genes and is commonly used, because it is technologically non-intensive and relatively inexpensive. Most of the older studies used candidate gene approach. However, recent studies have used a hybrid approach where a GWAS is used to identify genetic variation spaced throughout the human genome, followed by a candidate gene approach to examine genes within the region of interest. For example, GWAS may identify few SNPs on a gene are associated with outcome. Many of these SNPs may not be functional. Additional candidate gene studies could be conducted where SNPs from different haplotype blocks could be selected and genotyped and their association with the outcome could be confirmed. Alternatively, the entire gene could be sequenced to identify potential causal variants.

Statistical issues in gene association studies

Power

Irrespective of study design, it is critical to have sufficient power to detect association. The relative risk for critical illness for individual loci would be small, with relative risk ≤ 2. In general, association studies may be more likely to provide statistical evidence of a disease gene with low relative risks than linkage studies.[36] However, approximately 1000 cases and 1000 controls will be required to detect modest relative risks of 1.5.[37] Larger sample sizes would be necessary for rare alleles (frequency <10%), whereas smaller samples sizes would be required if the relative risks are larger. Numerous statistical tools are available to determine sample sizes.

Multiple testing

There is no easy statistical solution to the problem of multiple testing. One of the current approaches is to use a false discovery rate (FDR) statistic to decide what proportion of true positives to false positives is acceptable to the investigator, choose a level of significance based on this proportion, and follow up on all results that achieve this level of significance.[38] GWAS conduct large number of comparisons (up to 2 million comparisons). A P value $<0.05 \times 10^{-8}$ is often considered as threshold to account for multiple testing. Lower thresholds of P value, such as 10^{-6}, can be used if results are validated, especially in multiple cohorts.

The strongest evidence that a particular variant or candidate gene is associated with a trait, and thus may be causal, or in strong LD with a causal variant, is to replicate the result.[39] Replication is defined as doing the analyses in a different population, using different methods to avoid introduction of bias.

Population admixture

Subpopulations within a population may have a different genetic architecture. Differences in frequency of genetic variants within the population may lead to false positive results. False positive associations between genetic marker and disease can occur due to association of disease with a subpopulation, rather than the genetic marker. Self-reported race is used commonly to stratify subjects to avoid ethnic stratification. Population admixture is more common among self-identified African American subjects, compared to those identifying themselves as of Caucasian ethnic origin.[40] Although population admixture does occur in most genetic association studies, the extent to which results would be affected is less clear. Techniques have been developed to detect and correct for population stratification by typing unlinked markers.[41–43] Whether this approach is adequate is controversial.[44]

Epigenetics

Epigenetics is the study of heritable changes in gene expression that is caused by mechanisms other than changes in the underlying DNA sequence. The Greek term *epi* refers to over or above; thus, epigenetics refers to genetic changes outside of the DNA. Often these changes do not involve a change in the nucleotide sequence. Of the various molecular mechanisms underlying epigenetic changes, two mechanisms may be particularly important. These include DNA methylation of CpG residues and histone-3 (H3) acetylation.[44,45] These modifications cause remodelling of chromatin, a complex of DNA and the histone proteins with which DNA associates. Histone proteins are little spheres that DNA wraps around, and histone modifications lead to changes in gene expression.

Increasing evidence suggests that epigenetic changes may occur in severe sepsis due to exposure of cells to the inflammatory environment.[2] The role of epigenetic changes in several conditions that impair recovery after sepsis, such as atherosclerosis[3] and cancer,[4] and other chronic inflammatory conditions, such as rheumatoid arthritis,[5] has been well described. Epigenetics may play a role in the delayed resolution of immune response after severe sepsis. For example, peripheral blood leucocytes are activated during sepsis and may undergo epigenetic changes. These cells may thereby increase the expression of pro-inflammatory molecules, delay the resolution of immune response, and lead to persistent inflammation. Epigenetic changes can be assessed in the whole genome or within promoter regions of specific proteins. Drugs targeting epigenetic mechanisms are being studied and could be tested to improve immune resolution after sepsis to reduce long-term sequelae of sepsis.

Conclusion

The incidence of common critical illnesses, such as infection and sepsis, is rising with ageing of the US population.[46] Improvements in ICU care have reduced short-term mortality,[47] with a subsequent increase in a population with long-term sequelae. The mechanisms underlying long-term mortality and morbid sequelae remain unclear. Genetic studies may improve understanding of these mechanisms and allow targeting of therapies to reduce long-term sequelae.

References

1 Angus DC, Linde-Zwirble WT, Lidicker J, Clermont G, Carcillo J, Pinsky MR. Epidemiology of severe sepsis in the United States: analysis of incidence, outcome, and associated costs of care. *Crit Care Med* 2001;**29**:1303–10.

2 McCall CE, Yoza BK. Gene silencing in severe systemic inflammation. *Am J Respir Crit Care Med* 2007;**175**:763–7.

3 Lund G, Andersson L, Lauria M, et al. DNA methylation polymorphisms precede any histological sign of atherosclerosis in mice lacking apolipoprotein. *J Biol Chem* 2004;**279**:29147–54.

4 Vakkila J, Lotze MT. Inflammation and necrosis promote tumour growth. *Nat Rev Immunol* 2004; **4**:641–8.

5 Karouzakis E, Gay RE, Gay S, Neidhart M. Epigenetic control in rheumatoid arthritis synovial fibroblasts. *Nat Rev Rheumatol* 2009;**5**:266–72.

6 Kaplan V, Clermont G, Griffin MF, et al. Pneumonia: still the old man's friend? *Arch Intern Med* 2003; **163**:317–23.

7 Weycker D, Akhras KS, Edelsberg J, Angus DC, Oster G. Long-term mortality and medical care charges in patients with severe sepsis. *Crit Care Med* 2003;**31**:2316–23.

8 Yende S, Angus DC, Ali IS, et al. Influence of comorbid conditions on long-term mortality after pneumonia in older people. *J Am Geriatr Soc* 2007;**55**:518–25.

9 Angus DC, Laterre PF, Helterbrand J, et al. The effect of drotrecogin alfa (activated) on long-term survival after severe sepsis. *Crit Care Med* 2004;**32**:2199–206.

10 Quartin AA, Schein RM, Kett DH, Peduzzi PN. Magnitude and duration of the effect of sepsis on survival. Department of veterans Affairs systemic sepsis cooperative studies group. *JAMA* 1997;**277**: 1058–63.

11 Wunsch H, Guerra C, Barnato AE, Angus DC, Li G, Linde-Zwirble WT. Three-year outcomes for medicare beneficiaries who survive intensive care. *JAMA* 2010;**303**:849–56.

12 Hajnoczky G, Hoek JB. Mitochondrial longevity pathways. *Science* 2007;**315**:607–9.

13 Guarente L, Kenyon C. Genetic pathways that regulate ageing in model organisms. *Nature* 2000;**408**: 255–62.

14 Migliaccio E, Giorgio M, Mele S, et al. The p66shc adaptor protein controls oxidative stress response and life span in mammals. *Nature* 1999;**402**:309–13.

15 Napoli C, Martin-Padura I, de Nigris F, et al. Deletion of the p66Shc longevity gene reduces systemic and tissue oxidative stress, vascular cell apoptosis, and early atherogenesis in mice fed a high-fat diet. *Proc Natl Acad Sci USA* 2003;**100**:2112–16.

16 Rudolph V, Freeman BA. Cardiovascular consequences when nitric oxide and lipid signaling converge. *Circ Res* 2009;**105**:511–22.

17 Baker PR, Schopfer FJ, O'Donnell VB, Freeman BA. Convergence of nitric oxide and lipid signaling: anti-inflammatory nitro-fatty acids. *Free Radic Biol Med* 2009;**46**:989–1003.

18 Francia P, delli Gatti C, Bachschmid M, et al. Deletion of p66shc gene protects against age-related endothelial dysfunction. *Circulation* 2004;**110**:2889–95.

19 Boomer JS, To K, Chang KC, et al. Immunosuppression in patients who die of sepsis and multiple organ failure. *JAMA* 2011;**306**:2594–605.

20 Serhan CN, Chiang N, Van Dyke TE. Resolving inflammation: dual anti-inflammatory and pro-resolution lipid mediators. *Nat Rev Immunol* 2008;**8**:349–61.

21 Serhan CN, Oliw E. Unorthodox routes to prostanoid formation: new twists in cyclooxygenase-initiated pathways. *J Clin Invest* 2001;**107**:1481–9.

22 Epstein SE, Zhu J, Najafi AH, Burnett MS. Insights into the role of infection in atherogenesis and in plaque rupture. *Circulation* 2009;**119**: 3133–41.

23 Zwick ME, Cutler DJ, Chakravarti A. Patterns of genetic variation in Mendelian and complex traits. *Annu Rev Genomics Hum Genet* 2000;**1**:387–407.

24 Mira JP, Cariou A, Grall F, et al. Association of TNF2, a TNF-α promoter polymorphism, with septic shock susceptibility and mortality. *JAMA* 1999;**282**:561–8.

25 Yende S, Quasney MW, Tolley E, Zhang Q, Wunderink RG. Association of tumor necrosis factor gene polymorphisms and prolonged mechanical ventilation after coronary artery bypass surgery. *Crit Care Med* 2003;**31**:133–40.

26 Donn RP, Shelley E, Ollier WE, Thomson W. A novel 5'-flanking region polymorphism of macrophage migration inhibitory factor is associated with systemic-onset juvenile idiopathic arthritis. *Arthritis Rheum* 2001;**44**:1782–5.

27 Stein LD. Human genome End of the beginning. *Nature* 2004;**431**:915–16.

28 Bertina RM, Koeleman BPC, Koster T, et al. Mutation in blood coagulation factor V associated with resistance to activated protein C. *Nature* 1994;**369**:64–7.

29 Dawson SJ, Wiman B, Hamsten A, Green F, Humphries S, Henney AM. The two allele sequences of a common polymorphism in the promoter of the plasminogen activator inhibitor-1 (PAI-1) gene respond differently to interleukin-1 in HepG2 cells. *J Biol Chem* 1993;**268**:10739–45.

30 Eriksson P, Kallin B, 't Hooft FM, Bavenholm P, Hamsten A. Allele–specific increase in basal transcription of the plasminogen–activator inhibitor 1 gene is associated with myocardial infarction. *Proc Natl Acad Sci USA* 1995;**92**:1851–5.

31 Westendorp RG, Hottenga JJ, Slagboom PE. Variation in plasminogen–activator–inhibitor–1 gene and risk of meningococcal septic shock. *Lancet* 1999;**354**:561–3.

32 Hermans PW, Hibberd ML, Booy R, et al. 4G/5G promoter polymorphism in the plasminogen–activator–inhibitor–1 gene and outcome of meningococcal disease. Meningococcal Research Group. *Lancet* 1999;**354**:556–60.

33 Mignone F, Gissi C, Liuni S, Pesole G. Untranslated regions of mRNAs. *Genome Biol* 2002;**3**: reviews0004.

34 Gauderman WJ. Candidate gene association analysis for a quantitative trait, using parent–offspring trios. *Genet Epidemiol* 2003;**25**:327–38.

35 Hirschhorn JN, Daly MJ. Genome–wide association studies for common diseases and complex traits. *Nat Rev Genet* 2005;**6**:95–108.

36 Risch NJ. Searching for genetic determinants in the new millennium. *Nature* 2000;**405**:847–56.

37 Reich D, Patterson N, Jager PLD, et al. A whole–genome admixture scan finds a candidate locus for multiple sclerosis susceptibility. *Nat Genet* 2005;**37**:1113–18.

38 Hochberg Y, Benjamini Y. More powerful procedures for multiple significance testing. *Stat Med* 1990; **9**:811–18.

39 de Bakker PIW, Yelensky R, Pe'er I, Gabriel SB, Daly MJ, Altshuler D. Efficiency and power in genetic association studies. *Nat Genet* 2005;**37**:1217–23.

40 Sinha M, Larkin EK, Elston RC, Redline S. Self-reported race and genetic admixture. *N Engl J Med* 2006;**354**:421–2.

41 Pritchard JK, Stephens M, Rosenberg NA, Donnelly P. Association mapping in structured populations. *Am J Hum Genet* 2000;**67**:170–81.

42 Ardlie KG, Lunetta KL, Seielstad M. Testing for population subdivision and association in four case-control studies. *Am J Hum Genet* 2002;**71**:304–11.

43 Freedman ML, Reich D, Penney KL, et al. Assessing the impact of population stratification on genetic association studies. *Nat Genet* 2004;**36**:388–93.

44 Cardon LR, Palmer LJ. Population stratification and spurious allelic association. *Lancet* 2003;**361**:598–604.

45 Hake SB, Garcia BA, Duncan EM, et al. Expression patterns and post-translational modifications associated with mammalian histone H3 variants. *J Biol Chem* 2006;**281**:559–68.

46 Simonsen L, Conn LA, Pinner RW, Teutsch SM. Trends in infectious disease hospitalizations in the United States 1980–94. *Arch Intern Med* 1998;**158**:1923–8.

47 Martin GS, Mannino DM, Eaton S, Moss M. The epidemiology of sepsis in the United States from 1979 through 2000. *N Engl J Med* 2003;**348**:1546–54.

Chapter 28

Physiological Reserve and Frailty in Critical Illness

Robert C. McDermid and Sean M. Bagshaw

Introduction

Physicians have long desired for an operational definition of 'physiologic age'. This is borne out of the multitude of examples of patients with greater or lesser burdens of disease than is typical for their age and their uncertain responses to illness, making prognostication and therapeutic decision making challenging. This has led physicians to consider the concept 'physiologic reserve', rather than chronologic age, as a principal determinant of survival and functional outcomes following an episode of critical illness. In this model, the baseline state of health of an individual can be viewed as the interaction of one's individual genetic disposition with their cumulative exposures to acute and/or chronic illness occurring over their lifespan. In this chapter, we will explore the concept of the recently defined geriatric syndrome of frailty as a potential marker of 'physiologic age' and its relevance to the critical illness.

Loss of biologic complexity and the concept of physiologic reserve

The human body is a complex biologic system that has the ability to withstand and adapt to a multitude of external environmental stressors. This system is normally characterized by a highly elaborate response to such stressors, although its apparent internal randomness has an overall stability and structure to it.[1] Over the past two decades, the application of the discipline of non-linear dynamics ('chaos theory') to biologic systems has brought some clarity to, and understanding of, the processes underlying their function. The complexity of a system (which is a mathematical description of the number of ways the system can detect a change in its baseline state, process that change, and generate a distinct response) determines the system's ability to adapt to baseline changes and resiliency to catastrophic failure. When faced with a stimulus, the biologic system reacts to the change, mounting a focused, multi-modality adaptive response that temporarily reduces the variability evident within the system. A combination of the baseline level of complexity of a system and its capacity to reduce complexity in response to a stimulus seems to determine the ability of that system to adapt to the stimulus without experiencing catastrophic failure.

Conceptually, senescence, disease, or injury causes a reduction in the ability of a system to detect changes in the baseline state or induces limitations on the system's ability to adapt to those changes, with the effect that the output of the system is simplified, less complex, or less 'random'. Consequently, quantification of the changes in the complexity of a biologic system can provide useful information regarding its homeostatic functioning. Human data have confirmed this supposition, demonstrating that loss of output variability in the dynamics of healthy organ system

Table 28.1 Summary of changes in complexity to various organ systems that can occur in response to ageing or disease

Complexity change	Example condition(s)
Loss of heart rate variability[72–78]	Ageing, critical illness, trauma, ischaemic heart disease, CHF, prior to the onset of atrial fibrillation, and ventricular fibrillation
Loss of temperature curve complexity[79]	Critical illness
Fractal appearance of tumours[80,81]	Distinguish between benign and malignant breast masses
Respiratory rate complexity[82,83]	Ageing, CHF
Alterations in gait dynamics[84,85]	Ageing, Parkinson's disease
Pulsatile hormone release[86–88]	Ageing, sleep disturbance

function as an early sign of dysfunction. Both physiologic ageing and disease can lead to loss of complexity in various organ systems (see Table 28.1). Many of these changes have also been correlated with adverse outcomes of patients, including cardiovascular events, falls, fractures, and mortality. Loss of complexity leads to a reduction in the repertoire of possible physiologic responses to stressors, an impaired ability to adapt to perturbation, and a diminished threshold for decompensation (i.e. with less significant episodes of acute illness or injury).[2] Once a critical threshold level is exceeded, the aggregate system may no longer be able to maintain a steady state, and an accelerated and catastrophic dysregulation occurs.[3] This theoretical critical threshold can be interpreted as 'physiologic reserve'.

Frailty and its connection to physiologic reserve

A common phenotypic expression of this process is the clinical syndrome of frailty. Originally described in the geriatric populations, frailty is a syndrome in which small deficits accumulate, that individually may be insignificant but collectively may contribute to insurmountable burden of disease and a vulnerability to adverse events. Although closely correlated with age and ageing, the prevalence and severity of frailty varies greatly across age strata. Non-linear dynamics describe the phenomenon well, as the number of deficits seems to be more important than the specific deficits themselves. As the repertoire of physiologic responses to environmental stressors decreases, the ability to adapt and respond is reduced, leading to vulnerability to adverse clinical events and outcomes.[4] Also involved is the concept of 'punished inefficiency', in which the presence of several physiologic impairments leads to physiologic inefficiency.[5] In addition to a reduced complexity of physiologic responses, frail patients consume a greater proportion of their already diminishing energy reserves for maintaining homeostasis, with the result that the ability of the body to respond to new (and perhaps even trivial) stressors is further compromised. Examples illustrating this phenomenon are the findings that frail patients lose heart rate variability, balance dynamics are degraded, and antibody (Ab) response to annual trivalent inactivated influenza vaccination is decreased, potentially placing them at greater risk of cardiovascular insufficiency, falls, and influenza infection, respectively.[6–8] At some critical point in this vulnerable physiologic state, functional deficits begin to accumulate rapidly and eventually lead to a non-linear, 'avalanche-like destruction of the organism'.[9,10] The number of abnormal systems also appears to have more relevance than the nature of the specific abnormalities themselves, suggesting that a threshold loss of complexity is an important underlying mechanism of frailty.[11] The implication of these findings is that clinically evident frailty can be viewed as an expression of an organism near its tolerance threshold for perturbation, or at its upper limit of physiologic reserve.

A reduction in LBM, which is comprised mainly of visceral tissue and skeletal muscle, also seems to be a consistent feature of frailty.[12] One of the theories of ageing linking loss of lean mass with loss of complexity suggests that an excessively active pro-inflammatory immune response eventually overwhelms the system's capacity to contain the inflammatory response through depletion of this recruitable protein store. As a consequence, unbridled inflammation and unintended organ injury occur.[10] Data from the Cardiovascular Health Study supports this pro-inflammatory hypothesis. In this study of 4735 community-dwelling adults aged 65 or over, frail patients had significantly higher C-reactive protein (CRP), factor VIII, and D-dimer levels, even after controlling for cardiovascular disease, diabetes, age, sex, and race.[13] The inflammatory milieu is characterized by the generation of pro-inflammatory cytokines, which lead to an anorectic and catabolic state, culminating in a vicious cycle of inflammation, organ injury, and loss of LBM.[14–16] Many other factors also influence the rapidity of muscle loss, which include the adequacy of, and ability to, absorb and utilize nutrition, the ability to mobilize, and current neuromuscular function (including cognitive function). Additionally, the demands of concurrent disease can reduce existing protein stores and result in generalized wasting, similar to that seen in the advanced stages of cardiopulmonary disease, CKD, cancer, and HIV infection.[17,18] In several disease states, a loss of approximately 40% of LBM has been shown to be fatal.[19] Mechanistically, since muscle serves as a metabolic and protein reservoir that is mobilized when physiologic perturbation occurs, such as during states of critical illness or trauma, depletion of functional muscle stores may result in an inability to maintain homeostasis under stress.[20]

It should be noted that disagreement exists in the literature regarding the relative importance of muscle mass, muscle strength, and muscle power in determining outcome in elderly patients.[21] Studies of older adult outpatients have shown that the age-associated loss of muscle size and strength is closely linked to mortality and disability.[22–25] However, muscle size loses significant prognostic value after adjustment for muscle strength and power.[26,27] This may be due to an observed association with reduced cardiopulmonary function and an inability to increase oxygen delivery and utilization during periods of increased demand, as demonstrated both in healthy outpatients and in those with comorbid illness.[28,29] This specific loss of strength and power, independent of muscle mass, has been termed dynapenia and may simply be correlated with a generalized reduction in physiologic reserve that mediates the adverse morbidity and mortality in frail patients. However, it is also possible that the healthy functioning of the musculoskeletal system is linked, in a complex fashion, to the other organ systems, as demonstrated in an elegant study of the beneficial effects of exercise on cognitive function.[30] The implication may be that disease processes and therapy that effect muscular strength may ultimately have a deterministic effect on overall health and may be an essential component of modern treatment paradigms.

Although frailty was originally described in the elderly, features of frailty also arise in many disease states, irrespective of age strata, suggesting that frailty may be a process that develops in vulnerable populations, only one of which is the ageing and elderly. For example, the presence and duration of HIV infection is strongly associated with the frail phenotype (OR 3.4, 12.9, and 14.7 for HIV duration ≤4 years, 4–8 years, and >8 years, respectively).[31] Furthermore, the prevalence of frailty in HIV-infected men under the age of 55 was similar to that of non-HIV infected men over 65 years of age. This suggests that processes underlying a frail state may be more generalized than originally thought when the concept was developed in the elderly.

Operationalizing frailty

Unfortunately, the syndromic nature of frailty makes defining its presence and characterizing its severity potentially challenging. One of the most widely adopted tools used to measure frailty is the operational definition proposed by Fried and colleagues[4] (see Table 28.2). Despite its relative simplicity, there are limitations to this definition, which include the absence of cognitive and psychological domains, the limited stratification to one of frail, pre-frail, or non-frail categories, and the lack of validation of each of the five criteria used to define the syndrome. These limitations are underscored in a prospective trial evaluating the five 'Fried' criteria, in addition to the domains of cognitive impairment and depression, in a cohort of 754 independent elderly patients, followed for up to 7.5 years.[32] In this study, slow gait speed was the strongest predictor of adverse outcome (OR 3.8, 5.9, 2.5, and 2.7 for chronic disability, long-term nursing home stay, injurious fall, and death, respectively). The second strongest factor was low physical activity. Interestingly, cognitive impairment (defined as a score on the Folstein Mini-Mental Status Examination <24).[33] was found to have greater prognostic value than the other three criteria.

In an attempt to improve the recognition and treatment of frailty, many other scoring systems have been developed, all of which have advantages and drawbacks.[34] A recent systematic review of the various instruments highlighted eight of the most important domains of frailty: nutritional status, physical activity, mobility, energy, strength, cognition, mood, and psychosocial support.[34] Each of these domains was variably represented in the published scoring systems. In this review, the Frailty Index (FI), which utilizes a detailed 70-item inventory of clinical deficits to capture the presence and quantify the severity of frailty, was identified as the most comprehensive tool.[35] While useful in the context of research, its comprehensive nature does not easily lend itself to incorporation into the busy, and often chaotic, practice of clinical critical care medicine.

To this end, a number of clinical scales originally developed for outpatients may have more relevance to critical care, although none has, as yet, been validated in the critical care population. The Clinical Global Impression of Change in Physical Frailty (CGIC-PF) includes both patient- and surrogate-derived data, as well as clinical observation by a clinician, but has not been extensively validated.[36] The Groningen Frailty Indicator is a 15-item questionnaire originally mailed out to participants, which, to date, has not been validated for use with direct questioning of surrogates.[37] The third score (not included in the aforementioned systematic review) is the 7-point clinician judgement-based Clinical Frailty Scale (CFS), developed and validated by Rockwood et al.[38] The study involved 2305 patients aged 65 years or older participating in the Canadian Study on Health and Aging. In this study, the CFS correlated closely with the FI. In their multivariable analysis, each 1-point increase in the CFS translated into a significantly higher risk of death (OR 1.3) and

Table 28.2 A proposed clinical definition for the 'phenotype' of frailty

Presence of three or more of the following features
Decreased grip strength
Self-reported exhaustion
Unintentional weight loss >4.5 kg over the past year
Slow walking speed
Low physical activity

Adapted from Fried LP, Tangen CM, Walston J, Newman AB, Hirsch C, Gottdiener J, et al. 'Frailty in older adults: evidence for a phenotype', *Journals of Gerontology – Series A: Biological Sciences and Medical Sciences*, 2001, 56, 3, pp. M146–156, by permission of Oxford University Press and The Gerontological Society of America.

entry into an institutional facility (OR 1.5). Although the CFS is more generic and less detailed than the more comprehensive FI, it appears to be more clinically useful and no less valid, at least in an elderly outpatient population. While these frailty instruments have not been specifically utilized and validated in critically ill patients, there are studies currently ongoing.

Frailty as part of a critical care conceptual framework

Irrespective of the definition used, it is the concept of frailty as a marker of physiologic reserve that may have the most direct relevance to critical care across a broad range of age strata. Frailty has been shown to be associated with many diseases, including both clinical and subclinical cardiovascular disease,[39,40] cancer,[41] and CKD.[42] The Canadian Study of Health and Aging demonstrated the rising prevalence of frailty with increasing age, which may be as high as 43% in an elderly demographic.[38] When one considers the rising utilization of ICU resources by the elderly, the prevalence of pre-existing frailty in patients admitted to the ICU is also likely to be increasing.[43]

Additionally, critically ill patients may represent another group vulnerable to the development of frailty, and non-linear dynamics seem to explain many of these observed phenomena.[44] By definition, critical illness involves a catastrophic failure of homeostasis: acute stressors overwhelm physiologic reserve, and somatic support is required to maintain life. Similar to frail elderly patients, critically ill patients have heightened vulnerability to adverse events and outcomes. The short-term risks take the form of unpredictable life-threatening clinical deteriorations that occurs, independent of age or premorbid functional reserve. The severity of acute perturbation required to cause critical decompensation is variable, and it has been suggested to be a function of: (1) the rapidity with which the stressor affects change within the system, (2) the current level of physiologic instability, and (3) the degree to which somatic support can 'bolster' physiology.[45] Conceptually, life-supportive technology can be viewed as augmenting the output of the biologic system, providing the system with time to adapt and the opportunity to heal; however, in most circumstances, it does not directly affect the underlying process leading to the decompensation.

A more challenging problem is the subacute expression of critical illness. Catastrophic disruption of the system results in common patterns of organ dysfunction, but the specifics of which organs fail in a specific patient at a specific time and in a specific way remain unpredictable. A common finding in critical illness, however, is the rapid development of severe muscle wasting, motor weakness, and functional impairment over days to weeks, a process that would normally take years to develop in the outpatient setting. This critical illness-associated neuromuscular dysfunction occurs in 5–10% of critically ill patients and is associated with increased risk of ICU mortality, prolonged durations of hospitalization and rehabilitation, and reduced QoL after hospital discharge.[46–49] It has been suggested that critical illness may be a manifestation of the rapid development of varying levels of frailty due to the shared features of weakness, muscle wasting, poor functional status, and neurocognitive dysfunction, in addition to the psychological effects of depression and caregiver burnout.[50] Further supporting this is the fact that functional dependence after critical illness is correlated with two of the more prominent phenotypic features characterizing frailty: the inability to walk and poor upper extremity strength.[46] The strong association of muscle loss and weakness with complications in ICU also suggests that the processes leading to muscle wasting may be important therapeutic targets and interventions that prevent or minimize muscle wasting may improve outcomes. An implication of non-linearity is that therapy affecting only one aspect of the process may be more likely to fail, unless that treatment affects a single aetiological factor that leads to a cascade of decompensation or is able to affect multiple processes simultaneously.

The impact of premorbid functional status and frailty on outcome in ICU

Studies evaluating the contribution of chronological age in critically ill patients to predict outcomes seem to indicate that, while advancing age is associated with decreased survival and less favourable functional outcome, its independent predictive value is limited at best. The SAPS 3, a scoring system which utilizes data collected within the first hour of ICU admission, has been shown to have some discriminative value in terms of ICU survival and functional outcome, but it is neither sensitive nor specific enough to guide discussions regarding the utility of ongoing ICU support.[51] Additionally, a prospective multicentre study of 980 survivors of critical illness found that pre-existing comorbid disease was the strongest predictor of post-ICU QoL.[52] Small improvements in HRQoL, if any, were observed over the 3 years after ICU discharge. Furthermore, while not frailty per se, loss of lean muscle mass (i.e. sarcopenia) as a risk factor for poor clinical outcome in ICU has been examined in patients undergoing hepatic resection for colorectal liver metastases.[53] Peng et al. evaluated 259 patients, 41 of whom had significant muscle loss based on psoas muscle size on CT imaging. In this study, the finding of loss of psoas muscle size was associated with a longer duration of hospitalization and a higher risk of prolonged ICU stay (defined as more than 2 days). It was also associated with an OR of 3.3 for major postoperative complications but was not associated with disease-free or overall survival. Despite these and other provocative examples, there are no well-validated tools that will clearly discriminate survivors from non-survivors at the time of presentation to ICU with an episode of critical illness, nor do they reliably predict short- and long-term functional outcome and/or a patient's capacity to heal.[54] The high degree of confidence with which medical practitioners make predictions regarding the outcome of an individual patient and the effect of a specific intervention on that outcome lies in stark contrast to the limited accuracy of these predictions.[55,56] Consequently, although prognostication is something that is done on a daily basis by practitioners of critical care, this process is fraught with error.

Unfortunately, many other illness severity scoring systems, such as the APACHE score, are also not useful in the care of individual patients, as these tools were designed to compare patient populations, rather than to predict the probability of survival at the bedside. This was demonstrated in a systematic review that compared physicians' predictions to those of validated scoring systems; it found that, while physicians were twice as accurate at identifying patients who died prior to ICU discharge, both were only moderately precise.[57] One caveat with respect to physicians' predictions of outcome relates to perception: the prediction of low likelihood of survival by physicians is powerfully associated with the self-fulfilling prophecy of limitation or withdrawal of life-supportive measures and death, independent of the severity of illness.[58]

The role that frailty and physiologic reserve play in determining outcome in critical illness is yet to be clearly elucidated. Although there is some controversy regarding the independent prognostic value of premorbid functional status and ICU outcome, data support the hypothesis that physiologic reserve is important and that, when reserve is exhausted, recovery from critical illness may either be significantly prolonged or not possible. Studies are now attempting to identify biologic markers that, together with clinical prediction rules, can aid in reliably prognosticating more effectively, with the hope that some clinically useful measure of 'physiologic age' is discernable (see Table 28.3). In the non-critical illness literature, the detection of the syndrome of frailty in geriatric and perioperative populations appears to be gaining popularity as a strong potential 'biomarker' of prognosis. Unfortunately, the plethora of definitions, heterogeneity of patient populations, and paucity of critical care-specific data make firm conclusions regarding

Table 28.3 Biologic markers associated with states of 'chronic inflammation' and potential values as surrogate markers of frailty

Class	Biomarker
Acute phase proteins	CRP
	Pre-albumin/albumin
	Transthyretin (TTR)
	Alanine transaminase (ALT)
	Transferrin
	Retinol-binding protein (RBP)
	D-dimer
	Factor VIII
Immune activation/oxidative stress	Neopterin
	Pentraxin 3 (PTX3)
	Glutathione (GSH)/oxidized glutathione (GSSG)
	4-hydroxy-2,3-nonenal (HNE)
	Malonaldehyde (MDA)
	8-hydroxy-2'-deoxyguanosine (8-OHdG)
	CD8/CD28/CCR5 T cell expression
Inflammatory mediators	IL-6
	TNF-α
	Endotoxin (EA)/LPS
	CXC chemokine ligand 10 (CXCL-10)
Growth factors	IGF-1
	25-hydroxyvitamin D_3
Hormones	Hypothalamus-pituitary-gonadal axis

the prognostic or therapeutic implications of an existing or new development of a frail state not possible at present. However, data are emerging that suggest some of these measures of frailty may be useful in predicting not only mortality, but also intensity of support, adverse events, and functional outcome of elderly patients following hospitalization, including those requiring ICU admission.

Frailty and its association with mortality in, and morbidity after, ICU

In their study of 299 French octogenarians, Roch et al. found that premorbid functional status, as assessed by the McCabe, Knaus, and Karnovsky scores, did not seem to predict ICU mortality, in-hospital mortality, or mortality at 2 years post-discharge.[59] However, lack of identification of this effect may be partially explained by the high level of comorbid disease and functional limitation in this cohort; only 15% of enrolled patients had no functional limitation, and 57% of patients had diseases that were classified as fatal within 5 years. In contrast to these data, Goldstein et al. reported that mortality was strongly correlated with premorbid level of function and that changes in functional status were common amongst survivors.[60] (see Figure 28.1, Table 28.4) In this prospective study of 2213 patients admitted to ICU, those with a premorbid classification as 'severely limited' were substantially less likely to survive to hospitalization and when assessed 8 months after discharge when compared to patients with a premorbid activity level classified as 'active' or

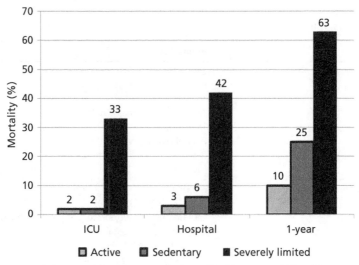

Fig. 28.1 Summary of short- and long-term survival stratified by premorbid activity status.

Reproduced from Goldstein RL, Campion EW, Thibault GE, Mulley AG, Skinner E, 'Functional outcomes following medical intensive care', *Critical Care Medicine*, 14, 9, pp. 783–788, copyright 1986, with permission from Wolters Kluwer and the Society of Critical Care Medicine.

Table 28.4 Summary of short- and long-term outcomes stratified by premorbid activity level

Baseline activity classification	Interventions during ICU stay (n, %)	Follow-up activity level (n, %)		
		Severely limited	Sedentary	Active
Active	137/917 (15)	12 (1.7)	524 (72.7)	185 (25.6)
Sedentary	174/1017 (17)	45 (6.7)	590 (88.2)	34 (5.1)
Severely limited	99/279 (35)	19 (29.8)	45 (68.1)	2 (3.0)

ICU, intensive care unit.

Reproduced from Goldstein RL, Campion EW, Thibault GE, Mulley AG, Skinner E, 'Functional outcomes following medical intensive care', *Critical Care Medicine*, 14, 9, pp. 783–788, copyright 1986, with permission from Wolters Kluwer and the Society of Critical Care Medicine.

'sedentary'. Interestingly, however, functional outcomes in surviving patients were not uniformly worse. Patients who were active often had a decline in function, but some of those classified as severely limited regained function if they survived. Unfortunately, this simple classification system did not have the discriminatory power to distinguish those with severe limitation who still have the capacity to recover.

Likewise, Sligl et al. demonstrated that mortality in critically ill patients with pneumonia was increased in those that were completely dependent for care when compared to functionally independent adults (OR 5.3 and 3.0 for 30-day and 1-year mortality, respectively).[61] Patients with less severe levels of dependency, identified by the use of a walking aid (such as a cane, walker, or wheelchair) had a non-significant trend towards increased risk. In a prospective observational study, Khouli et al. demonstrated that, in the 30 days prior to admission to ICU, each day described by the patient or proxy as 'physical health not good' was associated with an 8% increase in 6-month mortality.[62] Unfortunately, the authors do not report the proportion of QoL measures obtained from family members, rather than patients. This makes the data somewhat challenging to interpret, as the necessarily retrospective approach may introduce recall bias. Furthermore, a patient's QoL prior to ICU admission tends to be underestimated by family members, although the clinical relevance of the difference is debated.[63–65] In a study of 659 elderly patients admitted to ICU from the emergency department, dependence for care, moderate to severe cognitive impairment, and low BMI all independently predicted death prior to hospital discharge.[66] Similarly, the SUPPORT trial, which evaluated outcomes in severely ill hospitalized patients with an estimated mortality of 50% at 6 months, premorbid low BMI was independently predictive of mortality.[67] In fact, the U-shaped mortality curve of BMI characterizing healthy patients disappeared in the context of severe illness, suggesting that, during this period of physiologic stress, the benefits of moderate nutritional or caloric reserve outweighed the theoretical detrimental effects of moderate obesity.

To evaluate frailty in ICU, a useful group of patients to examine are those undergoing cardiac surgical procedures, as these patients are invariably supported in an ICU environment during the immediate post-operative period. Sundermann et al. examined an elderly cohort of these patients (over 75 years of age) and studied the predictive value of their previously validated Comprehensive Assessment of Frailty (CAF).[68] This score includes a combination of subjective weakness, objective measures of strength (rising from a chair and stair climbing), serum creatinine, and the CFS of Rockwood et al.[38] In the 1-year follow-up data, severe frailty, based on the CAF, was associated with significantly higher in-hospital, 30-day, and 1-year mortality when compared to non-frail or moderately frail patients.[69] In another observational study of 3826 patients undergoing cardiac surgery, Lee et al. demonstrated that frailty (defined as any impairment in ADLs, ambulation, or a documented history of dementia) was present in 4.1% preoperatively and was independently associated with higher in-hospital mortality (OR 1.8) and discharge to a long-term care facility (OR 6.3).[70] The patients in this study ranged from 57 to 78 years old. The median age of the patients exhibiting frailty was significantly older than their non-frail counterparts, but the youngest patient in the frail cohort was 61 years old, again demonstrating that the frail phenotype may develop in vulnerable patient populations, independent of age or ageing. Lastly, in a study of 594 elderly patients undergoing cardiac surgery, both intermediate frailty and frailty were associated with increased risks of post-operative complications (OR 2.06 and 2.54) and institutional discharge (OR 3.16 and 20.48).[71] This study modified the original operational definition of Fried,[4] with intermediate frailty defined as two or three of the criteria and frail as four or five of the criteria. ICU and hospital lengths of stay were significantly longer for those classified as either intermediate frailty or frail. In this study, the assessment of frailty had additive predictive value when used in conjunction with previously perioperative risk scores (i.e. American Society of Anesthesiologists).

Conclusion

The concept of 'physiologic reserve', defined simply as the critical threshold of physiologic adaptation that an individual can mount in response to acute illness and/or trauma before which failure to adapt predisposes to homeostatic failure and decompensation, is increasingly recognized as a potentially relevant prognostic determinant of survival and functional outcome for critically ill patients. Unfortunately, this concept can be challenging to translate to the bedside, as there is no discrete diagnostic test or measure for physiologic reserve. However, insight into the 'physiologic reserve' can be gained by evaluating surrogate clinical markers such as for the presence and severity of the frail phenotype. Frailty is a clinical syndrome defined by the accumulation of deficits that individually may be insignificant but collectively contribute to increased burden of chronic disease, vulnerability to adverse events, and diminished physiologic reserve. While the value of assessment of frailty has yet to be specifically evaluated in critically ill patients, the presence of a frail state has been shown to have associations with increased complexity of support, prolonged hospitalization, increased mortality, and long-term institutionalization for the elderly and those undergoing major cardiovascular surgery. The routine assessment of frailty in all patients developing critical illness may represent an additional prognostic tool that can be integrated into discussion with patients and/or families regarding decision making about the incremental benefit of ICU admission and support and/or withdrawal of support, following time-limited trials of advanced life support in the ICU. In addition, the frailty assessment could be used to target those patients that require intensive rehabilitative support peri- and post-critical care to optimize their outcome and potential recovery trajectory.

References

1 Varela M, Ruiz-Esteban R, De Juan M. Chaos, fractals, and our concept of disease. *Perspect Biology Med* 2010;**53**:584–95.

2 Lipsitz LA, Goldberger AL. Loss of 'complexity' and aging. Potential applications of fractals and chaos theory to senescence. *JAMA* 1992;**267**:1806–9.

3 Yates FE. Complexity of a human being: changes with age. *Neurobiol Aging* 2002;**23**:17–19.

4 Fried LP, Tangen CM, Walston J, et al. Frailty in older adults: evidence for a phenotype. *J Gerontol A Biol Sci Med Sci* 2001;**56**:M146–56.

5 Weiss CO. Frailty and chronic diseases in older adults. *Clin Geriatr Med* 2011;**27**:39–52.

6 Chaves PH, Varadhan R, Lipsitz LA, et al. Physiological complexity underlying heart rate dynamics and frailty status in community-dwelling older women. *J Am Geriatr Soc* 2008;**56**:1698–703.

7 Kang HG, Costa MD, Priplata AA, et al. Frailty and the degradation of complex balance dynamics during a dual-task protocol. *J Gerontol A Biol Sci Med Sci* 2009;**64**:1304–11.

8 Yao X, Li H, Leng SX. Inflammation and immune system alterations in frailty. *Clin Geriatr Med* 2011;**27**:79–87.

9 Mitnitski AB, Mogilner AJ, MacKnight C, Rockwood K. The mortality rate as a function of accumulated deficits in a frailty index. *Mech Ageing Dev* 2002;**123**:1457–60.

10 Franceschi C, Capri M, Monti D, et al. Inflammaging and anti-inflammaging: a systemic perspective on aging and longevity emerged from studies in humans. *Mech Ageing Dev* 2007;**128**:92–105.

11 Fried LP, Xue QL, Cappola AR, et al. Nonlinear multisystem physiological dysregulation associated with frailty in older women: implications for etiology and treatment. *J Gerontol A Biol Sci Med Sci* 2009;**64**:1049–57.

12 Kehayias JJ, Fiatarone MA, Zhuang H, Roubenoff R. Total body potassium and body fat: relevance to aging. *Am J Clin Nutr* 1997;**66**:904–10.

13 Walston J, McBurnie MA, Newman A, et al. Frailty and activation of the inflammation and coagulation systems with and without clinical comorbidities: results from the Cardiovascular Health Study. *Arch Inter Med* 2002;**162**:2333–41.

14 Grunfeld C, Feingold KR. Metabolic disturbances and wasting in the acquired immunodeficiency syndrome. *N Engl J Med* 1992;**327**:329–37.

15 Beutler B, Cerami A. Cachectin: more than a tumor necrosis factor. *N Engl J Med* 1987;**316**:379–85.

16 Bazar KA, Yun AJ, Lee PY. 'Starve a fever and feed a cold': feeding and anorexia may be adaptive behavioral modulators of autonomic and T helper balance. *Med Hypotheses* 2005;**64**:1080–4.

17 Lainscak M, Podbregar M, Anker SD. How does cachexia influence survival in cancer, heart failure and other chronic diseases? *Curr Opin Support Palliat Care* 2007;**1**:299–305.

18 **Tan BHL, Fearson CH.** Cachexia: prevalence and impact in medicine. *Curr Opin Clin Nutr Metab Care* 2008;**11**:400–7.

19 **Roubenoff R.** Sarcopenia: effects on body composition and function. *J Gerontol A Biol Sci Med Sci* 2003;**58**:1012–17.

20 **Manini TM, Clark BC.** Dynapenia and aging: an update. *J Gerontol A Biol Sci Med Sci* 2012;**67**: 28–40.

21 **Clark BC, Manini TM.** Sarcopenia =/= dynapenia. *J Gerontol A Biol Sci Med Sci* 2008;**63**:829–34.

22 **Cesari M, Pahor M, Lauretani F, et al.** Skeletal muscle and mortality results from the InCHIANTI Study. *J Gerontol A Biol Sci Med Sci* 2009;**64**:377–84.

23 **Janssen I.** Skeletal muscle cutpoints associated with elevated physical disability risk in older men and women. *Am J Epidemiol* 2004;**159**:413–21.

24 **Newman AB, Kupelian V, Visser M, et al.** Strength, but not muscle mass, is associated with mortality in the health, aging and body composition study cohort. *J Gerontol A Biol Sci Med Sci* 2006;**61**:72–7.

25 **Visser M, Simonsick EM, Colbert LH, et al.** Type and intensity of activity and risk of mobility limitation: the mediating role of muscle parameters. *J Am Geriatr Soc* 2005;**53**:762–70.

26 **Visser M, Newman AB, Nevitt MC, et al.** Reexamining the sarcopenia hypothesis. Muscle mass versus muscle strength. Health, Aging, and Body Composition Study Research Group. *Ann N Y Acad Sci* 2000;**904**:456–61.

27 **Studenski S, Perera S, Patel K, et al.** Gait speed and survival in older adults. *JAMA* 2011;**305**:50–8.

28 **Barbat-Artigas S, Dupontgand S, Fex A, Karelis AD, Aubertin-Leheudre M.** Relationship between dynapenia and cardiorespiratory functions in healthy postmenopausal women: novel clinical criteria. *Menopause* 2011;**18**:400–5.

29 **Cortopassi F, Divo M, Pinto-Plata V, Celli B.** Resting handgrip force and impaired cardiac function at rest and during exercise in COPD patients. *Respir Med* 2011;**105**:748–54.

30 **Colcombe SJ, Kramer AF, Erickson KI, et al.** Cardiovascular fitness, cortical plasticity, and aging. *Proc Natl Acad Sci USA* 2004;**101**:3316–21.

31 **Desquilbet L, Jacobson LP, Fried LP, et al.** HIV-1 infection is associated with an earlier occurrence of a phenotype related to frailty. *J Gerontol A Biol Sci Med Sci* 2007;**62**:1279–86.

32 **Rothman MD, Leo-Summers L, Gill TM.** Prognostic significance of potential frailty criteria. *J Am Geriatr Soc* 2008;**56**:2211–16.

33 **Folstein MF, Folstein SE, McHugh PR.** 'Mini-mental state'. A practical method for grading the cognitive state of patients for the clinician. *J Psychiatr Res* 1975;**12**:189–98.

34 **de Vries NM, Staal JB, van Ravensberg CD, Hobbelen JS, Olde Rikkert MG, Nijhuis-van der Sanden MW.** Outcome instruments to measure frailty: a systematic review. *Ageing Res Rev* 2011;**10**:104–14.

35 **Rockwood K, Andrew M, Mitnitski A.** A comparison of two approaches to measuring frailty in elderly people. *J Gerontol A Biol Sci Med Sci* 2007;**62**:738–43.

36 **Studenski S, Hayes RP, Leibowitz RQ, et al.** Clinical global impression of change in physical frailty: development of a measure based on clinical judgment. *J Am Geriatr Soc* 2004;**52**:1560–6.

37 **Schuurmans H, Steverink N, Lindenberg S, Frieswijk N, Slaets JP.** Old or frail: what tells us more? *J Gerontol A Biol Sci Med Sci* 2004;**59**:M962–5.

38 **Rockwood K, Song X, MacKnight C, et al.** A global clinical measure of fitness and frailty in elderly people. *CMAJ* 2005;**173**:489–95.

39 **Afilalo J, Karunananthan S, Eisenberg MJ, Alexander KP, Bergman H.** Role of frailty in patients with cardiovascular disease. *Am J Cardiol* 2009;**103**:1616–21.

40 **Newman AB, Gottdiener JS, McBurnie MA, et al.** Associations of subclinical cardiovascular disease with frailty. *J Gerontol A Biol Sci Med Sci* 2001;**56**:M158–66.

41 **Mohile SG, Xian Y, Dale W, et al.** Association of a cancer diagnosis with vulnerability and frailty in older Medicare beneficiaries. *J Natl Cancer Inst* 2009;**101**:1206–15.

42 Cook WL. The intersection of geriatrics and chronic kidney disease: frailty and disability among older adults with kidney disease. *Adv Chronic Kidney Dis* 2009;**16**:420–9.

43 Bagshaw SM, Webb SA, Delaney A, et al. Very old patients admitted to intensive care in Australia and New Zealand: a multi-centre cohort analysis. *Crit Care* 2009;**13**:R45.

44 Seely AJ, Christou NV. Multiple organ dysfunction syndrome: exploring the paradigm of complex nonlinear systems. *Crit Care Med* 2000;**28**:2193–200.

45 McDermid RC, Bagshaw SM. Frailty: a new conceptual framework in critical care medicine. In: Vincent JL (ed.) *Annual update in intensive care and emergency medicine*: Berlin: Springer; 2011. pp. 117–19.

46 van der Schaaf M, Dettling DS, Beelen A, Lucas C, Dongelmans DA, Nollet F. Poor functional status immediately after discharge from an intensive care unit. *Disabil Rehabil* 2008;**30**:1812–18.

47 De Jonghe B. Paresis acquired in the intensive care unit: a prospective multicenter study. *JAMA* 2002;**288**:2859–67.

48 Seneff MG, Zimmerman JE, Knaus WA, Wagner DP, Draper EA. Predicting the duration of mechanical ventilation: the importance of disease and patient characteristics. *Chest* 1996;**110**:469–79.

49 Garnacho-Montero J, Amaya-Villar R, Garcia-Garmendia JL, Madrazo-Osuna J, Ortiz-Leyba C. Effect of critical illness polyneuropathy on the withdrawal from mechanical ventilation and the length of stay in septic patients. *Crit Care Med* 2005;**33**:349–54.

50 McDermid RC, Bagshaw SM. ICU and critical care outreach for the elderly. *Best Pract Res Clin Anaesthesiol* 2011;**25**:439–49.

51 Capuzzo M, Moreno RP, Jordan B, Bauer P, Alvisi R, Metnitz PG. Predictors of early recovery of health status after intensive care. *Intensive Care Med* 2006;**32**:1832–8.

52 Orwelius L, Nordlund A, Nordlund P, et al. Pre-existing disease: the most important factor for health related quality of life long-term after critical illness: a prospective, longitudinal, multicentre trial. *Crit Care* 2010;**14**:R67.

53 Peng PD, van Vledder MG, Tsai S, et al. Sarcopenia negatively impacts short-term outcomes in patients undergoing hepatic resection for colorectal liver metastasis. *HPB (Oxford)* 2011;**13**:439–46.

54 Ferreira FL, Bota DP, Bross A, Melot C, Vincent JL. Serial evaluation of the SOFA score to predict outcome in critically ill patients. *JAMA* 2001;**286**:1754–8.

55 Copeland-Fields L, Griffin T, Jenkins T, Buckley M, Wise LC. Comparison of outcome predictions made by physicians, by nurses, and by using the Mortality Prediction Model. *Am J Crit Care* 2001;**10**:313–19.

56 Frick S, Uehlinger DE, Zuercher Zenklusen RM. Medical futility: predicting outcome of intensive care unit patients by nurses and doctors—a prospective comparative study. *Crit Care Med* 2003;**31**:456–61.

57 Sinuff T, Adhikari NK, Cook DJ, et al. Mortality predictions in the intensive care unit: comparing physicians with scoring systems. *Crit Care Med* 2006;**34**:878–85.

58 Rocker G, Cook D, Sjokvist P, et al. Clinician predictions of intensive care unit mortality. *Crit Care Med* 2004;**32**:1149–54.

59 Roch A, Wiramus S, Pauly V, et al. Long-term outcome in medical patients aged 80 or over following admission to an intensive care unit. *Crit Care* 2011;**15**:R36.

60 Goldstein RL, Campion EW, Thibault GE, Mulley AG, Skinner E. Functional outcomes following medical intensive care. *Crit Care Med* 1986;**14**:783–8.

61 Sligl WI, Eurich DT, Marrie TJ, Majumdar SR. Only severely limited, premorbid functional status is associated with short- and long-term mortality in patients with pneumonia who are critically ill: a prospective observational study. *Chest* 2011;**139**:88–94.

62 Khouli H, Astua A, Dombrowski W, et al. Changes in health-related quality of life and factors predicting long-term outcomes in older adults admitted to intensive care units. *Crit Care Med* 2011;**39**:731–7.

63 Gifford JM, Husain N, Dinglas VD, Colantuoni E, Needham DM. Baseline quality of life before intensive care: a comparison of patient versus proxy responses. *Crit Care Med* 2010;**38**:855–60.

64 Scales DC, Tansey CM, Matte A, Herridge MS. Difference in reported pre-morbid health-related quality of life between ARDS survivors and their substitute decision makers. *Intensive Care Med* 2006;**32**:1826–31.

65 Hofhuis J, Hautvast JL, Schrijvers AJ, Bakker J. Quality of life on admission to the intensive care: can we query the relatives? *Intensive Care Med* 2003;**29**:974–9.

66 Bo M, Massaia M, Raspo S, et al. Predictive factors of in-hospital mortality in older patients admitted to a medical intensive care unit. *J Am Geriatr Soc* 2003;**51**:529–33.

67 Galanos AN, Pieper CF, Kussin PS, et al. Relationship of body mass index to subsequent mortality among seriously ill hospitalized patients. SUPPORT Investigators. The Study to Understand Prognoses and Preferences for Outcome and Risks of Treatments. *Crit Care Med* 1997;**25**:1962–8.

68 Sundermann S, Dademasch A, Praetorius J, et al. Comprehensive assessment of frailty for elderly high-risk patients undergoing cardiac surgery. *Eur J Cardiothorac Surg* 2011;**39**:33–7.

69 Sundermann S, Dademasch A, Rastan A, et al. One-year follow-up of patients undergoing elective cardiac surgery assessed with the Comprehensive Assessment of Frailty test and its simplified form. *Interact Cardiovasc Thorac Surg* 2011;**13**:119–23; discussion 23.

70 Lee DH, Buth KJ, Martin BJ, Yip AM, Hirsch GM. Frail patients are at increased risk for mortality and prolonged institutional care after cardiac surgery. *Circulation* 2010;**121**:973–8.

71 Makary MA, Segev DL, Pronovost PJ, et al. Frailty as a predictor of surgical outcomes in older patients. *J Am Coll Surg* 2010;**210**:901–8.

72 Makikallio TH, Hoiber S, Kober L, et al. Fractal analysis of heart rate dynamics as a predictor of mortality in patients with depressed left ventricular function after acute myocardial infarction. TRACE Investigators. TRAndolapril Cardiac Evaluation. *Am J Cardiol* 1999;**83**:836–9.

73 Makikallio TH, Koistinen J, Jordaens L, et al. Heart rate dynamics before spontaneous onset of ventricular fibrillation in patients with healed myocardial infarcts. *Am J Cardiol* 1999;**83**:880–4.

74 Vikman S, Makikallio TH, Yli-Mayry S, et al. Altered complexity and correlation properties of R-R interval dynamics before the spontaneous onset of paroxysmal atrial fibrillation. *Circulation* 1999;**100**:2079–84.

75 Huikuri HV, Makikallio TH, Airaksinen KE, et al. Power-law relationship of heart rate variability as a predictor of mortality in the elderly. *Circulation* 1998;**97**:2031–6.

76 Mowery NT, Norris PR, Riordan W, Jenkins JM, Williams AE, Morris JA, Jr. Cardiac uncoupling and heart rate variability are associated with intracranial hypertension and mortality: a study of 145 trauma patients with continuous monitoring. *J Trauma* 2008;**65**:621–7.

77 Norris PR, Stein PK, Morris JA, Jr. Reduced heart rate multiscale entropy predicts death in critical illness: a study of physiologic complexity in 285 trauma patients. *J Crit Care* 2008;**23**:399–405.

78 Norris PR, Anderson SM, Jenkins JM, Williams AE, Morris JA, Jr. Heart rate multiscale entropy at three hours predicts hospital mortality in 3,154 trauma patients. *Shock* 2008;**30**:17–22.

79 Varela M, Churruca J, Gonzalez A, Martin A, Ode J, Galdos P. Temperature curve complexity predicts survival in critically ill patients. *Am J Respir Crit Care Med* 2006;**174**:290–8.

80 Velanovich V. Fractal analysis of mammographic lesions: a feasibility study quantifying the difference between benign and malignant masses. *Am J Med Sci* 1996;**311**:211–14.

81 Velanovich V. Fractal analysis of mammographic lesions: a prospective, blinded trial. *Breast Cancer Res Treat* 1998;**49**:245–9.

82 Peng CK, Mietus JE, Liu Y, et al. Quantifying fractal dynamics of human respiration: age and gender effects. *Ann Biomed Eng* 2002;**30**:683–92.

83 Kryger MH, Millar T. Cheyne-Stokes respiration: Stability of interacting systems in heart failure. *Chaos* 1991;**1**:265–9.

84 Hausdorff JM, Rios DA, Edelberg HK. Gait variability and fall risk in community-living older adults: a 1-year prospective study. *Arch Phys Med Rehabil* 2001;**82**:1050–6.

85 Hausdorff JM. Gait dynamics in Parkinson's disease: common and distinct behavior among stride length, gait variability, and fractal-like scaling. *Chaos* 2009;**19**:026113.

86 Brzezinski A. Melatonin in humans. *N Engl J Med* 1997;**336**:186–95.

87 Greenspan SL, Klibanski A, Rowe JW, Elahi D. Age-related alterations in pulsatile secretion of TSH: role of dopaminergic regulation. *Am J Physiol* 1991;**260**:E486–91.

88 Frank SA, Roland DC, Sturis J, et al. Effects of aging on glucose regulation during wakefulness and sleep. *Am J Physiol* 1995;**269**:E1006–16.

Chapter 29

Cognitive Reserve

Vanessa Raymont and Robert D. Stevens

Introduction

A significant body of evidence indicates that critical illness is associated with both acute brain dysfunction[1] and long-term impairments in cognition[2] and that these alterations could represent distinct patterns of neural damage.[3,4] Recent analyses in large cohorts of elderly subjects indicate a previously unrecognized relationship between accelerated cognitive decline and prior exposures, including delirium,[5] critical illness,[6] and severe sepsis.[7] It has long been observed that individuals differ remarkably in the face of neurological disease; that a direct, predictable relationship between the type and extent of neuropathological abnormality and the associated phenotypic expression is often difficult to identify. Hence, a pattern of brain damage with similar characteristics and magnitude can result in different levels of neurologic and cognitive impairment, and that impairment can vary in its rate of progression or recovery. The concept of cognitive reserve has been proposed to account for this variance.[8]

The cognitive reserve hypothesis emerged, following reports which indicated a remarkable discrepancy between the burden of Alzheimer's disease (AD) neuropathology, identified in postmortem samples, and the associated clinical manifestations; in addition, the brains of subjects with little or no clinical expression had increased weight and neuronal density when compared to those of age-matched controls.[9] Studies have reported that up to 25% of individuals with normal neuropsychological testing prior to death met full pathologic criteria for AD, suggesting that this degree of pathology does not invariably result in clinical dementia.[10] It has been speculated that these subjects may have had greater 'cognitive reserve', meaning a higher protective threshold before clinical impairment becomes detectable[11] (see Figure 29.1). However, additional work has indicated that, once clinical impairment becomes apparent, those with greater reserve have a propensity for more rapid cognitive decline, suggesting a failure of compensatory mechanisms.[12,13]

Models of reserve

Reserve may be modelled in terms of a passive mechanism or alternatively as an active process which more formally corresponds to the construct of cognitive reserve.[14] According to the **passive model**, 'brain reserve' is explained by inter-individual differences in the number of neurons or neuronal connectivity (e.g. synaptic density, dendritic arborization), thereby leading to differences in tolerance to pathology before a critical threshold for clinical symptoms is reached. At a very basic level, larger brains or regional differences in brain size might allow an individual to sustain more damage before clinical changes emerge, because sufficient neural substrate remains to support normal function.[15,16] The passive model recognizes that there are individual differences in overall brain reserve capacity (BRC), and clinical deficits emerge when

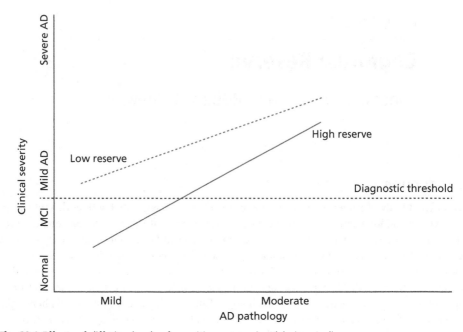

Fig. 29.1 Effects of differing levels of cognitive reserve in Alzheimer's disease.

Reprinted from *The Lancet Neurology*, 11, 11, Stern Y, 'Cognitive reserve in ageing and Alzheimer's disease', pp. 1006–1012, Copyright 2012, with permission from Elsevier.

reserve is depleted past a fixed threshold.[17] Individuals differ in their BRC, and brain damage is either sufficient or insufficient to deplete BRC beyond a critical threshold. Because reserve is seen as a factor modulating the relationship between pathology and its clinical outcome, the level of reserve also influences the severity of clinical symptoms after the threshold for their appearance has occurred. This model is illustrated in Figure 29.2 adapted from Satz et al.[17] A lesion of a particular size might result in a clinical deficit in a person with less reserve (patient B), because it exceeds the threshold of brain damage sufficient to produce a deficit. However, an individual with greater reserve (patient A) remains unaffected, because this threshold is not exceeded. The concept of BRC has been extensively studied in subjects with AD and other chronic degenerative disorders.[18] Validation in this population can be a challenge, because disease modelling must consider the multiplicity of variables which affect the risk for the disorder or the magnitude of BRC. On the other hand, the application of BRC could be more straightforward in acute brain injury where acquired pathology and BRC are independent; hence, BRC can be indirectly inferred by assessing the extent of pathology, compared to the extent of clinical symptoms.

However, passive/threshold brain reserve models do not account for differences in how the brain processes tasks when disease is present. In the **active** model, the brain compensates for damage by utilizing either pre-existing networks less susceptible to disruption in a more efficient manner ('neural reserve') or by recruiting new or alternative networks or cognitive strategies ('neural compensation').[14] The term cognitive reserve is increasingly used to denote this specific model of active neural reserve or compensation.[8] The active model does not assume that there is some fixed cut-off, at which functional impairment will occur, but emphasizes the way the brain uses its resources in the face of damage.[19] While this model implies the use of

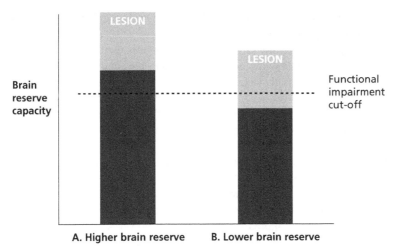

Fig. 29.2 The threshold or brain reserve model.

Adapted from Satz P, 'Brain reserve capacity on symptom onset after brain injury: A formulation and review of evidence for threshold theory', *Neuropsychology*, 7, pp. 273–295, copyright 1993, with permission from the American Psychological Society.

brain structures or networks to compensate for brain damage, healthy individuals use similar networks when coping with task demand.[19] Functional neuroimaging suggests that a common response to increasing task difficulty in normal individuals is increased activation of areas involved in an easier versions of the task or the recruitment of additional brain areas.[20] But there are individual differences in how this additional recruitment occurs; for any level of task difficulty, more skilled individuals typically show less task-related recruitment than less skilled individuals. Thus, this increased processing efficiency may represent a fundamental neural underpinning of cognitive reserve.

Active models of reserve imply variability at the level of brain networks, while passive models imply differences in the quantity of available neural substrate. However, the models might well be interdependent. A range of learning paradigms and other cognitively engaging tasks or experiences are known to induce lasting modifications in brain structure and function. It has been shown that an enriched environment and exercise, factors associated with reserve,[21,22] may be linked to neurogenesis and neuronal resistance to cell death.[23,24] For instance, there is evidence that environmental enrichment might act directly to prevent or slow the accumulation of AD pathology.[25] A comprehensive account of cognitive reserve must integrate complex interactions between genetic susceptibility, environmental influences on brain reserve and pathology, and the ability to actively compensate for the effects of such pathology.

Measurement of cognitive reserve

Given the different theories concerning cognitive reserve, efforts to measure and quantify it have been challenging. Anatomic measures such as volumetric analysis of the whole brain, individual lobes or Brodmann areas have all been linked to risk of age-related cognitive impairment or dementia.[15,26,27] Direct volumetric measurements of brain size can be obtained from imaging, and whole brain volume is correlated positively with cognitive function.[28] In biopsy or autopsy-based studies, neuronal density[29] or dendritic morphology[30] represent plausible, albeit less accessible, markers of reserve.

Variables descriptives of lifetime experience are commonly used as proxies for brain reserve, including social and economic status, occupational level, education, social networks, and leisure activities. In some populations, the degree of literacy is a better marker than the number of years of formal education.[31] The level of educational achievement might also be a marker for innate intelligence, which may, in turn, be genetically based, although some studies suggest that an estimate of premorbid intelligence quotient (IQ) might be a more accurate measure of reserve than educational attainment.[32,33]

Interestingly, education and other life experiences have been shown to increase reserve. Studies have demonstrated separate, additive, and synergistic effects for higher educational and occupational attainment and leisure activities, suggesting that each of these life experiences can contribute independently to reserve.[34–38] The prospective British 1946 Birth Cohort Study showed that reserve could be approximated to crystallized verbal ability and IQ at age 53 and was independently influenced by childhood cognitive level, educational attainment, and adult occupation.[39] While childhood intelligence provided the strongest contribution to the estimate of brain reserve, adult occupation was the weakest. However, these observations confirm that BRC is not fixed and that, at any point in the course of a lifetime, it results from a combination of exposures.[40]

Attempts to explain the beneficial effects of physical or mental activity on reserve have focused on factors such as CBF or greater synaptic plasticity.[41,42] Evidence suggests that neurogenesis may also be an important mechanism and that this can occur over an extended time in adult animals and humans.[23,24] It is well established that the adult mammalian brain is continuously generating new functioning neurons.[43] Animal studies suggest that aspects of life experience, including enriched environment[44] and exercise, can increase the amount of new neurons that are generated in mature animals.[24] Thus, a variable ostensibly associated with BRC, such as education, may dynamically influence the underlying neural substrate.

Another issue in measuring reserve is the challenge of the assessment of the nature and degree of any brain damage. Very often, proxy measures of pathology are used. For example, in studies of TBI, we have no direct measure of neuronal damage; instead, clinical indices have been established that appear to capture that severity. These include measures of the severity of the head trauma itself or measures of its sequelae, including the duration of loss of consciousness. In AD, there is no existing direct measure of pathologic severity in living humans. Snowdon et al. have demonstrated a relationship between measures of linguistic ability, acquired at an early age, and the presence of AD pathology noted post-mortem.[45] Other studies have used the characteristic reduction in parietotemporal and frontal blood perfusion and metabolism seen at rest in AD as an index of the severity of pathology.[46] The perfusion deficit correlates with disease severity, increases with disease progression, and its distribution overlaps with cortical areas with the greatest density of histopathological abnormalities.[48–50]

Physiologic neuroimaging studies have found that, in patients matched for overall severity of dementia, an inverse correlation exists between CBF and both the level of education[50] and occupational attainment.[38] This inverse relationship existed even after controlling for clinical dementia severity and was most prominently noted in prefrontal, premotor, and left superior parietal association areas. In a later study, a similar inverse relationship was found between regional CBF and increased engagement in leisure activities, even after controlling for educational and occupational attainment.[51] These observations have been replicated several times by other groups.[52,53]

Epidemiologic studies

A large body of epidemiological evidence has supported the concept of reserve. One systematic review identified 22 cohort studies published up to 2004 which evaluated the effects of education, occupation, premorbid IQ, and mental activities on the risk of developing dementia.[54] Ten out of 15 studies demonstrated a significant protective effect of education; nine out of 12 a protective effect of occupational attainment; two out of two a protective effect of premorbid IQ; and six out of six a protective effect of engaging in leisure activities. Studies that did not find a protective effect also had the lowest dementia rates. Integrating these studies, the authors reported that higher BRC was associated with significantly lowered risk for incident dementia.

There is also evidence for cognitive reserve in studies of normal age-related cognitive decline. In an ethnically diverse cohort of non-demented older subjects, Manly et al. found that increased literacy was associated with slower decline in memory, executive function, and language skills.[55] Several other studies of normal ageing reported slower cognitive and functional decline in individuals with higher educational attainment.[56,57] These studies suggest that the same education-related factors that delay the onset of dementia also allow individuals to cope more effectively with brain changes encountered in normal ageing. Because education and socio-economic status are highly correlated, large-scale studies have also been carried out to examine individuals who are highly educated but of low socio-economic status, and vice versa.[22,58] In one such study, the association between the risk of AD and low educational attainment remained significant, even when controlling for socio-economic status.[58] Lower childhood intelligence has been found to be a risk factor for late-onset dementia.[22] This association became stronger at later ages, suggesting childhood intelligence may well be a reliable proxy for brain reserve.

Conversely, a series of studies of patients with AD have suggested that, once AD emerges, those with higher reserve have poorer outcomes. In a prospective study of 593 community-based, non-demented individuals aged 60 years or older,[37] a higher level of education was associated with more rapid cognitive decline in patients with prevalent AD[12] and incident AD,[59] as it was in subjects who engaged in more leisure activities prior to dementia onset.[60] Building on this work, Hall et al. also examined memory test data collected at regular intervals from healthy older subjects who were followed prospectively until they became demented.[61] They modelled the data to determine the point of inflection at which memory began to decline more rapidly. They found that the point of inflection occurred later in patients with higher education but that the rate of memory decline after the point of inflection was more rapid in those with higher education.[61] In another study, longitudinal data were collected from 801 older Catholic nuns, priests, and brothers without dementia. Participation in cognitively stimulating tasks was shown to be associated with retention of cognitive function and a reduced risk of AD, after controlling for age, gender, and education. Leisure activities, irrespective of the extent of cognitive effort involved, surveyed in a non-demented general population sample have also been found to have a cumulatively protective effect on the likelihood of incident dementia.[51]

Biologic mechanisms of cognitive reserve: evidence from neuropathological and imaging studies

The concept of cognitive reserve arose from the observation that the degree of AD neuropathology may not completely explain the clinical manifestations of the disease.[9] Subsequent studies have confirmed that neuropsychological phenotypes in AD are dependent on factors distinct from lesion extent or density.[62–64] This paradigm has been explored *in vivo* by Kemppainen et al.

who found higher amyloid levels, as demonstrated by positron emission tomography (PET) imaging with Pittsburgh Compound B ([11C]PIB) uptake, in the lateral frontal cortex in AD subjects with higher educational level, compared with subjects whose educational level was lower.[65]

Anatomical neuroimaging

Studies in AD and other neurologic diseases suggest that, in the premorbid phase, subjects with higher cognitive reserve have greater whole and regional brain volumes, while, after the onset of clinical symptoms, theses volumes are smaller than in phenotypically matched subjects with lesser reserve.[26,27,66] Mori et al. used MRI to assess whole brain and intracranial volume and found that premorbid brain volume explained around 8–16% of the variance in cognitive decline during AD.[26] In a separate report, it was reported that the onset of AD occured at a later age in patients with larger premorbid brains.[67] In a recent study of patients with mild cognitive impairment, subjects with a higher education level had a significantly thinner cortex than less educated subjects with the same level of cognitive performance.[68] These results are at variance with a study which found that variance in cognitive performance was best explained by education and occupation, not intracranial volume.[22] Similarly, others have found limited or no difference in premorbid brain volume between healthy controls and dementia patients[69,70] and no association between premorbid brain size and age at onset.[70] However, in a high-resolution MRI study of 25 patients following a TBI, Kesler et al. found that larger brain size before injury decreased the extent of cognitive deficits, irrespective of injury severity.[66]

Physiological and functional neuroimaging

A correlation has been described between regional indices of CBF and neuropathological changes in patients with AD.[71] Subsequent studies have indicated that patients at risk for AD with higher education or occupation have, for comparable cognitive impairment, a more severe reduction in brain glucose metabolism than subjects with lower education/occupation.[72] Additionally, regional CBF within the parietotemporal lobes has been found to be significantly and inversely correlated with the level of education in patients with AD.[50] A similar pattern was shown with occupational attainment.[38]

Functional neuroimaging studies have also generally supported the active model of cognitive reserve, with evidence of both neural reserve and neural compensation.[73–76] Using functional MRI (fMRI), it has been shown that multiple sclerosis patients with greater intellectual enrichment require less deactivation of the brain's default mode network and less recruitment of prefrontal cortices to perform tasks, when compared to patients with lesser enrichment, suggesting that cognitive reserve is associated with greater task-activated cortical efficiency.[77] Scheibel et al. evaluated functional networks in 30 subjects with moderate to severe TBI, using fMRI and a visual cognitive control task.[78] They found that a higher level of education was associated with greater task-related activation in the left parietal lobe and posterior frontal lobe, suggesting that education may facilitate the ability of individuals with neuropathology to engage a left-sided network for verbal guidance or mediation as a form of compensation.

Cabeza et al. compared prefrontal cortex (PFC) activations in healthy younger and older adults when completing two memory tasks.[79] Younger adults were asymmetric in their recruitment of PFC regions during the source memory task relative to recall tasks, recruiting primarily from the right PFC. Low-performing older adults show similar patterns of activation as the younger adults, but high-performing older adults showed more bilateral engagement of PFC regions, thereby compensating for age-related cognitive impairment. Others have reported different examples of compensatory re-allocation. In one study, older subjects recruited compensatory networks not used by young subjects but also performed more poorly than younger subjects.[20,80]

This form of compensatory activation, in an attempt to maintain performance, may represent the use of compensatory networks that may then fail. Alternatively, this could represent dedifferentiation. The concept of dedifferentiation postulates that regional processing decreases with ageing due to increased levels of noise or decreased levels of functional integration.[81] If individuals who are performing more poorly activate areas that better performers do not, dedifferentiation is clearly a reasonable explanation. But, if an alternate network is used to compensate for the effects of age-related changes on the primary network, it may be possible to quantify these age-related changes using proxy measures such as atrophy or white matter hyperintensities. One would then predict that individuals with greater atrophy would be more likely to use the alternate network. Similarly, techniques, such as transcranial magnetic stimulation (TMS), will be helpful in testing these ideas by allowing direct manipulation of brain areas or networks.

Implications for prognostication and treatment

The concept of cognitive reserve explains why, in some individuals, cognitive disorders are less likely to be detected and are also less likely to impair daily function. Brain size and function are influenced by genetic factors, education, occupation, socio-economic environment, physical health, and lifestyle. It appears that these factors not only determine cognitive ability at any given age, but also are capable of augmenting cognitive reserve over time. As noted earlier, from the perspective of dementia, cognitive reserve and neuropathology are fully independent entities; education does not protect against the acquisition of AD neuropathology, only against its clinical expression. But, if brain size and function are determinants of premorbid cognitive ability, then the model of BRC is capable of working in a vicious cycle. Thus, negative influences on brain size and function, such as low educational and occupational attainment, are also risk factors for the development of CNS lesions, which, in turn, can deplete reserve and reduce protection against their clinical expression.

Determining the central mechanism for cognitive reserve is important in developing interventions to increase it, thereby slowing the effects of brain injury, advancing age, or dementia. Unfortunately, research suggests that cognitive training benefits only the task used in training itself and does not generalize to other tasks or behaviours. Nevertheless, imaging could be used as a meaningful endpoint in cognitive interventions. Imaging cognitive reserve would also be very useful for understanding any older adult's true clinical status, that is a combination of underlying disease-related brain changes and that individual's cognitive reserve in the face of those changes. Two individuals who appear the same clinically could differ widely on these underlying measures. This approach to characterizing patients could have strong implications for the prognostication and treatment of neurological disease and injury.

In fact, the concept of cognitive reserve has recently been applied to a wide range of disorders, including epilepsy,[82] multiple sclerosis,[83] sleep apnoea-related cognitive deficits,[84] and schizophrenia.[85] Patients presenting with better cognition after the onset of psychosis have better outcomes both in functional domains, such as work rehabilitation,[86] and in skills such as social problem solving.[87] Cognitive reserve may therefore moderate the impact of illness on patients' lives as well as modulate the likelihood of developing a disorder.

Conclusion

The cognitive reserve paradigm indicates that brain structure and function can provide a buffer against the expression of neurologic disease. Passive models of reserve focus on the protective potential of anatomical features, such as brain size, neural density, and synaptic connectivity, while active models emphasize the efficiency of neural networks and active compensation by alternative or more extensive networks after challenge. It is likely that both models represent unique features of a common biological substrate. Research is needed to delineate the latter and to identify targets which might be used to decrease the burden of neurological illness.

References

1   Ely EW, Shintani A, Truman B, et al. Delirium as a predictor of mortality in mechanically ventilated patients in the intensive care unit. *JAMA* 2004;**291**:1753–62.

2   Girard TD, Jackson JC, Pandharipande PP, et al. Delirium as a predictor of long-term cognitive impairment in survivors of critical illness. *Crit Care Med* 2010;**38**:1513–20.

3   Morandi A, Rogers BP, Gunther ML, et al; and Visions Investigation, V. I. S. N. S. The relationship between delirium duration, white matter integrity, and cognitive impairment in intensive care unit survivors as determined by diffusion tensor imaging: the VISIONS prospective cohort magnetic resonance imaging study. *Crit Care Med* 2012;**40**:2182–9.

4   Sharshar T, Carlier R, Bernard F, et al. Brain lesions in septic shock: a magnetic resonance imaging study. *Intensive Care Med* 2007;**33**:798–806.

5   Fong TG, Jones RN, Shi P, et al. Delirium accelerates cognitive decline in Alzheimer disease. *Neurology* 2009;**72**:1570–5.

6   Ehlenbach WJ, Hough CL, Crane PK, et al. Association between acute care and critical illness hospitalization and cognitive function in older adults. *JAMA* 2010;**303**:763–70.

7   Iwashyna TJ, Ely EW, Smith DM, Langa KM. Long-term cognitive impairment and functional disability among survivors of severe sepsis. *JAMA* 2010;**304**:1787–94.

8   Stern Y. Cognitive reserve in ageing and Alzheimer's disease. *Lancet Neurol* 2012;**11**:1006–12.

9   Katzman R, Terry R, Deteresa R, et al. Clinical, pathological, and neurochemical changes in dementia: a subgroup with preserved mental status and numerous neocortical plaques. *Ann Neurol* 1988;**23**:138–44.

10   Neuropathology Group. Medical Research Council Cognitive Function and Aging Study. Pathological correlates of late-onset dementia in a multicentre, community-based population in England and Wales. Neuropathology Group of the Medical Research Council Cognitive Function and Ageing Study (MRC CFAS). *Lancet* 2001;**357**:169–75.

11   Katzman R. Education and the prevalence of dementia and Alzheimer's disease. *Neurology* 1993;**43**: 13–20.

12   Stern Y, Albert S, Tang MX, Tsai WY. Rate of memory decline in AD is related to education and occupation: cognitive reserve? *Neurology* 1999;**53**:1942–7.

13   Wilson RS, Bennett DA, Gilley DW, Beckett LA, Barnes LL, Evans DA. Premorbid reading activity and patterns of cognitive decline in Alzheimer disease. *Arch Neurol* 2000;**57**:1718–23.

14   Stern Y. Cognitive reserve and Alzheimer disease. *Alzheimer Dis Assoc Disord* 2006;**20**:S69–74.

15   Chetelat G, Villemagne VL, Pike KE, et al. Larger temporal volume in elderly with high versus low beta-amyloid deposition. *Brain* 2010;**133**:3349–58.

16   Schofield PW, Logroscino G, Andrews HF, Albert S, Stern Y. An association between head circumference and Alzheimer's disease in a population-based study of aging and dementia. *Neurology* 1997;**49**:30–7.

17   Satz P. Brain reserve capacity on symptom onset after brain injury: A formulation and review of evidence for threshold theory. *Neuropsychology* 1993;**7**:273–95.

18 Meng X, D'arcy C. Education and dementia in the context of the cognitive reserve hypothesis: a systematic review with meta-analyses and qualitative analyses. *PLoS One* 2012;7:e38268.

19 Stern Y. What is cognitive reserve? Theory and research application of the reserve concept. *J Int Neuropsychol Soc* 2002;8:448–60.

20 Grady CL, Maisog JM, Horwitz B, et al. Age-related changes in cortical blood flow activation during visual processing of faces and location. *J Neurosci* 1994;14:1450–62.

21 Deary IJ, Whalley LJ, Batty GD, Starr JM. Physical fitness and lifetime cognitive change. *Neurology* 2006;67:1195–200.

22 Staff RT, Murray AD, Deary IJ, Whalley LJ. What provides cerebral reserve? *Brain* 2004;127:1191–9.

23 Brown J, Cooper-Kuhn CM, Kempermann G, et al. Enriched environment and physical activity stimulate hippocampal but not olfactory bulb neurogenesis. *Eur J Neurosci* 2003;17:2042–6.

24 Van Praag H, Kempermann G, Gage FH. Running increases cell proliferation and neurogenesis in the adult mouse dentate gyrus. *Nat Neurosci* 1999;2:266–70.

25 Lazarov O, Robinson J, Tang YP, et al. Environmental enrichment reduces Abeta levels and amyloid deposition in transgenic mice. *Cell* 2005;120:701–13.

26 Mori E, Hirono N, Yamashita H, et al. Premorbid brain size as a determinant of reserve capacity against intellectual decline in Alzheimer's disease. *Am J Psychiatry* 1997;154:18–24.

27 Sole-Padulles C, Bartres-Faz D, Junque C, et al. Brain structure and function related to cognitive reserve variables in normal aging, mild cognitive impairment and Alzheimer's disease. *Neurobiol Aging* 2009;30:1114–24.

28 Maclullich AM, Ferguson KJ, Deary IJ, Seckl JR, Starr JM, Wardlaw JM. Intracranial capacity and brain volumes are associated with cognition in healthy elderly men. *Neurology* 2002;59:169–74.

29 Valenzuela MJ, Matthews FE, Brayne C, et al. Multiple biological pathways link cognitive lifestyle to protection from dementia. *Biol Psychiatry* 2012;71:783–91.

30 Spires TL, Meyer-Luehmann M, Stern EA, et al. Dendritic spine abnormalities in amyloid precursor protein transgenic mice demonstrated by gene transfer and intravital multiphoton microscopy. *J Neurosci* 2005;25:7278–87.

31 Manly JJ, Schupf N, Tang MX, Stern Y. Cognitive decline and literacy among ethnically diverse elders. *J Geriatr Psychiatry Neurol* 2005;18:213–17.

32 Alexander GE, Furey ML, Grady CL, et al. Association of premorbid intellectual function with cerebral metabolism in Alzheimer's disease: implications for the cognitive reserve hypothesis. *Am J Psychiatry* 1997;154:165–72.

33 Teresi JA, Albert SM, Holmes D, Mayeux R. Use of latent class analyses for the estimation of prevalence of cognitive impairment, and signs of stroke and Parkinson's disease among African-American elderly of central Harlem: results of the Harlem Aging Project. *Neuroepidemiology* 1999;18: 309–21.

34 Evans DA, Beckett LA, Albert MS, et al. Level of education and change in cognitive function in a community population of older persons. *Ann Epidemiol* 1993;3:71–7.

35 Mortel KF, Meyer JS, Herod B, Thornby J. Education and occupation as risk factors for dementias of the Alzheimer and ischemic vascular types. *Dementia* 1995;6:55–62.

36 Rocca WA, Bonaiuto S, Lippi A, et al. Prevalence of clinically diagnosed Alzheimer's disease and other dementing disorders: a door-to-door survey in Appignano, Macerata Province, Italy. *Neurology* 1990;40:626–31.

37 Stern Y, Gurland B, Tatemichi TK, Tang MX, Wilder D, Mayeux R. Influence of education and occupation on the incidence of Alzheimer's disease. *JAMA* 1994;271:1004–10.

38 Stern Y, Alexander GE, Prohovnik I, et al. Relationship between lifetime occupation and parietal flow: implications for a reserve against Alzheimer's disease pathology. *Neurology* 1995;45:55–60.

39 Richards M, Sacker A. Lifetime antecedents of cognitive reserve. *J Clin Exp Neuropsychol* 2003;**25**: 614–24.

40 Richards M, Deary IJ. A life course approach to cognitive reserve: a model for cognitive aging and development? *Ann Neurol* 2005;**58**:617–22.

41 Rhyu IJ, Bytheway JA, Kohler SJ, et al. Effects of aerobic exercise training on cognitive function and cortical vascularity in monkeys. *Neuroscience* 2010;**167**:1239–48.

42 Rogers RL, Meyer JS, Mortel KF. After reaching retirement age physical activity sustains cerebral perfusion and cognition. *J Am Geriatr Soc* 1990;**38**:123–8.

43 Gould E, Reeves AJ, Graziano MS, Gross CG. Neurogenesis in the neocortex of adult primates. *Science* 1999;**286**:548–52.

44 Kempermann G, Kuhn HG, Gage FH. More hippocampal neurons in adult mice living in an enriched environment. *Nature* 1997;**386**:493–5.

45 Snowdon DA, Kemper SJ, Mortimer JA, Greiner LH, Wekstein DR, Markesbery WR. Linguistic ability in early life and cognitive function and Alzheimer's disease in late life. Findings from the Nun Study. *JAMA* 1996;**275**:528–32.

46 Prohovnik I, Mayeux R, Sackeim HA, Smith G, Stern Y, Alderson PO. Cerebral perfusion as a diagnostic marker of early Alzheimer's disease. *Neurology* 1988;**38**:931–7.48.

47 Brun A, Englund E. Regional pattern of degeneration in Alzheimer's disease: neuronal loss and histopathological grading. *Histopathology* 1981;**5**:549–64.

48 Pearson RC, Esiri MM, Hiorns RW, Wilcock GK, Powell TP. Anatomical correlates of the distribution of the pathological changes in the neocortex in Alzheimer disease. *Proc Natl Acad Sci USA* 1985;**82**:4531–4.

49 Rogers J, Morrison JH. Quantitative morphology and regional and laminar distributions of senile plaques in Alzheimer's disease. *J Neurosci* 1985;**5**:2801–8.

50 Stern Y, Alexander GE, Prohovnik I, Mayeux R. Inverse relationship between education and parietotemporal perfusion deficit in Alzheimer's disease. *Ann Neurol* 1992;**32**:371–5.

51 Scarmeas N, Levy G, Tang MX, Manly J, Stern Y. Influence of leisure activity on the incidence of Alzheimer's disease. *Neurology* 2001;**57**:2236–42.

52 Alexander GE, Furey ML, Grady CL, et al. Association of premorbid intellectual function with cerebral metabolism in Alzheimer's disease: implications for the cognitive reserve hypothesis. *Am J Psychiatry* 1997;**154**:165–72.

53 Perneczky R, Drzezga A, Diehl-Schmid J, et al. Schooling mediates brain reserve in Alzheimer's disease: findings of fluoro-deoxy-glucose-positron emission tomography. *J Neurol Neurosurg Psychiatry* 2006;**77**:1060–3.

54 Valenzuela MJ, Sachdev P. Brain reserve and dementia: a systematic review. *Psychol Med* 2006;**36**: 441–54.

55 Manly JJ, Touradji P, Tang MX, Stern Y. Literacy and memory decline among ethnically diverse elders. *J Clin Exp Neuropsychol* 2003;**25**:680–90.

56 Butler SM, Ashford JW, Snowdon DA. Age, education, and changes in the Mini-Mental State Exam scores of older women: findings from the Nun Study. *J Am Geriatr Soc* 1996;**44**:675–81.

57 Lyketsos CG, Chen LS, Anthony JC. Cognitive decline in adulthood: an 11.5-year follow-up of the Baltimore Epidemiologic Catchment Area study. *Am J Psychiatry* 1999;**156**:58–65.

58 Karp A, Kareholt I, Qiu C, Bellander T, Winblad B, Fratiglioni L. Relation of education and occupation-based socioeconomic status to incident Alzheimer's disease. *Am J Epidemiol* 2004;**159**:175–83.

59 Scarmeas N, Albert SM, Manly JJ, Stern Y. Education and rates of cognitive decline in incident Alzheimer's disease. *J Neurol Neurosurg Psychiatry* 2006;**77**:308–16.

60 Helzner EP, Scarmeas N, Cosentino S, Portet F, Stern Y. Leisure activity and cognitive decline in incident Alzheimer disease. *Arch Neurol* 2007;**64**:1749–54.

61 **Hall CB, Derby C, Levalley A, Katz MJ, Verghese J, Lipton RB.** Education delays accelerated decline on a memory test in persons who develop dementia. *Neurology* 2007;**69**:1657–64.

62 **Bennett DA, Wilson RS, Schneider JA, et al.** Apolipoprotein E epsilon4 allele, AD pathology, and the clinical expression of Alzheimer's disease. *Neurology* 2003;**60**:246–52.

63 **Koepsell TD, Kurland BF, Harel O, Johnson EA, Zhou XH, Kukull WA.** Education, cognitive function, and severity of neuropathology in Alzheimer disease. *Neurology* 2008;**70**:1732–9.

64 **Negash S, Xie S, Davatzikos C, et al.** Cognitive and functional resilience despite molecular evidence of Alzheimer's disease pathology. *Alzheimers Dement* 2013;**9**:e89–95.

65 **Kemppainen NM, Aalto S, Karrasch M, et al.** Cognitive reserve hypothesis: Pittsburgh Compound B and fluorodeoxyglucose positron emission tomography in relation to education in mild Alzheimer's disease. *Ann Neurol* 2008;**63**:112–18.

66 **Kesler SR, Adams HF, Blasey CM, Bigler ED.** Premorbid intellectual functioning, education, and brain size in traumatic brain injury: an investigation of the cognitive reserve hypothesis. *Appl Neuropsychol* 2003;**10**:153–62.

67 **Schofield PW, Mosesson RE, Stern Y, Mayeux R.** The age at onset of Alzheimer's disease and an intracranial area measurement. A relationship. *Arch Neurol* 1995;**52**:95–8.

68 **Querbes O, Aubry F, Pariente J, et al.** Early diagnosis of Alzheimer's disease using cortical thickness: impact of cognitive reserve. *Brain* 2009;**132**:2036–47.

69 **Edland SD, Xu Y, Plevak M, et al.** Total intracranial volume: normative values and lack of association with Alzheimer's disease. *Neurology* 2002;**59**:272–4.

70 **Jenkins R, Fox NC, Rossor AM, Harvey RJ, Rossor MN.** Intracranial volume and Alzheimer disease: evidence against the cerebral reserve hypothesis. *Arch Neurol* 2000;**57**:220–4.

71 **Friedland RP, Brun A, Budinger TF.** Pathological and positron emission tomographic correlations in Alzheimer's disease. *Lancet* 1985;**1**:228.

72 **Garibotto V, Borroni B, Kalbe E, et al.** Education and occupation as proxies for reserve in aMCI converters and AD: FDG-PET evidence. *Neurology* 2008;**71**:1342–9.

73 **Bosch B, Bartres-Faz D, Rami L, et al.** Cognitive reserve modulates task-induced activations and deactivations in healthy elders, amnestic mild cognitive impairment and mild Alzheimer's disease. *Cortex* 2010;**46**:451–61.

74 **Habeck C, Hilton HJ, Zarahn E, Flynn J, Moeller J, Stern Y.** Relation of cognitive reserve and task performance to expression of regional covariance networks in an event-related fMRI study of nonverbal memory. *Neuroimage* 2003;**20**:1723–33.

75 **Liao YC, Liu RS, Teng EL, et al.** Cognitive reserve: a SPECT study of 132 Alzheimer's disease patients with an education range of 0–19 years. *Dement Geriatr Cogn Disord* 2005;**20**:8–14.

76 **Scarmeas N, Zarahn E, Anderson KE, et al.** Cognitive reserve modulates functional brain responses during memory tasks: a PET study in healthy young and elderly subjects. *Neuroimage* 2003;**19**:1215–27.

77 **Sumowski JF, Wylie GR, Deluca J, Chiaravalloti N.** Intellectual enrichment is linked to cerebral efficiency in multiple sclerosis: functional magnetic resonance imaging evidence for cognitive reserve. *Brain* 2010;**133**:362–74.

78 **Scheibel RS, Newsome MR, Troyanskaya M, et al.** Effects of severity of traumatic brain injury and brain reserve on cognitive-control related brain activation. *J Neurotrauma* 2009;**26**:1447–61.

79 **Cabeza R.** Hemispheric asymmetry reduction in older adults: the HAROLD model. *Psychol Aging* 2002;**17**:85–100.

80 **Reuter-Lorenz P.** New visions of the aging mind and brain. *Trends Cogn Sci* 2002;**6**:394.

81 **Rajah MN, D'esposito M.** Region-specific changes in prefrontal function with age: a review of PET and fMRI studies on working and episodic memory. *Brain* 2005;**128**:1964–83.

82 **Oyegbile TO, Dow C, Jones J, et al.** The nature and course of neuropsychological morbidity in chronic temporal lobe epilepsy. *Neurology* 2004;**62**:1736–42.

83 Cader S, Cifelli A, Abu-Omar Y, Palace J, Matthews PM. Reduced brain functional reserve and altered functional connectivity in patients with multiple sclerosis. *Brain* 2006;**129**:527–37.

84 Alchanatis M, Zias N, Deligiorgis N, Amfilochiou A, Dionellis G, Orphanidou D. Sleep apnea-related cognitive deficits and intelligence: an implication of cognitive reserve theory. *J Sleep Res* 2005;**14**:69–75.

85 Koenen KC, Moffitt TE, Roberts AL, et al. Childhood IQ and adult mental disorders: a test of the cognitive reserve hypothesis. *Am J Psychiatry* 2009;**166**:50–7.

86 Bell MD, Bryson G. Work rehabilitation in schizophrenia: does cognitive impairment limit improvement? *Schizophr Bull* 2001;**27**:269–79.

87 Addington J, Addington D. Neurocognitive and social functioning in schizophrenia: a 2.5 year follow-up study. *Schizophr Res* 2000;**44**:47–56.

Chapter 30

Pathophysiology of Acute Kidney Injury, Repair, and Regeneration

Ching-Wei Tsai, Sanjeev Noel, and Hamid Rabb

Introduction

AKI is a common complication in hospitalized patients,[1-3] associated with significantly increased mortality, length of stay, and cost. Although AKI has largely been considered reversible, epidemiological studies have shown that a considerable number of patients with AKI have only partial renal recovery.[4] Animal studies have shown that AKI results in persistent and permanent structural and functional changes in the kidney, with renal fibrosis as an important contributor to the subsequent development of CKD.[5-7] Emerging evidence indicates that an AKI episode can lead to CKD and accelerate the progression to ESRD.[8-11] Coca et al.[12] conducted a systematic review and meta-analysis of the long-term outcomes after AKI and found that the mortality rate was 8.9 deaths/100 person-years in survivors of AKI. The CKD rate after an episode of AKI was 7.8 events/100 patient-years, and the ESRD rate was 4.9 events/100 patient-years. In a long-term follow-up study of 130 AKI patients who required dialysis, 41% developed CKD, of which 10% needed chronic dialysis. Patients who develop AKI can be divided into four groups: (1) complete recovery of renal function, (2) development of progressive CKD, (3) exacerbation of the rate of progression of pre-existing CKD, and (4) irreversible loss of kidney function that evolves to ESRD.[13] This chapter reviews the recent progress in understanding the pathophysiology of AKI in the injury, repair, and regeneration phases, including the progression to CKD.

Cellular changes during ischaemic AKI

The pathophysiology of kidney injury and repair is complicated. Ischaemia- reperfusion injury (IRI) is a major cause of AKI. Regardless of the aetiology of AKI (sepsis, ischaemia, or toxin), there are common features of injury process. Following the initial insults of AKI, reduction of effective renal perfusion leads to ATP depletion in vascular and tubular cells. Regions of kidney most prone to ischaemic injury are the S3 segment of the proximal tubule and the medullary thick ascending limb of the loop of Henle. During reperfusion, ATP depletion induces oxidative stress, and the ROS causes injury to the tubular epithelial cells (TECs). The ATP-depleted TECs, depending on the extent of injury, either undergo sublethal injury, characterized by functional and structural recovery, or lethal injury, characterized by apoptosis or necrosis.[14,15] Sublethal injury involves shedding of the brush border, changes in the actin cytoskeleton, disruption of tight junctions and adherens junctions, and loss of polarity with mislocalization of adhesion molecules and other polarized membrane proteins such as Na^+/K^+-ATPase and β-integrins.[16-20] The necrotic or apoptotic TECs shading from the basement membrane into the tubule lumen as well as protein, such as fibronectin, cause cast formation, which lead to intratubular obstruction and reduction in GFR.[16] Loss of TECs, destruction of tight junctions, and intratubular obstruction contribute to the tubular back-leakage, which further decreases effective GFR. Basolateral Na^+/K^+- ATPase mis-localization after ischaemia reduces the efficiency of transcellular sodium transport and increases intraluminal sodium delivery to the distal tubule, resulting in high fractional excretion of sodium in patients with acute tubular necrosis[18,19] (see Figure 30.1). During recovery from IRI, surviving TECs dedifferentiate and proliferate, eventually replacing the irreversibly injured TECs.[21] Under normal circumstances, proximal tubule cells divide at a low rate. Within 24–48 hours following IRI, the surviving TECs start to proliferate at a high rate, especially in the proximal tubules of the outer medulla.[22] However, recent reports indicate that bone marrow stem cells (BMSCs) and progenitor cells in the kidney contribute to new TECs in post-ischaemic kidney. Current evidence favours the view that restoration of the tubule epithelium after ischaemic AKI occurs predominantly from the proliferation of endogenous surviving TECs.[23] IRI interrupts the integrity of the renal vascular endothelium and increases microvascular permeability, enhances adhesion molecules' expression and leucocyte-endothelial interactions, and facilitates the extravasation of leucocytes. Increased expression of ICAM-1, P-selectin, and E-selectin on renal epithelium, and Toll-like receptors (TLR2 and TLR4) on TECs, activates immune response in the post-ischaemic

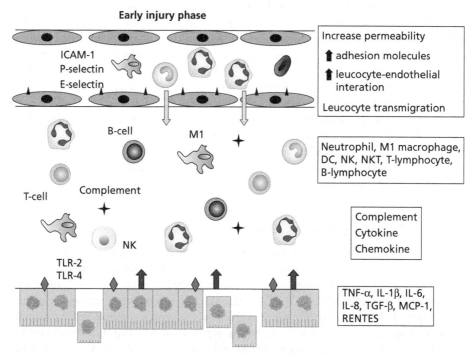

Fig. 30.1 Immune responses in the early injury phase of ischaemic AKI.
ICAM-1, intercellular adhesion molecule-1; DC, dendritic cell; M1, M1 macrophage; NK, natural killer cell; TLR, Toll-like receptor; TNF-α, tumour necrosis factor-α; IL-1β, interleukin-1β; IL-6, interleukin-6; IL-8, interleukin-8; TGF-β, transforming growth factor-β; RENTES, regulated and normal T cell expressed and secreted.

Reproduced from Jang HR, 'The interaction between ischemia-reperfusion and immune responses in the kidney', *Journal of Molecular Medicine*, 87, 9, 2009, pp. 859–864. With kind permission from Springer Science and Business Media.

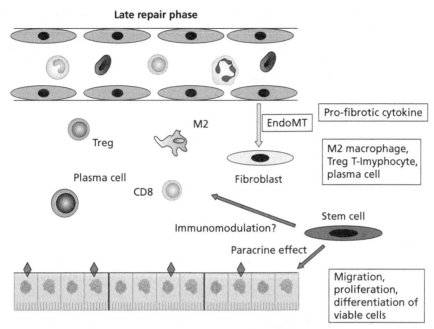

Fig. 30.2 Immune responses in the late repair phase of ischaemic AKI.
Treg, regulatory T cell; M2, M2 macrophage; CD8, cytotoxic T cell; EndoMT, endothelial-mesenchymal transformation.

Reproduced from: Jang HR, 'The interaction between ischemia-reperfusion and immune responses in the kidney', *Journal of Molecular Medicine*, 87, 9, 2009, pp. 859–864. With kind permission from Springer Science and Business Media.

kidneys. Complement activation further aggravates inflammation in the early phase of injury. Important effector cells in early injury phase include neutrophils, M1 macrophages (M1), natural killer (NK) cells, dendritic cells (DC), T lymphocytes, and possibly B cells. Soluble factors, including complement, pro-inflammatory cytokines, and chemokines, play an important role in the initiation phase of renal IRI (see Figure 30.2).

Microvascular changes during ischaemic AKI

Rarefaction of peritubular capillaries and endothelial-mesenchymal transition

The potential long-term effects of IRI on renal vascular structure were noted by Basile.[24] Post-ischaemic rat kidney manifested 30–50% reduction in microvessel density at 4, 8, and 40 weeks after injury.[5,6,25] Evidences from animal models and human have established a direct correlation between rarefaction of the peritubular capillaries and the development of tubulointerstitial fibrosis.[26,27,28] While exploring the mechanism of rarefaction of peritubular capillaries, it was demonstrated that renal IRI downregulates vascular endothelial cell growth factor (VEGF), an angiogenic factor, and upregulates ADAMTS-1, a novel VEGF inhibitor.[29] Treatment with VEGF-121 preserve vascular structure after ischaemia and influence chronic renal function.[30] Following repetitive administration of BrdU, no proliferating endothelial cells were identified up to 2 days after ischaemia and reperfusion and accounted for only ~1% of BrdU-positive cells after 7 days.

Furthermore, endothelial-mesenchymal transition (endoMT) was identified by co-localizing endothelial markers with the fibroblast marker. Utilizing labelled transgenic mice to trace the fate of endothelial cells following IRI, the yellow fluorescent protein (YFP)-positive endothelial cells were found to be a source of interstitial fibroblasts. This interstitial distribution of YFP-positive cells was attenuated by VEGF-121. These data indicate that reduction in renal microvascular density post-AKI results from limited regenerative capacity, combined with endoMT, which may contribute to progressive CKD.[31]

Chronic hypoxia and tubulointerstitial fibrosis

Either loss of peritubular capillaries or persistent vasoconstriction contributes to chronic hypoxia. Chronic hypoxia was proposed to trigger tubulointerstitial fibrosis, which is the hallmark of CKD of diverse aetiologies.[32] In fact, tubulointerstitial fibrosis provides the best predictive indicator of progression to ESRD.[33] *In vitro* studies on TECs and interstitial fibroblasts show that hypoxia can trigger a fibrotic response.[34] Activation of hypoxia-inducible factor (HIF) by hypoxia leads to the expression of a variety of adaptive genes.[35] Hypoxia induces the expression of fibrogenic factors, such as TGF-β,[26] promotes ECM accumulation, and suppresses matrix degradation via decreased expression of matrix metalloproteinases.[36] Furthermore, hypoxia may also induce endoMT and transdifferentiation of endothelial cells into (myo)fibroblasts.[31,37] Considering chronic hypoxia is an important mediator in CKD progression, therapeutic strategies, that either reverse vaso-constriction or preserve vascular structure, may prove beneficial. L-arginine treatment increases renal blood flow (RBF), reduces hypoxia, and attenuates the development of secondary renal scarring and proteinuria in post-ischaemic rats.[38] The renoprotective effect of administration of VEGF has been discussed previously. Several experimental studies demonstrated stabilization of HIF through cobalt chloride, carbon monoxide, and prolyl hydroxylase inhibitors attenuate IRI.[35,39,40] Strategies that restore microvasculature integrity and prevent hypoxia are potential targets for future therapy.

Inflammation

Inflammation and recruitment of leucocytes during ischaemia and reperfusion are now recognized as major mediators of endothelial and tubular cell injury.[14,41] Inflammation starts during renal ischaemia and accelerates upon reperfusion in post-ischaemic kidneys, with endothelial activation, leucocyte recruitment, upregulation of chemokines and cytokines, and activation of the comple-ment system. Both innate and adaptive immune responses are important contributors to IRI. Several reports demonstrate the renoprotective effects of therapy targeting immune components directly support the role of immunity in the pathogenesis of AKI.[42] Neutrophils are traditionally thought to be the first cells to accumulate at the site of ischaemic injury.[43] However, blockade of neutrophil function or neutrophil depletion provides only partial protection against injury, indi-cating that other leucocytes also mediate injury.[44] Later phases of AKI are characterized by infil-tration of monocyte and lymphocytes that predominate over neutrophils.[41,42,45,46] The activated leucocytes secrete pro-inflammatory cytokines, such as TNF-α, IL-1, and IFN-γ, which damage the proximal TECs and disrupt cell-matrix adhesion, inducing cell shedding into the lumen.[47–49]

Soluble molecules and immune cells in ischaemic AKI

Whilst many of the components in the early phase of AKI have been known, the immune reac-tions in the repair phase are not fully understood. Cell adhesion molecules as well as cytokines and chemokines produced by leucocytes may not only influence the level of injury, but also the migration, differentiation, and proliferation of renal epithelial cells during recovery phase.[21] Recent findings on M2 macrophage and regulatory T cell (Treg) in the recovery phase of IRI implicate the immune reactions also modulate the repair phase of AKI.

Macrophages

Macrophages are an important mediator in the initiation phase of IRI. Monocyte-derived macrophages have been reported to infiltrate in the kidney as early as 24 hours after reperfusion, mediated by CCR2 and CX3CR1 signalling pathways.[50,51,52] Depletion of macrophages by clodronate before renal IRI prevented AKI, whereas adoptive transfer of macrophages reconstituted AKI.[53,54] These results confirmed the role of macrophages in mediating injury in IRI. Recent evidences suggest that macrophages are also involved in renal repair and fibrosis after injury. Systemic macrophage depletion reduced renal fibrosis at 4 and 8 weeks in mice with I/R.[55] Reduction of macrophage infiltration in osteopontin knockout mice was correlated to less deposition of collagen types I and IV in the post-ischaemic kidney.[56]

However, the role of macrophages in kidney injury is far more complicated than previously thought. There are two distinct subsets of macrophages, classically activated (M1) or alternatively activated (M2). M2 macrophages are further subdivided into M2a (wound-healing macrophages), M2b, and M2c cells (regulatory macrophages).[57] Besides the well-known role in renal inflammation, macrophages also play a critical role in tissue remodelling and repair and immune regulation. M1 macrophages secrete pro-inflammatory cytokines, such as TNF-α, IFN-γ, and exacerbate renal injury. In contrast, M2 macrophages produce anti-inflammatory cytokines and inhibit T cell proliferation, which suppress inflammation and repair injury.[58] Furthermore, M1 and M2 macrophage also have different influences on fibrosis, profibrotic and anti-fibrotic, respectively.[59] Recently, Lee et al.[60] showed M1 macrophages are recruited into the kidney in the first 48 hours after IRI, whereas M2 macrophages predominate at later time points. Furthermore, when tracking fluorescently labelled macrophages that were injected after injury, they found that M1 macrophages can switch to an M2 phenotype in the kidney at the onset of kidney repair.[60]

DCs

DCs are not only involved in innate immunity, but also in antigen presention which can activate T cells. Dong et al. demonstrated that renal DCs are potent early producers of pro-inflammatory mediators, TNF-α, IL-6, MCP-1, and RANTES in the kidney following IRI. *In vivo* depletion of DCs before ischaemia substantially reduced the levels of TNF-α produced by the kidney.[61] Using CD11c-DTR transgenic mouse, kidney injury was significantly less in the DC-depleted mice than control mice which received mutant DT treatment.[62] However, in cisplatin-induced AKI model, DCs reduce cisplatin nephrotoxicity and its associated inflammation.[63] The roles of DCs in AKI need more studies.

NK cells

NK cells are important in the early stage of innate immune responses. One recent study showed that NK cells can directly kill renal TECs and contribute substantially to kidney IRI. NK cell depletion in wild-type mice was renoprotective, while adoptive transfer of NK cells worsened I/R renal injury in NK, T, and B cell null Rag2–/– γc–/– mice.[64]

Natural killer T (NKT) cells

NKT cells are a unique subset of T lymphocytes, with both T cell and NK cell receptors, and have the ability to promptly secrete large amounts of cytokines such as IFN-γ, TNF-α, and IL-4. They provide maturation signals to DCs, NK cells, and lymphocytes, thereby contributing to both innate and acquired immune responses.[65] CD1d-restricted NKT cells are significantly increased in the ischaemic kidney by 3 hours of reperfusion. Blockade of NKT cell activation with the anti-CD1d Ab, or NKT cell depletion with Ab, or using NKT cell-deficient mice (Jα18–/–) inhibited the accumulation of neutrophils after I/R and attenuated renal IRI. These results implicate the important contribution of NKT cells in kidney IRI.[66]

T lymphocytes

Numerous studies have shown that T lymphocytes are implicated in the pathogenesis of renal IRI.[46,67,68] CD4+ T cells infiltrate into the kidney following ischaemia.[69] CD4 knockout mice, but not CD8 knockout mice, were significantly protected from renal IRI, and adoptive transfer of CD4 T cells into CD4 knockout mice restored early post-ischaemic injury.[70] Blockade of the T cell CD28-B7 costimulatory pathway with CTLA4 Ig also attenuated renal dysfunction after IRI.[69]

T cell receptor (TCR) also plays a role in renal IRI. TCR αβ-deficient mice had a significant functional and structural protection from kidney IRI, which, in turn, was associated with a decreased level of TNF-α and IL-6 in post-ischaemic kidney, compared with wild-type mice.[71,72] One study investigating the CD4 T cell subsets Th1 or Th2 in a murine renal IRI model suggested that the Th1 phenotype is pathogenic whereas Th2 phenotype is protective. Mice deficient in STAT6 (the enzyme regulating Th2) showed more severe renal injury than wild-type mice, while mice deficient in STAT4 (the enzyme regulating Th1) had mild improvement in renal function after IRI.[73]

T cell trafficking was observed as early as 3 h after I/R and decrease at 24 hours.[74] T cell trafficking is also associated with increased vascular permeability in early ischaemic AKI.[75] More importantly, renal injury and permeability were attenuated in T cell-deficient mice, and the increased permeability was restored after T cell transfer.[76,77] Ascon et al.[74] showed infiltrating CD4+ and CD8+ T cells in injured kidney, up to 6 weeks after severe renal IRI. These T cells had increased expression of activation marker (CD69+) and effector memory (CD44hi CD62L–), and there was a significant upregulation of IL-1β, IL-6, TNF-α, IFN-γ, MIP-2, and RANTES expression.[78] Accordingly, moderate or severe kidney ischaemia may induce long-term T lymphocyte infiltration and cytokine/chemokine upregulation, which might contribute to the development of CKD.

Recently, Tregs were found to have a role in IRI. CD4+ CD25+ Treg cells are functionally mature T cell subpopulation that have been implicated in the maintenance of immunologic self-tolerance and negative control of a variety of physiological and pathological immune responses.[79] Gandolfo et al.[80] found that TCRβ+ CD4+ CD25+ Foxp3+ Treg cells trafficking into the kidneys were increased after 3 days and 10 days after IRI. Treg depletion after IRI, using anti-CD25 antibodies, aggravated renal injury and increased the production of pro-inflammatory cytokines. Treg transfer after IRI reduced cytokine production by T lymphocytes and promoted renal repair, evidenced by less tubules damage and more tubule proliferation. Kinsey et al. also revealed that Treg depletion resulted in more neutrophils, macrophages, and enhanced innate immune response in the kidney in the early phase of IRI.[81,82] They demonstrate that Tregs modulate kidney IRI through IL-10-mediated suppression of the innate immune system. These studies illustrated the important role of Tregs during renal repair.[82]

B lymphocytes

The role of B lymphocytes in IRI was first demonstrated when B cell-deficient (μMT) mice, compared with wild-type mice, had better renal function and reduced tubular injury at 24, 48, and 72 hours post-ischaemia.[83] Jang et al.[84] further showed that B cells limit repair after renal I/R. B cells infiltration peaked at day 3 in post-ischaemic kidneys and decreased over time. B cells subsequently activated and differentiated to plasma cells during the repair phase. Targeting infiltrating CD126-expressing plasma cells, using anti-CD126 Ab, led to diminished tubular atrophy, with enhanced tubular proliferation and reduced functional impairment in the late repair phase. Adoptive transfer of B cells into B cell-deficient (μMT) mice decreased tubular proliferation and increased tubular atrophy.

Renal regeneration and repair

Role of stem cells in renal repair and regeneration

The origin of proliferating cells during the repair/regeneration phase of AKI is currently not clear and remains debatable. Regenerative cell could be derived from three different types of cells: (1) bone marrow-derived stem cells that migrate into the injured kidney and differentiate into mature cells, (2) renal stem cells that move to the site of repair, and (3) surviving tubular cells that dedifferentiate, proliferate, and differentiate again. In the following sections, we list the current evidences from several novel studies (see Figure 30.3).

BMSCs do not directly replace renal epithelial cell

BMSCs include MSCs and haematopoietic stem cells (HSCs). BMSCs have been found to engraft into the liver, lung, gastrointestinal tract, and skin.[85,86] The multipotent properties of BMSCs raise great interest in whether the BMSCs directly participate in renal injury and repair and in the usage of BMSCs for treatment of AKI.[23] Several early studies claim that BMSCs transdifferentiated into tubule epithelia of the injured kidney.[87-90] However, later studies showed usually below 1% of circulating BMSCs engraft in a given organ.[91] Duffield et al.[92] used chimeric mice expressing green fluorescence protein (GFP) or bacterial β-gal exclusively in bone marrow-derived cells to track the fate of GFP-positive cell in renal IRI model. More than 99% of those GFP interstitial cells were leucocytes. Upon

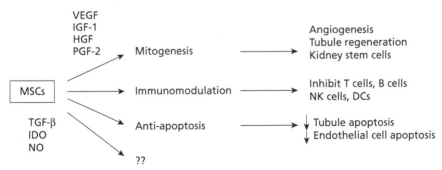

Fig. 30.3 The possible mechanisms of MSCs on renal repair and regeneration.
MSC, mesenchymal stem cells; VEGF, vascular endothelial growth factor; IGF-1, insulin like growth factor-1; HGF, hepatocyte growth factor; PGF-2, prostaglandin F2 alpha; IDO, indoleamine 2,3-dioxygenase; NO, nitric oxide.

IV injection of BMSCs, there was no evidence of differentiation of these MSCs into renal tubular cells, though a high proliferative rate at tubular cells was noted. These results indicated that BMSCs do not directly replace renal epithelia to a significant extent during renal repair.[92,93]

MSCs repair kidney by paracrine and endocrine mechanisms

Although endogenous BMSCs do not directly contribute to the replacement of renal epithelial cells, several studies show that exogenous administered MSCs are protective against renal injury.[94] Injection of MSCs remarkably protected cisplatin-induced mice from renal function impairment and severe tubular injury.[89] Similar renal protection from injected MSCs was found in a glycerol-induced pigment nephropathy model and in an IRI model.[95] Studies from Duffield et al.[92] and Lin et al.[91] showed protection from injury by exogenous MSCs but very little or no MSCs directly engraft into injured tubules. The mechanism of such protection may be due to immunomodulatory and paracrine effects of administered stem cells.[96]

MSCs secrete a variety of cytokines and growth factors that have both paracrine and autocrine activities, which can suppress the local immune system, inhibit fibrosis and apoptosis, enhance angiogenesis, and stimulate mitosis and differentiation of tissue-intrinsic reparative or stem cells.[97] Such paracrine effect is demonstrated by Togel et al.[96] They found intracarotid administration of MSCs either immediately or 24 hours after renal ischaemia resulted in significantly improved renal function, higher proliferative, and lower apoptotic indices, as well as lower renal injury, though infused MSCs were rarely engrafted. They further demonstrated that MSC-conditioned medium contains VEGF, hepatocyte growth factor (HGF), and IGF-1 and enhances endothelial cell growth and survival.[96,98] They concluded that the beneficial effects of MSCs in ischaemic kidney are primarily mediated via complex paracrine actions and not by their differentiation into target cells.

Bi et al. (2007) reported similar renal protective effects of either intraperitoneally or IV administered BMSCs, even though there were very few cells found in the kidney. Furthermore, conditioned media from cultured stromal cells induced proliferation of TECs and significantly diminished cisplatin-induced proximal tubule cell death *in vitro*. Intraperitoneal administration of the conditioned medium to mice injected with cisplatin diminished TECs apoptosis and limited renal injury. This means BMSCs protect the kidney from injury by secreting factors that limit apoptosis and enhance proliferation of the endogenous tubular cells.[99]

On the other hand, given the importance of inflammation in the pathophysiology of AKI, it is very important to consider the renoprotective effect of exogenously administered MSCs in term of immune modulation.[41,100] Human MSCs have been found to suppress immune responses, both *in vitro* and *in vivo*.[100-102] Immunosuppressive properties of MSCs have been reported to affect the function of a broad range of immune cells, including T cells, antigen-presenting cells, NK cells, and B cells.[100] The possible mechanisms of observed renoprotective effect of MSCs on IRI are illustrated in Figure 30.4. MSCs secrete a variety of cytokines and growth factors that have both paracrine and autocrine activities. These mediators include VEGF, IGF-1, HGF, and TGF-β. Through these factors, MSCs have mitogenic effect and promote angiogenesis, TEC repopulation, and probably kidney stem cell proliferation. In addition, MSCs can immunomodulate a broad range of immune cells, including T cells, antigen-presenting cells, NK cells, and B cells. MSCs also possess anti-apoptotic ability that decreases TEC and endothelial cell apoptosis.

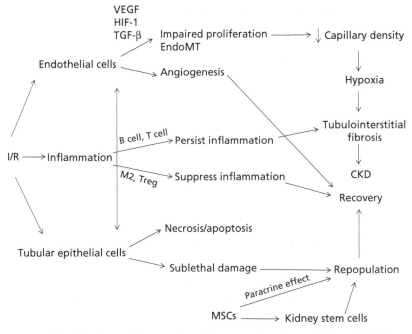

Fig. 30.4 Proposed mechanism in injury, repair, and regeneration phase of ischaemic AKI.

Role of growth factors in renal repair and regeneration

GH may play an important role in renal recovery. A number of growth factors, such as EGF, HGF, and IGF-1, are upregulated after AKI. Early studies showed administration of EGF, HGF, and IGF could accelerate the recovery of renal function and enhance tubule cell regeneration,[103,104] though clinical trials of IGF-I in patients with acute renal failure (ARF) have indeterminate or negative results. However, a recent study demonstrated that beneficial effects of MSCs on tubular cell repair in AKI are mediated by IGF-1.[105] VEGF, an angiogenic factor, was reduced in the initial post-ischaemic phase, and VEGF administration preserve microvascular density and attenuate CKD progression in rats with I/R.[30]

Many of these growth factors influence cells via autocrine or paracrine processes. They can stimulate cells to transit from G0 to G1 phase to initiate DNA synthesis and mitosis. Accordingly, to accelerate tubule cell re-entry into cell cycle during repair phase of AKI may be a important mechanism of these growth factors.[106] A recent study showed enhanced endothelial cell growth and survival using MSC-conditioned medium, containing VEGF, HGF, and IGF-1 in AKI.[96] This implies the possible role of growth factors in kidney repair and regeneration. It has been shown that surviving renal TECs secrete growth factors. The growth factors, irrespective of the cells that produce them, may participate in renal repair as paracrine regulators or chemoattractants to induce migration of regenerative cells.[107] Basic fibroblast growth factor (bFGF), which participates in early kidney development, re-expresses in the recovery phase of ARF. In rats with I/R, bFGF participates in the regeneration process. Treatment with bFGF has been shown to accelerate the regeneration process in ischaemic kidney.[108] HGF has mitogenic, motogenic, anti-apoptotic, and morphogenic activities for renal tubular cells, while it has angiogenic and angioprotective actions for endothelial cells. In AKI, HGF upregulates in the injured kidney and promotes renal regeneration.[109] In the late phases of recovery, HGF has anti-fibrotic effects, and the counterbalance between HGF and TGF-β influences the progression of CKD and renal fibrosis.[110,111]

Recently, Menke[112] found that colony-stimulating factor 1 (CSF-1), a macrophage growth factor, mediates renal repair by macrophage-dependent mechanism and direct autocrine/paracrine action on TECs. CSF-1 is generated predominantly by TECs during renal inflammation. Mice injected with CSF-1 following I/R had less tubular pathology, less fibrosis, and better renal function. In addition, CSF-1 treatment increased TEC proliferation and reduced TEC apoptosis.[112]

Erythropoietin (EPO) has been shown to promote renal functional recovery from ischaemic AKI.[113–115] These protective mechanisms come from multiple effects of EPO which is capable to inhibit cell apoptosis, increase HIF-1α expression, attenuate tubular hypoxia, and enhance TEC regeneration.[116,117] There are ongoing clinical trials testing the effect of EPO treatment on the development of AKI.

Maladaptive repair after AKI: tubulointerstitial fibrosis and progression to CKD

Several studies suggest renal injury and repair in AKI are a dynamic process in the spectrum of kidney disease regression or progression. AKI can result in complete repair or incomplete repair or worsen to maladaptive repair. Tubulointerstitial fibrosis is one kind of maladaptive repair. Persistent tubulointerstitial inflammation, with proliferation of fibroblasts and excessive deposition of ECM, lead to tubulointerstitial fibrosis, a common feature of many different kinds of kidney diseases and a primary determinant of progression to CKD or ESRD.[118]

The mechanism that triggers fibrogenic response after injury is not well understood. It has been proposed that epithelial cells may transform into a fibroblast, epithelial-mesenchymal transition (EMT) and contribute to fibrosis. However, recent studies by Humphreys et al. have challenged this concept. They performed fate-mapping, using genetically labelled renal epithelium, in models of kidney fibrosis to establish that epithelial cells do not contribute to the generation of myofibroblasts directly by transdifferentiation *in vivo*.[119] Lineage analysis showed that the majority of myofibroblasts differentiated from perivascular fibroblasts or pericytes. Basile et al.,[31] on the other hand, showed that EndoMT may be another source of fibroblasts.

Two new studies suggest that cell cycle arrest of epithelial cells and epigenetic modifications have key roles in the switch to chronic disease.[120,121] Using five AKI models, including ischaemic, toxic, and obstructive models, Yang et al.[122] showed a causal association between the development of fibrosis and the production of profibrotic cytokines correlated with the arrest of tubule epithelial cells in G2/M. G2/M arrest results in upregulation of profibrogenic growth factors. Abrogating the G2/M arrest markedly reduced fibrosis and cytokine production.[122]

Conclusion

AKI can lead to CKD and can accelerate the progression to ESRD. The pathophysiology of AKI involves a complex interplay among vascular, tubular, and inflammatory factors. Complete repair can often lead to a normal renal function, while incomplete repair or maladaptive repair may result in progression to CKD. Endothelial injury plays a critical role in the pathogenesis of AKI. Early phase involves the interplay among endothelial cells, TECs, and inflammatory cells. After IRI, endothelial damage causes endothelial dysfunction. Endothelial dysfunction induces the expression of cell adhesion molecules and enhances leucocyte-endothelial interactions. Inflammation further leads to apoptosis and necrosis of TECs, with subsequent secretion of inflammatory mediators. Activation of HIF-1, upregulation of TGF-β, and suppression of VEGF lead to impaired proliferation and EndoMT in the late phase. Decreased density of peritubular capillaries results in chronic hypoxia. Chronic hypoxia causes tubulointerstitial fibrosis and the onset of CKD. The exact repair mechanism of endothelium is unclear but appears to be mediated through efficient angiogenesis or involvement of endothelial progenitor cells. Depending on the severity of injury, the TECs may survive and proliferate. In the repair phase, surviving TECs repopulate the damaged tubule. MSCs do not directly contribute to the repopulation but help renal repair via paracrine effects. A concerted effort of M2 macrophages, Tregs, and various growth factors in the late phase suppresses inflammation and favours repair process. Inflammation mediates endothelial and tubular cell injury and repair. Both innate and adaptive immune components are involved in the early stage of kidney injury; however, others, such as M2 macrophage, Tregs, anti-inflammatory cytokines, and profibrogenic cytokines, may mediate the repair phase of AKI. Surviving renal TECs dedifferentiate, proliferate, and migrate to repair denuded areas of the tubule. The majority of cells that repopulate the tubules are believed to be derived from the surviving renal epithelial cells. BMSCs may not directly replace renal epithelial cells. Nevertheless, MSCs promote renal repair via paracrine and endocrine mechanisms. Adult renal stem cells have been firmly established in human kidney; however, its role in renal repair is not clear. GHs may play an important role in renal recovery; however, their applications in renal repair need more studies. The proper mechanism of endothelium or angiogenesis is unclear so far. Furthermore, tubulointerstitial fibrosis, as a result of maladaptive repair, appears to be the primary determinant of progression of AKI to CKD or ESRD. Understanding the mechanisms involved in kidney injury and repair is critical for the design of new therapeutic approaches to treat AKI and prevent its progression to CKD.[123]

References

1 **Ali T, Khan I, Simpson W, et al.** Incidence and outcomes in acute kidney injury: a comprehensive population-based study. *J Am Soc Nephrol* 2007;**18**:1292–8.

2 **Hoste EA, Kellum JA.** Incidence, classification, and outcomes of acute kidney injury. *Contrib Nephrol* 2007;**156**:32–8.

3 **Waikar SS, Liu KD, Chertow GM.** The incidence and prognostic significance of acute kidney injury. *Curr Opin Nephrol Hypertens* 2007;**16**:227–36.

4 **Macedo E, Bouchard J, Mehta RL.** Renal recovery following acute kidney injury. *Curr Opin Crit Care* 2008;**14**:660–5.

5 **Basile DP.** Rarefaction of peritubular capillaries following ischaemic acute renal failure: a potential factor predisposing to progressive nephropathy. *Curr Opin Nephrol Hypertens* 2004;**13**:1–7.

6 **Basile DP, Donohoe D, Roethe K, Osborn JL.** Renal ischaemic injury results in permanent damage to peritubular capillaries and influences long-term function. *Am J Physiol Renal Physiol* 2001;**281**:F887–99.

7 **Forbes JM, Hewitson TD, Becker GJ, Jones CL.** Ischaemic acute renal failure: long-term histology of cell and matrix changes in the rat. *Kidney Int* 2000;**57**:2375–85.

8 **Coca SG.** Long-term outcomes of acute kidney injury. *Curr Opin Nephrol Hypertens* 2010;**19**:266–72.

9 **Hsu CY, Chertow GM, McCulloch CE, Fan D, Ordonez JD, Go AS.** Nonrecovery of kidney function and death after acute on chronic renal failure. *Clin J Am Soc Nephrol* 2009;**4**:891–8.

10 **Lo LJ, Go AS, Chertow GM, et al.** Dialysis-requiring acute renal failure increases the risk of progressive chronic kidney disease. *Kidney Int* 2009;**76**:893–9.

11 Wald R, Quinn RR, Luo J, et al. Chronic dialysis and death among survivors of acute kidney injury requiring dialysis. *JAMA* 2009;**302**:1179–85.

12 Coca SG, Yusuf B, Shlipak MG, Garg AX, Parikh CR. Long-term risk of mortality and other adverse outcomes after acute kidney injury: a systematic review and meta-analysis. *Am J Kidney Dis* 2009;**53**:961–73.

13 Cerda J, Lameire N, Eggers P, et al. Epidemiology of acute kidney injury. *Clin J Am Soc Nephrol* 2008;**3**:881–6.

14 Sharfuddin AA, Molitoris BA. Pathophysiology of ischaemic acute kidney injury. *Nat Rev Nephrol* 2011;**7**:189–200.

15 Thadhani R, Pascual M, Bonventre JV. Acute renal failure. *N Engl J Med* 1996;**334**:1448–60.

16 Clarkson MF, Friedewald JJ, Eustace JA, Rabb H. Acute kidney injury. In: Brenner BM (ed.) *Brenner and Rector's The kidney*. Philadelphia, PA: Saunders, Elsevier; 2007. pp. 943–86.

17 Molitoris BA, Marrs J. The role of cell adhesion molecules in ischaemic acute renal failure. *Am J Med* 1999;**106**:583–92.

18 Molitoris BA. Ischemia-induced loss of epithelial polarity: potential role of the actin cytoskeleton. *Am J Physiol* 1991;**260**:F769–78.

19 Molitoris BA, Dahl R, Geerdes A. Cytoskeleton disruption and apical redistribution of proximal tubule Na(+)-K(+)-ATPase during ischemia. *Am J Physiol* 1992;**263**:F488–95.

20 Zuk A, Bonventre JV, Brown D, Matlin KS. Polarity, integrin, and extracellular matrix dynamics in the postischaemic rat kidney. *Am J Physiol* 1998;**275**:C711–31.

21 Bonventre JV. Dedifferentiation and proliferation of surviving epithelial cells in acute renal failure. *J Am Soc Nephrol* 2003;**14**(Suppl 1):S55–61.

22 Witzgall R, Brown D, Schwarz C, Bonventre JV. Localization of proliferating cell nuclear antigen, vimentin, c-Fos, and clusterin in the postischaemic kidney. Evidence for a heterogenous genetic response among nephron segments, and a large pool of mitotically active and dedifferentiated cells. *J Clin Invest* 1994;**93**:2175–88.

23 Humphreys BD, Valerius MT, Kobayashi A, et al. Intrinsic epithelial cells repair the kidney after injury. *Cell Stem Cell* 2008;**2**:284–91.

24 Basile DP. The endothelial cell in ischaemic acute kidney injury: implications for acute and chronic function. *Kidney Int* 2007;**72**:151–6.

25 Horbelt M, Lee SY, Mang HE, et al. Acute and chronic microvascular alterations in a mouse model of ischaemic acute kidney injury. *Am J Physiol Renal Physiol* 2007;**293**:F688–95.

26 Fine LG, Norman JT. Chronic hypoxia as a mechanism of progression of chronic kidney diseases: from hypothesis to novel therapeutics. *Kidney Int* 2008;**74**:867–72.

27 Ishii Y, Sawada T, Kubota K, Fuchinoue S, Teraoka S, Shimizu A. Injury and progressive loss of peritubular capillaries in the development of chronic allograft nephropathy. *Kidney Int* 2005;**67**: 321–32.

28 Kang DH, Kanellis J, Hugo C, et al. Role of the microvascular endothelium in progressive renal disease. *J Am Soc Nephrol* 2002;**13**:806–16.

29 Basile DP, Fredrich K, Chelladurai B, Leonard EC, Parrish AR. Renal ischemia reperfusion inhibits VEGF expression and induces ADAMTS-1, a novel VEGF inhibitor. *Am J Physiol Renal Physiol* 2008;**294**:F928–36.

30 Leonard EC, Friedrich JL, Basile DP. VEGF-121 preserves renal microvessel structure and ameliorates secondary renal disease following acute kidney injury. *Am J Physiol Renal Physiol* 2008;**295**: F1648–57.

31 Basile DP, Friedrich JL, Spahic J, et al. Impaired endothelial proliferation and mesenchymal transition contribute to vascular rarefaction following acute kidney injury. *Am J Physiol Renal Physiol* 2011;**300**: F721–33.

32 Fine LG, Orphanides C, Norman JT. Progressive renal disease: the chronic hypoxia hypothesis. *Kidney Int Suppl* 1998;**65**:S74–8.

33 Nath KA. Tubulointerstitial changes as a major determinant in the progression of renal damage. *Am J Kidney Dis* 1992;**20**:1–17.

34 Fine LG, Bandyopadhay D, Norman JT. Is there a common mechanism for the progression of different types of renal diseases other than proteinuria? Towards the unifying theme of chronic hypoxia. *Kidney Int Suppl* 2000;**75**:S22–6.

35 Nangaku M, Eckardt KU. Hypoxia and the HIF system in kidney disease. *J Mol Med (Berl)* 2007;**85**:1325–30.

36 Norman JT, Fine LG. Intrarenal oxygenation in chronic renal failure. *Clin Exp Pharmacol Physiol* 2006;**33**:989–96.

37 O'Riordan E, Mendelev N, Patschan S, et al. Chronic NOS inhibition actuates endothelial-mesenchymal transformation. *Am J Physiol Heart Circ Physiol* 2007;**292**:H285–94.

38 Basile DP, Donohoe DL, Roethe K, Mattson DL. Chronic renal hypoxia after acute ischaemic injury: effects of L-arginine on hypoxia and secondary damage. *Am J Physiol Renal Physiol* 2003;**284**:F338–48.

39 Bernhardt WM, Campean V, Kany S, et al. Preconditional activation of hypoxia-inducible factors ameliorates ischaemic acute renal failure. *J Am Soc Nephrol* 2006;**17**:1970–8.

40 Matsumoto M, Makino Y, Tanaka T, et al. Induction of renoprotective gene expression by cobalt ameliorates ischaemic injury of the kidney in rats. *J Am Soc Nephrol* 2003;**14**:1825–32.

41 Bonventre JV, Zuk A. Ischaemic acute renal failure: an inflammatory disease? *Kidney Int* 2004;**66**: 480–5.

42 Jang HR, Rabb H. The innate immune response in ischaemic acute kidney injury. *Clin Immunol* 2009;**130**:41–50.

43 Wu H, Chen G, Wyburn KR, et al. TLR4 activation mediates kidney ischemia/reperfusion injury. *J Clin Invest* 2007a;**117**:2847–59.

44 Thornton MA, Winn R, Alpers CE, Zager RA. An evaluation of the neutrophil as a mediator of in vivo renal ischaemic-reperfusion injury. *Am J Pathol* 1989;**135**:509–15.

45 Devarajan P. Update on mechanisms of ischaemic acute kidney injury. *J Am Soc Nephrol* 2006;**17**:1503–20.

46 Rabb H, Daniels F, O'Donnell M, et al. Pathophysiological role of T lymphocytes in renal ischemia-reperfusion injury in mice. *Am J Physiol Renal Physiol* 2000;**279**:F525–31.

47 Gailit J, Colflesh D, Rabiner I, Simone J, Goligorsky MS. Redistribution and dysfunction of integrins in cultured renal epithelial cells exposed to oxidative stress. *Am J Physiol* 1993;**264**:F149–57.

48 Goligorsky MS, Lieberthal W, Racusen L, Simon EE. Integrin receptors in renal tubular epithelium: new insights into pathophysiology of acute renal failure. *Am J Physiol* 1993;**264**:F1–8.

49 Lieberthal W, McKenney JB, Kiefer CR, Snyder LM, Kroshian VM, Sjaastad MD. Beta1 integrin-mediated adhesion between renal tubular cells after anoxic injury. *J Am Soc Nephrol* 1997;**8**:175–83.

50 Li L, Huang L, Sung SS, et al. The chemokine receptors CCR2 and CX3CR1 mediate monocyte/macrophage trafficking in kidney ischemia-reperfusion injury. *Kidney Int* 2008;**74**:1526–37.

51 Oh DJ, Dursun B, He Z, et al. Fractalkine receptor (CX3CR1) inhibition is protective against ischaemic acute renal failure in mice. *Am J Physiol Renal Physiol* 2008;**294**:F264–71.

52 Ysebaert DK, De Greef KE, Vercauteren SR, et al. Identification and kinetics of leukocytes after severe ischaemia/reperfusion renal injury. *Nephrol Dial Transplant* 2000;**15**:1562–74.

53 Day YJ, Huang L, Ye H, Linden J, Okusa MD. Renal ischemia-reperfusion injury and adenosine 2A receptor-mediated tissue protection: role of macrophages. *Am J Physiol Renal Physiol* 2005;**288**: F722–31.

54 Jo SK, Sung SA, Cho WY, Go KJ, Kim HK. Macrophages contribute to the initiation of ischaemic acute renal failure in rats. *Nephrol Dial Transplant* 2006;**21**:1231–9.

55 Ko GJ, Boo CS, Jo SK, Cho WY, Kim HK. Macrophages contribute to the development of renal fibrosis following ischaemia/reperfusion-induced acute kidney injury. *Nephrol Dial Transplant* 2008;**23**:842–52.

56 Persy VP, Verhulst A, Ysebaert DK, De Greef KE, De Broe ME. Reduced postischaemic macrophage infiltration and interstitial fibrosis in osteopontin knockout mice. *Kidney Int* 2003;**63**:543–53.

57 Ricardo SD, van Goor H, Eddy AA. Macrophage diversity in renal injury and repair. *J Clin Invest* 2008;**118**:3522–30.

58 Wang Y, Harris DC. Macrophages in renal disease. *J Am Soc Nephrol* 2011;**22**:21–7.

59 Nishida M, Hamaoka K. Macrophage phenotype and renal fibrosis in obstructive nephropathy. *Nephron Exp Nephrol* 2008;**110**:e31–6.

60 Lee S, Huen S, Nishio H, et al. Distinct macrophage phenotypes contribute to kidney injury and repair. *J Am Soc Nephrol* 2011;**22**:317–26.

61 Dong X, Swaminathan S, Bachman LA, Croatt AJ, Nath KA, Griffin MD. Resident dendritic cells are the predominant TNF-secreting cell in early renal ischemia-reperfusion injury. *Kidney Int* 2007;**71**:619–28.

62 Li L, Okusa MD. Macrophages, dendritic cells, and kidney ischemia-reperfusion injury. *Semin Nephrol* 2010;**30**:268–77.

63 Tadagavadi RK, Reeves WB. Renal dendritic cells ameliorate nephrotoxic acute kidney injury. *J Am Soc Nephrol* 2010;**21**:53–63.

64 Zhang ZX, Wang S, Huang X, et al. NK cells induce apoptosis in tubular epithelial cells and contribute to renal ischemia-reperfusion injury. *J Immunol* 2008;**181**:7489–98.

65 Diana J, Lehuen A. NKT cells: friend or foe during viral infections? *Eur J Immunol* 2009;**39**:3283–91.

66 Li L, Huang L, Sung SS, et al. NKT cell activation mediates neutrophil IFN-gamma production and renal ischemia-reperfusion injury. *J Immunol* 2007;**178**:5899–911.

67 Jang HR, Ko GJ, Wasowska BA, Rabb H. The interaction between ischemia-reperfusion and immune responses in the kidney. *J Mol Med (Berl)* 2009;**87**:859–64.

68 Ysebaert DK, De Greef KE, De Beuf A, et al. T cells as mediators in renal ischemia/reperfusion injury. *Kidney Int* 2004;**66**:491–6.

69 Takada M, Chandraker A, Nadeau KC, Sayegh MH, Tilney NL. The role of the B7 costimulatory pathway in experimental cold ischemia/reperfusion injury. *J Clin Invest* 1997a;**100**:1199–203.

70 Burne MJ, Daniels F, El Ghandour A, et al. Identification of the CD4(+) T cell as a major pathogenic factor in ischaemic acute renal failure. *J Clin Invest* 2001;**108**:1283–90.

71 Hochegger K, Schatz T, Eller P, et al. Role of alpha/beta and gamma/delta T cells in renal ischemia-reperfusion injury. *Am J Physiol Renal Physiol* 2007;**293**:F741–7.

72 Savransky V, Molls RR, Burne-Taney M, Chien CC, Racusen L, Rabb H. Role of the T-cell receptor in kidney ischemia-reperfusion injury. *Kidney Int* 2006;**69**:233–8.

73 Yokota N, Burne-Taney M, Racusen L, Rabb H. Contrasting roles for STAT4 and STAT6 signal transduction pathways in murine renal ischemia-reperfusion injury. *Am J Physiol Renal Physiol* 2003;**285**:F319–25.

74 Ascon DB, Lopez-Briones S, Liu M, et al. Phenotypic and functional characterization of kidney-infiltrating lymphocytes in renal ischemia reperfusion injury. *J Immunol* 2006;**177**:3380–7.

75 Liu M, Chien CC, Grigoryev DN, Gandolfo MT, Colvin RB, Rabb H. Effect of T cells on vascular permeability in early ischaemic acute kidney injury in mice. *Microvasc Res* 2009;**77**:340–7.

76 Ko GJ, Zakaria A, Womer KL, Rabb H. Immunologic research in kidney ischemia/reperfusion injury at Johns Hopkins University. *Immunol Res* 2010;**47**:78–85.

77 Burne-Taney MJ, Yokota N, Rabb H. Persistent renal and extrarenal immune changes after severe ischaemic injury. *Kidney Int* 2005;**67**:1002–9.

78 Ascon M, Ascon DB, Liu M, et al. Renal ischemia-reperfusion leads to long term infiltration of activated and effector-memory T lymphocytes. *Kidney Int* 2009;**75**:526–35.

79 Sakaguchi S, Ono M, Setoguchi R, et al. Foxp3 + CD25 + CD4 + natural regulatory T cells in dominant self-tolerance and autoimmune disease. *Immunol Rev* 2006;**212**:8–27.

80 Gandolfo MT, Jang HR, Bagnasco SM, et al. Foxp3+ regulatory T cells participate in repair of ischemic acute kidney injury. *Kidney Int* 2009;**76**:717–29.

81 Kinsey GR, Huang L, Vergis AL, Li L, Okusa MD. Regulatory T cells contribute to the protective effect of ischaemic preconditioning in the kidney. *Kidney Int* 2010;**77**:771–80.

82 Kinsey GR, Sharma R, Huang L, et al. Regulatory T cells suppress innate immunity in kidney ischemia-reperfusion injury. *J Am Soc Nephrol* 2009;**20**:1744–53.

83 Burne-Taney MJ, Ascon DB, Daniels F, Racusen L, Baldwin W, Rabb H. B cell deficiency confers protection from renal ischemia reperfusion injury. *J Immunol* 2003;**171**:3210–15.

84 Jang HR, Gandolfo MT, Ko GJ, Satpute SR, Racusen L, Rabb H. B cells limit repair after ischemic acute kidney injury. *J Am Soc Nephrol* 2010;**21**:654–65.

85 Krause DS, Theise ND, Collector MI, et al. Multi-organ, multi-lineage engraftment by a single bone marrow-derived stem cell. *Cell* 2001;**105**:369–77.

86 Petersen BE, Bowen WC, Patrene KD, et al. Bone marrow as a potential source of hepatic oval cells. *Science* 1999;**284**:1168–70.

87 Kale S, Karihaloo A, Clark PR, Kashgarian M, Krause DS, Cantley LG. Bone marrow stem cells contribute to repair of the ischaemically injured renal tubule. *J Clin Invest* 2003;**112**:42–9.

88 Lin F, Cordes K, Li L, et al. Hematopoietic stem cells contribute to the regeneration of renal tubules after renal ischemia-reperfusion injury in mice. *J Am Soc Nephrol* 2003;**14**:1188–99.

89 Morigi M, Imberti B, Zoja C, et al. Mesenchymal stem cells are renotropic, helping to repair the kidney and improve function in acute renal failure. *J Am Soc Nephrol* 2004;**15**:1794–804.

90 Poulsom R, Forbes SJ, Hodivala-Dilke K, et al. Bone marrow contributes to renal parenchymal turnover and regeneration. *J Pathol* 2001;**195**:229–35.

91 Lin F, Moran A, Igarashi P. Intrarenal cells, not bone marrow-derived cells, are the major source for regeneration in postischaemic kidney. *J Clin Invest* 2005;**115**:1756–64.

92 Duffield JS, Park KM, Hsiao LL, et al. Restoration of tubular epithelial cells during repair of the postischaemic kidney occurs independently of bone marrow-derived stem cells. *J Clin Invest* 2005;**115**:1743–55.

93 Duffield JS, Bonventre JV. Kidney tubular epithelium is restored without replacement with bone marrow-derived cells during repair after ischaemic injury. *Kidney Int* 2005;**68**:1956–61.

94 Humphreys BD, Bonventre JV. Mesenchymal stem cells in acute kidney injury. *Annu Rev Med* 2008;**59**:311–25.

95 Herrera MB, Bussolati B, Bruno S, Fonsato V, Romanazzi GM, Camussi G. Mesenchymal stem cells contribute to the renal repair of acute tubular epithelial injury. *Int J Mol Med* 2004;**14**:1035–41.

96 Togel F, Weiss K, Yang Y, Hu Z, Zhang P, Westenfelder C. Vasculotropic, paracrine actions of infused mesenchymal stem cells are important to the recovery from acute kidney injury. *Am J Physiol Renal Physiol* 2007;**292**:F1626–35.

97 Caplan AI, Dennis JE. Mesenchymal stem cells as trophic mediators. *J Cell Biochem* 2006;**98**:1076–84.

98 Togel F, Hu Z, Weiss K, Isaac J, Lange C, Westenfelder C. Administered mesenchymal stem cells protect against ischaemic acute renal failure through differentiation-independent mechanisms. *Am J Physiol Renal Physiol* 2005;**289**:F31–42.

99 Bi B, Schmitt R, Israilova M, Nishio H, Cantley LG. Stromal cells protect against acute tubular injury via an endocrine effect. *J Am Soc Nephrol* 2007;**18**:2486–96.

100 Stagg J. Immune regulation by mesenchymal stem cells: two sides to the coin. *Tissue Antigens* 2007;**69**:1–9.

101 McTaggart SJ, Atkinson K. Mesenchymal stem cells: immunobiology and therapeutic potential in kidney disease. *Nephrology (Carlton)* 2007;**12**:44–52.

102 Nauta AJ, Fibbe WE. Immunomodulatory properties of mesenchymal stromal cells. *Blood* 2007;**110**:3499–506.

103 Hammerman MR. Growth factors and apoptosis in acute renal injury. *Curr Opin Nephrol Hypertens* 1998;**7**:419–24.

104 Nigam S, Lieberthal W. Acute renal failure. III. The role of growth factors in the process of renal regeneration and repair. *Am J Physiol Renal Physiol* 2000;**279**:F3–11.

105 Imberti B, Morigi M, Tomasoni S, et al. Insulin-like growth factor-1 sustains stem cell mediated renal repair. *J Am Soc Nephrol* 2007;**18**:2921–8.

106 Wang S, Hirschberg R. Role of growth factors in acute renal failure. *Nephrol Dial Transplant* 1997;**12**:1560–3.

107 Baer PC, Geiger H. Mesenchymal stem cell interactions with growth factors on kidney repair. *Curr Opin Nephrol Hypertens* 2010;**19**:1–6.

108 Villanueva S, Cespedes C, Gonzalez A, Vio CP. bFGF induces an earlier expression of nephrogenic proteins after ischaemic acute renal failure. *Am J Physiol Regul Integr Comp Physiol* 2006;**291**:R1677–87.

109 Liu Y, Tolbert EM, Lin L, et al. Up-regulation of hepatocyte growth factor receptor: an amplification and targeting mechanism for hepatocyte growth factor action in acute renal failure. *Kidney Int* 1999;**55**:442–53.

110 Herrero-Fresneda I, Torras J, Franquesa M, et al. HGF gene therapy attenuates renal allograft scarring by preventing the profibrotic inflammatory-induced mechanisms. *Kidney Int* 2006;**70**:265–74.

111 Matsumoto K, Nakamura T. Hepatocyte growth factor: renotropic role and potential therapeutics for renal diseases. *Kidney Int* 2001 **59**: 2023–38.

112 Menke J, Iwata Y, Rabacal WA, et al. CSF-1 signals directly to renal tubular epithelial cells to mediate repair in mice. *J Clin Invest* 2009;**119**:2330–42.

113 Sharples EJ, Thiemermann C, Yaqoob MM. Mechanisms of disease: Cell death in acute renal failure and emerging evidence for a protective role of erythropoietin. *Nat Clin Pract Nephrol* 2005;**1**:87–97.

114 Vesey DA, Cheung C, Pat B, Endre Z, Gobe G, Johnson DW. Erythropoietin protects against ischaemic acute renal injury. *Nephrol Dial Transplant* 2004;**19**:348–55.

115 Yang CW, Li C, Jung JY, et al. Preconditioning with erythropoietin protects against subsequent ischemia-reperfusion injury in rat kidney. *FASEB J* 2003;**17**:1754–5.

116 Imamura R, Moriyama T, Isaka Y, et al. Erythropoietin protects the kidneys against ischemia reperfusion injury by activating hypoxia inducible factor-1alpha. *Transplantation* 2007;**83**:1371–9.

117 Moore E, Bellomo R. Erythropoietin (EPO) in acute kidney injury. *Ann Intensive Care* 2011;**1**:3.

118 Yang L, Humphreys BD, Bonventre JV. Pathophysiology of acute kidney injury to chronic kidney disease: maladaptive repair. *Contrib Nephrol* 2011;**174**:149–55.

119 Humphreys BD, Lin SL, Kobayashi A, et al. Fate tracing reveals the pericyte and not epithelial origin of myofibroblasts in kidney fibrosis. *Am J Pathol* 2010;**176**:85–97.

120 Bechtel W, McGoohan S, Zeisberg EM, et al. Methylation determines fibroblast activation and fibrogenesis in the kidney. *Nat Med* 2010;**16**:544–50.

121 Wynn TA. Fibrosis under arrest. *Nat Med* 2010;**16**:523–25.

122 Yang L, Besschetnova TY, Brooks CR, Shah JV, Bonventre JV. Epithelial cell cycle arrest in G2/M mediates kidney fibrosis after injury. *Nat Med* 2010;**16**:535–43.

123 Jo SK, Rosner MH, Okusa MD. Pharmacologic treatment of acute kidney injury: why drugs haven't worked and what is on the horizon. *Clin J Am Soc Nephrol* 2007;**2**:356–65.

Chapter 31

Myocardial Remodelling after Myocardial Infarction

Kavitha Vimalesvaran and Michael Marber

Introduction

Ventricular remodelling is defined as changes in the shape, structure, and function of the heart following myocardial injury. The process can affect the right and/or left ventricle. For the purposes of this chapter, the focus will be on the left ventricle alone. The left ventricular (LV) remodelling process after myocardial infarction (MI) is one that is complicated, active, and time-dependent and develops in parallel with a beneficial healing process.[1-4] The significant changes are best considered on a regional basis by separation into the infarct zone (IZ) and the non-infarcted, or remote, zone (NIZ). These changes comprise alterations in the: (1) LV structure, shape, and topography,[1,2] (2) constituent cell types, including myocytes and non-myocytes,[1,3,5-12] (3) secreted proteins, most notably cytokines, and growth factors,[1,3,13,14] and (4) the extracellular collagen matrix (ECCM).[1,3-9,11,12,15-18] Global LV structural remodelling after MI is notably affected by differential remodelling of the IZ and NIZ; a dominant feature in both these regions is an increase in the ECCM.[1,19,20]

The timing of remodelling

After coronary occlusion, the acute infarction process involves a march to necrosis, with transmural progression, along a wavefront from the endocardium to epicardium over several hours.[2,21] Early reperfusion or the availability of collateral blood flow[2,22,23] halts or impedes this transmural progression, respectively. Thus, the myocardial zone threatened with infarction often contains a spared or salvaged epicardial rim of viable heart tissue.[2,24] The epicardial rim of 'normal' myocardium is considered to offer a structural scaffold that hinders adverse remodelling.[2,19,25-27] An important physical determinant of resistance of the IZ to distension during early stages of healing is preservation of the integrity of the supporting collagen matrix in this salvaged epicardium.[2,27-29]

The healing process strives to mend the damaged ventricular wall to conserve integrity and to reinstate function.[2] It commences promptly after infarction and progresses over the ensuing weeks and months.[2,30-32] It is considered a dynamic process that is reliant on nutrient flow.[2] The sequence of adjustments occurring within the LV are orchestrated by humoral agents, growth factors, and cytokines of autocrine and paracrine origin.[2] The desired final outcome is a firm, non-compliant, contracted, and compacted scar. The interval between infarction and scar formation is about 3–6 weeks, with subsequent slower remodelling of the scar occurring over years.[2,30,32]

The post-MI heart shows exceptional capacity to adjust to the progressive changes occurring within the IZ and NIZ.[1] Consequently, MI results in time-dependent injury to myocytes, non-myocytes, and the ECCM in the IZ, whilst, in the NIZ, contractility is increased to compensate for the acute loss of contraction in the IZ. This recruitment of the NIZ causes reactive hypertrophy, with interstitial fibrosis, in turn, leading to ventricular dysfunction and increasing dilatation. Thus, collagen synthesis[1,33] and vascular remodelling are common to the IZ and NIZ.[1,3]

Collagen synthesis is affected by several endogenous molecules and is markedly increased after MI. Several agents that are used therapeutically for MI impact on collagen turnover and exert an anti-fibrotic effect.[1,20,31,34,35] This can alter ECCM remodelling in the IZ[1,20,34] and impede heal-ing,[1,36] and thereby encourage unfavourable remodelling, though the exact consequence likely relies on timing relative to pathophysiological stages of healing.

Post-MI remodelling can essentially be divided into three phases with initiation at the time of ischaemic injury. The first phase (0–72 hours) begins immediately during stages of evolution and completion of acute infarction. This phase involves acute infarct expansion over hours to days, with stretching, thinning, and dilatation of the IZ.[2] At cellular and structural levels, expansion is mediated by collagen matrix disruption and myocyte slippage.[2,26] Equilibrium between matrix metalloproteinases (MMPs), that degrade ECCM, and endogenous tissue inhibitors of MMPs (TIMPs), that inhibit MMPs,[1,37–39] preserves conventional/adaptive remodelling and function, and any disparity can effectively cause adverse remodelling.[1,13,14,37,40,41]

The second phase (72 hours to 6 weeks) comprises chronic inflammation with fibroblast prolif-eration and collagen deposition within the IZ. The normal response is a 2- to 3-fold expansion in myocardial collagen volume fraction, contributing to an increased LV stiffness and mild dysfunc-tion.[1,42] A failure of this response, even if localized, can have radical ramifications, including LV dilation[1,28,41] and rupture. In reperfused MI, decreased or damaged ECCM in the IZ[1,16,43,44] is related to cardiac rupture.[1,16,44]

The third and last phase (6 weeks and beyond) of ventricular remodelling includes further scar remodelling with contraction, maturation, and myofibroblast formation. This final phase of remodelling may cause progressive LV dilation, volume overload, and hypertrophy of the NIZ and is the most common cause of HF.

The stages of healing and remodelling after MI are summarized in Figure 31.1 and Table 31.1.

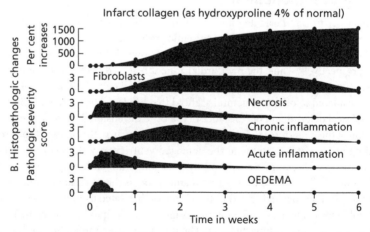

Fig. 31.1 The temporal sequence of, and interrelationship between, the pathophysiological process-es involved in healing and remodelling within the zone of myocardial infarction.

Reproduced from Jugdutt BI, 'Prevention of ventricular remodeling after myocardial infarction and in congestive heart failure', *Heart Failure Reviews*, 1, 2, pp. 115–129, copyright 1996. With kind permission from Springer Science and Business Media.

Table 31.1 Stages of healing and remodelling after MI

Stage/timing	Pathophysiologic process
Very early (~ first 24 hours)	Acute evolution and completion of MI; oedema increased glycosaminoglycans; necrosis, apoptosis; acute inflammation, neutrophils predominating; cytokine activation, ↑ MMPs, enhanced ECCM degradation. Infarct expansion observed.
Early (~ first 2 weeks)	Early IZ healing, before the collagen plateau, chronic inflammation with macrophages peaking after ~48 hours, and mononuclear cells; fibroblasts proliferation predominating after ~1 week; collagen deposition in IZ, 5-fold or more. Early LV dilation is noted with possible aneurysm formation and LV rupture.
Late (~3–6 weeks)	Late IZ healing to scar formation after the collagen plateau which leads to more collagen deposition and little cellular infiltration. Collagen remodelling with crosslinking and myofibroblast formation is observed. There is more LV dilation, volume overload, and hypertrophy.
Very late (~1.5 months to 1 year or more)	Late IZ scarring and NIZ fibrosis, with continued ECCM remodelling with contraction, maturation, and myofibroblast formation. The remodelling process consists of progressive LV dilation, further volume overload, and hypertrophy.

MMPs, matrix metalloproteinase; ECCM, extracellular collagen matrix; IZ, infarction zone; LV, left ventricle; NIZ, non-infarction zone.

Reproduced from Bodh I. Jugdutt, 'Ventricular remodeling after infarction and the extracellular collagen matrix: when is enough enough?', *Circulation*, 108, 11, pp. 1395–1403, copyright Wolters Kluwer, with permission. Data from Jugdutt BI. Prevention of ventricular remodelling post myocardial infarction: timing and duration of therapy. *Can J Cardiol* 1993 Jan–Feb;9(1):103–14.

Remodelling and hypertrophy

During post-infarction remodelling, hypertrophy is an adaptive response that compensates for the increased load, reduces the effect of progressive dilatation, and balances contractile function.[45,46] Neurohormonal activation, myocardial stretch, activation of the local tissue renin-angiotensin system (RAS), and paracrine/autocrine factors initiate myocyte hypertrophy. The RAS-aldosterone axis, alongside the production of catecholamines by the adrenal medulla, the spillover from sympathetic nerve terminals, and secretion of natriuretic peptides (atrial natriuretic peptide (ANP), BNP), are all increased due to relative hypoperfusion post-infarction. The hypertrophic response is affected, both directly and indirectly, by enhanced NE release. NE stimulates the α1-adrenoreceptors, which results in myocyte hypertrophy.[45] Renin release, which is induced by the activation of β1-adrenoreceptors in the juxtaglomerular apparatus, enhances the production of angiotensin II. The diminished stretch activation of vascular smooth muscle cells in the juxtaglomerular apparatus induces an increase in the production of angiotensin II that stimulates the presynaptic release of NE and its blocked reuptake, further increasing the post-synaptic action of NE[45] and contributing to the vicious cycles driving remodelling illustrated in Figure 31.2.

Heart failure (HF) progression

LV remodelling is, by and large, an unfavourable sign and is associated with HF progression. Gradual worsening of cardiac function has been established in patients with major remodelling which also underlies a sizeable proportion of cardiovascular morbidity and mortality.[47]

LV remodelling can be described as both an adaptive and a maladaptive process.[47] The heart is able to maintain function in response to pressure or volume overloading in the acute phase of

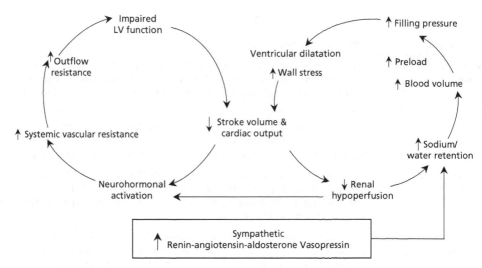

Fig. 31.2 Vicious cycles that drive progressive left ventricular remodelling.

cardiac injury through the adaptive process.[47,48] Initially, at least, the increase in preload is adaptive, maintaining the stroke volume through length-dependent recruitment of contractility via the Frank–Starling mechanism. However, through the actions of the Law of LaPlace, which is governed by the inverse relationship between pressure generation and radius, wall stress needs to increase to maintain equivalent intracavity pressure. This increases effective afterload, compromising contractility and initiating the vicious spiral depicted on the right of Figure 31.2. These two, and other vicious spirals, drive adverse remodelling and will result in progressive decompensation unless interrupted.[47]

Quantifying remodelling

Irrespective of the measurement criteria, progressive remodelling is always thought to be detrimental and to correlate with a poor prognosis.[47,49,50] The transition between adaptive and maladaptive remodelling cannot be precisely identified. However, the time course and occurrence of such a transition is expected to vary greatly. Therefore, appreciation of the extent of LV remodelling can assist in the assessment of prognosis.[47] Major independent increases in the risk of death in patients with coronary artery disease, recent MI, and HF[46,47,50,51] are related to the magnitude of the ventricular volume. The heart size, mass, ejection fraction, end-diastolic volume, end-systolic volume, and peak force of contraction[47,52] are all prognostically meaningful measures of LV remodelling. Each measure is representative of a varying characteristic of the disease state.[47] LV volumes, especially end-systolic volume, are associated with a poor prognosis.[47,50]

Despite the fact that heart size and shape may seem the most rational measures of remodelling, technical factors and varied modalities cause disparate results. For instance, only 38% of hypertensive patients with anatomic LV hypertrophy on M-mode echocardiography (ECHO) showed LV hypertrophy when evaluated using electrocardiography (ECG).[47,53] An increased risk of cardiac failure is indicated by the ECG manifestation of LV hypertrophy, irrespective of anatomical verification by ECHO.[47] The likely explanation is that measures of LV wall thickness, cavity size, and mass are relatively insensitive measures of ECCM accumulation, electrical coupling, and repolarization. Nonetheless, these pathological processes are key components of remodelling.[47]

The symptoms and signs of LV dysfunction lack both sensitivity and specificity,[47,54] as indicators of disease. The standard techniques to identify LV remodelling and systolic dysfunction are ECHO and radionuclide imaging.[47,54] Unfortunately, ECHO can lack reproducibility[47,55] and standardization,[47] and image quality is dependent on the availability of an acoustic window.[47,56] Cross-sectional imaging modalities, such as MRI and CT, offer superior precision and consistency[47,57] whilst allowing assessment of myocardial fibrosis and coronary anatomy, respectively. All these imaging modalities are expensive, and their use can be guided by measurement of circulating markers of LV strain such as BNP.

Therapeutic interventions to limit remodelling

The effects of therapies designed to prevent or attenuate post-infarction LV remodelling are best considered with reference to the pathophysiological mechanisms involved. Beyond the acute phase, ventricular remodelling is influenced mostly by infarct artery patency, ventricular loading conditions, neurohormonal activation, and local tissue growth factors.

Angiotensin-converting enzyme (ACE) inhibitors and angiotensin receptor blockers (ARBs)

For over 20 years, it has been known that mortality and morbidity in patients with HF due to systolic LV dysfunction[58,59] is improved through the use of ACE inhibitors. This has been supported by experimental and clinical data demonstrating their effectiveness in limiting remodelling, particularly in the post-infarction setting.[59–63] However, reports of the reversal of remodelling (i.e. reduction in size of an enlarged LV) in large patient cohorts, is rare. Instead, clinical trials involving ACE inhibitors against placebo suggest that the progress of remodelling is delayed, rather than prevented or reversed.[59,64]

ACE inhibitors only partially reduce angiotensin II production, because they do not act on alternative, ACE-independent pathways of conversion. Consequently, plasma levels of angiotensin II increase above initial values during long-term ACE inhibition. The effects of ACE inhibitors on cardiac remodelling and on sympathetic activity attenuate after 1 year of treatment.[59]

ARBs that act selectively on type 1 receptors (AT_1R) (mainly responsible for cardiac hypertrophy, aldosterone production, fibrosis, and vasoconstriction) can be used as a substitute for, or in combination with, an ACE inhibitor. ARBs work without inhibiting the possibly favourable activity of type 2 receptors (AT_2R) which mediate vasodilatation and probably inhibit myocardial fibrosis.[59,65,66]

Effects of an ACE inhibitor (enalapril) were compared with an ARB (candesartan) vs their combination in the Randomized Evaluation of Strategies for Left Ventricular Dysfunction (RESOLVD) trial where eligible patients were also randomized to receive a β-blocker (metoprolol) or a placebo.[59,67] Remodelling and a change in the neurohormonal profile were included as endpoints. The outcome showed an advantage to sequential blockade. After 1 year, the use of candesartan, in addition to enalapril, enhanced ejection fraction, hindered LV enlargement, and reduced plasma levels of BNP and aldosterone more than either single drug alone. Moreover, candesartan alone was not better than enalapril alone.

In summary, trials with ACE inhibitors and ARBs administered to patients with HF and LV systolic dysfunction demonstrated: (1) the usefulness of single-step angiotensin II antagonism (with an ACE inhibitor or with an ARB in patients who do not tolerate ACE inhibitors) for survival and for reducing the combined endpoint of mortality and morbidity, (2) the non-superiority of ARBs with respect to ACE inhibitors, and (3) the additional benefit of sequential blockade (ACE inhibitor plus ARB) on morbidity and on cardiovascular mortality.[59]

β-adrenoreceptor blockers

The proof that β-adrenoreceptor blockers decrease morbidity and mortality in HF due to LV systolic dysfunction, both of ischaemic or non-ischaemic aetiology and ranging over all grades of severity, is overwhelming. A more permanent benefit is achieved from β-blockers than from that obtained with ACE inhibitors alone.[59]

Sizeable and continued improvement in ejection fraction and reverse remodelling, with reductions in LV sphericity and functional mitral regurgitation, have been shown with β-blockers of proven clinical benefit in HF such as metoprolol, carvedilol, and bisoprolol.[59,68–71] In this aspect, the effectiveness of β-blockers seems to be greater than that of ACE inhibitors and ARBs. Nonetheless, it has to be considered that patients enrolled in clinical trials of β-blockers were already taking an ACE inhibitor. Hence, on a background of ACE inhibition, β-blockers result in significant reverse remodelling. It is unknown whether the same results would have been achieved in the absence of inhibition of the RAS.[59]

The discrete role of β-blockers in reversal of remodelling has been reinforced by a small study in which metoprolol was withdrawn. This caused worsening of LV function, which recovered once therapy was reinstated.[59,72] In addition, the causal relationship between β-blocker treatment and reverse remodelling is strengthened by the dose-response relationship between β-blocker and LV volume or ejection fraction.[59,73–76] The carvedilol dose, in particular, was inversely related to mortality, reinforcing the relationship between reverse remodelling and survival.[59,76] The significance of β-blocker therapy in promoting reverse remodelling is also emphasized by an 'observational study, in which carvedilol therapy and carvedilol dose were found to be among the predictors of normalization of cardiac size and function on multivariate analysis. Notably, in this study, normalization of size and function was associated with a 100% event-free survival at a median follow-up of 17 months, compared with a 24% mortality and a <60% event-free survival in patients whose conditions did not normalize'.[59,74]

In summary, regardless of functional class and aetiology, trials of β-blockers in patients with HF and LV systolic dysfunction demonstrate the advantage of metoprolol, carvedilol, and bisoprolol in reducing mortality and morbidity in patients already medicated with an ACE inhibitor. The value of β-blockers in achieving reverse remodelling is evidently greater and more clearly dose-related than that of ACE inhibitors.[59]

Aldosterone receptor antagonists (ARAs)

ARAs decrease mortality and morbidity in patients with advanced HF (New York Heart Association (NYHA) functional classes III and IV), due to systolic LV dysfunction of any cause,[59,77] as well as in patients with recent MI, LV dysfunction, and symptomatic HF or diabetes mellitus.[59,78] In the Randomised Aldactone Evaluation Study (RALES), which enrolled patients with advanced HF and hence at high risk for clinical events, survival curves separated early, a difference that persisted for at least 3 years.[59,77] A similar observation was made in Eplerenone Post-Acute Myocardial Infarction Heart Failure Efficacy and Survival Study (EPHESUS). This observation presages a cardinal influence of treatment on disease mechanism. In particular, aldosterone is a significant keystone of the RAS pathway and is responsible for numerous maladaptations other than sodium and water retention. Most significant amongst these is its ability to drive hypertrophy, fibrosis, and sympathetic nervous system activation.[59,79]

Conclusion

The remodelling process after myocardial infarction is complex, time-dependent, and inexorably intertwined with the process of healing. Nonetheless, based on their pathophysiological role and, in particular, on the results of randomized controlled intervention studies, beta 1 receptor agonists, angiotensin II, and aldosterone drive maladaptive responses. Inhibiting these pathways both attenuates the remodelling process and reduces morbidity and mortality, reinforcing their inexorable link.

References

1 **Jugdutt BI.** Ventricular remodeling after infarction and the extracellular collagen matrix: when is enough enough? *Circulation* 2003;**108**:1395–403.

2 **Jugdutt BI.** Prevention of ventricular remodeling after myocardial infarction and in congestive heart failure. *Heart Fail Rev* 1996;**1**:115–29.

3 **Jugdutt BI.** Remodeling of the myocardium and potential targets in the collagen degradation and synthesis pathways. *Curr Drug Targets Cardiovasc Haematol Disord* 2003;**3**:1–30.

4 **Jugdutt BI.** Identification of patients prone to infarct expansion by the degree of regional shape distortion on an early two-dimensional echocardiogram after myocardial infarction. *Clin Cardiol* 1990;**13**: 28–40.

5 **Cleutjens JP.** The role of matrix metalloproteinases in heart disease. *Cardiovasc Res* 1996;**32**:816–21.

6 **Eghbali M, Blumenfeld OO, Seifter S, et al.** Localization of types I, III and IV collagen mRNAs in rat heart cells by *in situ* hybridization. *J Mol Cell Cardiol* 1989;**21**:103–13.

7 **Eghbali M, Czaja MJ, Zeydel M, et al.** Collagen chain mRNAs in isolated heart cells from young and adult rats. *J Mol Cell Cardiol* 1988;**20**:267–76.

8 **Nag AC.** Study of non-muscle cells of the adult mammalian heart: a fine structural analysis and distribution. *Cytobios* 1980;**28**:41–61.

9 **Weber KT, Anversa P, Armstrong PW, et al.** Remodeling and reparation of the cardiovascular system. *J Am Coll Cardiol* 1992;**20**:3–16.

10 **Zak R.** Development and proliferative capacity of cardiac muscle cells. *Circ Res* 1974;**35**:17–26.

11 **Weinberg E, Schoen F, George D, et al.** Angiotensin-converting enzyme inhibition prolongs survival and modifies the transition to heart failure in rats with pressure overload hypertrophy due to ascending aortic stenosis. *Circulation* 1994;**90**:1410–22.

12 **Eghbali M, Tomek R, Woods C, Bhambi B.** Cardiac fibroblasts are predisposed to convert into myocyte phenotype: specific effect of transforming growth factor beta. *Proc Natl Acad Sci* 1991;**88**:795–9.

13 **Mann DL, Spinale FG.** Activation of matrix metalloproteinases in the failing human heart: breaking the tie that binds. *Circulation* 1998;**98**:1699–702.

14 **Mann DL.** Inflammatory mediators and the failing heart. *Circulation Res* 2002;**91**:988–98.

15 **Beltrami C, Finato N, Rocco M, et al.** Structural basis of end-stage failure in ischemic cardiomyopathy in humans. *Circulation* 1994;**89**:151–63.

16 **Factor SM, Robinson TF, Dominitz R, Cho SH.** Alterations of the myocardial skeletal framework in acute myocardial infarction with and without ventricular rupture. A preliminary report. *Am J Cardiovasc Pathol* 1987;**1**:91–7.

17 **Jugdutt BI.** Effect of reperfusion on ventricular mass, topography, and function during healing of anterior infarction. *Am J Physiol* 1997;**272**:H1205–11.

18 **Marijianowski M, Teeling P, Becker A.** Remodeling after myocardial infarction in humans is not associated with interstitial fibrosis of noninfarcted myocardium. *J Am Coll Cardiol* 1997;**30**:76–82.

19 **Jugdutt B, Tang S, Khan M, Basualdo C.** Functional impact of remodeling during healing after non-Q wave versus Q wave anterior myocardial infarction in the dog. *J Am Coll Cardiol* 1992;**20**:722–31.

20 Zannad F, Alla Fo, Dousset B, Perez A, Pitt B. Limitation of excessive extracellular matrix turnover may contribute to survival benefit of spironolactone therapy in patients with congestive heart failure: insights from the Randomized Aldactone Evaluation Study (RALES). *Circulation* 2000;**102**:2700–6.

21 Reimer KA, Lowe JE, Rasmussen MM, Jennings RB. The wavefront phenomenon of ischemic cell death. 1. Myocardial infarct size vs duration of coronary occlusion in dogs. *Circulation* 1977;**56**:786–94.

22 Jugdutt BI, Becker LC, Hutchins GM. Early changes in collateral blood flow during myocardial infarction in conscious dogs. *Am J Physiol* 1979;**237**:H371–80.

23 Jugdutt BI, Hutchins GM, Bulkley BH, Becker LC. Myocardial infarction in the conscious dog: three-dimensional mapping of infarct, collateral flow and region at risk. *Circulation* 1979;**60**:1141–50.

24 Reimer KA, Jennings RB. The 'wavefront phenomenon' of myocardial ischemic cell death. II. Transmural progression of necrosis within the framework of ischemic bed size (myocardium at risk) and collateral flow. *Lab Invest* 1979;**40**:633–44.

25 Hutchins GM, Bulkley BH. Infarct expansion versus extension: two different complications of acute myocardial infarction. *Am J Cardiol* 1978;**41**:1127–32.

26 Weisman HF, Healy B. Myocardial infarct expansion, infarct extension, and reinfarction: pathophysiologic concepts. *Prog Cardiovasc Dis* 1987;**30**:73–110.

27 Jugdutt BI, Khan MI. Impact of increased infarct transmurality on remodeling and function during healing after anterior myocardial infarction in the dog. *Can J Physiol Pharmacol* 1992;**70**:949–58.

28 Caulfield JB, Borg TK. The collagen network of the heart. *Lab Invest* 1979;**40**:364–72.

29 Jugdutt BI, Tang SB, Khan MI, Basualdo CA. Functional impact of remodeling during healing after non-Q wave versus Q wave anterior myocardial infarction in the dog. *J Am Coll Cardiol* 1992;**20**: 722–31.

30 Fishbein MC, Maclean D, Maroko PR. The histopathologic evolution of myocardial infarction. *Chest* 1978;**73**:843–9.

31 Jugdutt BI. Prevention of ventricular remodelling post myocardial infarction: timing and duration of therapy. *Can J Cardiol* 1993;**9**:103–14.

32 Jugdutt BI, Amy RW. Healing after myocardial infarction in the dog: changes in infarct hydroxyproline and topography. *J Am Coll Cardiol* 1986;**7**:91–102.

33 Jugdutt BI, Joljart MJ, Khan MI. Rate of collagen deposition during healing and ventricular remodeling after myocardial infarction in rat and dog models. *Circulation* 1996;**94**:94–101.

34 Jugdutt BI, Lucas A, Khan MI. Effect of angiotensin-converting enzyme inhibition on infarct collagen deposition and remodelling during healing after transmural canine myocardial infarction. *Can J Cardiol* 1997;**13**:657–68.

35 Cohn JN, Tognoni G. A randomized trial of the angiotensin-receptor blocker valsartan in chronic heart failure. *N Engl J Med* 2001;**345**:1667–75.

36 Nguyen QT, Cernacek P, Calderoni A, et al. Endothelin a receptor blockade causes adverse left ventricular remodeling but improves pulmonary artery pressure after infarction in the rat. *Circulation* 1998;**98**:2323–30.

37 Tyagi SC. Proteinases and myocardial extracellular matrix turnover. *Mol Cell Biochem* 1997;**168**:1–12.

38 Woessner JF, Jr. Role of matrix proteases in processing enamel proteins. *Connect Tissue Res* 1998;**39**: 69–73; discussion 141–9.

39 Tyagi SC, Kumar SG, Banks J, Fortson W. Co-expression of tissue inhibitor and matrix metalloproteinase in myocardium. *J Mol Cell Cardiol* 1995;**27**:2177–89.

40 Heymans S, Luttun A, Nuyens D, et al. Inhibition of plasminogen activators or matrix metalloproteinases prevents cardiac rupture but impairs therapeutic angiogenesis and causes cardiac failure. *Nat Med* 1999;**5**:1135–42.

41 Fedak PW, Altamentova SM, Weisel RD, et al. Matrix remodeling in experimental and human heart failure: a possible regulatory role for TIMP-3. *Am J Physiol Heart Circ Physiol* 2003;**284**:H626–34.

42 Covell JW. Factors influencing diastolic function. Possible role of the extracellular matrix. *Circulation* 1990;**81**(2 Suppl):III155–8.

43 Zhao M, Zhang H, Robinson T, Factor S, Sonnenblick E, Eng C. Profound structural alterations of the extracellular collagen matrix in postischemic dysfunctional ('stunned') but viable myocardium. *J Am Coll Cardiol* 1987;**10**:1322–34.

44 Becker RC, Hochman JS, Cannon CP, et al. Fatal cardiac rupture among patients treated with thrombolytic agents and adjunctive thrombin antagonists: Observations from the Thrombolysis and Thrombin Inhibition in Myocardial Infarction 9 Study. *J Am Coll Cardiol* 1999;**33**:479–87.

45 Sutton MG, Sharpe N. Left ventricular remodeling after myocardial infarction: pathophysiology and therapy. *Circulation* 2000;**101**:2981–8.

46 Pfeffer M, Braunwald E. Ventricular remodeling after myocardial infarction. Experimental observations and clinical implications. *Circulation* 1990;**81**:1161–72.

47 Cohn JN, Ferrari R, Sharpe N. Cardiac remodeling—concepts and clinical implications: a consensus paper from an international forum on cardiac remodeling. Behalf of an International Forum on Cardiac Remodeling. *J Am Coll Cardiol* 2000;**35**:569–82.

48 Sabbah HN, Goldstein S. Ventricular remodelling: consequences and therapy. *Eur Heart J* 1993; **14**(suppl C):24–9.

49 Gaudron P, Eilles C, Kugler I, Ertl G. Progressive left ventricular dysfunction and remodeling after myocardial infarction. Potential mechanisms and early predictors. *Circulation* 1993;**87**:755–63.

50 White H, Norris R, Brown M, Brandt P, Whitlock R, Wild C. Left ventricular end-systolic volume as the major determinant of survival after recovery from myocardial infarction. *Circulation* 1987;**76**: 44–51.

51 Hammermeister K, DeRouen T, Dodge H. Variables predictive of survival in patients with coronary disease. Selection by univariate and multivariate analyses from the clinical, electrocardiographic, exercise, arteriographic, and quantitative angiographic evaluations. *Circulation* 1979;**59**:421–30.

52 Cohn JN, Johnson G, Ziesche S, et al. A comparison of enalapril with hydralazine-isosorbide dinitrate in the treatment of chronic congestive heart failure. *N Engl J Med* 1991;**325**:303–10.

53 Carr A, Prisant L, Watkins L. Detection of hypertensive left ventricular hypertrophy. *Hypertension* 1985;**7**:948–54.

54 No authors listed. Guidelines for the diagnosis of heart failure. The Task Force on Heart Failure of the European Sociey of Cardiology. *Eur Heart J* 1995;**16**:741–51.

55 Gottdiener JS. Left ventricular mass, diastolic dysfunction, and hypertension. *Adv Intern Med* 1993; **38**:31–56.

56 Francis CM, Caruana L, Kearney P, et al. Open access echocardiography in management of heart failure in the community. *BMJ* 1995;**310**:634–6.

57 Krzesinski JM, Rorive G, Van Cauwenberge H. Hypertension and left ventricular hypertrophy. *Acta Cardiol* 1996;**51**:143–54.

58 Effects of enalapril on mortality in severe congestive heart failure. Results of the Cooperative North Scandinavian Enalapril Survival Study (CONSENSUS). The CONSENSUS Trial Study Group. *N Engl J Med* 1987;**316**:1429–35.

59 Frigerio M, Roubina E. Drugs for left ventricular remodeling in heart failure. *Am J Cardiol* 2005; **96**:10L–8L.

60 Greenberg B, Quinones MA, Koilpillai C, et al. Effects of long-term enalapril therapy on cardiac structure and function in patients with left ventricular dysfunction. Results of the SOLVD echocardiography substudy. *Circulation* 1995;**91**:2573–81.

61 St John Sutton M, Pfeffer MA, Plappert T, et al. Quantitative two-dimensional echocardiographic measurements are major predictors of adverse cardiovascular events after acute myocardial infarction. The protective effects of captopril. *Circulation* 1994;**89**:68–75.

62 Lopez-Sendon J, Swedberg K, McMurray J, et al. Expert consensus document on angiotensin converting enzyme inhibitors in cardiovascular disease. *Eur Heart J* 2004;**25**:1454–70.

63 Quinones MA, Greenberg BH, Kopelen HA, et al. Echocardiographic predictors of clinical outcome in patients with left ventricular dysfunction enrolled in the SOLVD registry and trials: significance of left ventricular hypertrophy. Studies of Left Ventricular Dysfunction. *J Am Coll Cardiol* 2000;**35**:1237–44.

64 Fedak PW, Verma S, Weisel RD, Li RK. Cardiac remodeling and failure: from molecules to man (Part I). *Cardiovasc Pathol* 2005;**14**:1–11.

65 Azizi M, Ménard JL. Combined blockade of the renin-angiotensin system with angiotensin-converting enzyme inhibitors and angiotensin II type 1 receptor antagonists. *Circulation* 2004;**109**:2492–9.

66 Opie LH, Sack MN. Enhanced angiotensin II activity in heart failure: reevaluation of the counterregulatory hypothesis of receptor subtypes. *Circulation Res* 2001;**88**:654–8.

67 McKelvie RS, Yusuf S, Pericak D, et al. Comparison of candesartan, enalapril, and their combination in congestive heart failure: Randomized Evaluation of Strategies for Left Ventricular Dysfunction (RESOLVD) Pilot Study: The RESOLVD Pilot Study Investigators. *Circulation* 1999;**100**:1056–64.

68 Dubach P, Myers J, Bonetti P, et al. Effects of bisoprolol fumarate on left ventricular size, function, and exercise capacity in patients with heart failure: analysis with magnetic resonance myocardial tagging. *Am Heart J* 2002;**143**:676–83.

69 Hall SA, Cigarroa CG, Marcoux L, Risser RC, Grayburn PA, Eichhorn EJ. Time course of improvement in left ventricular function, mass and geometry in patients with congestive heart failure treated with beta-adrenergic blockade. *J Am Coll Cardiol* 1995;**25**:1154–61.

70 Lowes BD, Gill EA, Abraham WT, et al. Effects of carvedilol on left ventricular mass, chamber geometry, and mitral regurgitation in chronic heart failure. *Am J Cardiol* 1999;**83**:1201–5.

71 Zugck C, Haunstetter A, Kruger C, et al. Impact of beta-blocker treatment on the prognostic value of currently used risk predictors in congestive heart failure. *J Am Coll Cardiol* 2002;**39**:1615–22.

72 Khattar RS, Senior R, Soman P, van der Does R, Lahiri A. Regression of left ventricular remodeling in chronic heart failure: comparative and combined effects of captopril and carvedilol. *Am Heart J* 2001;**142**:704–13.

73 Packer M, Colucci WS, Sackner-Bernstein JD, et al. Double-blind, placebo-controlled study of the effects of carvedilol in patients with moderate to severe heart failure. The PRECISE Trial. Prospective Randomized Evaluation of Carvedilol on Symptoms and Exercise. *Circulation* 1996;**94**:2793–9.

74 Cioffi G, Stefenelli C, Tarantini L, Opasich C. Chronic left ventricular failure in the community: Prevalence, prognosis, and predictors of the complete clinical recovery with return of cardiac size and function to normal in patients undergoing optimal therapy. *J Card Fail* 2004;**10**:250–7.

75 Bristow MR, O'Connell JB, Gilbert EM, et al. Dose-response of chronic beta-blocker treatment in heart failure from either idiopathic dilated or ischemic cardiomyopathy. Bucindolol Investigators. *Circulation* 1994;**89**:1632–42.

76 Bristow MR, Gilbert EM, Abraham WT, et al. Carvedilol produces dose-related improvements in left ventricular function and survival in subjects with chronic heart failure. MOCHA Investigators. *Circulation* 1996;**94**:2807–16.

77 Pitt B, Zannad F, Remme WJ, et al. The effect of spironolactone on morbidity and mortality in patients with severe heart failure. Randomized Aldactone Evaluation Study Investigators. *N Engl J Med* 1999;**341**:709–17.

78 Pitt B, Remme W, Zannad F, et al. Eplerenone, a selective aldosterone blocker, in patients with left ventricular dysfunction after myocardial infarction. *N Engl J Med* 2003;**348**:1309–21.

79 White PC. Aldosterone: direct effects on and production by the heart. *J Clin Endocrinol Metab* 2003;**88**:2376–83.

Chapter 32

Sepsis-Associated Encephalopathy

Eric Magalhaes, Angelo Polito, Andréa Polito, and Tarek Sharshar

Introduction

Sepsis represents the most frequent and severe form of systemic illness that can trigger an acute form of brain dysfunction in critically ill patients in the absence of any CNS infection. This acute brain dysfunction, termed sepsis-associated encephalopathy (SAE),[1] occurs in patients with sepsis, most of the time in relation to documented bacterial or fungal infections.[2,3] SAE is independently associated with decreased hospital and intensive care survival[3,4,5] and with long-term cognitive disability.[6] SAE presents as a global alteration of cognitive function and by an altered level of consciousness (ranging from hyper-alertness to lethargy), thus constituting a clinical continuum with delirium. However, focal neurological signs may also be identified and should prompt consideration for a localized brain lesion that is most often of ischaemic origin.[7] The diagnosis of SAE requires a systematic approach which considers the contribution of multiple systemic perturbations that can lead to brain dysfunction. In this chapter, we describe the pathophysiology of SAE and propose a rational diagnostic approach.

Pathophysiology

From systemic inflammation to sickness behaviour

The inflammatory response generated by sepsis is a major source of signalling to the brain, leading to changes in mood and cognition. These changes are part of a physiological behavioural response called 'sickness behaviour' (see Figure 32.1). It is stereotypically characterized by weakness, malaise, listlessness, inability to concentrate, apathy, lethargy, and anorexia. It should be distinguished from encephalopathy that symptomatically ranges from confusion (or delirium) to coma.[8]

Two main neurological structures are involved in brain signalling.[8] The vagus nerve detects visceral inflammation by its terminal cytokine receptors and relays the signal to autonomic and neuroendocrine centres that control baroreflex and adrenal axis or vasopressin secretion, respectively. The vagal nerve also reduces inflammation by releasing acetylcholine which will bind nicotinic receptors of macrophages.[9] The circumventricular organs (CVOs) are midline structures bordering the third and fourth ventricles that are located near neuroendocrine and neurovegetative nuclei. As they lack BBB and express receptors for innate and adaptive immune systems,[10,11] CVOs detect and allow the passage of circulating mediators that will indirectly signal deeper areas involved in controlling behavioural, neuroendocrine, and neurovegetative responses.[8] Various mediators are involved in this brain signalling, notably pro- and anti-inflammatory cytokines, prostaglandins, and NO.[12–15]

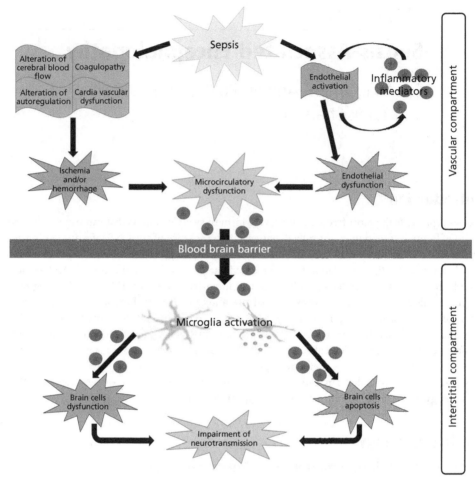

Fig. 32.1 Representation of the two main pathogenic processes involved in sepsis-associated brain dysfunction. These two processes are not exclusive, and both include microcirculatory dysfunction. In the ischaemic process on the left, the combination of macrocirculatory dysfunction and coagulopathy impairs oxygen and nutriment supply and leads finally to ischaemia and haemorrhage. In the neuroinflammatory process on the right, the key step is endothelial activation that induces production of excessive pro-inflammatory mediators, leading to endothelial dysfunction. Both processes alter microcirculation and induce BBB dysfunction, allowing the passage of neurotoxic mediators into the brain, notably inflammatory mediators. The main consequence of these processes is activation of microglial cells, leading to brain cells dysfunction and apoptosis. Impairment of neurotransmission is the endpoint of this pathophysiological process and explains the observed clinical features.

Pathophysiological cerebral processes

SAE results from neuroinflammatory and ischaemic processes that are not mutually exclusive and that will end up by cellular dysfunction and impair neurotransmission. Microcirculatory alteration is common to both processes.

Acute neuroinflammatory process during sepsis

Endothelial activation and blood-brain barrier dysfunction

This process encompasses endothelial activation that subsequently alters microcirculation and the BBB, thus compromising oxygen supply and allowing the passage of neurotoxic and inflammatory mediators into the CNS.

Endothelial activation is considered one the main pathophysiological mechanisms of organ failures in sepsis and involves the cerebral vasculature. This endothelial activation is characterized by the expression of various adhesion molecules,[16–19] Toll-like and cytokine receptors[20] as well as the production of pro-inflammatory cytokines and NO by endothelial and inducible nitric oxide synthase (iNOS)[21] and synthesis of type 2 cyclo-oxygenase.[22] The activated endothelium sustains brain inflammation by releasing pro-inflammatory cytokines and NO[21] into the parenchyma and by recruiting activated leucocytes.[18,20,23]

BBB dysfunction is a consequence of endothelial activation, along with the alteration of vascular tone and microcirculation.[24] MRI supports the presence of BBB alteration by showing vasogenic oedema in patients with septic shock.[7] This BBB disruption can sometimes affect the whole white matter[7] or be localized in posterior lobes as in posterior reversible encephalopathy syndrome.[25] It has been recently reported that BBB alteration is reduced by intravenous immunoglobulin (IvIg), given before the onset of experimental sepsis.[26] Experimental studies indicate that BBB dysfunction is characterized by the detachment of pericytes,[27] increased permeability at the level of tight junction proteins, or via a transcellular pathway.[26,28–30] Factors involved in this alteration include mainly complement,[31,32,33] TNF-α,[34] ROS, and reactive nitrogen species (RNS).[35] This increased permeability allows the passage of leucocytes[20] and various inflammatory, metabolic, pharmacologic, and neurotoxic mediators within brain parenchyma.[13,14,24,36,37] Then brain cells exhibit cytokine receptors and release inflammatory mediators, amplifying the neuroinflammatory process.[37–39]

Microglial activation

Experimental and human neuropathological studies reported microglial activation during sepsis.[40,41,42] It seems that activated microglial cells are involved in the recruitment of leucocytes[43] and are preferentially situated in the vicinity of brain blood vessels.[27] Various factors can directly affect these cells in sepsis like TNFα, iNOS,[13,14,24,36,44] or glucose.[41] Activated microglial cells, like astrocytes, can amplify the neuroinflammatory process by releasing NO and pro-inflammatory cytokines.[45] It has been suggested that pathological microglial activation may be a key mechanism of delirium in septic patients. Thus, minocycline, by inhibiting microglial cells, has been shown to facilitate the recovery from sickness behaviour, along with a reduction in cortical and hippocampal expression of mRNA levels of IL-1β and IL-6.[37] Statins could also modulate microglial activation.[46] There are arguments for a role of microglial activation in the transition from delirium to cognitive decline and also of sepsis-induced microglial activation in neurodegenerative diseases. These two points are discussed in the following sections.

Ischaemic process during sepsis

Small case series have reported ischaemic stroke in patients with septic shock.[7] Neuropathological studies have noted ischaemia in brain areas susceptible to low CBF.[42] Ischaemia might be related to the impairment of cerebral perfusion. Data are mixed regarding cerebral perfusion during septic shock. While some studies did not show impaired perfusion,[47] others have indicated a decrease in cerebral perfusion pressure or in CBF and also an alteration in the regulation of cerebral perfusion, including impaired CO_2 reactivity and cerebrovascular pressure autoregulation.[48] It is not known, however, to what extent these disturbances might account for ischaemia. Our group failed to find an association between the duration or severity of hypotension and cerebral ischaemia in previous neuropathological studies.[42] It has been shown that disturbances in cerebral autoregulation were associated with delirium.[49] One way to determine the importance of cerebral perfusion in septic shock would be to determine whether perfusion monitoring and optimization reduce the incidence of stroke. This approach might be limited by two factors: microcirculatory dysfunction and coagulopathy.

Cerebral microcirculatory dysfunction has been documented in various experimental models of sepsis but not yet in humans.[2,50] It may account for diffuse ischaemic damages and microhaemorrhages observed in the brain of patients who died from septic shock.[42]

Disturbances of haemostasis, especially disseminated intravascular coagulation (DIC), that can involve the brain may also play a role in the development of SAE.[7] A neuropathological study reported that 10% of patients with septic shock have haemorrhagic lesions associated with clotting disorders.[42] Moreover, ischaemic stroke is associated with low platelets count and high activated clotting time.[51]

Finally, another mechanism might be represented by cardiac embolism. It has been recently shown that new-onset atrial fibrillation is associated with an increased risk of stroke and mortality in septic patients.[52]

Cellular dysfunction and apoptosis

After gaining entry into the brain, pro-inflammatory mediators will induce cellular oxidative stress.[53,54,55] Various brain areas of septic rats, especially in the hippocampus and cortex, are liable to an early, but transitory, oxidative stress.[53,54] It results from peroxinitrite formation (NO pathway),[56,57,58] decrease in antioxidant factors (heat shock proteins[58] or ascorbate),[59] impairment of superoxide dismutase pathway,[53] mitochondrial dysfunction,[55,56,57,60] and maybe from hyperglycaemia and hypoxaemia.[61] Mitochondrial dysfunction might be at the origin of the neuronal bioenergetic failure.[55,62] However, this mechanism was not confirmed in healthy volunteers challenged with LPS.[35,63,64]

Apoptosis is one of the main consequences of oxidative stress. The expression of iNOS seems involved in mitochondrial-mediated apoptosis found in sepsis.[56,60,65] Human data have shown that the intensity of neuronal apoptosis is correlated with the expression of endothelial iNOS.[66] In addition to NO, there are various pro-apoptotic molecules that may be involved such as TNF-α, glucose, or glutamate.[67] The identification of multifocal necrotizing leukoencephalopathy in a patient with septic shock supports the pro-apoptotic role of TNF-α.[68] We recently reported a correlation between blood glucose level and the intensity of microglial apoptosis, whose mechanism might be the lack of downregulation of GLUT5.[41] Finally, glutamate neurotoxicity has been incriminated in several neurological disorders.[69] Large amounts of this neuromediator are released by activated microglial cells.[56] Recycling and glutamate export of ascorbate by astrocytes are inhibited during sepsis,[59,70] accounting for its decrease in plasma and cerebrospinal fluid (CSF) in patients with SAE.[71]

Impairment of neurotransmission

The final consequence of these neuroinflammatory and ischaemic processes is an impairment of neurotransmission which can directly explain clinical signs of encephalopathy.[72] The β-adrenergic system,[73] GABA receptor system,[74] and cholinergic release[75] are affected during sepsis.

The imbalance between dopaminergic and cholinergic neurotransmission is considered a major mechanism of delirium in critically ill patients.[44] Nonetheless, the administration of rivastigmine did not decrease the duration of delirium.[76] The use of GABA agonists, such as benzodiazepines, is associated with an increased risk of brain dysfunction in critically ill patients.[77] Noradrenergic neurotransmission might be also involved in SAE, as dexmedetomidine, an α2-adrenergic receptor agonist which is believed to modulate activity in the locus coeruleus, is associated with reduced brain dysfunction in septic patients when compared to midazolam.[78,79]

NO[32] and neurotoxic amino acids are particularly incriminated in the alteration of neurotransmission. Neurotoxic amino acids, such as ammonium, tyrosine, tryptophan, and phenylalanine, are released in excess by liver and muscles during sepsis and easily reach the brain in the setting of BBB alteration.[80-82] The concomitant decrease in branched-chain amino acids might potentiate their neurotoxic effect.[80-82] Metabolic disorders, notably related to kidney and liver failure, contribute to neurotransmitter alteration, as well as various drugs that are administered in septic patients (i.e. sedatives, analgesics, antibiotics).

Patterns of brain injury in SAE

One may argue that neuroinflammatory process will be widely distributed, as opposed to the more localized process in focal ischaemia. Indeed, ischaemic stroke is often revealed by a focal neurological sign. On the other hand, the brain of septic patients is liable to multiple lacunae,[42] and the report of multifocal necrotizing leukoencephalopathy indicates that some regions of the brain are more sensitive to neuroinflammatory process.[68]

The prevalence of delirium, long-term psychological disorders (such as PTSD), and cognitive decline (especially memory and attention) suggests that the hippocampus is particularly affected during sepsis. This might be explained by its vulnerability to inflammatory, but also ischaemic, hypoxic, or dysglycaemic, insults.

There is evidence for brainstem dysfunction during sepsis. Indeed, we found that some brainstem responses in sedated critically ill patients are associated with poor outcome, including death and the occurrence of delirium.[83] Impaired sympathetic control of heart rate is frequent and associated with increased mortality in septic patients, suggesting a central autonomic regulatory impairment.[84] The brainstem exerts a significant influence on the immune response through the sympathetic[85] and parasympathetic nervous system.[9] Brainstem nuclei are liable to apoptosis,[66] and the use of dexmedetomidine, which have anti-apoptotic properties, results in less delirium in septic patients.[78] Brainstem dysfunction could then account for alteration of awareness (which is controlled by reticular ascending activating substance) and autonomic control of cardiovascular and immune system in septic patients.

Diagnosis and differential diagnosis

Clinical examination of the acutely confused critically ill patient

Detection of acute brain dysfunction in ICU is based on neurological examination. SAE is characterized by acute changes in mental status, cognition, alteration of sleep/wake cycle, disorientation, impaired attention, and/or disorganized thinking. Sometimes, exaggerated motor activity with agitation and/or hallucinations can be observed. Alternatively, agitation and drowsiness can occur. Less frequent motor symptoms, such as paratonic rigidity, asterixis, tremor, and multifocal myoclonus, may be present. Physicians may consider the use of validated clinical instruments for the detection of brain dysfunction in critically ill patients such as the confusion assessment method for the ICU (CAM-ICU) and the intensive care delirium screening checklist (ICDSC).

Both CAM-ICU and ICDSC are validated tools for the detection of ICU delirium in mechanically ventilated patients.[86] The risk to develop delirium can be evaluated by the PRE-DELERIC score[87] and, if sedated, by testing oculocephalic response that, when abolished, is associated with increased risk of delirium.[83] The GCS,[88] FOUR coma scale,[89] the Richmond Agitation and Sedation Scale (RASS), or the Assessment to Intensive Care Environment (ATICE) can be used for the assessment of awareness.[90] Once brain dysfunction is identified, an exhaustive neurological examination, assessing neck stiffness, motor responses, muscular strength, plantar and deep tendon reflexes, and cranial nerves, is mandatory to search for focal neurological signs.

Other tests

Unexplained, sudden fluctuations in mental status or attention or the occurrence of focal neurological signs, seizure, or neck stiffness should prompt the physician to consider neuroimaging, EEG, and/or lumbar puncture. Whenever meningitis or encephalitis is suspected, a CSF analysis must be considered before or after neuroimaging.

In case of focal neurological signs, brain imaging is indicated. Brain MRI has a higher sensitivity than CT for the detection of acute CNS disorders such as recent ischaemic or haemorrhagic stroke, white matter disorders, brain abscess. Nonetheless, the risks and benefits of transporting a critically ill patient in order to perform brain imaging should always be carefully considered.

In the absence of focal sign or when neuroimaging is normal, physicians should carefully rule out a common metabolic disturbance that can impair consciousness such as hypoglycaemia, hypercalcaemia, hypo- or hypernatraemia. Adrenal insufficiency can be revealed by altered consciousness, and sepsis can also worsen hepatic or uraemic encephalopathy. Physicians should consider the discontinuation of neurotoxic drugs such as some antibiotics, steroids, and cardiovascular drugs. Plasma levels of potentially toxic drugs in the presence of liver and/or renal failure should always be checked. Critically ill patients are also susceptible to drug withdrawal, in particular, of benzodiazepines and opioids. The chronological link and neurological improvement after their re-administration may suggest a withdrawal syndrome. Tobacco dependency is a risk factor for delirium in critically ill patients; it may be prevented by the use of nicotine patch in chronic smokers.[91] Alcohol withdrawal-related delirium represents a potentially fatal, but not frequent, complication that occurs in 5% of hospitalized alcohol-dependent patients within 48–72 hours from the last drink. In malnourished or alcoholic patients, Wernicke's encephalopathy must always be suspected, especially if there is evidence of ophthalmoplegia or ataxia.[92] Endocarditis is also often associated with brain dysfunction and has to be suspected in the presence of microbleeds on MRI.

EEG is required in the case of abnormal movement with altered consciousness to diagnose seizures but also in the case of isolated alteration of consciousness that remain unexplained, as it can be secondary to non-convulsive seizures. It has been recently shown that sepsis can be associated with electroencephalographic abnormalities: epileptic discharge, periodic epileptiform discharge,[93] increased theta rhythms, triphasic waves, or burst suppression.[94]

Finally, assessments of plasma levels of brain injury biomarkers, such as neuron-specific enolase and S-100 β-protein, have been proposed for detecting brain dysfunction in sedated septic patients.[95,96]

Treatment

At the moment, no specific treatment for SAE is available, and treatment should focus on supportive interventions aiming at the control of sepsis, the management of organ failure and metabolic disturbances, and the discontinuation of neurotoxic drugs. Preventive and curative treatment that has been assessed for delirium might be proposed for SAE, although almost all studies have not assessed their effect on septic patients in subgroup analyses.

It is interesting to note that treatment with activated protein C in septic shock patients with a GCS <13 significantly reduces the plasma level of S-100 β-protein;[97] however, this drug is no more available. Steroids have been shown to reduce post-traumatic stress syndrome and to reduce BBB alteration and brain oedema.[98] Benefit of blood glucose control for the prevention of sepsis-related brain dysfunction has not yet been demonstrated, although experimental data support this therapeutic approach.[99] Experimental studies show that the use of IvIg,[26] magnesium,[28] riluzole,[100] calcium channel blockers, steroids, or anti-cytokine antibodies has a protective effect on the integrity of the BBB.[101] Moreover, treatment with the antioxidant drugs N-acetylcysteine and deferoxamine prevents cognitive impairment in septic mice.[54] Finally, the correction of the aliphatic amino acid defect may allow regression of signs of encephalopathy, probably stimulating an increased neurotransmitter synthesis.[82]

Outcome and long-term cognitive decline

The impact of SAE on outcomes is not known but is certainly close to that reported for delirium (see Figure 32.2). It is clearly established that delirium in critically ill patients is associated with a

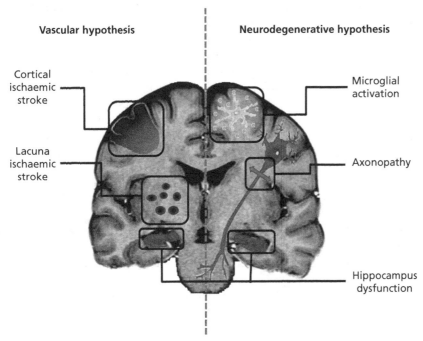

Fig. 32.2 Two hypotheses regarding long-term cognitive decline after SAE. On the left, the vascular hypothesis is the most described in neuroradiological studies. Multiple lacunar or cortical strokes may have a role in long-term cognitive decline. On the right, a representation of the neurodegenerative hypothesis with microglial activation and axonopathy. Chronic microglial activation may produce neurotoxic mediators, leading to a chronic impairment of neurotransmission. These mechanisms are not exclusive. The hippocampus seems to be the most frequent anatomical structure involved in long-term cognitive decline.

prolonged length of stay in ICU,[102] a longer duration of MV,[103] extra costs,[77] in-hospital mortality,[104] and its duration to 1-year mortality.[105]

At admission, about one-third of patients with sepsis have a GCS <12. A GCS <8 in septic patients is independently associated with increased mortality.[5] Risk of death also increases with severity of electrophysiological abnormalities, ranging from 0 when EEG is interpreted as normal to 67% when it shows burst suppressions.[93,106,107] Electrographic seizures and periodic epileptic discharges have been shown to be associated with increased mortality in septic patients monitored with continuous EEG.[93] The prognostic value of MRI findings remains to be determined,[7] but preliminary results indicate that ischaemic stroke is associated with increased mortality.[108]

As reported in critically patients who developed delirium in the ICU[109] and in survivors from ARDS,[110] sepsis survivors suffer from residual deficits in cognitive function up to 8 years after hospitalization for infection.[6] This cognitive decline is proportional to the severity of sepsis and can affect patients with absence to moderate pre-existing functional limitations.[6] There are mainly two hypotheses regarding this long-term cognitive decline observed in survivors of sepsis: a neurodegenerative process involving microglial activation and a vascular process related to diffuse ischaemic damage.

Microglial activation has been suggested to be a key mechanism linking delirium with cognitive decline.[44] This hypothesis is supported by the identification of microglial activation in neurodegenerative disorders, especially Alzheimer's disease.[111] During chronic CNS disease, microglia is primed and shows exaggerated response to repeated systemic or central inflammatory stimulations.[112,113] Weberpals et al.[114] reported that cognitive impairment in LPS-treated mice was associated with activation of microglial cells and not neuronal death; Semmler et al. noted that septic rats that developed cognitive dysfunction have a reduced cholinergic innervation.[75] According to this hypothesis, the decrease in cholinergic inhibition of the microglial cells would make them neurotoxic.[44] However, this hypothesis has been challenged by a clinical trial of the acetylcholinesterase inhibitor rivastigmine showing no benefit in terms of prevention of post-operative delirium.[76] Finally, it has been recently shown that elevated level of amyloid-beta in intensive care patients with delirium is correlated with long-term cognitive impairment.[115]

A vascular process related to diffuse ischaemic damage may be a second link between SAE and long-term cognitive decline. Neuropathological and neuroradiological reports support this hypothesis.[7,42,108] A preliminary neuroradiological study suggests that white matter lesions induced by sepsis are associated with cognitive decline.[116] It seems that insults of the hippocampus would account for the pattern of long-term psychological disorders and cognitive dysfunction.[53] Indeed, the hippocampus is involved in PTSD pathophysiology as well as in attention and memory, which are the two cognitive domains most frequently altered in SAE and delirium.[117] It has been shown that reduction of oxidative stress in the hippocampus is associated with less cognitive dysfunction in septic rats.[53] Other structures can be involved, notably cholinergic innervation of the parietal cortex.[75] Once again, iNOS seems to be involved, as NOS2 gene deficiency protects from sepsis-induced long-term cognitive deficits.[114]

Finally, it is conceivable that an axonopathy could account to long-term cognitive alteration. Axonal damages can be involved in white matter hyperdensities that preliminary neuroradiological data suggest to be associated with subsequent cognitive decline in critically patients who developed delirium.[118] This hypothesis also links SAE with CIP, another major neurology complication of sepsis. It is likely that these two diseases have common pathophysiological mechanisms.

Conclusion

Sepsis represents the most frequent and severe cause of brain dysfunction in critically ill patients. The pathophysiology of SAE is complex and results from both inflammatory and ischaemic processes that affect all types of brain cells. The diagnosis of encephalopathy relies essentially on neurological examination and brain imaging. In daily clinical practice, it is of foremost importance to rule out brain infection. At the moment, the treatment of SAE is mainly based on the resolution of sepsis.

References

1 Consales G, De Gaudio AR. Sepsis associated encephalopathy. *Minerva Anestesiol* 2005;**71**:39–52.

2 Iacobone E, Bailly-Salin J, Polito A, Friedman D, Stevens RD, Sharshar T. Sepsis-associated encephalopathy and its differential diagnosis. *Crit Care Med* 2009;**37**:S331–6.

3 Sprung CL, Peduzzi PN, Shatney CH, et al. Impact of encephalopathy on mortality in the sepsis syndrome. The Veterans Administration Systemic Sepsis Cooperative Study Group. *Crit Care Med* 1990;**18**:801–6.

4 Akrout N, Sharshar T, Annane D. Mechanisms of brain signaling during sepsis. *Curr Neuropharmacol* 2009;**7**:296–301.

5 Eidelman LA, Putterman D, Putterman C, Sprung CL. The spectrum of septic encephalopathy. Definitions, etiologies, and mortalities. *JAMA* 1996;**275**:470–3.

6 Iwashyna TJ, Ely EW, Smith DM, Langa KM. Long-term cognitive impairment and functional disability among survivors of severe sepsis. *JAMA* 2010;**304**:1787–94.

7 Sharshar T, Carlier R, Bernard F, et al. Brain lesions in septic shock: a magnetic resonance imaging study. *Intensive Care Med* 2007;**33**:798–806.

8 Dantzer R, O'connor JC, Freund GG, Johnson RW, Kelley KW. From inflammation to sickness and depression: when the immune system subjugates the brain. *Nat Rev Neurosci* 2008;**9**:46–56.

9 Tracey KJ. Reflex control of immunity. *Nat Rev Immunol* 2009;**9**:418–28.

10 Lacroix S, Rivest S. Effect of acute systemic inflammatory response and cytokines on the transcription genes encoding cyclooxygenase enzymes (COX-1 and COX-2) in the rat brain. *J Neurochem* 1998;**70**:452–66.

11 Laflamme N, Souci G, Rivest S. Circulating cell wall components derived from Gram-negative and not gram-positive bacteria cause of a profound transcriptionnal activation of the gene Toll-like receptor 2 in the CNS. *J Neurochem* 2001;**70**:648–57.

12 Konsman JP, Kelley K, Dantzer R. Temporal and spatial relationships between lipopolysaccharide-induced expression of Fos, interleukin-1beta and inducible nitric oxide synthase in rat brain. *Neuroscience* 1999;**89**:535–48.

13 Wong ML, Bongiorno PB, Al-Shekhlee A, Esposito A, Khatri P, Licinio J. IL-1 beta, IL-1 receptor type I and iNOS gene expression in rat brain vasculature and perivascular areas. *Neuroreport* 1996;**7**, 2445–8.

14 Wong ML, Rettori V, Al-Shekhlee A, et al. Inducible nitric oxide synthase gene expression in the brain during systemic inflammation. *Nat Med* 1996;**2**:581–4.

15 Wong ML, Bongiorno PB, Rettori V, Mccann SM, Licinio J. Interleukin (IL)-1ß, IL-1 receptor antagonist, IL-10, and IL-13 gene expression in the central nervous system during systemic inflammation: pathophysiological implications. *Proc Natl Acad Sci USA* 1997;**94**:227–32.

16 Hess DC, Bhutwala T, Sheppard JC, Zhao W, Smith J. ICAM-1 expression on human brain microvascular endothelial cells. *Neurosci Lett* 1994;**168**:201–4.

17 Hess DC, Thompson Y, Sprinkle A, Carroll J, Smith, J. E-selectin expression on human brain microvascular endothelial cells. *Neurosci Lett* 1996;**213**:37–40.

18 Hofer S, Bopp C, Hoerner C, et al. Injury of the blood brain barrier and up-regulation of icam-1 in polymicrobial sepsis. *J Surg Res* 2008;**146**:276–81.

19 Omari KM, Dorovini-Zis K. CD40 expressed by human brain endothelial cells regulates CD4 + T cell adhesion to endothelium. *J Neuroimmunol* 2003;**134**:166–78.

20 Zhou H, Andonegui G, Wong CH, Kubes P. Role of endothelial TLR4 for neutrophil recruitment into central nervous system microvessels in systemic inflammation. *J Immunol* 2009;**183**:5244–50.

21 Freyer D, Manz R, Ziegenhorn A, et al. Cerebral endothelial cells release TNF-alpha after stimulation with cell walls of Streptococcus pneumoniae and regulate inducible nitric oxide synthase and ICAM-1 expression via autocrine loops. *J Immunol* 1999;**163**:4308–14.

22 Matsumura K, Cao C, Ozaki M, Morii H, Nakadate K, Watanabe Y. Brain endothelial cells express cyclooxygenase-2 during lipopolysaccharide-induced fever: light and electron microscopic immunocy-tochemical studies. *J Neurosci* 1998;**18**:6279–89.

23 Bohatschek M, Werner A, Raivich G. Systemic LPS injection leads to granulocyte influx into normal and injured brain: effects of ICAM-1 deficiency. *Exp Neurol* 2001;**172**:137–52.

24 Semmler A, Hermann S, Mormann F, et al. Sepsis causes neuroinflammation and concomitant decrease of cerebral metabolism. *J Neuroinflammation* 2008;**5**:38.

25 Bartynski WS, Boardman JF, Zeigler ZR, Shadduck RK, Lister J. Posterior reversible encephalopathy syndrome in infection, sepsis, and shock. *AJNR Am J Neuroradio* 2006;**27**:2179–90.

26 Esen F, Senturk E, Ozcan PE, et al. Intravenous immunoglobulins prevent the breakdown of the blood-brain barrier in experimentally induced sepsis. *Crit Care Med* 2012;**40**:1214–20.

27 Nishioku T, Dohgu S, Takata F, et al. Detachment of brain pericytes from the basal lamina is involved in disruption of the blood-brain barrier caused by lipopolysaccharide-induced sepsis in mice. *Cell Mol Neurobiol* 2009;**29**:309–16.

28 Esen F, Erdem T, Aktan D, et al. Effect of magnesium sulfate administration on blood-brain bar-rier in a rat model of intraperitoneal sepsis: a randomized controlled experimental study. *Crit Care* 2005;**9**:R18–23.

29 Mayhan G. Effect of lipopolysaccharide on the permeability and reactivity of the cerebral microcircula-tion: role of inducible nitric oxide synthase. *Brain Res* 1998;**792**:353–7.

30 Yi X, Wang Y, Yu FS. Corneal epithelial tight junctions and their response to lipopolysaccharide chal-lenge. *Invest Ophthalmol Vis Sci* 2000;**41**:4093–100.

31 Flierl MA, Stahel PF, Rittirsch D, et al. Inhibition of complement C5a prevents breakdown of the blood-brain barrier and pituitary dysfunction in experimental sepsis. *Crit Care* 2009;**13**:R12.

32 Jacob A, Brorson JR, Alexander JJ. Septic encephalopathy: inflammation in man and mouse. *Neurochem Int* 2011;**58**:472–6.

33 Jacob A, Hack B, Chiang E, Garcia JG, Quigg RJ, Alexander JJ. C5a alters blood-brain barrier integ-rity in experimental lupus. *FASEB J* 2012;**24**:1682–8.

34 Tsao N, Hsu HP, Wu CM, Liu CC, Lei HY. Tumour necrosis factor-alpha causes an increase in blood-brain barrier permeability during sepsis. *J Med Microbiol* 2001;**50**:812–21.

35 Berg RM, Moller K, Bailey DM. Neuro-oxidative-nitrosative stress in sepsis. *J Cereb Blood Flow Metab* 2011;**31**:1532–44.

36 Alexander JJ, Jacob A, Cunningham P, Hensley L, Quigg RJ. TNF is a key mediator of septic enceph-alopathy acting through its receptor, TNF receptor-1. *Neurochem Int* 2008;**52**:447–56.

37 Henry CJ, Huang Y, Wynne AM, Godbout JP. Peripheral lipopolysaccharide (LPS) challenge pro-motes microglial hyperactivity in aged mice that is associated with exaggerated induction of both pro-inflammatory IL-1beta and anti-inflammatory IL-10 cytokines. *Brain Behav Immun* 2009;**23**: 309–17.

38 Bi XL, Yang JY, Dong YX, et al. Resveratrol inhibits nitric oxide and TNF-alpha production by lipopolysaccharide-activated microglia. *Int Immunopharmacol* 2005;**5**:185–93.

39 Gavillet M, Allaman I, Magistretti PJ. Modulation of astrocytic metabolic phenotype by pro-inflammatory cytokines. *Glia* 2008;**56**:975–89.

40 Lemstra AW, Groen In' T, Woud JC, et al. Microglia activation in sepsis: a case-control study. *J Neuroinflammation* 2007;**4**:4.

41 Polito A, Brouland JP, Porcher R, et al. Hyperglycaemia and apoptosis of microglial cells in human septic shock. *Crit Care* 2011;**15**:R131.

42 Sharshar T, Annane D, De La Grandmaison GL, Brouland JP, Hopkinson NS, Francoise G. The neuropathology of septic shock. *Brain Pathol* 2004;**14**:21–33.

43 Zhou H, Lapointe BM, Clark SR, Zbytnuik L, Kubes P. A requirement for microglial TLR4 in leukocytes recruitment in response to lipopolysaccharide. *J Immunol* 2006;**177**:8103–10.

44 Van Gool WA, Van De Beek D, Eikelenboom P. Systemic infection and delirium: when cytokines and acetylcholine collide. *Lancet* 2010;**375**:773–5.

45 Cheret C. Neurotoxic activation of microglia is promoted by a nox1-dependent NADPH oxidase. *J Neurosci* 2008;**28**:12039–51.

46 Morandi A, Hughes CG, Girard TD, Mcauley DF, Ely EW, Pandharipande PP. Statins and brain dysfunction: a hypothesis to reduce the burden of cognitive impairment in patients who are critically ill. *Chest* 2011;**140**:580–5.

47 Matta BF, Stow P. Sepsis-induced vasoparalysis does not involve the cerebral vasculature: indirect evidence from autoregulation and carbon dioxide reactivity studies. *Br J Anaesth* 1996;**76**:790–4.

48 Burkhart, C. S., Siegemund, M. & Steiner, L. A. Cerebral perfusion in sepis. *Crit Care* 2010;**14**, 215.

49 Pfister D, Siegemund M, Dell-Kuster S, et al. Cerebral perfusion in sepsis-associated delirium. *Crit Care* 2008;**12**:R63.

50 Taccone FS, Su F, Pierrakos C, et al. Cerebral microcirculation is impaired during sepsis: an experimental study. *Crit Care* 2010;**14**:R140.

51 Polito A, Eischwald F, Maho AL, et al. Pattern of Brain Injury in the Acute Setting of Human Septic Shock. *Crit Care* 2013;**17**(5):R204.

52 Walkey AJ, Wiener RS, Ghobrial JM, Curtis LH, Benjamin EJ. Incident stroke and mortality associated with new-onset atrial fibrillation in patients hospitalized with severe sepsis. *JAMA* 2011;**306**:2248–54.

53 Barichello T, Fortunato JJ, Vitali AM, et al. Oxidative variables in the rat brain after sepsis induced by cecal ligation and perforation. *Crit Care Med* 2006;**34**:886–9.

54 Barichello T, Machado RA, Constantino L, et al. Antioxidant treatment prevented late memory impairment in an animal model of sepsis. *Crit Care Med* 2007;**35**:2186–90.

55 D'avila JC, Santiago AP, Amancio RT, Galina A, Oliveira MF, Bozza FA. Sepsis induces brain mitochondrial dysfunction. *Crit Care Med* 2008;**36**:1925–32.

56 Brown GC, Bal-Price A. Inflammatory neurodegeneration mediated by nitric oxide, glutamate, and mitochondria. *Mol Neurobiol* 2003;**27**:325–55.

57 Chan JY, Chang AY, Wang LL, Ou CC, Chan SH. Protein kinase C-dependent mitochondrial translocation of proapoptotic protein Bax on activation of inducible nitric-oxide synthase in rostral ventrolateral medulla mediates cardiovascular depression during experimental endotoxemia. *Mol Pharmacol* 2007;**71**:1129–39.

58 Li FC, Chan JY, Chang AY. In the rostral ventrolateral medulla, the 70-kDA heat shock protein (HSP70), but not HSP90, confers neuroprotection against fatal endotoxemia via augmentation of nitric-oxide synthase I (NOS I)/protein kinase G signaling pathway and inhibition of NOS II/peroxinitite cascade. *Mol Pharmacol* 2005;**68**:179–92.

59 Korcok J, Wu F, Tyml K, Hammond RR, Wilson JX. Sepsis inhibits reduction of dehydroascorbic acid and accumulation of ascorbate in astroglial cultures: intracellular ascorbate depletion increases nitric oxide synthase induction and glutamate uptake inhibition. *J Neurochem* 2002;**81**:185–93.

60 Messaris E, Memos N, Chatzigianni E, et al. Time-dependent mitochondrial-mediated programmed neuronal cell death prolongs survival in sepsis. *Crit Care Med* 2004;**32**:1764–70.

61 Won SJ, Tang XN, Suh SW, Yenari MA, Swanson RA. Hyperglycemia promotes tissue plasminogen activator-induced hemorrhage by Increasing superoxide production. *Ann Neurol* 2011;**70**: 583–90.

62 Maekawa T, Fujii Y, Sadamitsu D, et al. Cerebral circulation and metabolism in patients with septic encephalopathy. *Am J Emerg Med* 1991;**9**:139–43.

63 Hotchkiss RS, Karl IE. Reevaluation of the role of cellular hypoxia and bioenergetic failure in sepsis. *JAMA* 1992;**267**:1503–10.

64 Moller K, Strauss GI, Qvist J, et al. Cerebral blood flow and oxidative metabolism during human endotoxemia. *J Cereb Blood Flow Metab* 2002;**22**:1262–70.

65 Semmler A, Okulla T, Sastre M, Dumitrescu-Ozimek L, Heneka MT. Systemic inflammation induces apoptosis with variable vulnerability of different brain regions. *J Chem Neuroanat* 2005;**30**:144–57.

66 Sharshar T, Gray F, Lorin De La Grandmaison G, et al. Apoptosis of neurons in cardiovascular autonomic centres triggered by inducible nitric oxide synthase after death from septic shock. *Lancet* 2003;**362**:1799–805.

67 Yuan J, Yankner BA. Apoptosis in the nervous system. *Nature* 2000;**407**:802–9.

68 Sharshar T, Gray F, Poron F, Raphael JC, Gajdos P, Annane D. Multifocal necrotizing leukoencephalopathy in septic shock. *Crit Care Med* 2002;**30**:2371–5.

69 Villmann C, Becker CM. On the hypes and falls in neuroprotection: targeting the NMDA receptor. *Neuroscientist* 2007;**13**:594–615.

70 Wilson JX, Dragan M. Sepsis inhibits recycling and glutamate-stimulated export of ascorbate by astrocytes. *Free Radic Biol Med* 2005;**39**:990–8.

71 Voigt K, Kontush A, Stuerenburg HJ, Muench-Harrach D, Hansen HC, Kunze K. Decreased plasma and cerebrospinal fluid ascorbate levels in patients with septic encephalopathy. *Free Radic Res* 2002;**36**:735–9.

72 Stevens RD, Nyquist PA. Coma, delirium, and cognitive dysfunction in critical illness. *Crit Care Clin* 2006;**22**:787–804; abstract x.

73 Kadoi Y, Saito S, Kunimoto F, Imai T, Fujita T. Impairment of the brain beta-adrenergic system during experimental endotoxemia. *J Surg Res* 1996;**61**:496–502.

74 Kadoi Y, Saito S. An alteration in the gamma-aminobutyric acid receptor system in experimentally induced septic shock in rats. *Crit Care Med* 1996;**24**:298–305.

75 Semmler A, Frisch C, Debeir T, et al. Long-term cognitive impairment, neuronal loss and reduced cortical cholinergic innervation after recovery from sepsis in a rodent model. *Exp Neurol* 2007;**204**:733–40.

76 Van Eijk MM, Roes KC, Honing ML, et al. Effect of rivastigmine as an adjunct to usual care with haloperidol on duration of delirium and mortality in critically ill patients: a multicentre, double-blind, placebo-controlled randomised trial. *Lancet* 2010;**376**:1829–37.

77 Pandharipande P, Jackson J, Ely EW. Delirium: acute cognitive dysfunction in the critically ill. *Curr Opin Crit Care* 2005;**11**:360–8.

78 Pandharipande PP, Sanders RD, Girard TD, et al. Effect of dexmedetomidine versus lorazepam on outcome in patients with sepsis: an a priori-designed analysis of the MENDS randomized controlled trial. *Crit Care* 2007;**14**:R38.

79 Pandharipande PP, Sanders RD, Girard TD, et al. Effect of dexmedetomidine versus lorazepam on outcome in patients with sepsis: an a priori-designed analysis of the MENDS randomized controlled trial. *Crit Care* 2010;**14**:R38.

80 Basler T, Meier-Hellmann A, Bredle D, Reinhart K. Amino acid imbalance early in septic encephalopathy. *Intensive Care Med* 2002;**28**:293–8.

81 Berg RM, Taudorf S, Bailey DM, et al. Cerebral net exchange of large neutral amino acids after lipopolysaccharide infusion in healthy humans. *Crit Care* 2010;**14**:R16.

82 Freund HR, Ryan JA, Jr, Fischer JE. Amino acid derangements in patients with sepsis: treatment with branched chain amino acid rich infusions. *Ann Surg* 1978;**188**:423–30.

83 Sharshar T, Porcher R, Siami S, et al. Brainstem responses can predict death and delirium in sedated patients in intensive care unit. *Crit Care Med* 2011;**39**:1960–7.

84 Annane D, Trabold F, Sharshar T, et al. Inappropriate sympathetic activation at onset of septic shock: a spectral analysis approach. *Am J Respir Crit Care Med* 1999;**160**:458–65.

85 Kumar V, Sharma A. Neutrophils: Cinderella of innate immune system. *Int Immunopharmacol* 2010;**10**:1325–34.

86 Ely EW, Inouye SK, Bernard GR, et al. Delirium in mechanically ventilated patients: validity and reliability of the confusion assessment method for the intensive care unit (CAM-ICU). *JAMA* 2001;**286**:2703–10.

87 Boogaard M, Pickkers P, Slooter AJ, et al. Development and validation of PRE-DELIRIC (PREdiction of DELIRium in ICu patients) delirium prediction model for intensive care patients: observational multicentre study. *BMJ* 2012;**344**:e420.

88 Teasdale G, Jennett B. Assessment of coma and impaired consciousness. A practical scale. *Lancet* 1974;**2**:81–4.

89 Wijdicks EF, Bamlet WR, Maramattom BV, Manno EM, Mcclelland RL. Validation of a new coma scale: the FOUR score. *Ann Neurol* 2005;**58**:585–93.

90 De Jonghe B, Cook D, Griffith L, et al. Adaptation to the Intensive Care Environment (ATICE): development and validation of a new sedation assessment instrument. *Crit Care Med* 2003;**31**: 2344–54.

91 Lucidarme O, Seguin A, Daubin C, et al. Nicotine withdrawal and agitation in ventilated critically ill patients. *Crit Care* 2010;**14**:R58.

92 Sechi G, Serra A. Wernicke's encephalopathy: new clinical settings and recent advances in diagnosis and management. *Lancet Neurol* 2007;**6**:442–55.

93 Oddo M, Carrera E, Claassen J, Mayer SA, Hirsch LJ. Continuous electroencephalography in the medical intensive care unit. *Crit Care Med* 2009;**37**:2051–6.

94 Watson PL, Shintani AK, Tyson R, Pandharipande PP, Pun BT, Ely EW. Presence of electroencephalogram burst suppression in sedated, critically ill patients is associated with increased mortality. *Crit Care Med* 2008;**36**:3171–7.

95 Nguyen DN, Spapen H, Su F, et al. Elevated serum levels of S-100beta protein and neuron-specific enolase are associated with brain injury in patients with severe sepsis and septic shock. *Crit Care Med* 2006;**34**:1967–74.

96 Piazza O, Russo E, Cotena S, Esposito G, Tufano R. Elevated S100B levels do not correlate with the severity of encephalopathy during sepsis. *Br J Anaesth* 2007;**24**:24.

97 Spapen H, Nguyen DN, Troubleyn J, Huyghens L, Schiettecatte J. Drotrecogin alfa (activated) may attenuate severe sepsis-associated encephalopathy in clinical septic shock. *Crit Care* 2010;**14**:R54.

98 Schelling G, Roozendaal B, Krauseneck T, Schmoelz M, Briegel J. Efficacy of hydrocortisone in preventing posttraumatic stress disorder following critical illness and major surgery. *Ann N Y Acad Sci* 2006;**1071**:46–53.

99 Espinoza-Rojo M, Iturralde-RodríguezK I, Chanez-Cardenas ME, Ruiz-Tachiquín ME, Aguilera P. Glucose transporters regulation on ischemic brain: possible role as therapeutic target. *Cent Nerv Syst Agents Med Chem* 2010;**10**:317–25.

100 Toklu HZ, Uysal MK, Kabasakal L, Sirvanci S, Ercan F, Kaya M. The effects of riluzole on neurological, brain biochemical, and histological changes in early and late term of sepsis in rats. *J Surg Res* 2009;**152**:238–48.

101 **Wratten ML.** Therapeutic approaches to reduce systemic inflammation in septic-associated neurologic complications. *Eur J Anaesthesiol Suppl,*2008;**42**:1–7.

102 **Salluh JI, Soares M, Teles JM, et al.** Delirium epidemiology in critical care (DECCA): an international study. *Crit Care* 2010;**14**:R210.

103 **Lin SM, Huang CD, Liu CY, et al.** Risk factors for the development of early-onset delirium and the subsequent clinical outcome in mechanically ventilated patients. *J Crit Care* 2008;**23**:372–9.

104 **Ely EW, Shintani A, Truman B, et al.** Delirium as a predictor of mortality in mechanically ventilated patients in the intensive care unit. *JAMA* 2004;**291**:1753–62.

105 **Pisani MA, Kong SY, Kasl SV, Murphy TE, Araujo KL, Van Ness PH.** Days of delirium are associated with 1-year mortality in an older intensive care unit population. *Am J Respir Crit Care Med* 2009;**180**:1092–7.

106 **Young GB, Bolton CF, Archibald YM, Austin TW, Wells GA.** The electroencephalogram in sepsis-associated encephalopathy. *J Clin Neurophysiol* 1992;**9**:145–52.

107 **Young GB, Bolton CF, Austin TW, Archibald YM, Gonder J, Wells GA.** The encephalopathy associated with septic illness. *Clin Invest Med* 1990;**13**, 297–304.

108 **Le Maho AL, Polito A, Eischwald F, Annane D, Carlier R, Sharshar T.** Cerebral magnetic resonance imaging in septic shock patients with acute brain dysfunction. *ESICM Congress* Berlin; 2011.

109 **Girard TD, Jackson JC, Pandharipande PP, et al.** Delirium as a predictor of long-term cognitive impairment in survivors of critical illness. *Crit Care Med* 2010;**38**:1513–20.

110 **Hopkins RO, Weaver LK, Pope D, Orme JF, Bigler ED, Larson LV.** Neuropsychological sequelae and impaired health status in survivors of severe acute respiratory distress syndrome. *Am J Respir Crit Care Med* 1999;**160**:50–6.

111 **Ho GJ, Drego R, Hakimian E, Masliah E.** Mechanisms of cell signaling and inflammation in Alzheimer's disease. *Curr Drug Targets Inflamm Allergy* 2005;**4**:247–56.

112 **Cunningham C, Wilcockson DC, Campion S, Lunnon K, Perry VH.** Central and systemic endotoxin challenges exacerbate the local inflammatory response and increase neuronal death during chronic neurodegeneration. *J Neurosci* 2005;**25**:9275–84.

113 **Perry VH, Cunningham C, Holmes C.** Systemic infections and inflammation affect chronic neurodegeneration. *Nat Rev Immunol* 2007;**7**:161–7.

114 **Weberpals M, Hermes M, Hermann S, et al.** NOS2 gene deficiency protects from sepsis-induced long-term cognitive deficits. *J Neurosci* 2009;**29**:14177–84.

115 **Van den Boogaard M, Kox M, Quinn KL, et al.** Biomarkers associated with delirium in critically ill patients and their relation with long-term subjective cognitive dysfunction; indications for different pathways governing delirium in inflamed and noninflamed patients. *Crit Care* 2011;**15**:R297.

116 **Morandi A, Rogers BP, Gunther ML, et al.** The relationship between delirium duration, white matter integrity, and cognitive impairment in intensive care unit survivors as determined by diffusion tensor imaging: the Visions prospective cohort magnetic resonance imaging study. *Crit Care Med* 2012;**40**:2182–9.

117 **Hopkins RO, Weaver LK, Collingridge D, Parkinson RB, Chan KJ, Orme JF, Jr.** Two-year cognitive, emotional, and quality-of-life outcomes in acute respiratory distress syndrome. *Am J Respir Crit Care Med* 2005;**171**:340–7.

118 **Morandi A, Gunther ML.** Neuroimaging. *Psychiatry* 2010;**7**:28–33.

Chapter 33

Critical Illness Neuropathy, Myopathy, and Sodium Channelopathy

Mark M. Rich

Introduction

Skeletal muscle weakness following critical illness is a common problem that complicates recovery from critical illness. In affected patients, the primary cause of weakness is dysfunction of the peripheral nervous system, also known as neuromuscular dysfunction. The first report of neuromuscular dysfunction in the setting of critical illness was over 30 years ago in a patient treated for status asthmaticus.[1] Since that time, there have been many reports of debilitating weakness that develop in various ICU settings.[2,3,4] Early reports of weakness during critical illness found that, in some patients, the prolonged presence of NMBAs was the cause of weakness.[5] However, with awareness of this syndrome and careful dosing of NMBAs it has become less common for continued neuromuscular blockade to be the cause of prolonged weakness in the ICU.[6] Despite awareness and avoidance of prolonged neuromuscular blockade, weakness in the ICU continues to be a frequent complication of critical illness.

Critical illness neuropathy, myopathy, and sodium channelopathy

Critical illness neuropathy

The primary causes of weakness include neuropathy, also known as CIP, and myopathy. The myopathy is now termed CIM,[7] although it has been variably referred to as acute quadriplegic myopathy, thick filament myopathy, or acute myopathy of critical illness. CIP is a generalized neuropathy that was first described two decades ago in the setting of sepsis and MOF.[2,8,9] Physical examination reveals weakness, loss of sensation, and loss of reflexes. NCS in patients with CIP demonstrate reduced sensory and motor amplitudes, whilst the EMG exhibits evidence of denervation. The EMG findings of denervation change with time such that, in the acute setting, there is spontaneous activity of muscle and normal motor unit amplitudes but a reduction in the number of units recruited. In the chronic setting, spontaneous activity is still present, but motor unit amplitudes become increased, as the remaining axons sprout and innervate muscle fibres denervated due to neuropathy. Nerve biopsy reveals death of axons. All of the above findings are consistent with axonal polyneuropathy as the mechanism underlying weakness in patients with CIP.

CIM

CIM is a myopathy that occurs in the setting of treatment with high-dose corticosteroids and NMBAs.[10,11] The myopathy becomes evident when the NMBAs are stopped and the patient remains severely weak. Physical examination reveals weakness, with intact sensation and preserved reflexes. NCS show that the motor amplitudes are reduced, but sensory responses are normal. EMG studies demonstrate spontaneous activity, along with the recruitment of small motor units with atrophied myofibres on muscle biopsy and loss of myosin and disorganization of sarcomeres.

The above descriptions suggest that CIP and CIM can be easily distinguished by the clinical setting, the physical examination, electrophysiologic findings on nerve conduction, and EMG as well as biopsies of muscle and nerve.[4] However, in clinical practice, differentiating CIP and CIM is often difficult.

Critical illness sodium channelopathy

The first description of a defect in membrane excitability in the setting of critical illness was in patients with CIM.[12-16] It was found that, in severely affected patients, there was no electrical response to direct electrical stimulation (ES) of muscle. In both neuropathy and diseases of the neuromuscular junction, muscle retains its excitability, so the only explanation that could account for the result was inexcitability of muscle. Loss of muscle electrical excitability had previously been described only in rare inherited diseases of ion channels, known as the periodic paralyses. The finding of muscle inexcitability in patients with no history of ion channel disease suggested that this was a novel type of disease that is due to a defect in regulation of genetically normal channels, rather than a mutation of ion channels.

More recently, it has been found that the peripheral nerve has a similar defect of excitability during the acute phase of sepsis.[17,18] In both skeletal muscle and peripheral nerve, the primary defect underlying the loss of excitability appears to be the inactivation of sodium channels. Inactivation of sodium channels is a voltage-dependent process such that either depolarization of the resting potential or a hyperpolarized shift in the voltage dependence of sodium channel sensitivity to inactivation could underlie the increase in inactivation. In both skeletal muscle and peripheral nerve, it appears that both depolarization of the resting potential and a shift in the sensitivity of sodium channels to inactivation appear to contribute to the increase in inactivation.[17-21] These data demonstrate that, in addition to CIP and CIM, there is a sodium channelopathy that occurs in the acute phase of critical illness.

There are nine different sodium channel isoforms.[22] The sodium channel isoform normally expressed in skeletal muscle is Nav1.4. In the animal model of CIM, a second sodium channel isoform (Nav1.5) is also expressed.[23] Both the Nav1.4 and Nav1.5 isoforms appear to function abnormally in the rat model of CIM.[24] In the peripheral nerve, a different sodium channel (Nav 1.6) is the primary isoform expressed.[25,26] With the finding that the peripheral nerve is affected, it thus appears that three different sodium channel isoforms are all affected by critical illness. The Nav 1.5 sodium channel isoform is normally expressed in cardiac tissue. The finding that the cardiac sodium channel isoform malfunctions in skeletal muscle raises the possibility that there might be malfunction of sodium channels in the heart during sepsis. A study looking at ECGs in patients with sepsis found a reversible reduction in ECG amplitude that was consistent with a reduction in cardiac sodium current density[27] but could alternatively be accounted for by anasarca.[28] If there is a reduction in cardiac sodium current, it would provide a mechanism to account for the decrease in cardiac contractility that underlies the high-output cardiac failure during sepsis.[29] Further studies will be required to determine if sodium channelopathy contributes to cardiac dysfunction during sepsis. The primary sodium channel isoforms expressed in the CNS are Nav1.1 and Nav1.2.[22] It is not known whether function of these sodium channel isoforms is affected by sepsis. If inactivation of these sodium channel isoforms is increased during sepsis, this could provide an explanation for septic encephalopathy.

CIP, CIM, and sodium channelopathy as causes of neuromuscular failure

From the work previously described, it has become clear that there are at least three major contributors to neuromuscular failure in patients with weakness following critical illness: CIP, CIM, and a sodium channelopathy affecting both nerve and muscle. An important question is whether these three disorders are distinct and are triggered by different aspects of critical illness and occur in distinct patient populations or whether they represent different manifestations of a single disorder.

In their classic forms, after patients have recovered from the acute stage of critical illness, CIP and CIM are easy to distinguish and appeared to occur in distinct patient populations. CIP occurred in patients with sepsis, and CIM occurred in patients treated with corticosteroids and NMBAs. However, as more studies have been performed, it has become clear that some patients with CIM have sepsis and SIRS and have not been treated with either corticosteroids or NMBAs.[13,15,16,30] Thus, both CIP and CIM can be triggered by sepsis and SIRS. Furthermore, in the acute setting, it has been difficult to distinguish between CIP and CIM. There are a number of reasons for this: (1) critically ill patients are difficult to examine in detail to distinguish between CIP and CIM. Patients are often sedated or encephalopathic such that they cannot cooperate with sensory examination; (2) because patients cannot cooperate, they are unable to voluntarily recruit motor units during the EMG portion of electrophysiologic studies. The inability to study motor unit amplitude and recruitment has been a major hurdle in many studies in distinguishing between CIP and CIM; and (3) many studies have used the presence of spontaneous activity on EMG as an indicator of denervation and thus the presence of CIP. However, spontaneous activity on EMG is also present in CIM, and thus the use of spontaneous activity to categorize patients is a mistake. Thus, most studies performed during the acute phase of critical illness have not accurately distinguished between CIP and CIM.

In smaller studies, in which there was careful evaluation of CIP and CIM, it appears that the syndromes often occur together.[13,16,30,31,32,33] The co-occurrence of CIP and CIM has led to the terms polyneuromyopathy or CRIMYNE.[31,34] The mechanism underlying the co-occurrence of CIP and CIM was unclear but favoured the possibility that they are part of a single syndrome. However, the finding that sodium channelopathy affects both nerve and muscle raises the possibility that what was interpreted as co-occurrence of CIP and CIM is really sodium channelopathy that affects nerve and muscle. It thus remains unclear whether CIP, CIM, and sodium channelopathy are distinct syndromes. When patients with what is likely the acute sodium channelopathy are followed with serial NCS they evolve into CIP, CIM, or both.[31,33,35] This suggests that sodium channelopathy is an early stage of both CIP and CIM and that it recovers more rapidly than either CIP or CIM. This leaves unresolved the question of whether CIP and CIM are part of a single syndrome and coexist in many patients during the early phase of recovery from critical illness.

Prognosis of CIP, CIM, and sodium channelopathy

The development of neuromuscular dysfunction worsens both the short-term and long-term prognosis of patients. Acutely, the development of neuromuscular dysfunction may increase mortality.[32–34,36–39] Both CIM and CIP are associated with PMV and increased length of hospital and ICU stay.[38,40,41] The development of neuromuscular dysfunction during the acute phase of illness also worsens long-term prognosis. Weakness often persists for months to years.[35,39,42–45] The mechanism underlying chronic weakness is unknown. It might be expected that functional outcome in CIP would be determined by the extent of axonal degeneration, as axons regrow very slowly. Given the slow regrowth of axons, recovery would be expected to gradually spread from more proximal to distal muscles and that reinnervation of distal muscles might be incomplete, as reinnervation of muscles that are denervated for prolonged periods is not complete.[46]

In theory, patients with CIM should have a better prognosis and recover faster than patients with CIP, since muscle, unlike nerve, regenerates relatively rapidly. However, some studies suggest they have similar functional outcomes.[35,47] There are reasons that recovery in CIM might be limited. In CIM, there is extreme atrophy of muscle that is accompanied by apoptosis of muscle nuclei.[48] The loss of muscle nuclei may make it difficult for muscle bulk to recover following atrophy, as there will be fewer muscle nuclei to direct protein synthesis. Another potential contributor to chronic myopathy could be the extreme loss of myosin that occurs during the acute phase of CIM.[11,49,50] Loss of myosin is likely a contributor to the disorganization of sarcomeres occurring in CIM.[11,51] It is not known whether myosin loss is fully reversed after recovery from CIM or whether the disorganization of sarcomeres is reversed. For these reasons, the prognosis of CIM may be worse than the prognosis for recovery that might be expected for a necrotic myopathy, in which the only factor limiting recovery is regeneration of muscle fibres. At this point in time, it is not clear whether CIP, CIM, or another mechanism is the primary cause of chronic functional impairment.

Although there are limited data, the rapid recovery of nerve conduction amplitudes in some patients suggest that sodium channelopathy is reversible and does not contribute to long-term dysfunction.[17,34] It is the author's impression that encephalopathy rapidly improves during this same time period. One interpretation of these data is that sodium channels in all tissues revert to normal function over a period of several days following recovery from the acute illness.

Work-up of skeletal muscle weakness following critical illness

Neuromuscular dysfunction is often recognized by difficulty in weaning from MV and by the presence of diffuse weakness in a cooperative patient. Early signs of development of neuromuscular dysfunction are non-specific and may simply include a reduction in spontaneous movement of the limbs. Clinically, patients with CIM and CIP appear similar; both have a flaccid quadriparesis or quadriplegia. The cranial nerves, including extraocular movements, typically remain intact. Laboratory assessment of patients with neuromuscular dysfunction, including CK, is usually unrevealing. Abnormalities typically reflect the systemic illness and do not alert the clinician to the presence of myopathy or neuropathy. However, when identified, elevated CK levels should raise the possibility of a toxic or an inflammatory myopathy.

Despite the limitations of interpretation previously described, electrodiagnostic testing can be informative in patients with severe weakness following critical illness. Electrophysiologic testing entails simple procedures, which may easily be performed at the bedside and can definitively localize the cause of weakness to the peripheral nervous system, thereby excluding the possibility of CNS dysfunction as well as non-neurological aetiologies for diffuse weakness such as malnutrition and deconditioning. It is important to note that there are cases in which technical issues limit interpretation. Examinations performed in the presence of significant peripheral oedema can produce low-amplitude or absent sensory nerve evoked responses in the absence of pathology. Furthermore, sensory and motor responses may be obscured by interference from electrical equipment commonly found in the ICU environment such as IV pumps, monitors, and beds. For these reasons, it is preferable to have an examiner who is familiar with technical issues associated with performing NCS in the ICU.

Definitive diagnoses of CIP and CIM are made by nerve and muscle biopsy, respectively. However, the routine use of nerve and muscle biopsy is not warranted. Since the prognosis of CIP and CIM are not clearly different and there is currently no therapy for either disorder, there is no prognostic or therapeutic information to be obtained from a biopsy. Nerve and muscle biopsies remain extremely valuable for research studies of CIP and CIM.

Conclusion

The understanding of mechanisms underlying weakness triggered by critical illness is still rapidly evolving. New mechanisms that contribute to weakness continue to be identified. Determining and eliminating the risk factors for each mechanism underlying weakness will hopefully allow us to reduce the frequency and severity of weakness in critically ill patients. In addition, determining specific molecular mechanisms that contribute to weakness will provide therapeutic targets to reverse weakness in affected patients.

References

1 Macfarlane IA, Rosenthal FD. Severe myopathy after status asthmaticus [letter]. *Lancet* 1977;**2**:615.

2 Bolton CF. Neuromuscular manifestations of critical illness. *Muscle Nerve* 2005;**32**:140–63.

3 Stevens RD, Dowdy DW, Michaels RK, Mendez-Tellez PA, Pronovost PJ, Needham DM. Neuromuscular dysfunction acquired in critical illness: a systematic review. *Intensive Care Med* 2007;**33**:1876–91.

4 Stevens RD, Marshall SA, Cornblath DR, et al. A framework for diagnosing and classifying intensive care unit-acquired weakness. *Crit Care Med* 2009;**37**:S299–308.

5 Segredo V, Caldwell JE, Matthay MA, Sharma ML, Gruenke LD, Miller RD. Persistent paralysis in critically ill patients after long-term administration of vecuronium. *N Engl J Med* 1992;**327**:524–8.

6 Puthucheary Z, Rawal J, Ratnayake G, Harridge S, Montgomery H, Hart N. Neuromuscular blockade and skeletal muscle weakness in critically ill patients: time to rethink the evidence? *Am J Respir Crit Care Med* 2012;**185**:911–17.

7 Lacomis D, Zochodne DW, Bird SJ. Critical illness myopathy. *Muscle Nerve* 2000;**23**:1785–8.

8 Bolton CF, Gilbert JJ, Hahn AF, Sibbald WJ. Polyneuropathy in critically ill patients. *J Neurol Neurosurg Psychiatry* 1984;**47**:1223–31.

9 Zochodne DW, Bolton CF, Wells GA, et al. Critical illness polyneuropathy. A complication of sepsis and multiple organ failure. *Brain* 1987;**110**:819–41.

10 Danon MJ, Carpenter S. Myopathy with thick filament (myosin) loss following prolonged paralysis with vecuronium during steroid treatment. *Muscle Nerve* 1991;**14**:1131–9.

11 Lacomis D, Giuliani MJ, Van Cott A, Kramer DJ. Acute myopathy of intensive care: clinical, electromyographic, and pathological aspects [see comments]. *Ann Neurol* 1996;**40**:645–54.

12 Allen DC, Arunachalam R, Mills KR. Critical illness myopathy: further evidence from muscle-fiber excitability studies of an acquired channelopathy. *Muscle Nerve* 2008;**37**:14–22.

13 Lefaucheur JP, Nordine T, Rodriguez P, Brochard L. Origin of ICU acquired paresis determined by direct muscle stimulation. *J Neurol Neurosurg Psychiatry* 2006;**77**:500–6.

14 Rich MM, Teener JW, Raps EC, Schotland DL, Bird SJ. Muscle is electrically inexcitable in acute quadriplegic myopathy [see comments]. *Neurology* 1996;**46**:731–6.

15 Rich MM, Bird SJ, Raps EC, Mccluskey LF, Teener JW. Direct muscle stimulation in acute quadriplegic myopathy. *Muscle Nerve* 1997;**20**:665–73.

16 Trojaborg W, Weimer LH, Hays AP. Electrophysiologic studies in critical illness associated weakness: myopathy or neuropathy—a reappraisal. *Clin Neurophysiol* 2001;**112**:1586–93.

17 Novak KR, Nardelli P, Cope TC, et al. Inactivation of sodium channels underlies reversible neuropathy during critical illness in rats. *J Clin Invest* 2009;**119**:1150–8.

18 Z'graggen WJ, Lin CS, Howard RS, Beale RJ, Bostock H. Nerve excitability changes in critical illness polyneuropathy. *Brain* 2006;**129**:2461–70.

19 Rich MM, Pinter MJ. Sodium channel inactivation in an animal model of acute quadriplegic myopathy. *Ann Neurol* 2001;**50**:26–33.

20 Rich MM, Pinter MJ. Crucial role of sodium channel fast inactivation in muscle fibre inexcitability in a rat model of critical illness myopathy. *J Physiol* 2003;**547**:555–66.

21 Rich MM, Pinter MJ, Kraner SD, Barchi RL. Loss of electrical excitability in an animal model of acute quadriplegic myopathy. *Ann Neurol* 1998;**43**:171–9.

22 Goldin AL. Resurgence of sodium channel research. *Annu Rev Physiol* 2001;**63**:871–94.

23 Rich MM, Kraner SD, Barchi RL. Altered gene expression in steroid-treated denervated muscle. *Neurobiol Dis* 1999;**6**:515–22.

24 Filatov GN, Rich MM. Hyperpolarized shifts in the voltage dependence of fast inactivation of Nav1.4 and Nav1.5 in a rat model of critical illness myopathy. *J Physiol* 2004;**559**:813–20.

25 Angaut-Petit D, Mcardle JJ, Mallart A, Bournaud R, Pincon-Raymond M, Rieger F. Electrophysiological and morphological studies of a motor nerve in 'motor endplate disease' of the mouse. *Proc R Soc Lond B Biol Sci* 1982;**215**:117–25.

26 Caffrey JM, Eng DL, Black JA, Waxman SG, Kocsis JD. Three types of sodium channels in adult rat dorsal root ganglion neurons. *Brain Res* 1992;**592**, 283–97.

27 Rich MM, Mcgarvey ML, Teener JW, Frame LH. ECG changes during septic shock. *Cardiology* 2002;**97**:187–96.

28 Madias JE, Bazaz R. On the mechanism of the reduction in the ECG QRS amplitudes in patients with sepsis. *Cardiology* 2003;**99**:166–8.

29 Merx MW, Weber C. Sepsis and the heart. *Circulation* 2007;**116**:793–802.

30 Latronico N, Fenzi F, Recupero D, et al. Critical illness myopathy and neuropathy. *Lancet* 1996;**347**:1579–82.

31 Bednarik J, Lukas Z, Vondracek P. Critical illness polyneuromyopathy: the electrophysiological components of a complex entity. *Intensive Care Med* 2003;**29**:1505–14.

32 De Jonghe B, Sharshar T, Lefaucheur JP, et al. Paresis acquired in the intensive care unit: a prospective multicenter study. *JAMA* 2002;**288**:2859–67.

33 Khan J, Harrison TB, Rich MM, Moss M. Early development of critical illness myopathy and neuropathy in patients with severe sepsis. *Neurology* 2006;**67**:1421–5.

34 Latronico N, Bertolini G, Guarneri B, et al. Simplified electrophysiological evaluation of peripheral nerves in critically ill patients: the Italian multi-centre CRIMYNE study. *Crit Care* 2007;**11**:R11.

35 Guarneri B, Bertolini G, Latronico N. Long-term outcome in patients with critical illness myopathy or neuropathy: the Italian multicentre CRIMYNE study. *J Neurol Neurosurg Psychiatry* 2008;**79**:838–41.

36 Berek K, Margreiter J, Willeit J, Berek A, Schmutzhard E, Mutz NJ. Polyneuropathies in critically ill patients: a prospective evaluation [see comments]. *Intensive Care Med* 1996;**22**:849–55.

37 Coakley JH, Nagendran K, Yarwood GD, Honavar M, Hinds CJ. Patterns of neurophysiological abnormality in prolonged critical illness. *Intensive Care Med* 1998;**24**:801–7.

38 Garnacho-Montero J, Madrazo-Osuna J, Garcia-Garmendia JL, et al. Critical illness polyneuropathy: risk factors and clinical consequences. A cohort study in septic patients. *Intensive Care Med* 2001;**27**:1288–96.

39 Leijten FS, Harinck-De Weerd JE, Poortvliet DC, De Weerd AW. The role of polyneuropathy in motor convalescence after prolonged mechanical ventilation. *JAMA* 1995;**274**:1221–5.

40 **De Jonghe B, Bastuji-Garin S, Durand MC, et al.** Respiratory weakness is associated with limb weakness and delayed weaning in critical illness. *Crit Care Med* 2007;**35**:2007–15.

41 **Garnacho-Montero J, Amaya-Villar R, Garcia-Garmendia JL, Madrazo-Osuna J, Ortiz-Leyba C.** Effect of critical illness polyneuropathy on the withdrawal from mechanical ventilation and the length of stay in septic patients. *Crit Care Med* 2005;**33**:349–54.

42 **Cheung AM, Tansey CM, Tomlinson G, et al.** Two-year outcomes, health care use, and costs of survivors of acute respiratory distress syndrome. *Am J Respir Crit Care Med* 2006;**174**:538–44.

43 **Fletcher SN, Kennedy DD, Ghosh IR, et al.** Persistent neuromuscular and neurophysiologic abnormalities in long-term survivors of prolonged critical illness. *Crit Care Med* 2003;**31**:1012–16.

44 **Herridge MS, Cheung AM, Tansey CM, et al.** One-year outcomes in survivors of the acute respiratory distress syndrome. *N Engl J Med* 2003;**348**:683–93.

45 **Zifko UA.** Long-term outcome of critical illness polyneuropathy. *Muscle Nerve Suppl,*2000;**9**:S49–52.

46 **Gordon T, Tyreman N, Raji MA.** The basis for diminished functional recovery after delayed peripheral nerve repair. *J Neurosci* 2011;**31**:5325–34.

47 **Lacomis D, Petrella JT, Giuliani MJ.** Causes of neuromuscular weakness in the intensive care unit: a study of ninety-two patients. *Muscle Nerve* 1998;**21**:610–77.

48 **Di Giovanni S, Mirabella M, D'amico A, Tonali P, Servidei S.** Apoptotic features accompany acute quadriplegic myopathy. *Neurology* 2000;**55**:854–8.

49 **Larsson L.** Acute quadriplegic myopathy: an acquired 'myosinopathy'. *Adv Exp Med Biol* 2008;**642**: 92–8.

50 **Larsson L, Li X, Edstrom L, et al.** Acute quadriplegia and loss of muscle myosin in patients treated with nondepolarizing neuromuscular blocking agents and corticosteroids: mechanisms at the cellular and molecular levels. *Crit Care Med* 2000;**28**:34–45.

51 **Stibler H, Edstrom L, Ahlbeck K, Remahl S, Ansved T.** Electrophoretic determination of the myosin/actin ratio in the diagnosis of critical illness myopathy. *Intensive Care Med* 2003;**29**:1515–27.

Chapter 34

The Impact of Critical Illness on Skeletal Muscle Structure

Catherine L. Hough

Introduction: critical illness and physical functional outcomes

Patients with critical illness, particularly those with acute respiratory failure and syndromes of overwhelming systemic inflammatory response, such as sepsis, are at risk of developing profound weakness and skeletal muscle loss. Early in the course of critical illness, this ICUAW is associated with increased risk of hospital mortality, PMV, increased ICU and hospital length of stay, and decreased likelihood of returning to independent living at hospital discharge. Importantly, neuromuscular sequelae are not limited to the acute phase of critical illness. Survivors continue to experience physical functional impairment for years after initial hospitalization, with reduced performance on standardized physical performance tests, such as the 6-minute walk test, with persistent decrements in physical aspects of HRQoL for at least 5 years.

While it is clear that pre-existing comorbid disease and antecedent physical functional decline are indeed risk factors for post-ICU physical functional impairment, it is also apparent that critical illness is an independent risk for neuromuscular dysfunction. Critically ill patients may be at risk of developing myriad abnormalities of muscle and nerve, including changes of skeletal muscle structure, loss of muscle mass, muscle membrane inexcitability, polyneuropathy, prolonged neuromuscular blockade, and mitochondrial dysfunction with bioenergetic failure. These abnormalities could be associated—perhaps causally—with impaired short- and long-term physical function. While many of these potential aetiologies will be discussed in other chapters, this chapter will focus on changes in skeletal muscle structure found in critically ill patients. This chapter will begin with a review of normal muscle structure and function. Next, we will present histological and ultrastructural findings in critically ill patients. Finally, we conclude with a brief discussion of potential risk factors and aetiologic mechanisms involved in the development of muscle pathology in the ICU.

Normal skeletal muscle structure and function

Skeletal muscle has a unique structure that is tightly related to its contractile function. Each muscle is a syncytium comprising hundreds of long, cylindrical, multinucleated cells which are formed by the fusion of myoblasts. Muscle cells—called myocytes, myofibres, or muscle fibres—are oriented parallel to one another and separated by connective tissue, blood vessels, and nerves. The plasma membrane of the myocyte is called the sarcolemma, covering the cell in its folds and penetrating through the muscle fibre at regular intervals in tunnels called the transverse (or T) tubules. The cell's many nuclei are located peripherally, just beneath the sarcolemma, along the entire length of the myocyte. The intracellular fluid is called the sarcoplasm, which is filled with myofibrils—the main contractile apparatus of muscle. Also in the sarcoplasm are mitochondria,

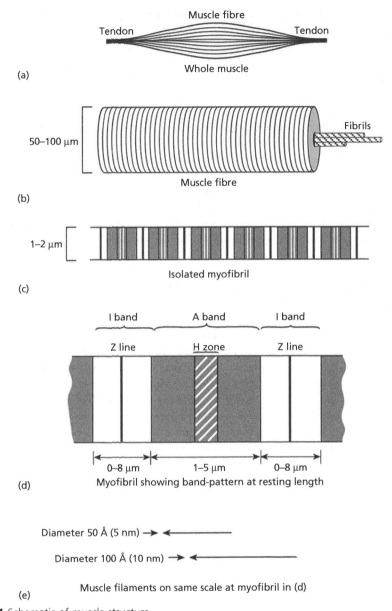

Fig. 34.1 Schematic of muscle structure.

Reproduced from David A. Warrell, Timothy M. Cox, and John D. Firth, *Oxford Textbook of Medicine* (5 ed.), Figure 24.24.1.1, with permission from Oxford University Press.

which are interspersed among the myofibrils to provide energy for contraction, and a series of channels, called the sarcoplasmic reticulum. At the ends of each myocyte, the sarcoplasmic reticulum ends in terminal cisternae, which associate with the T-tubules to form triads; these triads are involved in the propagation of action potentials (see Figure 34.1).

Myofibrils are long polymers which form the myofilaments: myosin and actin. Myosin filaments, also called 'thick filaments', are composed of a few hundred myosin molecules that cleave

ATP to move and form cross-bridges with actin. Actin filaments, also called 'thin filaments', are polymers of three proteins: actin, tropomyosin, and troponin. Polymerized helices of actin molecules make up the majority of structure of the actin filament and carries adenosine diphosphate (ADP). Tropomyosin winds around the actin helices and covers the ADP, which is the site where myosin and actin bind. Troponin regulates this interaction by binding to actin, tropomyosin, and calcium, which is sequestered in the sarcoplasmic reticulum. Myosin and actin filaments interdigitate, forming dark and light bands (called A-bands and I-bands, respectively) in repeating units called the sarcomere. Each sarcomere is bound by Z-discs, to which the actin filaments anchor. Z-discs connect across all the myofilaments in each muscle fibre. In the middle of the sarcomere is the M-line, which crosslinks the myosin filaments to provide stability for the sarcomere during contraction.[1] The striated appearance of the alternating light and dark filaments is visible in longitudinal section on light microscopy, but visualization of individual myofilaments and additional elements of the muscle ultrastructure requires electron microscopy (EM).

Contraction begins as an action potential travels down a nerve, depolarizes the neuromuscular junction, and spreads across the sarcolemma. The action potential is propagated along muscle by opening voltage-gated sodium channels and extends through the T-tubule system, which leads to release of calcium ions from the sarcoplasmic reticulum. Calcium ions bind to troponin, which induces a conformational change in tropomyosin which allows actin and myosin to bind. Upon binding to the ADP on actin, the myosin head undergoes a conformational change which slides the myosin along the actin, shortening the sarcomere as the Z-discs are pulled closer together. Continued contraction requires repetitive action potentials and a supply of ATP.[2]

There are two primary types of muscle fibres: type I and type II. Type I fibres are red in colour due to myoglobin which allows for aerobic activity, have a high density of mitochondria, contract more slowly, and are resistant to fatigue. Type II fibres are white, since they lack myoglobin, and are primarily anaerobic, have fewer mitochondria, contract more quickly (called 'fast twitch'), and fatigue within minutes. Type II fibres use glycolytic pathways to generate ATP. The histology of type I and II fibres can be differentiated under light microscopy by staining for the myosin ATPase activity at different pHs; type I fibres stain dark in acid (pH 4.3) and type II in base (pH 10).

Loss of function may precede changes in structure

While normal muscle structure is required for muscle function, the converse is not necessarily true. Early in the course of critical illness, skeletal muscle may lose its ability to contract normally and generate full force. Electrodiagnostic studies performed within the first 96 hours of critical illness show marked reduction or absence of compound motor action potential amplitudes as the muscle membrane becomes electrically inexcitable[3] (see Chapter 33 for further details). It appears that membrane inexcitability may be due to post-translational modification to the voltage-gated sodium channels that prevents its ability to propagate an action potential,[4] which, in the early phase, is not associated with structurally visible pathology.[5,6] However, it may be that membrane inexcitability may potentiate further myopathic changes. In a recent study of patients with severe sepsis, those with membrane inexcitability had more atrophy of type II fibres than did patients with normal membrane function.[7]

Muscle biopsy of ICU patients: an overview of study designs

In 1977, MacFarlane and colleagues reported a case of severe myopathy in a patient with status asthmaticus.[8] Their investigation did not include a peripheral muscle biopsy but reported significant weakness and electrophysiologic findings consistent with myopathy. A few years later, Bolton reported a series of five patients who developed severe weakness in the ICU.[9] Electrophysiologic studies were interpreted as consistent with polyneuropathy, with severe reduction in both motor and SNAPs. Three patients died and had autopsies performed, with nerve histopathology that revealed a primary axonal neuropathy and muscle histopathology that showed both neurogenic atrophy and myopathic features, including cytoarchitectural disorganization of muscle fibres. Bolton noted that this '. . . may have been secondary to denervation or may represent primary muscle damage,' suggesting that myopathy might be a significant contributor to ICUAW, in addition to the contribution of polyneuropathy.[9]

Since these two early reports of what would eventually become termed as CIM,[10] there have been many studies of critically ill patients which included muscle biopsies. There are two most common types of study designs used in these reports, which are summarized in Tables 34.1 and 34.2. Most reports are case series of patients found to have developed severe weakness in the ICU or who were unable to be weaned from MV.[11-20] There are cohort studies that identify a population at risk for ICUAW such as requirement for 7 days of intensive care, presence of MOF, or receipt of MV.[6,19,21-24] The primary outcome measure of this group of studies was the identification of ICUAW, either by clinical examination or electrophysiologic assessment. In most of these studies, muscle biopsy was only obtained on selected subjects with either clinical or electrophysiologic evidence of weakness. Only in two studies did patients with normal clinical and electrophysiologic evaluations have muscle biopsies performed.[6,23] Additionally, there are two studies derived from cohorts of ICU patients who had muscle biopsies performed for an investigation unrelated to ICUAW.[25,26] No information was systematically collected regarding strength or other markers of nerve or muscle function.

It is relevant to review details of the study designs before discussing the muscle biopsy findings. Most studies obtained muscle from the lower extremities, either by biopsy or via autopsy. Few studies included biopsies at multiple time points, and most obtained muscle samples later in the course of critical illness (generally after 14 days). Patients with the highest severity of illness were likely to have contraindications to biopsy, such as DIC or other coagulopathies, and may have thus been underrepresented in the population studied.[23] Only two studies had the potential to investigate the associations between muscle biopsy findings and clinical presentation,[6,23] since these are the only investigations to obtain muscle biopsies on patients without the clinical syndrome of ICUAW. However, these studies evaluated few patients and are thus underpowered to investigate such associations with confidence. It may well be that muscle histopathology is much more widespread in the ICU population (and perhaps in other acutely or chronically ill populations) than the existing literature represents. Muscle histopathology may be present in many patients who are not recognized clinically; future studies enrolling cohorts of patients, both with and without ICUAW, are needed to understand the significance of these findings.

Spectrum of muscle histopathology in patients with ICUAW

As discussed in previous chapters, critical illness associated neuromuscular disorders include overlapping aetiologies that may affect both muscle and nerve.[27,28] ICU-acquired pathology of either muscle or nerve can affect the muscle histology. In general, three major patterns of abnormalities are seen in muscle of critically ill patients: atrophy, loss of the thick myosin filaments, and necrosis. Tables 34.1 and 34.2 summarize results of studies of muscle histopathology in critical illness.

Atrophy

Atrophy is defined by a reduction in the cross-sectional area of a muscle fibre, often presenting as an increased variability of size among muscle fibres. Muscle fibre atrophy is among the most common muscle pathologies in general and is omnipresent in patients with ICUAW. Several different

Table 34.1 Cohort studies

Author	Population	Biopsy criteria	Number (%)	Atrophy	Myosin loss	Necrosis	Neurogenic atrophy	Normal muscle	Comments
Amaya-Villar (2005)[21]	MV >48 hours, COPD	Clinical evidence of AQM	3/25 (12%)	Yes (type II)	Yes	Yes	No	No	
Bednarik (2005)[22]	MOF (>2 organs)	Electrophysiologic evidence of CIPM	11/46 (24%)	Yes (type II)	Yes	Yes	Yes	No	Included EM on 4/11 samples
Coakley (1998)[23]	ICU >7 days	No contraindications	24/44 (55%)	Yes (mixed, and type II)		Yes	Yes	Yes	Normal muscle in 2/24, both with normal electrophysiologic studies
De Jonghe (2002)[24]	MV >7 days	Persisting weakness after 14 days	10/95 (11%)	Yes (type II)	Yes	Yes	Yes	No	
Ahlbeck (2009)[6]	MV >3 days	All	10/10 (100%)	No	Yes	No	No	Yes	Normal muscle in 10/10 on day 4, 5/10 day 14

MV, mechanical ventilation; COPD, chronic obstructive pulmonary disease; MOF, multiple organ failure; AQM, acute quadriplegic myopathy; CIPM, critical illness polyneuropathy/myopathy; EM: electron microscopy.

Table 34.2 Case series of patients with ICUAW

Author	Number	Atrophy	Myosin loss	Necrosis	Neurogenic atrophy	Normal muscle	Additional findings
Lacomis (1996)[11]	14	Yes (types I and II)	Yes	Yes	Rare	No	Z-band streaming on EM
Sander (2002)[12]	8	Yes (type II predominant)	Yes	No	No	No	Core-like lesions and patchy myofibrillar pallor Abundance of fibres with fat droplets Glycogen in fibres with contractile filament loss. Preservation of actin and Z-discs
Latronico (1996)[13]	24	Yes	No	Yes	Yes	No	Increased intracellular lipids
Larsson (2000)[14]	7	Yes	Yes	Yes	Yes	No	Disorganized myofibrils Lysosomal activation
Hanson (1997)[15]	4	Yes	Yes	Yes	No	No	Enlarged cisternae of the sarcoplasmic reticulum Enlarged and accumulating mitochondria Increase in glycogen and lipid Shortened I-bands
Matsumoto (2000)[16]	4	Yes	Yes	Yes	No	No	
Hund (1996)[17]	3	Yes	No	No	Yes	No	
Lopate (1998)[18]	1	Yes	Yes	No	No	No	Describes prominent N-lines, caused by detachment of titin from myosin
Wokke (1988)[19]	2	Yes (type II more than I)	Yes	No	No	No	Z-band streaming
Showalter (1997)[20]	5	Yes	Yes	Yes	No	No	Perimysial and endomysial mononuclear cells Dilated tubular profiles

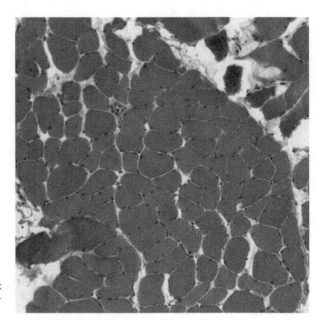

Fig. 34.2 Muscle atrophy, seen on deltoid muscle biopsy of a critically ill patient with H & E stain.

The contributor would like to thank Dr D. Born for his assistance in producing this image.

patterns of muscle atrophy may be seen. Perhaps most commonly, the atrophy is non-selective, affecting both type 1 and type 2 fibres. These atrophic fibres are often round, rather than having the normal polygonal shape. Next is type 2 fibre atrophy in which the fibres may be either round or angular. The third pattern reported is when the patient is afflicted by a concomitant neuropathy and is called **neurogenic atrophy**. Fibres affected by neurogenic atrophy are usually angular in shape. Neurogenic atrophy with denervation may display fibre-type grouping, wherein groups of the same type of fibre are found together, rather than displaying the typical checkerboard pattern mixing type 1 and 2 fibres. Atrophic muscle fibres may display an increased density on modified Gomori trichrome staining.[20,29]

Figures 34.2 and 34.3 demonstrates myofibre atrophy in a patient with ARDS on day 10 of critical illness. There are small, rounded, and angular fibres, seen with haematoxylin and eosin stain (H & E) and then with myosin ATPase stain at alkaline pH. Most atrophic fibres stained darkly at alkaline pH; this represents type 2 predominance. Studies that obtained sequential muscle biopsies demonstrated that muscle fibre atrophy is progressive over time, with rates of loss between 1.5% and 13.8% of the cross-sectional area for each additional day in the ICU.[25]

Thick filament loss

The selective loss of myosin is a classic finding in weak patients with critical illness and is considered by many to be diagnostic. In fact, a suggested definition of CMI requires 'muscle histopathologic findings of myopathy with myosin loss'.[10] Selective myosin loss may also be called 'thick filament myopathy'[30] or 'acquired myosinopathy'.[31] There are several ways that myosin loss can be recognized using light microscopy. Focal loss might be recognized as basophilic staining on H & E[32] but, more commonly, requires enzymatic stains. Fibres with myosin loss may demonstrate incomplete or no staining with myosin ATPase at either acid or alkaline pH.[11] Staining for myosin heavy chain (which include slow and fast myosin isoforms)[11] is disrupted but less affected than the myosin ATPase. This finding provides evidence for the theory that, as myosin is selectively lost, it is first disaggregated, but the myosin monomers remain intact.[33]

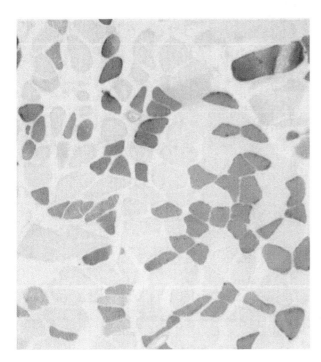

Fig. 34.3 Predominant type II muscle atrophy, seen on deltoid muscle biopsy of a critically ill patient with alkaline ATPase stain.

The contributor would like to thank Dr D. Born for his assistance in producing this image.

Light microscopy is not sensitive to myosin loss, which may easily be unrecognized or confused with entirely neuropathic patterns of atrophy.[12] For this reason, it has been suggested 'that future studies of critically ill quadriplegic patients incorporate either muscle EM or biochemical quantification of myosin'.[12] Since actin is generally undisturbed in the process of thick filament loss until very advanced stages, one approach to recognizing myosin loss is to use gel electrophoresis to isolate actin and myosin from muscle biopsies and calculate the myosin/actin ratio.[14,16,34] Normal myosin/actin ratios in healthy controls have been measured in the range of 1.3–1.4; patients in the acute phase of CIM have ratios well under 1 (0.37 ± 0.17,[34] 0.55 ± 0.9[16])

EM is the gold standard for the evaluation of muscle ultrastructure and the most sensitive approach to the identification of myosin loss.[12] In isolated thick filament loss, EM may reveal intact Z-discs and I-bands, with reduced or absent A-bands and the disappearance of the M-lines. Thick filament loss might spare some fibres (either by fibre type or non-selective) or might be present in most sampled muscle fibres. Hypercontraction with shortening of the I-band is common, as is Z-disc streaming. In more severely affected fibres, particularly those with necrotic findings as well, thick filament loss is associated with significant architectural disruption, with shattering of the sarcomere. Figure 34.4 presents an example of these EM findings of thick filament loss. Of note, thick filament loss is not unique to CIM but has been reported in other conditions such as cancer cachexia.[35]

Necrosis

The third category includes necrosis, degeneration, and regeneration. Since each muscle cell is a syncytium, most necrosis is segmental, affecting only a portion of the muscle fibre. The necrozing portion becomes electrically isolated from the motor end plate until regeneration is complete. Large amounts of necrosis are called rhabdomyolysis. Regeneration of myopathic muscle fibres

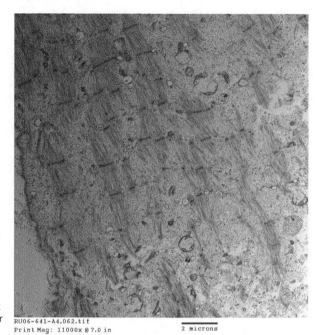

Fig. 34.4 CIM with myosin loss and architectural disarray, seen on deltoid muscle biopsy of a critically ill patient with EM.

The contributor would like to thank Dr D. Born and Dr C. Miller for their assistance in producing this image.

RU06-641-A4.062.tif
Print Mag: 11000x @ 7.0 in   2 microns

may lead to the abnormal finding of central nuclei, as satellite cells proliferate, migrate, differentiate, and fuse. Necrosis may be identified by rounded fibres, with obscuration of the myofibrillar network and influx of macrophages. Necrotic fibres may become pale or hypercontracted. On EM, severely necrotic fibres have no identifiable A-bands or I-bands; instead, the cytoplasm is filled with granular material.[33] Regenerating muscle fibres are often small and filled with basophilic cytoplasm[33] and are usually seen contemporaneously with findings of necrosis. Figures 34.5 and 34.6 presents H & E light micrographs demonstrating a regenerating fibre and central nuclei, both evidence of necrosis and regeneration.

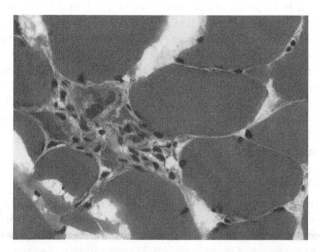

Fig. 34.5 Muscle cell regeneration (a marker of necrosis), seen on deltoid muscle biopsy of a critically ill patient with H & E stain.

The contributor would like to thank Dr D. Born for his assistance in producing this image.

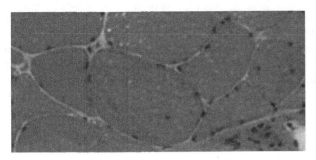

Fig. 34.6 Central nuclei (a marker of necrosis), seen on deltoid muscle biopsy of a critically ill patient with H & E stain.

The contributor would like to thank Dr D. Born for his assistance in producing this image.

Necrosis is a less common finding in series of patients with CIM than atrophy or thick filament loss. If present, necrosis typically occurs in very few fibres[25] but can be severe and widespread, as is the case in rhabdomyolysis. Potential risk factors for muscle necrosis include number of organs failed as well as renal failure.[25] Muscle necrosis can be detected by elevations of serum CK and myoglobin, as sarcolemmal integrity is lost and lysosomes break down the sarcoplasmic proteins, releasing them into the circulation. Since the presence and degree of muscle necrosis is variable across cases of CIM, elevations of CK and myoglobin support diagnosis but are not required.[10,29]

Pathogenesis of skeletal muscle pathology in critical illness

Clinical risk factors

To date, there have been no published studies evaluating the clinical risk factors for CIM nor its pathologic components: atrophy, thick filament loss, or necrosis. In fact, there are few established clinical risk factors for the broader category of critical illness associated neuromuscular abnormalities. Only three factors—MOF, SIRS, and PMV—have been shown to be associated with neuromuscular abnormalities in more than one cohort study that included adjustment for potential confounders in multivariable analyses.[27] Despite myriad papers suggesting a causal relationship between treatment with GCs and/or NMBAs and neuromuscular abnormalities, these epiphenomenologic associations may indeed be the result of confounding in the setting of indication bias. That is, the sickest patients were both at highest risk to develop neuromuscular abnormalities and most likely to receive these pharmacologic therapies. Indeed, RCTs of GCs[36] and NMBAs[37] (which use randomization to prevent indication bias) have not shown overwhelming relationships between these exposures and neuromuscular outcomes.

Pathogenesis

Similar to the histologic studies, early investigations seeking to understand the pathobiology of skeletal muscle in critical illness have focused on single cases or case series of weak patients. These early clinical reports used immunostaining to understand the pathways that were active in the development of atrophy and myosin loss. Focusing on proteolytic pathways, investigators found evidence of activation of calcium-activated proteases (calpain),[20] the ATP-ubiquitin system,[26] and lysosomal proteases (cathepsin B)[26] (see Chapter 35 for full details). It was hypothesized that these pathways work in tandem, first resulting in myosin loss with fibre atrophy, potentially progressing to degradation of other cytoskeletal proteins, and leading to, in some cases, the activation of lysosomes and ubiquitin as fibre necrosis.[26] Others suggested that the activation of apoptotic pathways is more significant and demonstrated the presence of overexpression of caspase and apoptotic nuclei in the majority of affected fibres.[38] More recently, studies have used mRNA expression to look beyond pathways involved in protein breakdown[39] to understand the potential role for decreased production of myosin, looking at myosin heavy chain[40] and MyoD,[41] a key protein regulating muscle differentiation and repair. These studies have suggested complicated relationships between MPB and MPS that are altered by common factors in critical illness such as immobility[39] and inflammation.[41]

It has been suggested that understanding of the effects of critical illness on skeletal muscle has been hampered by the lack of animal models that can mimic the conditions of the ICU.[42] Very recently, investigators have cultivated such models using mice,[43] rats,[42] and pigs,[5] subjected to critical illness conditions such as ALI, MV, and immobilization. These studies are beginning to confirm previous suspicions—such as the importance of the ubiquitin proteasome pathway (UPP)[42] to identify key players in regulation such as muscle-specific RING finger proteins,[42,43] and to describe the complicated and elegant temporal sequence of events[44] leading to myopathy in critical illness. It is anticipated that this novel information will lead to clinical approaches to prevent and/or treat the neuromuscular sequelae of critical illness.

Conclusion

Amongst critically ill patients with profound weakness, abnormalities of skeletal muscle are ubiquitous. Atrophy and myosin loss are the most common, with muscle necrosis a less generalizable finding. The balance between myosin breakdown and production may be at the core of CIM, with intricate relationships between aspects of critical illness and its treatments. While existing clinical studies have provided provocative pilot data, there is great need for well-designed translational research studies that can elucidate the incidence, risk factors, mechanisms, and outcomes of CIM.[45] Without this knowledge, understanding of the role of myopathy in clinical ICUAW and important, patient-centred long-term outcomes will remain weak.

References

1 Schoenauer R, Lange S, Hirschy A, Ehler E, Perriard JC, Agarkova I. Myomesin 3, a novel structural component of the M-band in striated muscle. *J Mol Biol* 2008;**376**:338–51.

2 Dumitru D. *Electrodiagnostic medicine*. Philadelphia, SL: Hanley & Belfus, Mosby; 1995.

3 Rich MM, Teener JW, Raps EC, Schotland DL, Bird SJ. Muscle is electrically inexcitable in acute quadriplegic myopathy. *Neurology* 1996;**46**:731–6.

4 Rich MM, Pinter MJ. Crucial role of sodium channel fast inactivation in muscle fibre inexcitability in a rat model of critical illness myopathy. *J Physiol* 2003;**547**:555–66.

5 Ochala J, Ahlbeck K, Radell PJ, Eriksson LI, Larsson L. Factors underlying the early limb muscle weakness in acute quadriplegic myopathy using an experimental ICU porcine model. *PLoS One* 2011;**6**:e20876.

6 Ahlbeck K, Fredriksson K, Rooyackers O, et al. Signs of critical illness polyneuropathy and myopathy can be seen early in the ICU course. *Acta Anaesthesiol Scand* 2009;**53**:717–23.

7 Bierbrauer J, Koch S, Olbricht C, et al. Early type II fiber atrophy in intensive care unit patients with nonexcitable muscle membrane. *Crit Care Med* 2012;**40**:647–50.

8 MacFarlane IA, Rosenthal FD. Severe myopathy after status asthmaticus. *Lancet* 1977;**2**:615.

9 Bolton CF, Gilbert JJ, Hahn AF, Sibbald WJ. Polyneuropathy in critically ill patients. *J Neurol Neurosurg Psychiatry* 1984;**47**:1223–31.

10 **Lacomis D, Zochodne DW, Bird SJ.** Critical illness myopathy. *Muscle Nerve* 2000;**23**:1785–8.

11 **Lacomis D, Giuliani MJ, Van Cott A, Kramer DJ.** Acute myopathy of intensive care: clinical, electro-myographic, and pathological aspects. *Ann Neurol* 1996;**40**:645–54.

12 **Sander HW, Golden M, Danon MJ.** Quadriplegic areflexic ICU illness: selective thick filament loss and normal nerve histology. *Muscle Nerve* 2002;**26**:499–505.

13 **Latronico N, Fenzi F, Recupero D, et al.** Critical illness myopathy and neuropathy. *Lancet* 1996;**347**: 1579–82.

14 **Larsson L, Li X, Edstrom L, et al.** Acute quadriplegia and loss of muscle myosin in patients treated with nondepolarizing neuromuscular blocking agents and corticosteroids: mechanisms at the cellular and molecular levels. *Crit Care Med* 2000;**28**:34–45.

15 **Hanson P, Dive A, Brucher JM, Bisteau M, Dangoisse M, Deltombe T.** Acute corticosteroid myopathy in intensive care patients. *Muscle Nerve* 1997;**20**:1371–80.

16 **Matsumoto N, Nakamura T, Yasui Y, Torii J.** Analysis of muscle proteins in acute quadriplegic myo-pathy. *Muscle Nerve* 2000;**23**:1270–6.

17 **Hund EF, Fogel W, Krieger D, DeGeorgia M, Hacke W.** Critical illness polyneuropathy: clinical findings and outcomes of a frequent cause of neuromuscular weaning failure. *Crit Care Med* 1996;**24**: 1328–33.

18 **Lopate G, Pestronk A, Yee WC.** N lines in a myopathy with myosin loss. *Muscle Nerve* 1998;**21**:1216–9.

19 **Wokke JH, Jennekens FG, van den Oord CJ, Veldman H, van Gijn J.** Histological investigations of muscle atrophy and end plates in two critically ill patients with generalized weakness. *J Neurol Sci* 1988;**88**:95–106.

20 **Showalter CJ, Engel AG.** Acute quadriplegic myopathy: analysis of myosin isoforms and evidence for calpain-mediated proteolysis. *Muscle Nerve* 1997;**20**:316–22.

21 **Amaya-Villar R, Garnacho-Montero J, Garcia-Garmendia JL, et al.** Steroid-induced myopathy in patients intubated due to exacerbation of chronic obstructive pulmonary disease. *Intensive Care Med* 2005;**31**:157–61.

22 **Bednarik J, Vondracek P, Dusek L, Moravcova E, Cundrle I.** Risk factors for critical illness polyneuro-myopathy. *J Neurol* 2005;**252**:343–51.

23 **Coakley JH, Nagendran K, Yarwood GD, Honavar M, Hinds CJ.** Patterns of neurophysiological abnormality in prolonged critical illness. *Intensive Care Med* 1998;**24**:801–7.

24 **De Jonghe B, Sharshar T, Lefaucheur JP, et al.** Paresis acquired in the intensive care unit: a prospective multicenter study. *JAMA* 2002;**288**:2859–67.

25 **Helliwell TR, Coakley JH, Wagenmakers AJ, et al.** Necrotizing myopathy in critically-ill patients. *J Pathol* 1991;**164**:307–14.

26 **Helliwell TR, Wilkinson A, Griffiths RD, McClelland P, Palmer TE, Bone JM.** Muscle fibre atrophy in critically ill patients is associated with the loss of myosin filaments and the presence of lysosomal enzymes and ubiquitin. *Neuropathol Appl Neurobiol* 1998;**24**:507–17.

27 **Stevens RD, Dowdy DW, Michaels RK, Mendez-Tellez PA, Pronovost PJ, Needham DM.** Neuromuscular dysfunction acquired in critical illness: a systematic review. *Intensive Care Med* 2007; **33**:1876–91.

28 **Khan J, Harrison TB, Rich MM, Moss M.** Early development of critical illness myopathy and neuropa-thy in patients with severe sepsis. *Neurology* 2006;**67**:1421–5.

29 **Bolton CF.** Neuromuscular manifestations of critical illness. *Muscle Nerve* 2005;**32**:140–63.

30 **Bolton CF.** Sepsis and the systemic inflammatory response syndrome: neuromuscular manifestations. *Crit Care Med* 1996;**24**:1408–16.

31 **Laing NG (ed.).** *The sarcomere and skeletal muscle disease.* New York, NY: Springer *Science* + Business Media; LLC Landes Bioscience; 2008.

32 **Neuromuscular Disease Center.** Available at: http://neuromuscular.wustl.edu.

33 Dubowitz V, Brooke MH, Neville HE. *Muscle biopsy: a practical approach.* 2nd ed. London: Bailliere Tindall; 1985.

34 Stibler H, Edstrom L, Ahlbeck K, Remahl S, Ansved T. Electrophoretic determination of the myosin/actin ratio in the diagnosis of critical illness myopathy. *Intensive Care Med* 2003;**29**:1515–27.

35 Acharyya S, Ladner KJ, Nelsen LL, et al. Cancer cachexia is regulated by selective targeting of skeletal muscle gene products. *J Clin Invest* 2004;**114**:370–8.

36 Hough CL, Steinberg KP, Taylor Thompson B, Rubenfeld GD, Hudson LD. Intensive care unit-acquired neuromyopathy and corticosteroids in survivors of persistent ARDS. *Intensive Care Med* 2009;**35**:63–8.

37 Papazian L, Forel JM, Gacouin A, et al. Neuromuscular blockers in early acute respiratory distress syndrome. *N Engl J Med* 2010;**363**:1107–16.

38 Di Giovanni S, Mirabella M, D'Amico A, Tonali P, Servidei S. Apoptotic features accompany acute quadriplegic myopathy. *Neurology* 2000;**55**:854–8.

39 Di Giovanni S, Molon A, Broccolini A, et al. Constitutive activation of MAPK cascade in acute quadriplegic myopathy. *Ann Neurol* 2004;**55**:195–206.

40 Norman H, Zackrisson H, Hedstrom Y, et al. Myofibrillar protein and gene expression in acute quadriplegic myopathy. *J Neurol Sci* 2009;**285**:28–38.

41 Guttridge DC, Mayo MW, Madrid LV, Wang CY, Baldwin AS, Jr. NF-kappaB-induced loss of MyoD messenger RNA: possible role in muscle decay and cachexia. *Science* 2000;**289**:2363–6.

42 Ochala J, Gustafson AM, Diez ML, et al. Preferential skeletal muscle myosin loss in response to mechanical silencing in a novel rat intensive care unit model: underlying mechanisms. *J Physiol* 2011;**589**:2007–26.

43 Files DC, D'Alessio FR, Johnston LF, et al. A critical role for muscle ring finger-1 in acute lung injury-associated skeletal muscle wasting. *Am J Respir Crit Care Med* 2012;**185**:825–34.

44 Llano-Diez M, Gustafson AM, Olsson C, Goransson H, Larsson L. Muscle wasting and the temporal gene expression pattern in a novel rat intensive care unit model. *BMC Genomics* 2011;**12**:602.

45 Hough CL, Needham DM. The role of future longitudinal studies in ICU survivors: understanding determinants and pathophysiology of weakness and neuromuscular dysfunction. *Curr Opin Crit Care* 2007;**13**:489–96.

Chapter 35

Skeletal Muscle Mass Regulation in Critical Illness

Zudin Puthucheary, Hugh Montgomery, Nicholas Hart, and Stephen Harridge

Introduction

Whilst outcome from critical illness is improving, survival is associated with impaired skeletal muscle function, a phenomenon known as ICUAW.[1,2] Muscle is a dynamic, plastic, and malleable tissue that is highly sensitive to the mechanical and metabolic signals provided by muscle loading, exercise, and feeding. Immobilization, bed rest, and prolonged exposure to a microgravity environment will, independent of any other factors, result in a loss in muscle mass (wasting/atrophy).[3] Conversely, activity of a muscle which causes mechanical overload, e.g. high-resistance strength training, will result in an adaptation whereby a muscle will increase in mass or hypertrophy.[4] This chapter will discuss the effect of critical illness on skeletal muscle mass (Figure 35.1).[5] Specifically, the focus will be on the unique challenges to which muscle is exposed in this environment. These include inflammation, sepsis, sedation, and feeding, all of which combine with the disuse signals of immobilization and bed rest to negatively affect peripheral skeletal muscle.

Skeletal muscle

Structure and function

Skeletal muscle is the largest tissue in the body, accounting for approximately 20–40% of the total body mass.[6] Each muscle, depending on its size, is made up of many hundreds, and, in some cases, hundreds of thousands, of elongated muscle fibres. Each fibre is made up of an array of different proteins required for: (1) contraction, e.g. actin and myosin, (2) activation, e.g. sarcoplasmic reticulum, (3) metabolism, e.g. mitochondria, (4) structural integrity, e.g. titin, and (5) maintenance and repair, e.g. satellite cells.[6] Muscle fibres are not homogeneous, as the expression of different protein isoforms results in their exhibiting markedly different contractile and metabolic properties. Fibres containing the slow myosin heavy chain isoform (MHC-I) are slow-contracting and oxidative in their metabolic profile; MHC-IIa fibres are fast-contracting with some oxidative potential, whereas the fastest contracting MHC-IIX fibres are fast-contracting glycolytic fibres with poor resistance to fatigue. Although it has numerous other functions, such as an endogenous source of heat,[7] a dynamic metabolic store, and a metabolic regulator,[7] the prime function of muscle is to convert chemical energy into mechanical work.[8] The strength of a muscle (the maximal force that can be produced during a single maximal voluntary isometric contraction) and its power (the product of speed of movement and force of contraction) are determined in large part by muscle size.[8] A loss of muscle mass therefore has deleterious consequences for contractile function.

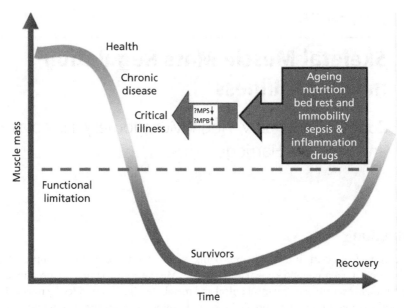

Fig. 35.1 Schematic representation of factors regulating muscle mass and function in critically ill patients. MPS, muscle protein synthesis; MPB, muscle protein breakdown.

Reproduced with permission from Puthucheary Z., et al., 'Structure to function: muscle failure in critically ill patients', *Journal of Physiology*, 588, 23, pp. 4641–4648, Wiley, © 2010 The Authors. Journal compilation © 2010 The Physiological Society.

Muscle mass regulation

Muscle is a dynamic tissue, in which continuous protein synthesis and breakdown occur. For a muscle to alter its size, either the rate of synthesis or the rate of breakdown, or both, must be modified. Rodent and cell-based models have previously been used to study the mechanisms which drive the processes of synthesis and breakdown,[9] with technological developments in stable isotope use, in conjunction with mass spectrometry, increasingly augmenting these with human data. Translational skeletal muscle research in critically ill patients has been technically challenging, with limited data available, which has led to specific ICU rodent models being developed.[10]

Measuring muscle protein synthesis and breakdown

In human beings, the measurement of MPS is achieved through the constant infusion of stable isotope-labelled amino acids, such as leucine ($(1,2-{}^{13}C_2)$ leucine), and measurement of its incorporation into muscle, samples of which are obtained through biopsy. The measurement of MPB is less robust, relying on the measurement of the arteriovenous difference of constantly infused (D_5) phenylalanine, coupled with measurements of blood flow across a limb. In healthy young humans, the basal fractional rate of myofibrillar protein synthesis is in the region of 0.02–0.06% per hour.[11] MPS is stimulated transiently by feeding (and, specifically, exclusively by essential amino acids, particularly leucine)[12] and exercise, but, in healthy young adults, a balance is maintained with MPB such that muscle mass is maintained.[12]

Molecular regulation of protein turnover

Both MPS and MPB are the end-products of complex interdependent series of intracellular processes. MPS and MPB do not function in complete isolation from one another but, for convenience and simplicity, are considered separately.

MPS

Three main stages occur in the synthesis of new amino acids and proteins from encoded DNA. Each stage is controlled, in part, by three groups of proteins which drive: (1) **initiation** (controlled by eukaryotic initiation factors, EIFs), (2) **elongation** (by eukaryotic elongation factors, EEFs), and (3) **termination** (by eukaryotic release factors, ERFs). Following termination, proteins undergo tertiary and quaternary structure development folding.

These groups of regulatory proteins are controlled by upstream signalling pathways, whose activity is modulated by a variety of proteins and stimuli. MPS is mediated by several pathways, convergent on protein kinase B (**also known as AKT**) in the main, with some independent activity via IRS-1[13] (Figure 35.2). Regulation of activity of these pathways is not completely understood, and, although commonly referred to as the IGF-1/P13K protein kinase B (IGF-1/PI3K/AKT) pathway, anabolism can also occur via other pathways such as those downstream of nuclear factor kappa beta (NFκβ).[13,14]

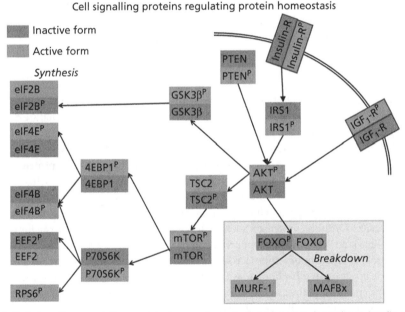

Fig. 35.2 Cell signalling regulating protein homeostasis. P, phosphorylated; insulin-R, insulin receptor; IGF-1R, insulin-like growth factor-1 receptor; IRS-1, insulin receptor substrate 1; PTEN, phosphatase and tensin homolog; AKT, protein kinase B; FOXO, forkhead box class O-1; MuRF-1, muscle ring finger protein-1;, MAFBX, muscle atrophy F-Box-1;TSC2, tuberous sclerosis complex 2; mTOR, mammalian target of rapamycin; 4EBP-1, eukaryotic initiation factor 4E binding protein 1; P70s6K, 70-kDa S6 protein kinase; GSK3B, glycogen synthetase kinase 3 beta; Elf2B, eukaryotic initiation factor 2-B; EIF4e, eukaryotic initiation factor 4e; EEF2, eukaryotic elongation factor 2; RPS6, ribosomal protein S6.

Two components of the pathways worth highlighting are mTOR and the 70-kDa S6 protein kinase (p70s6k). mTOR regulates protein synthesis by controlling two important proteins P70S6K and EIF 4E binding protein 1 (E4BP-1). Whilst it is a downstream target of AKT, mTOR can be activated independently of the AKT pathway by infusions of amino acids and, in particular, branched-chain amino acids such as leucine.[15] Further evidence of the central role of mTOR in the regulation of metabolism is emerging, defining the role of mTOR in mitochondrial biogenesis and in the regulation of ROS generation.[16] P70s6k is an important regulator of translation (Figure 35.2). Not only has P70s6k been demonstrated to be upregulated by resistance exercise, but a direct relationship between the activation of p70s6K and muscle mass has been demonstrated in animals.[17] In addition to P70s6K being a marker of MPS, it has also been found to respond appropriately when exercise is coupled with amino acid loading.[18]

Whilst a pathway directed though IGF-1 is attractive, the reality is more complex. For example, rodent studies have shown hypertrophic adaptation and activation of the pathway despite IGF-1 receptors being mutated.[19] During growth and development, the GH and IGF-1 axis plays a key role in driving muscle growth, and recombinant GH is a treatment for deficiency. However, its role in regulating normal adult muscle mass remains unclear.

Physiological elevations of anabolic hormones, such as GH, combined with resistance exercise, fails to enhance training-induced muscle hypertrophy. This was demonstrated in a study that investigated the effect on upper limb muscles trained in a 'natural' hormonally enhanced environment where GH, IGF-I, and testosterone were elevated by prior high-volume lower limb resistance exercise. There was no enhancement to growth or strength observed in comparison to training in the basal hormonal milieu.[20]

MPB

MPB is an essential component of protein homeostasis. In energy-deficient states, MPB provides amino acids necessary for gluconeogenesis and energy production.[21] This dual nature contributes to the complex physiology of the process of MPB. Three pathways have been described, controlling MPB in humans: (1) the autophagy-lysosomal pathway, (2) the cytosolic proteases, and (3) the UPP. In the autophagy-lysosomal pathway, extracellular and cytosolic proteins are taken up by endocytosis and degraded within the lysosome by acid-based proteases such as cathepsins and acid hydrolases.[9,21] Currently, the lysosomal pathway is considered to control the extracellular and membrane surface protein turnover, rather than the intracellular turnover under normal circumstances.[9,22] Cytosolic proteases, such as the calpains,[23] are required for calcium-activated proteolysis. This is an ATP-independent process which responds to a rise in intracellular calcium and plays a role in tissue injury and necrosis.[9,23] However, their role in normal skeletal muscle remains unclear. Caspases (**also known as Interleukin-β converting enzyme related proteases**) are part of the apoptotic pathways and respond to DNA damage and noxious stimuli, leading to programmed cell death.[9] Finally, the UPP is an ATP-dependent pathway that is considered to be the mechanism by which the majority of intracellular proteins are degraded.[9,24–26] The ubiquitin-activating enzymes (E1 ligases) create an active form of ubiquitin and bind it to ubiquitin carrier proteins (E2 ligases). The ubiquitin is then transferred to the substrate by ubiquitin protein ligases (E3 ligases, e.g. muscle ring finger-1 (MuRF-1) or muscle atrophy factor (Mafbx)). This occurs repeatedly until a polyubiquitin chain is formed, which is recognized by the 26s proteasome and degraded by the 20s core.

The UPP has been demonstrated to be the final common proteolysis pathway in disease models of starvation,[27] diabetes,[28] acidosis,[29] cancer cachexia,[21] sepsis,[30] disuse,[27] and GC therapy).[31] In health, blocking of other pathways leads to only a minor reduction in MPB.[32] An important caveat to the acceptance of the UPP as the only mechanism of proteolysis is our limited knowledge of all components of the UPP and their influences on each other. Although MuRF-1 is frequently measured,[9,25] MuRF-2 and MuRF-3 are less so, resulting in limited data detailing the actions and interactions of these E3 ligases.[33,34] A key feature of the UPP which is wholly relevant to critically ill patients is that it is ATP-dependent.[34,35] Mitochondrial dysfunction has been demonstrated in critically ill patients, and the ATP availability of cells in such patients is unknown.[36,37] Many of the studies reported in this section were carried out using animal models, either *ex vivo* or *in vivo*. Whilst there are numerous issues with interpreting such data in the clinical context, it is worth noting that upregulation of the UPP has been documented in many disease states in humans, including COPD,[38] sepsis,[39,40] trauma,[41] statin myopathy,[42] cancer cachexia,[43] and burns,[44] and in human experimental models of immobilization[45] as well as in response to exercise.[46]

A parallel pathway to IGF-1 is the NFκβ pathway, which is also likely to be involved in muscle atrophy in the critically ill. It is activated by members of the tumour necrosis factor (TNF) family, with upregulation demonstrated in sepsis and disuse.[47,48] A specific member of the TNF family TWEAK (TNF-related weak inducer of apoptosis) has been shown to induce muscle atrophy.[49] Animal studies have linked the NFκβ pathway to ubiquitinization as a mode of promoting protein breakdown.[14]

Myostatin

Myostatin (otherwise known as GDF-8) is a protein that is member of the TGF-β family, which is a negative regulator of muscle mass. High expression promotes muscle atrophy and inhibits satellite cell renewal.[50] Knockout and mutation animal studies exhibit extreme muscle hypertrophy,[51,52] with supporting evidence in a child with clinical features of significant muscle hypertrophy in which a myostatin mutation was identified.[53] Myostatin binds to the type IIB activin receptor and acts via phosphorylation of Smad2 and Smad3 (mothers against decapentaplegic homolog), in turn dephosphorylating and activating FOXO[54] which inhibits MPS by inhibiting mTOR.[55,56] Myostatin also acts via non-Smad pathways, including the mitogen-activated protein kinase (MAPK),[57] extracellular signal regulated kinase (ERK),[58] and c-Jun N-terminal kinases (JNK) pathways.[59] Whilst promising results from blockade of this pathway exist, translation into human studies has yet to occur.[60] Furthermore, myostatin per se may not be a key regulator but one of a group of proteins acting on the activin receptor.[61] Like many highly conserved proteins, myostatin has pleiotropic effects in metabolic modulation,[55] and its exact role at this stage remains to be defined.

Extracellular regulation of myostatin occurs by a variety of proteins. Follistatin, a glycoprotein similar to the TGF-β family, binds to myostatin and prevents receptor binding.[61] Myostatin circulates in a latent form, bound to a pro-peptide. Its release from the pro-peptide can be inhibited by TGF-β binding protein 3 and also by growth and differentiation serum factor associated protein-1 (GASP-1).[62] Micro-RNA (miR), which are short 22-sequence non-coding RNA (**previously called junk RNA**) that regulate gene expression via post-transcriptional modification of mRNA,[63] have also been shown to regulate myostatin expression. Specifically, animal studies have demonstrated the involvement of miR-1 and miR-206 in myostatin inhibition,[64] whilst human studies have shown that ingestion of essential amino acids results in the upregulation on miR-499, miR-1, miR-208b, and miR-23a, with a corresponding decrease in myostatin.[65]

In human models of immobilization, the association between myostatin activity and muscle mass remains unclear.[45,66] In a single study, rehabilitation following cast immobilization was associated with low myostatin mRNA expression, with a parallel gain in muscle mass.[45] Exercise and GH studies have demonstrated a decrease in myostatin mRNA,[67–69] though conflicting results exist.[70] Both sarcopenia and cigarette smoking have been associated with an increase in myostatin mRNA expression.[71,72]

Animal models

Animal models have distinct attractions. Researchers are able to perform longitudinal observational and interventional studies with adequately matched controls. Different insults and stimuli can be delivered individually and dose-titrated to develop a model of human disease. Indeed, much of our mechanistic understanding of biomedical science has been derived in this fashion. Ochala et al.[10] have used an experimental rat model designed to mimic the human critical illness condition, with animals being sedated and paralysed with post-synaptic neuromuscular blockade and MV. In this rodent model, muscle atrophy is observed, with downregulation of myosin synthesis, an upregulation of UPP, and a sequential change in the localization of MuRF-1 and MuRF-2. However, caution must be exercised when extrapolating animal models to human disease. Specifically, total protein turnover in adult rats is 3–4 times greater than in humans, with a 2.5-fold higher protein synthetic rate.[73] This is likely to be related to the differences in metabolic stability (the ability to maintain homeostasis) between rodents and humans. The basal metabolic rate per gram body weight is 7 times greater in rats,[74] with different ageing rates between the two species.[75] Rodents used in studies are often immature and still growing, which is in contrast to the middle-aged and elderly critically ill patients that are admitted into the ICU. A recent review of animal studies has highlighted the difference between the animal model and human condition. In particular, 5 hours of muscle unloading initiate a muscle proteolytic response in animals, whereas humans regularly unload their muscles for at least 5 hours during sleep with no such effect.[76] Conceptually, animal studies would indicate that breakdown is the driving force in muscle homeostasis, yet, for the reasons previously outlined, caution should be taken in extrapolating these data to humans. Furthermore, these conclusions are, in the main, drawn from studies on the UPPs, rather than actual measures of breakdown, which is a further limitation. Finally, many studies are performed in the *ex-vivo* setting where normal rat muscle displays lower muscle synthetic rates and higher muscle breakdown rates than that *in vivo*, leading to the false assumption that alterations in MPS affect MPB directly. Despite these limitations, animal studies remain invaluable for the mechanistic and structural understanding of muscle physiology. In respect to translation into clinically novel and innovative ideas, their contribution needs to be carefully considered. If we are to clearly understand the effect of critical illness on muscle physiology, and thereby develop molecules and other interventions to prevent muscle wasting, human studies are needed.

Muscle protein regulation in critically ill patients

Performing invasive physiological experiments on critically ill patients has many challenges. Aside from the practical difficulties of obtaining assent from the relatives and retrospective consent from the patient, there are obvious technical difficulties of performing muscle biopsies in physiologically unstable patients, with the inherent risks of bleeding and infection. Therefore, to gain further insight into the pathophysiological condition of muscle wasting, data have been extrapolated from similar scenarios in **healthy** humans such as leg cast immobilization.[77] Such studies help to define which factors associated with muscle wasting might be **causative** in this process. However, limitations again apply to such studies: (1) many purported insults are difficult ethically to recreate in healthy volunteers (e.g. prolonged neuromuscular blockade without sedation) and (2) the cumulative effect of multiple insults cannot be measured for the same reasons.

Several studies have examined the alterations in anabolic and catabolic signalling in critically ill patients. Interpretation of these studies is difficult as a result of significant methodological flaws with sample sizes to date. Whilst a single study has suggested homogeneity in the metabolic response to critical illness,[78] there are currently limited data reporting the impact of sex, age, and presenting illness affecting muscle mass loss in the critically ill. These studies lack measurements of actual alterations in muscle mass, which hinders the investigation of temporal and effect associations. Standardization of biopsy time points has not occurred. Critical illness is a dynamic process,[79–82] with common secondary complications such as ventilator-acquired pneumonia. Biopsies taken at a single time point are unlikely to reflect the complex metabolic adaptation that occurs during the early acute and later recovery phases in the critically ill. Longitudinal data, including objective measures of muscle mass, deep phenotyping of patients, and simultaneous measures of dynamic protein turnover, are required but have yet to be published.

Within these limitations, cross-sectional data do exist. Twelve critically ill patients, compared with healthy age- and sex-matched controls, were shown to have increased signalling of the downstream pathway components of AKT, suggesting increased anabolic signalling with blunted proteolysis.[83] In a group of eight patients with seven healthy controls, stable isotope studies demonstrated variable rates of MPS with high rates of MPB, accompanied by upregulation of catabolic signalling.[84] The same group has demonstrated similar findings with further small-group experiments, although both studies were limited by lack of anabolic signalling measurements.[39] In a recent study, 64 long-stay patients were biopsied at a median of 15 days,[85] results demonstrating that there was no increase in gene expression of E3 ligases or myostatin, compared to controls. The only study to examine the relationship between gene expression and protein concentration in ten critically ill patients observed dissociation.[86] The same study found a suppression of anabolic signalling, paralleled by an upregulation of breakdown pathways. Crucially, mRNA expression of anabolic signalling was increased, without translation into protein production, implying an initiation of a synthetic programme at the transcriptional level. As regards myostatin, two conflicting cross-sectional studies in the critically ill, with non-standardized biopsy time points, have demonstrated low[83] and high[86] myostatin mRNA expression. Equivocal findings have been repeatedly observed in patients with COPD,[87,88] with a single study reporting lower levels of myostatin following rehabilitation, albeit in a cross-sectional, rather than longitudinal, study.[89]

Loss of muscle function

As stated at the beginning of the chapter, muscle function (strength and power) is related to muscle size. Thus, it might be reasonable to assume that the loss of function is directly proportional to the loss in size. For obvious reasons, whole muscle function measurements are difficult, if not impossible, to perform in the critical care setting. However, it is possible to study objectively the function of individual fibres which have been dissected from biopsy samples. These fibres are permeabilized and can be activated chemically *in vitro*. Here, the forces produced can be related to the cross-sectional area of the fibre. Such studies have been undertaken in healthy young individuals to evaluate the effects of bed rest and suggest that there is not only a loss of fibre size, but also a loss in 'quality'. This is indicated by a decreased force produced per unit area of muscle, otherwise known as a loss in specific force.[90] Specific force loss has also been demonstrated in muscle fibres taken from frail elderly people and has been attributed, in part, to a selective loss of the thick filament protein myosin.[91] In the sedated, paralysed mechanically-ventilated rat, a similar loss of specific force has been observed, also with a selective loss of myosin.[10] A selective loss of myosin has been also been described in muscle samples taken from critically ill patients.[92] This suggests that specific force loss is a phenomenon that is present in critically ill patients, and longitudinal studies are needed to confirm this. It would be hypothesized that the loss of muscle mass underestimates the loss in muscle function.

Conclusion

During critical illness, skeletal muscle is challenged with immobilization and inflammation, with the addition of sedatives superimposed on the primary illness and organ failure. Under these conditions, it is not surprising that muscle homeostasis is severely disrupted and that there is a loss in muscle mass. The mechanisms regulating muscle loss during critical illness are starting to be understood, but many questions remain unanswered. Detailed understanding of these mechanisms is essential if we are to develop strategies to minimize, or even prevent, muscle wasting, intensive care-acquired muscle weakness, and the long-term functional debility experienced by ICU survivors.

References

1 De Jonghe B, Sharshar T, Lefaucheur JP, et al. Paresis acquired in the intensive care unit: a prospective multicenter study. *JAMA* 2002;**288**:2859–67.

2 Herridge MS, Tansey CM, Matté A, et al. Functional disability 5 years after acute respiratory distress syndrome. *N Engl J Med* 2011;**364**:1293–304.

3 Murton AJ, Greenhaff PL. Muscle atrophy in immobilization and senescence in humans. *Curr Opin Neurol* 2009;**22**:500–5.

4 Aagaard P, Andersen JL, Dyhre-Poulsen P, et al. A mechanism for increased contractile strength of human pennate muscle in response to strength training: changes in muscle architecture. *J Physiol* 2001;**534**:613–23.

5 Puthucheary Z, Montgomery H, Moxham J, Harridge S, Hart N. Structure to function: muscle failure in critically ill patients. *J Physiol* 2010;**588**:4641–8.

6 Lieber R. *Skeletal muscle structure, function, and plasticity: the physiological basis of rehabilitation.* Philadelphia, PA: Lippincott Williams & Wilkins; 2002.

7 Edwards R, Hill D, Jones D. Heat production and chemical changes during isometric contractions of the human quadriceps muscle. *J Physiol* 1975;**251**:303–15.

8 Billeter R, Hoppeler H. Muscular basis of strength. In: **Komi PV** (ed.) *Strength and power in sport.* 2nd ed. Oxford: Blackwell Science; 2003. pp. 50–72.

9 Lecker SH, Solomon V, Mitch WE, Goldberg AL. Muscle protein breakdown and the critical role of the ubiquitin-proteasome pathway in normal and disease states. *J Nutr* 1999;**129**:227S–37S.

10 Ochala J, Gustafson AM, Diez ML, et al. Preferential skeletal muscle myosin loss in response to mechanical silencing in a novel rat intensive care unit model: underlying mechanisms. *J Physiol* 2011;**589**:2007–26.

11 Emery PW, Edwards RH, Rennie MJ, Souhami RL, Halliday D. Protein synthesis in muscle measured in vivo in cachectic patients with cancer. *Br Med J (Clin Res Ed)* 1984;**289**:584–6.

12 Rennie MJ. Muscle protein turnover and the wasting due to injury and disease. *Br Med Bull* 1985;**41**:257–64.

13 Glass DJ. Skeletal muscle hypertrophy and atrophy signaling pathways. *Int J Biochem Cell Biol* 2005;**37**:1974–84.

14 Cai D, Frantz JD, Tawa NE, Jr, et al. IKKbeta/NF-kappaB activation causes severe muscle wasting in mice. *Cell*, 2004;119:285–98.

15 Tato I, Barton R, Ventura F, Rosa JL. Amino Acids activate mammalian target of rapamycin complex 2 (mTORC2) via PI3K/AKT signalling. *J Biol Chem* 2011;286:6128–42.

16 Watanabe R, Wei L, Huang J. mTOR signalling, function, novel inhibitors and therapeutic targets. *J Nuclear Med* 2011;52:497–500.

17 Baar K, Esser K. Phosphorylation of p70(S6k) correlates with increased skeletal muscle mass following resistance exercise. *Am J Physiol* 1999;276:C120–127.

18 Karlsson HK, Nilsson PA, Nilsson J, Chibalin AV, Zierath JR, Blomstrand E. Branched-chain amino acids increase p70S6k phosphorylation in human skeletal muscle after resistance exercise. *Am J Physiol Endocrinol Metab* 2004;287:E1–7.

19 Wojtaszewski JF, Higaki Y, Hirshman MF, et al. Exercise modulates postreceptor insulin signaling and glucose transport in muscle-specific insulin receptor knockout mice. *J Clin Invest* 1999;104: 1257–64.

20 West DWD, Burd NA, Tang JE, et al. Elevations in ostensibly anabolic hormones with resistance exercise enhance neither training-induced muscle hypertrophy nor strength of the elbow flexors. *J App Physiol* 2010;108:60–7.

21 Temparis S, Asensi M, Taillandier D, et al. Increased ATP-ubiquitin-dependent proteolysis in skeletal muscles of tumor-bearing rats. *Cancer Res* 1994;54:5568–73.

22 Mitch WE, Goldberg AL. Mechanisms of muscle wasting. The role of the ubiquitin-proteasome pathway. *N Engl J Med* 1996;335:1897–905.

23 Puthucheary Z, Rawal J, Connolly B, et al. Serial Muscle Ultrasound Can Detect Acute Muscle Loss In Multi-Organ Failure. *Am J Respir Crit Care Med* 2011;183:A2376.

24 Cahill NE, Murch L, Jeejeebhoy K, et al. When early enteral feeding is not possible in critically ill patients: results of a multicenter observational study. *JPEN J Parenter Enteral Nutr* 2011;35:160–8.

25 Lecker SH, Jagoe RT, Gilbert A, et al. Multiple types of skeletal muscle atrophy involve a common program of changes in gene expression. *FASEB J* 2004;18:39–51.

26 Novak P, Vidmar G, Kuret Z, Bizovicar N. Rehabilitation of critical illness polyneuropathy and myopathy patients: an observational study. *Int J Rehabil Res* 2011;34:336–42.

27 Medina R, Wing SS, Goldberg AL. Increase in levels of polyubiquitin and proteasome mRNA in skeletal muscle during starvation and denervation atrophy. *Biochem J* 1995;307:631–7.

28 Price SR, Bailey JL, Wang X, et al. Muscle wasting in insulinopenic rats results from activation of the ATP-dependent, ubiquitin—proteasome proteolytic pathway by a mechanism including gene transcription. *J Clin Invest* 1996;98:1703–8.

29 Vanhorebeek I, Gunst J, Derde S, et al. Mitochondrial Fusion, Fission, and Biogenesis in Prolonged Critically Ill Patients. *J Clin Endocrinol Metab* 2011;97:E59–64.

30 Voisin L, Breuille D, Combaret L, et al. Muscle wasting in a rat model of long-lasting sepsis results from the activation of lysosomal, Ca2-activated, and ubiquitin-proteasome proteolytic pathways. *J Clin Invest* 1996;97:1610–7.

31 Auclair D, Garrel DR, Chaouki Zerouala A, Ferland LH. Activation of the ubiquitin pathway in rat skeletal muscle by catabolic doses of glucocorticoids. *Am J Physiol* 1997;272:c1007–16.

32 Furuno KGA. The activation of protein degradation in muscle by Ca2 + or muscle injury does not involve a lysosomal mechanism. *Biochem J* 1986;237:859–64.

33 Gregorio CC, Perry CN, Mcelhinny AS. Functional properties of the titin/connectin-associated proteins, the muscle-specific RING finger proteins (MURFs), in striated muscle. *J Muscle Res Cell Motil*, 2005;26:389–400.

34 Jagoe RT, Goldberg AL. What do we really know about the ubiquitin-proteasome pathway in muscle atrophy? *Curr Opin Clin Nutr Metab Care* 2001;4:183–90.

35 Coux O, Tanaka K, Goldberg AL. Structure and functions of the 20S and 26S proteasomes. *Annu Rev Biochem* 1996;65:801–47.

36 Brealey D, Brand M, Hargreaves I, et al. Association between mitochondrial dysfunction and severity and outcome of septic shock. *Lancet* 2002;360:219–23.

37 Carre JE, Orban J-C, Re L, et al. Survival in Critical Illness Is Associated with Early Activation of Mitochondrial Biogenesis. *Am J Respir Crit Care Med* 2010;182:745–51.

38 Doucet M, Russell AP, Leger B, et al. Muscle Atrophy and Hypertrophy Signaling in Patients with Chronic Obstructive Pulmonary Disease. *AJRCCM* 2007;176:261–9.

39 Klaude M, Fredriksson K, Tjader I, et al. Proteasome proteolytic activity in skeletal muscle is increased in patients with sepsis. *Clin Sci (Lond)* 2007;112:499–506.

40 Tiao G, Hobler S, Wang JJ, et al. Sepsis is associated with increased mRNAs of the ubiquitin—proteasome proteolytic pathway in human skeletal muscle. *J Clin Invest*, 1997;99:163–8.

41 Mansoor O, Beaufrere B, Boirie Y, et al. Increased mRNA levels for components of the lysosomal, Ca2-activated, and ATP-ubiquitin-dependent proteolytic pathways in skeletal muscle from head trauma patients. *Proc Natl Acad Sci USA* 1996;93:2714–18.

42 Mallinson JE, Constantin-Teodosiu D, Sidaway J, Westwood FR, Greenhaff PL. Blunted Akt/FOXO signalling and activation of genes controlling atrophy and fuel use in statin myopathy. *J Physiol* 2009;587:219–30.

43 Bossola M., Muscaritoli M, Costelli P, et al. Increased muscle ubiquitin mRNA levels in gastric cancer patients. *Am J Physiol Regul Integr Comp Physiol* 2001;280:R1518–23.

44 Biolo G, BosuttiA, Iscra F, Toigo G, Gullo A, Guarnieri G. Contribution of the ubiquitin-proteasome pathway to overall muscle proteolysis in hypercatabolic patients. *Metabolism* 2000;49:689–91.

45 Jones SW, Hill RJ, Krasney PA, O'conner B, Peirce N, Greenhaff PL. Disuse atrophy and exercise rehabilitation in humans profoundly affects the expression of genes associated with the regulation of skeletal muscle mass. *FASEB J* 2004;18:1025–7.

46 Murton AJ, Constantin D, Greenhaff PL. The involvement of the ubiquitin proteasome system in human skeletal muscle remodelling and atrophy. *Biochim Biophys Acta* 2008;1782:730–43.

47 Hunter RB, Stevenson E, Koncarevic A, Mitchell-Felton H, Essig DA, Kandarian SC. Activation of an alternative NF-kappaB pathway in skeletal muscle during disuse atrophy. *FASEB J* 2002;16:529–38.

48 Penner CG, Gang G, Wray C, Fischer JE, Hasselgren PO. The transcription factors NF-kappab and AP-1 are differentially regulated in skeletal muscle during sepsis. *Biochem Biophys Res Commun* 2001;281:1331–6.

49 Dogra C, Changotra H, Wedhas N, Qin X, Wergedal JE, Kumar A. TNF-related weak inducer of apo-ptosis (TWEAK) is a potent skeletal muscle-wasting cytokine. *Faseb J.* 2007;21:1857–69.

50 Mccroskery S, Thomas M, Platt L, et al. Improved muscle healing through enhanced regeneration and reduced fibrosis in myostatin-null mice. *J Cell Sci* 2005;118:3531–41.

51 Mcpherron, A. C. & Lee, S. J. Double muscling in cattle due to mutations in the myostatin gene. *Proc Natl Acad Sci USA* 1997;94:12457–61.

52 Mcpherron AC, Lawler AM, Lee SJ. Regulation of skeletal muscle mass in mice by a new TGF-beta superfamily member. *Nature*, 1997;387:83–90.

53 Schuelke M, Wagner KR, Stolz LE, et al. Myostatin mutation associated with gross muscle hypertrophy in a child. *N Engl J Med* 2004;350:2682–8.

54 Wing SS, Lecker SH, Jagoe RT. Proteolysis in illness-associated skeletal muscle atrophy: from pathways to networks. *Crit Rev Clin Lab Sci* 2011;48:49–70.

55 Lebrasseur NK, Walsh K, Arany Z. Metabolic benefits of resistance training and fast glycolytic skeletal muscle. *Am J Physiol Endocrinol Metab* 2011;300:E3–10.

56 Zhu X, Topouzis S, Liang LF, Stotish RL. Myostatin signaling through Smad2, Smad3 and Smad4 is regulated by the inhibitory Smad7 by a negative feedback mechanism. *Cytokine* 2004;26:262–72.

57 Philip B, Lu Z, Gao Y. Regulation of GDF-8 signaling by the p38 MAPK. *Cellular Signalling*, 2005;**17**:365–375.

58 Yang W, Chen Y, Zhang Y, Wang X, Yang N, Zhu D. Extracellular signal-regulated kinase 1/2 mitogen-activated protein kinase pathway is involved in myostatin-regulated differentiation repression. *Cancer Res* 2006;**66**:1320–6.

59 Huang Z, Chen D, Zhang K, Yu B, Chen X, Meng J. Regulation of myostatin signaling by c-Jun N-terminal kinase in C2C12 cells. *Cellular Signalling*, 2007;**19**:2286–95.

60 Zhou X, Wang JL, Lu J, et al. Reversal of cancer cachexia and muscle wasting by ActRIIB antagonism leads to prolonged survival. *Cell* 2010;**142**:531–43.

61 Lee SJ, Lee YS, Zimmers TA, et al. Regulation of Muscle Mass by Follistatin and Activins. *Mol Endocrinol* 2010;**24**:1998–2008.

62 Elkina Y, Von Haehling S, Anker SD, Springer J. The role of myostatin in muscle wasting: an overview. *J Cachexia Sarcopenia Muscle* 2011;**2**:143–51.

63 Lee SJ. Regulation of muscle mass by myostatin. *Annu Rev Cell Dev Biol* 2004;**20**:61–86.

64 Clop A, Marcq F, Takeda H, et al. A mutation creating a potential illegitimate microRNA target site in the myostatin gene affects muscularity in sheep. *Nat Genet* 2006;**38**:813–8.

65 Drummond MJ, Glynn EL, Fry CS, Dhanani S, Volpi E, Rasmussen BB. Essential Amino Acids Increase MicroRNA-499, -208b, and -23a and Downregulate Myostatin and Myocyte Enhancer Factor 2C mRNA Expression in Human Skeletal Muscle. *J Nutr* 2009;**139**:2279–84.

66 De Boer MD, Selby A, Atherton P, et al. The temporal responses of protein synthesis, gene expression and cell signalling in human quadriceps muscle and patellar tendon to disuse. *J Physiol* 2007;**585**:241–51.

67 Hulmi JJ, Ahtiainen JP, Kaasalainen T, et al. Postexercise myostatin and activin IIb mRNA levels: effects of strength training. *Med Sci Sports Exerc* 2007;**39**:289–97.

68 Louis E, Raue U, Yang Y, Jemiolo B, Trappe S. Time course of proteolytic, cytokine, and myostatin gene expression after acute exercise in human skeletal muscle. *J Appl Physiol* 2007;**103**:1744–51.

69 Lui JC, Baron J. Mechanisms limiting body growth in mammals. *Endocr Rev* 2011;**32**:422–40.

70 Willoughby DS. Effects of heavy resistance training on myostatin mRNA and protein expression. *Med Sci Sports Exerc* 2004;**36**:574–82.

71 Leger B, Derave W, De Bock K, Hespel P, Russell AP. Human sarcopenia reveals an increase in SOCS-3 and myostatin and a reduced efficiency of Akt phosphorylation. *Rejuvenation Res* 2008;**11**:163–75B.

72 Petersen AM, Magkos F, Atherton P, et al. Smoking impairs muscle protein synthesis and increases the expression of myostatin and MAFbx in muscle. *Am J Physiol Endocrinol Metab* 2007;**293**:E843–8.

73 Waterlow JC, Garlick PJ, Millward DJ. *Protein turnover in mammalian tissues and in the whole body.* Amsterdam: Elsevier North-Holland; 1978.

74 Demetrius L. Of mice and men. *EMBO Reports* 2005;**6**:39–44.

75 Demetrius L. Caloric restriction, metabolic rate, and entropy. *J Gerontol A Biol Sci Med Sci* 2004;**59**:902–15.

76 Phillips SM, Glover EI, Rennie MJ. Alterations of protein turnover underlying disuse atrophy in human skeletal muscle. *J Appl Physiol* 2009;**107**:645–54.

77 Glover EI, Phillips SM, Oates BR, et al. Immobilization induces anabolic resistance in human myofibrillar protein synthesis with low and high dose amino acid infusion. *J Physiol* 2008;**586**:6049–61.

78 Gamrin L, Essen P, Forsberg AM, Hultman E, Wernerman J. A descriptive study of skeletal muscle metabolism in critically ill patients: free amino acids, energy-rich phosphates, protein, nucleic acids, fat, water, and electrolytes. *Crit Care Med* 1996;**24**:575–83.

79 Finfer S. Corticosteroids in Septic Shock. *N Engl J Med* 2008;**358**:188–90.

80 Sprung CL, Annane D, Keh D, et al. Hydrocortisone Therapy for Patients with Septic Shock. *N Engl J Med* 2008;**358**:111–24.

81 **The Acute Respiratory Distress Syndrome Network.** Ventilation with Lower Tidal Volumes as Compared with Traditional Tidal Volumes for Acute Lung Injury and the Acute Respiratory Distress Syndrome. *N Engl J Med* 2000;**342**:1301–8.

82 **The National Heart, L., and Blood Institute Acute Respiratory Distress Syndrome (ARDS) Clinical Trials Network*.** Comparison of Two Fluid-Management Strategies in Acute Lung Injury. *N Engl J Med* 2006;**354**:2564–75.

83 **Jespersen JG, Nedergaard A, Reitelseder S, et al.** Activated protein synthesis and suppressed protein breakdown signaling in skeletal muscle of critically ill patients. *PLoS One* 2011;**6**:e18090.

84 **Klaude M, Mori M.** Protein metabolism and gene expression in skeletal muscle of critically ill patients with sepsis. *Clin Sci (Lond)* 2011;**122**:133–42.

85 **Derde S, Hermans G, Derese I, et al.** Muscle atrophy and preferential loss of myosin in prolonged critically ill patients. *Crit Care Med* 2012;**40**:79–89.

86 **Constantin D, Mccullough J, Mahajan RP, Greenhaff PL.** Novel events in the molecular regulation of muscle mass in critically ill patients. *J Physiol* 2011;**589**:3883–95.

87 **Ju CR, Chen RC.** Serum myostatin levels and skeletal muscle wasting in chronic obstructive pulmonary disease. *Respir Med* 2012;**106**:102–8.

88 **Vogiatzis I, Simoes DC, Stratakos G, et al.** Effect of pulmonary rehabilitation on muscle remodelling in cachectic patients with COPD. *Eur Respir J* 2010;**36**:301–10.

89 **Troosters T, Probst VS, Crul T, et al.** Resistance training prevents deterioration in quadriceps muscle function during acute exacerbations of chronic obstructive pulmonary disease. *Am J Respir Crit Care Med* 2010;**181**:1072–7.

90 **Larsson L, Li X, Berg HE, Frontera WR.** Effects of removal of weight-bearing function on contractility and myosin isoform composition in single human skeletal muscle cells. *Pflugers Arch* 1996;**432**:320–8.

91 **D'antona G, Pellegrino MA, Adami R, et al.** The effect of ageing and immobilization on structure and function of human skeletal muscle fibres. *J Physiol* 2003;**552**:499–511.

92 **Derde S, Hermans G, Derese I, et al.** Muscle atrophy and preferential loss of myosin in prolonged critically ill patients. *Crit Care Med* 2011;**40**:79–89.

Chapter 36

Malnutrition in Critical Illness: Implications, Causes, and Therapeutic Approaches

Daren K. Heyland and Marina Mourtzakis

Introduction

Malnutrition is generally defined as an inadequate intake of nutrients or calories for appropriate physiological functioning. **Undernourishment** specifically refers to hypocaloric intake, as well as reduced macro- and micronutrient intakes, relative to the calculated recommendation for a patient. Although these terms are often used interchangeably, this chapter will focus on undernourishment of the critically ill patient, its attendant physiological and clinical consequences, and strategies to counter its effects. Undernourishment in the ICU may be secondary to iatrogenic malnutrition where a patient presents with a healthy body composition and nutritional status at the time of ICU admission but may become undernourished during their ICU and hospital stay. Patients who are malnourished prior to ICU admission, such as patients with pre-existing malnutrition, may exhibit exacerbated tissue losses when combined with iatrogenic malnutrition.

Consequences of undernourishment

Change in body composition

Iatrogenic undernourishment contributes to accelerated weight loss in critically ill patients. Although weight loss has essentially been used as a surrogate marker of nutritional status, it cannot distinguish changes of specific tissues such as adipose and lean tissue losses. Moreover, it is an inaccurate representation of losses, given the massive fluid loads and shifts that occur in critically ill patients. Loss of lean tissue, such as skeletal muscle mass, is specifically associated with morbidity, increased length of hospital stay, and mortality.[1-3] From a physiological perspective, muscle atrophy may impair cytokine signalling and result in increased risk of infections[4] and may also impair insulin signalling and result in glucose intolerance.[5,6] Skeletal muscle plays a significant role in immune function and cytokine metabolism[7] and is the largest depot (> 75%) for glucose handling;[8,9] thus, changes in the integrity of skeletal muscle may further complicate the metabolic management of ICU patients. For patients who survive hospitalization, low muscularity would compromise functional status in recovery. Despite that, most of the weight lost during hospitalization is regained within a year following ICU discharge[10] the weight regained is distributed as fat mass, rather than lean tissue,[11] which would compromise recovery of functional status and may also lead to future comorbidities. The potential multifactorial causes of lean tissue losses in critically ill patients include prolonged bed rest,[12] various metabolic disturbances, including pro-inflammation and insulin resistance,[13] as well as undernourishment from low caloric and protein intakes.[14,15] Any combination of these features may attenuate protein synthesis and may simultaneously accelerate protein degradation.

Muscle protein homeostasis

Caloric deficit can lead to significant proteolysis in patients undergoing elective surgery where total body protein losses can reach 16%, with the majority (67%) of this loss comprising skeletal muscle. While there is limited research in this area, it is possible that AMP-activated protein kinase (AMPK), which is an energy sensor that is activated when ATP supply is reduced, may be partly responsible for inducing muscle proteolysis during a caloric deficit.[17] Pasiakos et al. supported this notion with their findings that 80% reduction in caloric intake in weight-stable, physically active, healthy individuals resulted in reduced protein synthesis rates, attributed to reduced muscle AMPK.[18]

Distinct reduction in protein intake leads to inadequate amino acid availability, also known as hypoaminoacidaemia, which can have profound negative effects on protein synthesis.[19] Amino acid availability for protein synthesis is particularly important in facilitating immune and other physiological functions in the critically ill patient. To provide the needed amino acids to build proteins necessary for these functions, skeletal muscle degradation is triggered, compounding the metabolic complications of a critically ill patient. Protein degradation is driven by proteasome and lysosomal systems, whereas calpain and caspase activities are virtually unchanged in critically ill patients.[20,21] A reduction in glutamine[22,23] specifically can negatively alter glutathione status.[24,25] Decreased glutathione concentrations reflect oxidative stress and have a potentially causative role in insulin resistance[26] and increased inflammation.[25] Low glutamine can also impair lymphocyte[27] and monocyte[28] function as well as the ability to use glutamine for glucose production.[29] In contrast, glutamine supplementation may positively influence glucose utilization and reduce infection and pneumonia rates.[30] Increased availability of essential amino acids,[31] particularly leucine, may stimulate MPS, independent of increases in insulin with feeding.[31,32]

Clinical complications

In several studies, negative cumulative energy balance has been associated with increased total number of complications,[33,34] bloodstream infections,[35] ARDS,[33] renal failure,[33] greater length of ICU stay,[34] and more days on MV.[34] Thus, undernourishment has been a significant concern in critically ill patients. Since cumulative energy deficit not only entails hypocaloric intakes, but also encompasses reduced protein intakes, the accelerated loss of lean tissue is expected. With hypocaloric and reduced protein intakes, patient metabolic and energy needs are unmet, leading to impeded recovery. Tsai et al. demonstrated that patients receiving less that 60% of caloric requirements were 2.4 times more likely to die in the first 7 days of ICU admission, demonstrating the vital importance of early nutrition intervention.[36]

Iatrogenic undernourishment

Prevalence

A recent international survey involving more than 150 ICUs further characterized the nature of this problem.[37] In mechanically ventilated patients that remain in ICU for at least 3 days, the majority of patients received EN (67% patients), with EN supplemented with parenteral nutrition (PN) being provided to 16.8% of patients and PN alone only being used in

7.6% of patients. A total of 8.5% of patients did not receive any artificial nutrition. On average, EN was started 46.5 hours after ICU admission (site average ranged from 8.2 to 149.1 hours). Overall, the actual amounts of energy and protein delivered by standard ICU EN protocols was only 45.3% and 42.1%, respectively, and the adoption of strategies to optimize the delivery of EN were low. Only 58.7% and 14.7% patients with high gastric residual volumes received motility agents and small bowel feeding, respectively. Iatrogenic malnutrition and poor compliance with nutrition best practices is a global problem.

Contrasting management strategies and similar clinical outcomes

Contrast these observations with the accumulating evidence that better fed patients have better clinical outcomes. In another international, prospective, observational cohort study of nutrition practices in ICU, Heyland and colleagues analysed the relationship between nutrition intake and subsequent clinical outcomes.[38] It was hypothesized in this study that this relationship may be modified by the premorbid nutritional status of the patient. BMI was used as a surrogate marker of nutritional status prior to ICU admission. Regression models were developed to explore the relationship between nutrition received and 60-day mortality and VFDs and investigate the influence of admission BMI on this relationship. Overall, study patients received a mean of 1034 kcal/day and 47 g protein/day. There was a significant inverse linear relationship between the odds of mortality and total daily calories received. An increase of 1000 calories per day was associated with an overall reduction in mortality (OR for 60-day mortality 0.76, 95% CI 0.61–0.95, $P = 0.014$) and an increase in VFDs (3.5 VFD, 95% CI 1.2–5.9, $P = 0.003$). Similar results were obtained when comparing increasing protein intake and its effect on mortality, but no effect of increasing protein on VFD was observed. The investigators subsequently used the same methodology in a different dataset to demonstrate that 1000 kcal/day or 30 g of protein/day more is also associated with reduced infectious complications.[39]

In contrast, other observational studies suggest that feeding less than goal calories is associated with optimal outcomes.[40,41] Krishnan et al. performed a prospective cohort study of 187 critically ill adult medical patients with an ICU stay of at least 96 hours prior to being able to eat by mouth.[40] Patients were categorized into tertiles, according to percentage levels of energy intake achieved over the entire ICU stay until patients began feeding orally, and no statistical adjustment was made for the widely varying number of days used in the calculation of overall nutritional intake for each patient (range 4–41 days). Patients in the highest tertile (receiving ≥66% of recommended calories) were less likely to be discharged from the hospital alive and to achieve spontaneous ventilation before ICU discharge when compared with patients in the lowest tertile. This is supported by data from Arabi et al. who conducted a post hoc analysis of a dataset of 523 patients from a single centre, investigating the relationship between nutritional intake over the first 7 days and subsequent clinical outcomes. Patients who tolerated >64% of their caloric goal had the highest hospital mortality, higher risk of ICU-acquired infections, and longer lengths of stay, even after adjustment for ICU length of stay and known confounding variables.[41]

Whilst there may be differences in study methods, patients included, and the use of nutrition between the various studies, the discordant results observed are largely explained by the different statistical approach used across studies, in particular, the method of accounting for the duration of exposure to nutrition or length of stay in the ICU. Since most feeding protocols recommend gradually increasing nutrition over the first several days of ICU stay, with little or none given on the first few days, the daily average amount of calories received would be lower for patients with fewer days of artificial nutrition or shorter stays in ICU. Hence, patients discharged alive early after a short stay who received little, if any, feeds may significantly influence the results of these observational analysis. All of the prior analyses have attempted to account for the confounding effect of duration of nutrition exposure by use of sample restriction (e.g. only including patients with a minimum or the same lengths of stay) and/or statistical adjustment through regression models. Thus, the nuanced differences in the methodological approach amongst these studies largely explain the contradictory conclusions.

Optimal calorie delivery

In a prospective, multi-institutional survey of nutrition practices involving 352 ICUs and 7872 mechanically ventilated, critically ill patients who remained in ICU for at least 96 hours, Heyland and colleagues examined the relationship between the amount of calories administered and clinical outcomes and compared different statistical methodologies used in published observational studies, attempting to associate the amount of calories administered and mortality.[42] In the initial unadjusted analysis, a significant association was observed between increased caloric intake and increased mortality (OR 1.28, 95% CI 1.12–1.48 for patients receiving > 2/3 of their caloric prescription vs those receiving < 1/3 of their prescription). When the days after permanent progression to oral intake were excluded, the estimates of harm were attenuated (unadjusted analysis: OR 1.04, 95% CI 0.90–1.20). Restricting the analysis to patients with at least 4 days in ICU prior to progression to oral intake and excluding the days of observation after progression to oral intake resulted in a significant benefit to increased caloric intake (unadjusted OR 0.73, 95% CI 0.63–0.85). When further adjusting for both evaluable days and other important covariates, patients that received > 2/3 of their caloric prescription are much less likely to die than those receiving < 1/3 of their prescription (OR 0.67, 95% CI 0.56–0.79, $P < 0.0001$). When treated as a continuous variable, the overall association between the percentage of caloric prescription received and mortality is highly statistically significant, with increasing calories associated with decreasing mortality ($P < 0.0001$). It would appear from these analyses that the published association between the amount of calories and its relationship to outcome is significantly influenced by data handling in terms of accurate categorization of the data as well as the statistical methodology. The optimal approach suggests that attempting to meet caloric targets (> 80%) is associated with improved clinical outcomes in critically ill patients (see Figure 36.1).

Although observational studies do not define causality, the relationship between nutritional delivery and outcome is supported by the results of RCTs comparing different routes of delivery and timing of feeding[43–45] and a recent trial of supplemental PN.[46] These data are consistent with the data from large-scale observational studies,[38,39,42] indicating enhancing nutritional delivery results in improved clinical and economic outcomes. However, a recent single-center trial of trophic enteral feeding, compared with enteral feeding to goal calories observed no difference in outcomes,[47] whilst another single-centre trial of permissive underfeeding (60–70% caloric goal), compared to feeding 90–100% of caloric goal, concluded that permissive underfeeding may be associated with lower mortality.[48] Interestingly, the average BMI in both these studies was 28–29 kg/m², the average age was in low 50s, and the majority of patients had a short ICU stay (< 5 days), suggesting that younger, overweight patients with short ICU stays do not receive a mortality benefit from goal-directed calories and protein delivery. However, there may be other patient cohorts, such older patients with high or low BMI who have protracted ICU stays, that

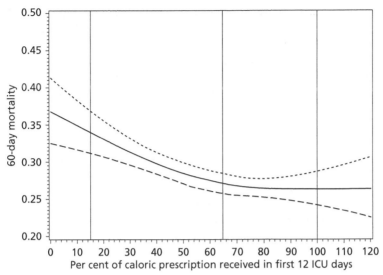

Fig. 36.1 Relationship between hospital mortality at 60 days and 12-day caloric delivery. The solid line is the model fit by a restricted cubic spline, with knots placed at the 5th, 50th, and 95th percentiles. The dashed lines provide 95% confidence bands, and the horizontal lines provide the location of the knots.[42]

Reproduced from Heyland DK, Cahill N, Day A. Optimal amount of calories for critically ill patients: Depends on how you slice the cake! *Critical Care Medicine* 39(12), pp. 2619–2626, copyright 2011, with permission from Wolters Kluwer and the Society of Critical Care Medicine.

benefit from receiving the target amounts of calories and protein. This hypothesis is supported by observational studies that have shown that patients with BMI less than 25 kg/m^2 and greater than 35 kg/m^2 with prolonged stay receive greatest benefit from aggressive nutrition intake.[38,49] Moreover, even if there is no significant mortality benefit, patients receiving targeted feeding regimes possibly exhibit enhanced functional status at ICU discharge.[47] Clinicians must consider functional status at discharge as a key outcome of nutritional intervention, as it is considered that functional status is correlated with muscle mass. This outcome could be much more important in a patient population over the age of 65 years, as sarcopenia is an active process, even before the onset of their critical illness.[43] Nevertheless, these contrasting observations highlight the importance of a thorough nutrition risk assessment at admission to ICU to identify patients that are likely to benefit the most from aggressive feeding or, on the other hand, be harmed the most by iatrogenic underfeeding.

Nutrition risk assessment in critically ill patients

Various screening tools currently exist for use in hospitalized patients that are based on criteria, including: (1) history of unplanned weight loss, (2) decreased oral intake, (3) BMI, (4) severity of acute illness, (5) gastrointestinal symptoms, (6) mobility, and (7) physical assessment.[50–55] None of these screening tools have been developed and validated specifically for the critically ill population. A novel approach to quantifying risk in the critically ill patient is therefore warranted, especially one that accounts for systemic inflammatory response as well as acute and chronic starvation.

Consistent with the definitions of malnutrition by Jensen and colleagues,[56] the NUTrition Risk in the Critically ill score (NUTRIC score) was developed, in which the risk of adverse events that may be modifiable by nutrition therapy were quantified.[57] In a secondary analysis of a prospective observational study, data for key variables considered for inclusion in the score were collected in 598 critically ill patients. Variables included age, baseline APACHE II, baseline sequential organ failure (SOFA) score, number of comorbidities, days from hospital admission to ICU admission, BMI < 20 kg/m², estimated oral intake in the week prior, weight loss in the last 3 months, and serum IL-6, procalcitonin (PCT), and CRP levels. After multivariable modelling, the final NUTRIC score consisted of six variables, including age, baseline APACHE II score, baseline SOFA score, number of comorbidities, days from hospital admission to ICU admission, and serum IL-6. These specific variables were found to be highly predictive of outcomes, such as mortality and duration of MV, with higher NUTRIC scores predicting poor outcome. More importantly, patients with a higher NUTRIC score benefited from meeting their estimated nutrition needs, compared to patients with lower NUTRIC score that did not have any benefit from more nutrition (see Figure 36.2). This novel scoring tool will enable practitioners in identifying the critically ill patients that are more likely to benefit from aggressive nutrition.

Determination of caloric requirements is important on the initial nutritional evaluation, as it enables the calorie requirement goal to be set. This is estimated using simple equations (25–30 kcal/kg per day), more sophisticated predictive equations (such as the Harris–Benedict), or calculated by specific measurement using indirect calorimetry.[58] There is no strong evidence to support any one method of determining protein-energy requirements. It is, however, important that the targets are achieved in a timely fashion.

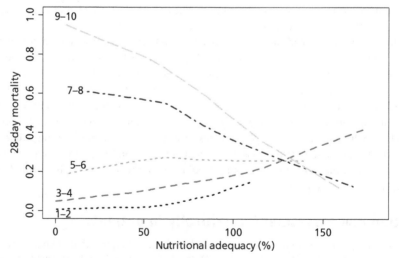

Fig. 36.2 Relationship between NUTRIC score, nutritional adequacy, and 28-day mortality. The NUTRIC scores ranges from 1 to 10. Each line numbered 1–10 represents a patient group with a certain NUTRIC score: 1 = low risk, 10 = high risk. The figures shows that, for patients with a high NUTRIC score, the 28-day mortality decreases with increasing nutritional adequacy, whereas this relationship is not observed in patients with low nutritional adequacy. Nutritional adequacy is defined as the amount of calories received over the amount of calories prescribed.

Strategies to maximize the benefits and minimize the risks of EN

Timing of EN

Enteral feeding is the preferred route of nutrient administration, and the evidence suggests that it should be started as soon as possible after admission to ICU. In critically ill patients, there have been 14 RCTs comparing early EN (started within 24–48 hours of admission to the ICU) to delayed nutrient intake (delayed EN or oral diet).[59] When results from these studies were aggregated, early EN was associated with a trend towards a reduction in mortality (RR 0.60; 95% CIs 0.46, 1.01; $P = 0.06$) and a significant reduction in infectious complications (RR 0.76; 95% CIs 0.59, 0.98; $P = 0.04$) when compared to delayed nutrient intake. Although the mortality results lack statistical significance, these data suggest an improvement in clinical outcome. In addition, a significant increase in nutrient delivery was associated with early enteral feeding.

Before endorsing the concept of early enteral feeding, one must consider the potential risks of such a strategy. Two recent non-randomized studies of early enteral feeding delivered into the stomach was associated with increased complications.[60,61] In contrast, Taylor and colleagues combined an aggressive early feeding protocol with the use of small bowel feedings and observed that head-injured patients fed aggressively, compared to standard (slower) provision of EN, not only had better nutritional status, but also had fewer complications and a more rapid recovery from their illness.[43] Moreover, in a large multicentre observational study, Artinian and colleagues demonstrated that early EN (within 48 hours) was associated with a small increase in pneumonia rates, but notwithstanding these patients who were fed early had a lower mortality rate, compared to patients who received delayed EN.[62] Recent data from the same group suggest that even patients on vasopressors may benefit from early EN. They used a multi-institutional database to identify mechanically ventilated patients on vasopressors and compared the outcomes of those who received early EN to those patient who were received delayed EN, using propensity-matching analysis to adjust for confounding variables.[63] They demonstrated that the group of patients that received early EN had a much lower mortality rate than those that received delayed EN. Moreover, they described that the sickest patients, in particular, those patients on multiple vasopressors, had the greatest benefit. This is the strongest available evidence to support the safety and efficacy of feeding the haemodynamically challenged patient. By no means are we advocating that EN has any role in the unresuscitated, unstable patient, but, once fully resuscitated, EN should be initiated, even if the patient is on inotropes and vasopressors. If there are concerns about tolerating high-volume intragastric nutrition in such patients, either direct jejunal feeding or initiating low-volume feeds (trophic feeds) at 10–20 mL/hour for the first 24 hours, with regular reassessment of absorption rate, should be considered.

Reducing the risk of aspiration: role for small bowel feeding

Aspiration may occur from the antegrade passage of contaminated oropharyngeal secretions or the retrograde passage of contaminated gastric contents into the larynx. Regurgitation occurs more frequently than aspiration.[64] By delivering enteral feeds into the small bowel, beyond the pylorus, the frequency of regurgitation and aspiration, and possibly the risk of pneumonia, is decreased, while, at the same time, nutrient delivery is maximized.[65] There are 11 randomized trials that evaluated the effect of route of feeding on rates of VAP.[66] When these results were aggregated, there was a significant reduction in VAP associated with small bowel feedings (RR 0.77; 95% CIs 0.60, 1.00; $P = 0.05$) compared to gastric feeding. One has to balance this evidence with consideration of the difficulties in obtaining small bowel access, in particular, placement of jejunal tubes. It would not be acceptable to delay initiating of EN for days until small bowel access can be arranged. Given that the majority of patients will absorb intragastric feeds, it seems more prudent to reserve small bowel feeds for patients at high risk for intolerance to EN. This would include patients on high-dose inotropes and vasopressors, prolonged requirement for continuous infusions of sedatives and muscle relaxants, high gastric residual volumes, patients with high nasogastric drainage, and patients at high risk for regurgitation and aspiration, being nursed in a prolonged supine position.[58]

Body position

Several studies document that elevation of the head of the bed is associated with less gastric regurgitation and pulmonary aspiration. An RCT by Drakulovic and colleagues demonstrated that the frequency of pneumonia in critically ill patients managed in the supine position receiving EN into the stomach was associated with a higher risk of pneumonia, compared to feeding patients with the head of the bed elevated to 45° (23% vs 5%; $P < 0.05$).[67] However, van Nieuwenhoven et al.[68] were not able to repeat these findings. In particular, these investigators were not able to achieve 45° elevation in the intervention group, and the supine group was nursed at approximately 20°. Although these methodological issues may explain, in part, the negative findings associated with this study, a pragmatic approach is to elevate the head of the bed to an angle of between 30° and 45° to reduce the risks associated with enteral feedings.

Motility agents

Gastrointestinal prokinetic agents improve gastric emptying, improve tolerance to EN, reduce gastro-oesophageal reflux and pulmonary aspiration and therefore may have the potential to improve outcomes in critically ill patients.[69] While no study has demonstrated an impact from the use of these agents on clinical outcomes, their low probability of harm and favourable feasibility and cost considerations warrant their use as a strategy to optimize nutritional intake and minimize regurgitation. Due to concerns of bacterial resistance with the use of the macrolide antibiotic erythromycin, metoclopramide is preferable. It can be prescribed with the initiation of enteral feeds or reserved for patients who experience persistently high gastric residuals. It can be discontinued after four doses if there is no benefit observed or when tolerance to EN is established. For refractory cases, metoclopramide can be used, in combination with erythromycin, with good effect.[70] Reducing narcotic drug doses may also be effective in improving gastric function and tolerance to EN while reducing risk of aspiration.

Feeding protocols

Several observational studies document that EN is frequently interrupted for reasons related to gastrointestinal intolerance, such as high gastric residual volumes, nausea, and vomiting, and interruptions related to essential procedures.[71] Over the duration of the ICU stay, these interruptions result in inadequate delivery of EN, with associated complications of inadequate nutrition. Nurse-directed feeding protocols have been shown to increase daily EN delivered[72] and include the use of motility agents in response to gastrointestinal intolerance and minimize interruptions. Withholding EN is a controversial subject, but recent studies have shown that inappropriately low cessation thresholds provide no protection against gastric aspiration. Higher thresholds (> 400 mL/hour gastric residual volume) appear as safe as lower thresholds (< 250 mL/hour gastric residual volume).[73,74] Second-generation protocols, such as the PEP uP protocol, have been shown to be very effective in achieving goal calories and protein by the second day of ICU admission.[75]

Use of combined EN and PN

Whilst EN is the preferred method for providing nutrition intake, some critically ill patients will not tolerate adequate amounts of EN to reach their nutritional needs. To increase protein and calorie intake in these patients, some practitioners may prescribe supplemental PN. However, there has been considerable controversy regarding the timing of supplemental PN in the critical care setting. Guideline recommendations range from continued underfeeding with EN alone for up to 7–10 days[76] to the addition of supplemental PN within 24–48 hours in patients who are expected to be intolerant of EN within 72 hours of admission.[77] Data have demonstrated the adverse clinical outcome of cumulative energy deficit and caloric debt has to be balanced against the adverse events experienced in patients who receive PN during their ICU stay,[33–35] with a recent observational study and RCT failing to support the use of PN.[78,79] Despite this, it is not clear whether 'supplemental PN' should be added to 'insufficient EN' early in the course of nutritionally high-risk patients such as those patients with a low BMI. There are ongoing trials that will address this important question.[80,81]

The synergistic effects of nutrition and rehabilitation

Short-term immobilization can have profound effects on skeletal muscle wasting, an effect which is potentially exacerbated by iatrogenic malnutrition. Following 14 days of immobilization in healthy individuals, MPS is reduced, regardless of elevated amino acid availability, indicating that muscle anabolism is inhibited.[82,83] Thus, not only does bed rest result in a disturbance of muscle mass homeostasis, with a consequent loss in muscle loss at a rate of 1.5–2% per day during the first 2–3 weeks, but muscle has a resultant inability to utilize circulating amino acids for protein synthesis. This has been termed as anabolic resistance. However, there is evidence to suggest that essential amino acid supplementation during prolonged bed rest can stimulate protein synthesis and this physiological targeting of the anabolic signalling network, rather than targeting individualized components, may have a beneficial outcome in terms of limiting, or even preventing, muscle loss.[84] Merging nutrition and rehabilitation as synergistic strategies may further limit loss in muscle mass during critical illness. Further details can be found in Chapters 37 and 45.

In health, exercise can promote positive protein balance and insulin sensitivity.[85–87] For clinical populations, exercise also presents the benefit of reducing systemic inflammation. For example, although IL-6 is commonly associated with muscle atrophy, it is also elevated with exercise and works to counter the muscle wasting effects of TNF-α, CRP, and IL-1 while increasing anti-inflammatory mediators like IL-10.[88] The exercise-related rise in IL-6 is also linked to insulin-sensitizing effects on muscle following exercise.[2] While these physiological benefits have not been explored in critical care, early mobilization in critically ill patients has demonstrated reduced length of ICU and hospital stay,[89] as well as increased physical function at discharge, highlighting the potential beneficial effects on skeletal muscle.[90–95]

Several forms of rehabilitation or exercise have been used in the hospital setting to assess its benefits on clinical outcomes;[96] these include EMS,[89–91,97] PT,[96] and cycle ergometry,[88,93,94,98] the latter two having been assessed in critically ill patients. The use of passive and active range-of-motion exercises that were progressively followed by bedside functioning training and ambulation resulted in improved physical and respiratory function.[96] In this study, 53% of patients were able to complete a 2-minute walk test at 6 weeks, whereas there were no patients in the usual care group that could perform this task at 6 weeks.[96] The most impressive protocols and findings stem from studies that used bedside cycle ergometry for passive assisted exercise.[88,93,94] Morris et al.[88] demonstrated improvements in the number of days to the first day out of bed as well as improved ICU and hospital length of stay in the group who underwent cycle ergometry, compared to those patients who received usual care. However, these early mobilization studies have largely ignored nutritional status and nutrition intake. Furthermore, in those studies that have documented nutritional intake, this has been inadequate, with patients receiving only 34–37% of their prescribed nutritional requirement.[88,92]

Conclusion

Malnutrition adversely affects physiological and clinical outcomes. Although iatrogenic under-nourishment is widespread across the globe and occurs in many patients following admission to intensive care, data are available that demonstrate delivery of between 80 and 90% nutritional requirement in a subset of these ICUs.[37] Achieving 80–90% nutritional delivery is therefore achievable and is associated with the beneficial physiological and clinical outcomes.[42] Strategies to maximize these benefits as well as minimize the risk of EN are essential. These should include early initiation of EN (within 24–48 hours), adoption of second-generation feeding protocols (PEP uP protocol), use of motility agents, small bowel feeding tubes, and elevation of the head of the bed. Given the positive results on early mobilization, it could be hypothesized that combining early mobilization and nutrition interventions would limit muscle mass loss and maintaining muscle integrity and function. We have learned from the discipline of sports medicine that the interactions between sports nutrition and exercise are powerful interventions to optimizing size, function, and metabolism of muscle. Although adaptations are required to accommodate the effect of critical illness on skeletal muscle structure and biology, these lessons can be translated to the critically ill population to improve clinical outcomes and recovery.

References

1 **Gruther W, Benesch T, Zorn C, et al.** Muscle wasting in intensive care patients: ultrasound observed of m. quadriceps femoris muscle layer. *J Rehabil Med* 2008;**40**:185–9.

2 **Lightfoot A, McArdle A, Griffiths RD.** Muscle in defense. *Crit Care Med* 2009;**37**:S384–90.

3 **Mourtzakis M, Fan C, Heyland DK.** Skeletal muscle measured at the time of ICU admission may be a determinant of clinical outcomes. Abstract. *Critical Care Canada Forum* 2009.

4 **Cosquéric G, Sebag A, Ducolombier C, Thomas C, Piette F, Weill-Engerer S.** Sarcopenia is predictive of nosocomial infection in care of the elderly. *Br J Nutr* 2006;**96**:895–901.

5 **Blanc S, Normand S, Pachiaudi C, Fortrat JO, Laville M, Gharib C.** Fuel homeostasis during physical inactivity induced by bed rest. *J Clin Endocrinol Metab* 2000;**85**:2223–33.

6 **Mikines KJ, Richter EA, Dela F, Galbo H.** Seven days of bed rest decrease inuslin action on glucose uptake in leg and whole body. *J Appl Physiol* 1991;**70**:1245–54.

7 **Brandt C and Pedersen BK.** The role of exercise-induced myokines in muscle homeostasis and the defense against chronic diseases. *J Biomed Biotechnol* 2010;**2010**:520258.

8 **DeFronzo RA, Jacot E, Jequier E, Wahren J, Felber JP.** The effect of insulin on the disposal of intravenous glucose: results from indirect calorimetry and hepatic and femoral venous catheterization. *Diabetes* 1981;**30**:1000–7.

9 **Shulman GI, Rothman DL, Jue T, Stein P, DeFronzo RA, Shulman RG.** Quantitation of muscle glycogen synthesis in normal subjects and subjects with non-insulin dependent diabetes by ^{13}C nuclear magnetic resonance spectroscopy. *N Engl J Med* 1990;**322**:223–8.

10 Herridge MS, Cheung AM, Tansey CM, et al; Canadian Critical Care Trials Group. One-year outcomes in survivors of the acute respiratory distress syndrome. *N Engl J Med* 2003;**348**:683–93.

11 Reid CL, Murgatroyd PR, Wright A, Menon DK. Quantification of lean and fat tissue repletion following critical illness: a case report. *Critical Care* 2008;**12**:R79.

12 Brower RG. Consequence of bed rest. *Crit Care Med* 2009;**37**:S422–8.

13 Glass DJ. Signaling pathways perturbing muscle mass. *Curr Opin Clin Nutr Metab Care* 2010;**13**:225–9.

14 Rubinson L, Diette GB, Song X, Brower RG, Krishnan JA. Low caloric intake is associated with nosocomial bloodstream infections in patients in the medical intensive care unit. *Crit Care Med* 2004;**32**:350–7.

15 Heyland DK, Schroter-Noppe D, Drover JW, et al. Nutrition support in the critical care setting: current practice in canadian ICUs—opportunities for improvement? *JPEN J Parenter Enteral Nutr* 2003;**27**:74–83.

16 Monk DN, Plank LD, Franch-Arcas G, Finn PJ, Streat SJ, Hill GL. Sequential changes in the metabolic response in critically injured patients during the first 25 days after blunt trauma.*Ann Surg* 1996;**223**:395–405.

17 Bolster DR, Crozier SJ, Kimball SR, Jefferson LS. AMP-activated protein kinase suppresses protein synthesis in rat skeletal muscle through down-regulated mammalian target of rapamycin (mTOR) signaling. *J Biol Chem* 2002;**27**:23977–80.

18 Pasiakos SM, Vislocky LM, Carbone JW, et al. Acute energy deprivation affects skeletal muscle protein synthesis and associated intracellular signaling proteins in physically active adults. *J Nutr* 2010;**140**: 745–51.

19 Kobayashi H, Børsheim E, Anthony TG, et al. Reduced amino acid availability inhibits muscle protein synthesis and decreases activity of initiation factor eIF2B. *Am J Physiol Endocrinol Metab* 2003;**284**: 488–98.

20 Klaude M, Mori M, Tjäder I, Gustafsson T, Wernerman J, Rooyackers O. Protein metabolism and gene expression in skeletal muscle of critically ill patients with sepsis. *Clin Sci (Lond)* 2011;**122**:133–42.

21 Klaude M, Fredriksson K, Tjäder I, et al. Proteasome proteolytic activity in skeletal muscle is increased in patients with sepsis. *Clin Sci* 2007;**112**:499–506.

22 Luo JL, Hammarqvist F, Andersson K, Wernerman J. Surgical trauma decreases glutathione synthetic capacity in human skeletal muscle tissue. *Am J Physiol Endocrinol Metab* 1998;**275**:359–65.

23 Gamrin L, Essen P, Forsberg AM, Hultman E, Wernerman J. A descriptive study of skeletal muscle metabolism in critically ill patients: Free amino acids, energy-rich phosphates, protein, nucleic acids, fat, water, and electrolytes. *Crit Care Med* 1996;**24**:575–83.

24 Biolo G, Antonione R, De Cicco M. Glutathione metabolism in sepsis. *Crit Care Med* 2007;**35**:S591–5.

25 Reid M, Badaloo A, Forrester T, et al. In vivo rates of erythrocyte glutathione synthesis in children with severe protein-energy malnutrition. *Am J Physiol Endocrinol Metab* 2000;**278**:405–12.

26 Khamaisi M, Kavel O, Rosenstock M, et al. Effect of inhibition of glutathione synthesis on insulin action: in vivo and in vitro studies using buthionine sulfoximine. *Biochem J* 2000;**349**:579–86.

27 Juretic A, Spagnoli GC, Hörig H, et al. Glutamine requirements in the generation of lumphokine-activated killer cells. *Clin Nutr* 1994;**13**:42–9.

28 Spittler A, Winkler S, Götzinger P, et al. Influence of glutamine on the phyenotype and function of human monocytes. *Blood* 1995;**86**:1564–9.

29 Meyer C, Woerle HJ, Gerich J. Paradoxical changes of muscle glutamine release during hyperinsulinemia euglycemia and hypoglycemia in humans: further evidence for the glucose-glutamine cycle. *Metabolism* 2004;**53**:1208–14.

30 Déchelotte P, Hasselmann M, Cynober L, et al. L-alanyl-L-glutamine dipeptide-supplemented total parenteral nutrition reduces infectious complications and glucose intolerance in critically ill patients: the French controlled, ramdomized, double-blind, multi-center study. *Crit Care Med* 2006;**34**:598–604.

31 Cuthbertson D, Smith K, Babraj J, et al. Anabolic signaling deficits underlie amino acid resistance of wasting, aging muscle. *FASEB J* 2005;**19**:422–44.

32 Vary T, Lynch CJ. Nutrient signaling components controlling protein synthesis in striated muscle. *J Nutr* 2007;**137**:1835–43.

33 Dvir D, Cohen J, Singer P. Computerized energy balance and complications in critically ill patients: an observational study *Clin Nutr* 2006;**25**:37–44.

34 Villet S, Chiolero RL, Bollmann MD, et al. Negative impact of hypocaloric feeding and energy balance on clinical outcome in ICU patients. *Clin Nutr* 2005;**24**:502–9.

35 Rubinson L, Diette GB, Song X, Brower RG, Krishnan JA. Low caloric intake is associated with nosocomial bloodstream infections in patients in the medical intensive care unit. *Crit Care Med* 2004;**32**:350–7.

36 Tsai JR, Chang WT, Sheu CC, et al. Inadequate energy delivery during early critical illness correlates with increased risk of mortality in patients who survive at least seven days: a retrospective study. *Clin Nutr* 2011;**30**:209–14.

37 Jones N, Dhaliwal RD, Day A, Jiang X, Heyland DK. Nutrition therapy in the critical care setting: What is 'Best Achievable' practice? An international multicenter observational study. *Crit Care* 2010;**38**:395–401.

38 Alberda C, Gramlich L, Jones N, et al. The relationship between nutritional intake and clinical outcomes in critically ill patients: results of an international multicenter observational study. *Intensive Care Med* 2009;**35**:1728–37.

39 Heyland DK, Stephens KE, Day AG, McClave SA. The success of enteral nutrition and ICU-acquired infections: a multicenter observational study. *Clin Nutr* 2011;**30**:148–55.

40 Krishnan JA, Parce PB, Martinez A, Diette GB, Brower RG. Caloric intake in medical ICU patients: consistency of care with guidelines and relationship to clinical outcomes. *Chest* 2003;**124**:297–305.

41 Arabi YM, Haddad SH,Tamim HM, et al. Near-target caloric intake in critically ill medical-surgical patients is associated with adverse outcomes. *JPEN J Parenter Enteral Nutr* 2010;**34**;280.

42 Heyland DK, Cahill N, Day A. Optimal amount of calories for critically ill patients: Depends on how you slice the cake! *Crit Care Med* 2011;**39**:2619–26.

43 Taylor SJ, Fettes SB, Jewkes C, Nelson RJ. Prospective, randomized, controlled trial to determine the effect of early enhanced enteral nutrition on clinical outcome in mechanically ventilated patients suffering head injury. *Crit Care Med* 1999;**27**:2525–31.

44 Martin CM, Doig GS, Heyland DK, Morrison T, Sibbald WJ. Multicenter, cluster-randomized clinical trial of algorithms for critical-care enteral and parenteral therapy (ACCEPT). *CMAJ* 2004;**170**:197–204.

45 McClave SA, Heyland DK. The physiologic response and associated clinical benefits from provision of early enteral nutrition. *Nutr Clin Pract* 2009;**24**:305–15.

46 Singer P, Anbar R, Cohen J, et al. The tight calorie control study (TICACOS): a prospective, randomized, controlled pilot study of nutritional support in critically ill patients *Intensive Care Med* 2011;**37**:601–9.

47 Rice T, Mogan S, Hays MA, Bernard GR, Jensen GL, Wheeler AP. Randomized trial of initial trophic versus full-energy enteral nutrition in mechanically ventilated patients with acute respiratory failure *Crit Care Med* 2011;**39**:967–74.

48 Arabi Y M, Tamin HM, Dhar GS, et al. Permissive underfeeding and intensive insulin therapy in critically ill patients:a randomized controlled trial *Am J Clin Nutr* 2011;**93**:569–77.

49 Faisy C, Lerolle N, Dachraoui F, et al. Impact of energy deficit calculated by a predictive method on outcome in medical patients requiring prolonged acute mechanical ventilation. *Br J Nutr* 2009;**101**:1079–87.

50 Detsky AS, McLaughlin JR, Baker JP, et al. What is subjective global assessment of nutritional status? 1987. Classical article. *Nutr Hosp* 2008;**23**:400–7.

51 **Malnutrition Advisory Group.** A consistent and reliable tool for malnutrition screening. Nurs Times 2003;**99**:26–7.

52 **Nestle Nutrition Institute.** *MNA® mini nutritional assessment.* Available at: http://www.mna-elderly.com (accessed October 2010).

53 **Kruizenga HM, Seidell JC, de Vet HC, Wierdsma NJ, van Bokhorst-de van derSchueren MA.** Development and validation of a hospital screening tool for malnutrition: the short nutritional assessment questionnaire (SNAQ). *Clin Nutr* 2005;**24**:75–82.

54 **Ferguson M, Capra S, Bauer J, Banks M.** Development of a valid and reliable malnutrition screening tool for adult acute hospital patients. *Nutrition* 1999;**15**:458–64.

55 **Lim SL, Tong CY, Ang E, et al.** Development and validation of 3-Minute Nutrition Screening (3-MinNS) tool for acute hospital patients in Singapore. *Asia Pac J Clin Nutr* 2009;**18**:395–403.

56 **Jensen GL, Mirtallo J, Compher C, et al.**; International Consensus Guideline Committee. Adult starvation and disease-relatedmalnutrition: a proposal for etiology-based diagnosis in the clinical practicesetting from the International Consensus Guideline Committee. *JPEN J ParenterEnteral Nutr* 2010;**34**:156–9.

57 **Heyland DK, Dhaliwal R, Jiang X, Day A.** Quantifying nutrition risk in the critically ill patient: The development and initial validation of a novel risk assessment tool. *Crit Care* 2011;**15**:R268.

58 **Boullata J, Williams J, Cottrell F, Hudson L, Compher C.** Accurate determination of energy needs in hospitalized patients. *J Am Diet Assoc* 2007;**107**:393–401.

59 **Critical Care Nutrition.** *Clinical practice guidelines.* Available at: http://www.criticalcarenutrition.com/ index.php?option=com_content&view=article&id=18&Itemid=10 (accessed 3 October 2011).

60 **Ibrahim EH, Mehringer L, Prentice D, et al.** Early versus late enteral feeding of mechanically ventilated patients: Results of a clinical trial. *JPEN* 2002;**26**:174–81.

61 **Mentec H, Dupont H, Bocchetti M, Cani P, Ponche F, Bleichner G.** Upper digestive intolerance during enteral nutrition in critically ill patients: frequency, risk factors, and complications. *Crit Care Med* 2001;**29**:1955–96.

62 **Artinian V, Krayem H, DiGiovine B.** Effects of early enteral feeding on the outcome of critically ill mechanically ventilated medical patients. *Chest* 2006;**129**:960–7.

63 **Khalid I, Doshi P, DiGiovine B.** Early enteral nutrition and outcomes of critically ill patients treated with vasopressors and mechanical ventilation. *Am J Crit Care* 2010;**19**:261–8.

64 **Lukan JK, McClave SA, Stefater AJ, et al: Poor validity of residual volumes as a marker for risk of aspiration.** *Amer J Clin Nutrit* 2002;75:417–18S.

65 **Heyland DK, Drover JW, MacDonald S, Novak F, Lam M.** Effect of postpyloric feeding on gastroesophageal regurgitation and pulmonary microaspiration: results of a randomized controlled trial. *Crit Care Med* 2001;**29**:1495–501.

66 **Critical Care Nutrition.** *Clinical practice guidelines.* Available at: http://www.criticalcarenutrition.com/ index.php?option=com_content&view=article&id = 18&Itemid=10 (accessed: 23 March 2011).

67 **Drakulovic MB, Torres A, Bauer TT, Nicolas JM, Nogue S, Ferrer M.** Supine body position as a risk factor for nosocomial pneumonia in mechanically ventilated patients: a randomised trial. *Lancet* 1999;**354**:1851–8.

68 **van Nieuwenhoven CA, Vandenbroucke-Grauls C, van Tiel FH, et al.** Feasibility and effects of the semirecumbent position to prevent ventilator-associated pneumonia: a randomized study.*Crit Care Med* 2006;**34**:396–402.

69 **Booth CM, Heyland DK, Paterson WG.** Gastrointestinal promotility drugs in the critical care setting: A systematic review of the evidence. *Crit Care Med* 2002;**30**:1429–35.

70 **Nguyen NQ, Chapman M, Fraser RJ, Bryant LK, Burgstad C, Holloway RH.** Prokinetic therapy for feed intolerance in critical illness: one drug or two? *Crit Care Med* 2007;**35**:2561–7.

71 Heyland DK, Konopad E, Alberda C, Keefe L, Cooper C, Cantwell B. How well do critically ill patients tolerate early, intragastric enteral feeding? Results of a prospective multicenter trial. *Nutr Clin Pract* 1999;**14**:23–8.

72 Heyland DK, Cahill NE, Dhaliwal R, Sun X, Day AG, McClave SA. Impact of enteral feeding protocols on enteral nutrition delivery: results of a multicenter observational study. *JPEN J Parenter Enteral Nutr* 2010;**34**:675–84.

73 Montejo JC, Miñambres E, Bordejé L, et al. Gastric residual volume during enteral nutrition in ICU patients: the REGANE study. *Intensive Care Med* 2010;**36**:1386–93.

74 McClave SA, Lukan JK, Stefater JA, et al. Poor validity of residual volumes as a marker for risk of aspiration in critically ill patients. *Crit Care Med* 2005;**33**:324–30.

75 Heyland DK, Cahill NE, Dhaliwal R, et al. Enhanced protein-energy provision via the enteral route in critically ill patients: a single center feasibility trial of the PEP uP protocol. *Crit Care* 2010;**14**:R78.

76 McClave SA, Martindale RG, Vanek VW, et al. Guidelines for the provision and assessment of nutrition support therapy in the adult critically ill patient: Society of Critical Care MEdicien (SCCM) and Americal Society for Enteral and Parenteral Nutrition (ASPEN). *J PEN* 2009;**33**:277–316.

77 Singer P, Berger MM, Van den Berghe G, et al. Parenteral Nutrition in the ICU: Guidelines. *Clin Nutr* 2009;**28**:387–400.

78 Casaer MP, Mesotten D, Hermans G, et al. Early versus late parenteral nutrition in critically ill adults. *N Engl J Med* 2011;**365**:506–17.

79 Kutsogiannis J, Alberda C, Gramlich L, et al. Early use of supplemental parenteral nutrition in critically ill patients: Results of an international multicenter observational study. *Crit Care Med* 2011;**39**: 2691–9.

80 ClinicalTrials.gov. *Trial of supplemental parenteral nutrition in under and over weight critically ill patients (TOP-UP).* Available at: http://www.clinicaltrials.gov/ct2/show/NCT01206166. NLM Identifier: NCT01206166.

81 ClinicalTrials.gov. *Impact of SPN on infection rate, duration of mechanical ventilation and rehabilitation in ICU patients.* Available at: http://www.clinicaltrials.gov/ct2/show/NCT00802503. NLM Identifier: NCT00802503.

82 Glover EI, Phillips SM, Oates BR, et al. Immobilization induces anabolic resistance in human myofibrillar protein synthesis with low and high dose amino acid infusion. *J Physiol* 2008;**586**:6049–61.

83 Biolo G, Beniamino C, Lebenstedt M, et al. Short-term bed rest impairs amino acid-induced protein anabolism in humans. *J Physiol* 2004;**558**:381–8.

84 Paddon-Jones D, Sheffield-Moore M, Urban RJ, et al. Essential amino acid and carbohydrate supplementation ameliorates muscle protein loss in humans during 28 days bedrest. *J Clin Endocrinol Metab* 2004;**89**:4351–8.

85 Biolo G, Williams BD, Fleming RYD, Wolfe RR. Insulin action on muscle protein kinetics and amino acid transport during recovery after resistance exercise. *Diabetes* 1999;**48**:949–57.

86 Ferrando AA, Tipton KD, Bamman MM, Wolfe RR. Resistance exercise maintains skeletal muscle protein synthesis during bed rest. *J Appl Physiol* 1997;**82**:807–10.

87 Richter EA, Mikines KJ, Galbo H, Kiens B. Effect of exercise on insulin action in human skeletal muscle. *J Appl Physiol* 1989;**66**:876–85.

88 Price SR, Mitch WE. Mechanisms stimulating protein degradation to cause muscle atrophy. *Curr Opin Clin Nutr Metab Care* 1998;**1**:79–83.

89 Morris PE, Goad A, Thompson C, et al. Early intensive care unit mobility therapy in the treatment of acute respiratory failure. *Crit Care Med* 2008;**36**:2238–43.

90 Zanotti E, Felicetti G, Maini M, Fracchia C. Peripheral muscle strength training in bed-bound patients with COPD receiving mechanical ventilation: effect of electrical stimulation. *Chest* 2003;**124**: 292–6.

91 Vivodtzev I, Pépin JL, Vottero G, et al. Improvement in quadriceps strength and dyspnea in daily tasks after 1 month of electrical stimulation in severely deconditioned and malnourished COPD. *Chest* 2006;**129**:1540–8.

92 Nuhr MJ, Pette D, Berger R, et al. Beneficial effects of chronic low-frequency stimulation of thigh muscles in patients with advanced chronic heart failure. *Eur Heart J* 2004;**25**:136–43.

93 Schweickert WD, Pohlman MC, Pohlman AS, et al. Early physical and occupational therapy in mechanically ventilated, critically ill patients: a randomized controlled trial. *Lancet* 2009;**373**:1874–82.

94 Burtin C, Clerckx B, Robbeets C, et al. Early exercise in critically ill patients enhances short-term functional recovery. *Crit Care Med* 2009;**37**:2499–505.

95 Needham D, Truong AD, Fan E. Technology to enhance physical rehabilitation of critically ill patients. *Crit Care Med* 2009;**37**:S436–41.

96 Gibson JN, Smith K, Rennie MJ. Prevention of disuse muscle atrophy by means of electrical stimulation: maintenance of protein synthesis. *Lancet* 1988;**2**:767–70.

97 Chiang LL, Wang LY, Wu CP, Wu HD, Wu YT. Effects of physical training on functional status in patients with prolonged mechanical ventilation. *Phys Ther* 2006;**86**:1271–81.

98 Porta R, Vitacca M, Gilè LS, et al. Supported arm training in patients recently weaned from mechanical ventilation. *Chest* 2005;**128**:2511–20.

Part 6

Therapeutic and Rehabilitation Strategies in the ICU

Chapter 37

Introduction: Therapeutic and Rehabilitation Strategies in the ICU

Nicholas Hart

In recent years, there has been a substantial change in the approach of the clinician toward the critically ill patient. Previously, the critical care team has been wholly focused on the preservation of life, but attention has now shifted to include both the intermediate and the long-term outcome of an expanding cohort of complex patients. Seminal work evaluating the physical consequences of critical illness (see Chapters 23 and 24, respectively) has driven clinical researchers to develop methods to diagnose critical illness-induced neuromyopathic dysfunction, which is a major factor determining long-lasting impairment in physical function. Recent work has been directed toward developing strategies that will improve muscle weakness and subsequently enhance physical performance.

Although one would rationally consider the use of passive muscle exercises and active exercise therapy early in the course of critical illness to be clinically useful in limiting critical illness-induced muscle wasting and weakness, there is a biological, as well as clinical logistic, reason for opposing such a treatment strategy. From a biological viewpoint, the use of passive or active mobilization during early critical illness may be ineffective, or even harmful, to the muscle, as this is a time when the muscle is exposed to increased MPB and reduced MPS, combined with a loss in mitochondrial function, all of which may result in anabolic resistance (see Chapter 35). Furthermore, it is a major task to undertake exercise therapy in the critically ill patient early in the course of critical illness when there is cardiovascular and respiratory instability, with a complete dependence on organ support systems. Despite these concerns, observational data have demonstrated an adequate safety profile of performing early mobilization therapy within the ICU, albeit that there are still inherent personnel as well as non-personnel barriers to providing these physical treatments. In addition to confirming the safety profile of exercise therapy as an intervention, clinical trial data support the use of exercise therapy early in the course of critical illness to improve functional outcome. These data have not only driven the revolution in the management of critically ill patients, but, by necessity, they have led to a greater collaborative multidisciplinary environment to facilitate the delivery of care, with integration of efforts between physicians, nurses, and physical and occupational therapists.

These approaches have been integrated into the other established strategies, which have aimed to reduce the morbidity of critical illness. Regarding liberation from invasive mechanical ventilation (IMV), there are data to support both reduction in PSV and SBTs as the most clinically effective modes to effect weaning (see Chapter 39). These strategies may be particularly effective when combined with sedation-sparing (see Chapter 40) and sleep-promoting strategies (see Chapter 41). Although the primary goal of insulin therapy was to mitigate the effects of stress hyperglycaemia during critical illness, it has been shown that anabolic and anti-catabolic actions of insulin facilitate preservation of the neuromuscular integrity. This represents an important beneficial long-term 'side effect' that clinicians should weigh carefully when considering gly-caemic management strategies and their limitations. Other clinical strategies that have indirect actions on muscle function include the use of RRT, which has been shown to reduce the risk of muscle weakness, consistent with studies indicating the toxic effect on muscle in chronic renal failure of the accumulation of renally excreted waste products. Finally, neuromuscular stimulation has been shown to have a direct action in reducing muscle wasting in critically ill populations, but results of large clinical trials are needed before recommending this as a treatment.

Chapter 38

Choice of Renal Replacement Therapy and Renal Recovery

Antoine G. Schneider, Neil J. Glassford, and Rinaldo Bellomo

Introduction

Severe AKI is a major complication of critical illness, with an incidence of 5.7% in a recent multicentre study of close to 30 000 patients.[1] Severe AKI is associated with major metabolic disturbances, such as metabolic acidosis, hyperkalaemia, or fluid overload, that, if left untreated, might lead to death. Therefore, treatment in the form of RRT is sometimes necessary.

RRT relies on two different physical principles: convection and diffusion. These two principles can be used separately (haemofiltration or haemodialysis) or in combination (haemodiafiltration). More importantly and more relevant to clinical practice, RRT can be applied continuously or intermittently. Continuous modern therapies applied in intensive care include continuous veno-venous haemofiltration (CVVH) and continuous veno-venous haemodiafiltration (CVVHDF), while intermittent therapy includes IHD and sustained low-efficiency dialysis (SLED).

Both intermittent and continuous therapies achieve a degree of metabolic control, and, to date, despite numerous observational studies and RCTs[2–9] and two meta-analyses,[2,10] no modality has been shown superior to the other in terms of in-hospital mortality. However, some data suggest that CRRT could be associated with better renal recovery and less long-term RRT dependency. Since long-term RRT dependency is associated with high costs and decreased QoL, such an outcome difference could be very important.

In this chapter, we present physiological and experimental evidence suggesting that renal recovery might be better with CRRT as opposed to IHD.

Evidence from basic science and clinical studies

RBF and GFR are normally autoregulated when systemic mean arterial pressure (MAP) is between 70 and 100 mmHg. This autoregulation is dependent on the sodium chloride concentration in the macula densa.[11] A decrease in this concentration triggers an increased secretion of renin and activation of the RAS, which acts to increase systemic blood pressure and to induce efferent arteriolar vasoconstriction. Simultaneously, the resistance in the afferent arterioles is decreased. Both these effects aim to maintain RBF and GFR.

In the setting of AKI, however, as demonstrated by Kelleher et al.[12] in an animal model, autoregulation of RBF is lost, and decreases in systolic blood pressure are associated with marked decreases in RBF and inulin clearance (a marker of GFR). Biopsies taken after moderate hypotension (within the normal autoregulation range) revealed areas of tubular necrosis, consistent with fresh tubular damage. These findings were consistent with those of other models[13,14] and with further work showning that abnormal post-ischaemic vascular reactivity can be seen in different models of ischaemic AKI.[15]

Hypotension is a common event during IHD. In patients with AKI, it has been reported to occur in 20–50% of all acute IHD treatments and results in the interruption of the treatment in 5–10% of the cases.[16–19] This is particularly true in AKI in critical illness, as illustrated by the Acute Renal Failure Trial Network (ATN) trial,[20] which will be discussed in details later. In this study, 37% of the IHD sessions were complicated by hypotension. Given the experimental findings, it seems biologically plausible that repeated episodes of hypotension, as induced by repeated IHD sessions, might compromise the recovery of kidneys that have lost their blood flow regulation. This notion is further supported by work by Conger et al.[21] These investigators performed renal biopsies 3–4 weeks after the initial insults in a group of soldiers receiving IHD for AKI. Histological examination revealed areas of fresh tubular necrosis, which seemed to only be logically explained by the multiple hypotensive episodes that occurred during the treatment.

In addition to hypotension, IHD can also trigger a reduction in cardiac index in the first hour[22] as well as an increased oxygen consumption.[23] Both these effects can delay or compromise renal recovery. For all these reasons, in the context of RRT, to optimize the chances of renal recovery, it would seem wise to choose a modality that can limit haemodynamic instability. Several clinical studies provide evidence that this may be true in man.

Clinical studies presenting renal recovery data

Data from clinical studies are summarized in Table 38.1. The first clinical study (see Figure 38.1), suggesting a difference in renal recovery between the two modalities, was reported in 2001 by Mehta et al.[24] These investigators reported the result of an RCT in which patients with AKI were randomly assigned to either CRRT or IHD. This study was designed and powered to demonstrate an expected decrease in mortality of 27% in the CRRT arm. Overall, 718 patients were screened and 166 randomized. Despite the fact that randomization failed to deliver balance of allocation (patients allocated to CRRT were more severely ill, according to APACHE scoring), renal recovery seemed better in those survivors who had received CRRT. On intention-to-treat analysis, 17% of patients in the IHD arm had some degree of chronic renal impairment at hospital discharge or death, as compared with only 4% of those treated with CRRT ($P = 0.01$). Moreover, 92.3% of patients only receiving CRRT, with no crossover to IHD, achieved complete renal recovery, as compared with 59.4% of those treated with only IHD ($P < 0.01$). The initial choice of therapy was also crucial: 44.7% of those crossing from CRRT to IHD achieved complete renal recovery, as compared with only 6.7% of those swapping from IHD to CRRT ($P < 0.01$).

The study described in the previous paragraph provides strong evidence that IHD delays renal recovery. However, it also carries several important limitations. The randomized process was not successful, since patients randomized to CRRT had higher illness severity scores, included significantly more males than female and more patients with limitations of medical therapy, and the IHD group included more patients with chronic renal failure (P not significant). The design of the study similarly allowed for crossovers, and many patients did not get the treatment to which they were randomized, which makes interpretation of the data difficult. However, the difference in renal recovery was striking and of great concern.

A small Canadian retrospective observational study on 93 critically ill patients requiring RRT was published by Jacka et al. in 2005.[25] In this study, only 13% of the patients that received CRRT remained RRT-dependent at hospital discharge vs 63% of those that received IHD. These results

Table 38.1 Studies summary

	Number of patients		Year of publication	Country	Type of study	Max follow-up	Main findings
	CRRT	IHD					
Mehta (2001)[24]	84	82	2001	USA	RCT	Hospital discharge	CRRT-treated patients have a higher in-hospital mortality, but complete recovery of renal function was more common
Jacka (2005)[25]	65	25	2005	Canada	Retrospective cohort study	Hospital discharge	Renal recovery was substantially higher in the patients treated with CRRT
SWING (2007)[26]	1911	291	2007	Sweden	Retrospective cohort study	90 days	Patients treated with IHD end up requiring long-term haemodialysis more often than those treated with CRRT
BEST (2007)[27]	1006	212	2007	23 countries	Retrospective cohort study	Hospital discharge	The choice of CRRT as initial treatment is not a predictor of survival or of dialysis-free hospital survival but strong predictor of dialysis independence at hospital discharge among survivors
ATN (2008)[20]	783	313	2008	USA	RCT	60 days	No difference in mortality between high- and low-intensity RRT
RENAL (2009)[28]	1464	0	2009	Australia, New Zealand	RCT	90 days	No difference in mortality between low- (25 mL/kg) and high- (40 mL/kg) intensity CVVHDF

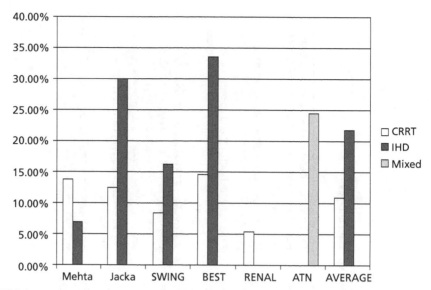

Fig. 38.1 Percentage of patients treated with either CRRT or IHD in different studies, who survived to hospital discharge but remained haemodialysis-dependent. The term 'mixed', in reference to the ATN trial,[20] refers to the fact that most of these patients also received some CRRT. For abbreviations and names of studies, see text.

were criticized, because the renal recovery was considered too low in the IHD group. Nonetheless, these findings provide further support for the notion that IHD delays or prevents renal recovery.

These findings were confirmed, although to a lesser magnitude, by the much larger SWING study published in 2007.[26] The SWING study was a retrospective observational study examining 2202 patients treated with RRT in 32 Swedish ICUs over 10 years. It demonstrated no difference in mortality between those treated with CRRT and those with IHD. However, amongst the 1102 patients who survived to 90 days, only 8.3% of the 944 patients treated with CRRT developed a need for chronic haemodialysis vs 16.5% of the 158 treated with IHD. The OR for inability to achieve dialysis independence at 90 days' dependence in IHD-treated patients was 2.19 and rose to 2.60 when corrected for comorbidities, calendar year, hospital type, and diagnosis in ICU. Obviously, due to its observational design, this study was subject to confounders. Its interpretation is also limited by the absence of ICU illness severity scores, dialysis dose, time on dialysis, and, importantly, underlying renal disease. However, from the pre-ICU data, it seems likely that patients were quite similar, and, if anything, sicker patients were treated with CRRT, as they presented with slightly more diabetes and HF. Also, a higher percentage of CRRT patients had more severe diagnoses, such as sepsis (17 vs 10%) and pancreatitis (13 vs 9%), while intoxications were more frequent in the IHD patients (9 vs 2%). Finally, a time period bias is also possible since, from 2000 to 2004, 90% of the patients were treated with CRRT vs 76% in the earlier period. However, the OR remained larger than 2 after correction for the time period effect.

Similar data have been returned from an international study, the Beginning and Ending Supportive Therapy for the Kidney (BEST Kidney) study. This was a prospective epidemiological study involving 54 ICUs in 23 countries. In an additional analysis,[27] 1218 patients were stratified, depending on the initial strategy of RRT employed during their ICU admission, with 1006 patients initially receiving CRRT and 212 patients receiving IHD. Those receiving CRRT as the initial mode of therapy had higher SAPS II scores, were more likely to be hypotensive, and required vasoactive medication and MV, with worse pulmonary gas exchange. RRT was commenced earlier in their admission, and they were more acidotic and tended to have more furosemide given in the period before RRT commencement. This suggests that sicker patients were commenced on CRRT in the majority of cases. The reported rate of intra-treatment hypotension was 27.9% in the IHD arm vs 18.8% in the CRRT arm. The BEST kidney investigators found that the initial mode of RRT did not influence in-hospital mortality (OR 1.005, 95% CI 0.673–1.502, $P = 0.98$). However, among patients treated with CRRT who survived to hospital discharge, 5.2% were dialysis-dependent at discharge vs 17.5% of those treated with IHD (P <0.0001). Despite a higher number of patients with chronic renal dysfunction in the IHD-treated group, on multivariable logistic regression analysis, CRRT, as an initial RRT modality, remained an independent predictor of renal recovery, with ORs strikingly similar to those of the SWING study (OR 2.653, 95% CI 0.523–1.238, $P = 0.0008$). This association was maintained and, in fact, strengthened when a propensity score, using the ten variables significantly related to the choice of initial mode of RRT, was calculated and included in the analysis (OR 3.365, 95%CI 1.942–6.804, P <0.0001).

Finally, two recent large, well-conducted, randomized multicentre trials have provided high-quality data to help us understand the impact of RRT on renal recovery: the Randomized Evaluation of Normal versus Augmented Level Renal Replacement Therapy (RENAL) study[28] and the Veterans Administration/National Institutes of Health (VA/NIH) Acute renal failure Trial Network (ATN) study.[20] Together, these studies demonstrated that there is no patient survival or renal recovery benefit from increasing the intensity of RRT. Although this was the primary hypothesis tested, both studies provide interesting additional information on how the choice of therapy may affect renal recovery.

The RENAL study was a large, multicentre RCT performed in Australian and New Zealand centres where all 1508 patients meeting the inclusion criteria received CRRT in the form of CVVHDF. They were randomized to one of two 'doses' (25 vs 40 mL/kg/hour), determined by the rate of effluent flow. In the US ATN study, 1124 patients were randomized to either a high-intensity or low-intensity RRT group. Haemodynamically stable patients received IHD—three (low-intensity group) or six (high-intensity group) times per week. Haemodynamically unstable patients received CRRT in the form of CVVHDF at an efferent flow of 20 or 35 mL/kg/hour. The protocol allowed modality changes to adapt to the patient's cardiovascular status. Both these studies failed to demonstrate any statistically significant difference between the groups in either patient or renal outcome. Hence, as confirmed by a subsequent meta-analysis,[29] these studies showed that increasing the dose of RRT does not affect outcome or renal recovery. However, apart from the geographical areas, these two studies differed greatly by the number of patients treated with IHD: all patients enrolled in the RENAL study received CRRT, while 313 (27.8%) enrolled in the ATN trial received IHD as initial modality, for a total of >5000 IHD treatments during the study period.

As might be expected, the rates of renal recovery differed substantially between the two studies. At day 28, 45.2% of the survivors were RRT-dependent in the ATN study vs only 13.3% in the RENAL study. Similarly, at the end of the follow-up, 24.6% of ATN survivors remained on RRT (at day 60),[30] as compared with only 5.6% of RENAL survivors (at day 90). This is a >3 times relative difference in RRT dependence. Additionally, the mean number of RRT-free days at 28 days in the ATN trial was 6.5 vs 17 in the RENAL trial. This translates to a >2.5 times increase in RRT-free days at day 28 when CRRT was used, compared with a combination of CRRT and IHD. These findings are strikingly consistent with those of the SWING and BEST studies. These differences might be explained by differences in baseline disease severity. However, although slightly more patients in the ATN trial required MV (80.6% vs 73.6%) at admission, the patients in the RENAL study were older (64.5 vs 59.6 years old) and required inotropes more frequently (72.3% vs 45%), and a higher percentage of them had chronic renal impairment (58% vs 34.4%).

Conclusion

Although there is no definitive level I evidence, experimental studies, observational studies, and data from RCTs from multiple countries in multiple conditions and in a very large number of patients all consistently seem to point to the fact that IHD delays and, in some patients, prevents renal recovery. Until any convincing high-level contrary evidence shows that IHD is not a risk factor for the lack of renal recovery, it would seem prudent for clinicians to prescribe CRRT as the preferred modality of RRT in critically ill patients with AKI.

References

1 Uchino S, Kellum JA, Bellomo R, et al. Acute renal failure in critically ill patients: a multinational, multicenter study. *JAMA* 2005;**294**:813–18.

2 Kellum JA, Angus DC, Johnson JP, et al. Continuous versus intermittent renal replacement therapy: a meta-analysis. *Intensive Care Med* 2002;**28**:29–37.

3 Kierdorf H. Continuous versus intermittent treatment: clinical results in acute renal failure. *Contrib Nephrol* 1991;**93**:1–12.

4 Bosworth C, Paganini EP, Cosentino F, Heyka RJ. Long-term experience with continuous renal replacement therapy in intensive-care unit acute renal failure. *Contrib Nephrol* 1991;**93**:13–16.

5 Kruczynski K, Irvine-Bird K, Toffelmire EB, Morton AR. A comparison of continuous arteriovenous hemofiltration and intermittent hemodialysis in acute renal failure patients in the intensive care unit. *Asaio J* 1993;**39**:M778–81.

6 Rialp G, Roglan A, Betbese AJ, et al. Prognostic indexes and mortality in critically ill patients with acute renal failure treated with different dialytic techniques. *Ren Fail* 1996;**18**:667–75.

7 Swartz RD, Messana JM, Orzol S, Port FK. Comparing continuous hemofiltration with hemodialysis in patients with severe acute renal failure. *Am J Kidney Dis* 1999;**34**:424–32.

8 Uehlinger DE, Jakob SM, Ferrari P, et al. Comparison of continuous and intermittent renal replacement therapy for acute renal failure. *Nephrol Dial Transplant* 2005;**20**:1630–7.

9 Augustine JJ, Sandy D, Seifert TH, Paganini EP. A randomized controlled trial comparing intermittent with continuous dialysis in patients with ARF. *Am J Kidney Dis* 2004;**44**:1000–7.

10 Rabindranath K, Adams J, Macleod AM, Muirhead N. Intermittent versus continuous renal replacement therapy for acute renal failure in adults. *Cochrane Database Syst Rev* 2007;3:CD003773.

11 Singh P, Thomson SC. Renal homeostasis and tubuloglomerular feedback. *Curr Opin Nephrol Hypertens* 2010;**19**:59–64.

12 Kelleher SP, Robinette JB, Miller F, Conger JD. Effect of hemorrhagic reduction in blood pressure on recovery from acute renal failure. *Kidney Int* 1987;**31**:725–30.

13 Adams PL, Adams FF, Bell PD, Navar LG. Impaired renal blood flow autoregulation in ischemic acute renal failure. *Kidney Int* 1980;**18**:68–76.

14 Matthys E, Patton MK, Osgood RW, Venkatachalam MA, Stein JH. Alterations in vascular function and morphology in acute ischemic renal failure. *Kidney Int* 1983;**23**:717–24.

15 Conger JD, Hammond WS. Renal vasculature and ischemic injury. *Ren Fail* 1992;**14**:307–10.

16 Davenport A. Intradialytic complications during hemodialysis. *Hemodial Int* 2006;**10**:162–7.

17 Lameire N, Van Biesen W, Vanholder R, Colardijn F. The place of intermittent hemodialysis in the treatment of acute renal failure in the ICU patient. *Kidney Int Suppl* 1998;**66**:S110–19.

18 Abdeen O, Mehta RL. Dialysis modalities in the intensive care unit. *Crit Care Clin* 2002;**18**:223–47.

19 Manns M, Sigler MH, Teehan BP. Intradialytic renal haemodynamics—potential consequences for the management of the patient with acute renal failure. *Nephrol Dial Transplant* 1997;**12**:870–2.

20 Palevsky PM, Zhang JH, O'Connor TZ, et al. Intensity of renal support in critically ill patients with acute kidney injury. *N Engl J Med* 2008;**359**:7–20.

21 Conger JD. Does hemodialysis delay recovery from acute renal failure? *Sem Dial* 1990;**3**:146–8.

22 Davenport A, Will EJ, Davidson AM. Improved cardiovascular stability during continuous modes of renal replacement therapy in critically ill patients with acute hepatic and renal failure. *Crit Care Med* 1993;**21**:328–38.

23 Van der Schueren G, Diltoer M, Laureys M, Huyghens L. Intermittent hemodialysis in critically ill patients with multiple organ dysfunction syndrome is associated with intestinal intramucosal acidosis. *Intensive Care Med* 1996;**22**:747–51.

24 Mehta RL, McDonald B, Gabbai FB, et al. Collaborative Group for Treatment of ARFitICU: a randomized clinical trial of continuous versus intermittent dialysis for acute renal failure. *Kidney Int* 2001;**60**:1154–63.

25 Jacka MJ, Ivancinova X, Gibney RTN. Continuous renal replacement therapy improves renal recovery from acute renal failure. *Can J Anaesth* 2005;**52**:327–32.

26 Bell M, Granath F, Schon S, Ekbom A, Martling CR. Continuous renal replacement therapy is associated with less chronic renal failure than intermittent haemodialysis after acute renal failure. *Intensive Care Med* 2007;**33**:773–80.

27 Uchino S, Bellomo R, Kellum JA, et al. Patient and kidney survival by dialysis modality in critically ill patients with acute kidney injury. *Int J Artif Organs* 2007;**30**:281–92.

28 Bellomo R, Cass A, Cole L, et al. Intensity of continuous renal-replacement therapy in critically ill patients. *N Engl J Med* 2009;**361**:1627–38.

29 Jun M, Lambers Heerspink HJ, Ninomiya T, et al. Intensities of renal replacement therapy in acute kidney injury: a systematic review and meta-analysis. *Clin J Am Soc Nephrol* 2010;**5**:956–63.

30 Ronco C, Honore P. Renal support in critically ill patients with acute kidney injury. *N Engl J Med* 2008;**359**:1959; author reply 1961–52.

Chapter 39

Ventilator Liberation Strategies

Stefano Nava and Luca Fasano

Introduction

Discontinuing MV is a process which begins as soon as a patient with acute respiratory failure (ARF) who needs a ventilatory support is connected to the ventilator and encompasses the entire process of liberating the patient from the ventilator, including post-extubation NIV support and/or post-extubation monitoring to assess weaning success. In the ICU, the weaning process must be aggressively pursued in order to prevent delays in extubation and minimize adverse effects of MV.[1] The 'good' outcome of self-extubated patients, of whom almost 50% do not need reintubation,[2] suggests that, in many subjects, extubation is unduly delayed. Weaning failure is defined as either the failure of SBT or the need for reintubation within 48 hours following extubation. In this chapter, we will therefore discuss not only the strategy of liberation from MV, but also the causes, consequences, and treatment of weaning failure.

Weaning

Weaning accounts for approximately 40% of the total time spent on MV,[3] and PMV is associated with increased risk of complications and mortality[4,5] and with increased costs. PMV is therefore not only a 'medical' problem, but it has also a social and economical impact. US costs for MV were estimated to be $27 billion, representing 12% of all hospital costs. Incidence, mortality, and cumulative population costs rise significantly with age.[6] In the US, every year, about 300 000 receive prolonged life support in ICU, and this number is likely to double within a decade, with associated costs of more than US $50 billion.[7]

The weaning process includes the treatment of ARF, aimed to support the ventilatory pump and gas exchange, and the assessment of readiness to wean, so that the support given to the patient by the mechanical ventilator can be progressively and rationally decreased and finally discontinued. Readiness to breathe spontaneously can only be achieved once the acute illness which induced ARF has been treated, thereby reducing the respiratory and cardiac workload. MV is associated with a number of complications: VAP, other intensive care-related infections, critical illness neuromuscular abnormalities (CINMA), insufficient nutritional support, sleep deprivation, delirium, anxiety, and depression, all of which can significantly impair the weaning process.

Usually, weaning means liberation from invasive MV (IMV), but, as NIV may permit extubation while continuing MV, the concept of 'weaning in progress' has been proposed.[1] An International Consensus Conference[1] was held in 2005 to provide recommendations regarding the management of this process. An 11-member international jury answered five predefined questions.

(1) What is known about the epidemiology of weaning problems? (2) What is the pathophysiology of weaning failure? (3) What is the usual process of initial weaning from the ventilator? (4) Is there a role for different ventilator modes in more difficult weaning? (5) How should patients with

prolonged weaning failure be managed? According to this International Task Force, three groups of patients can be identified:[1]

- Simple weaning (successful extubation at the first attempt after a single SBT)
- Difficult weaning (patients with up to three SBTs and up to 7 days from the first SBT)
- Prolonged weaning (more than three SBTs and more than 7 days after the first SBT).

Simple–to-wean patients are about 70% of all the ventilated subjects and have a 5% ICU mortality; difficult-to-wean patients and those with prolonged weaning have together a 25% ICU mortality.[8,9] A recent study showed that prolonged weaning is associated with increased mortality and morbidity in the ICU, while difficult weaning was associated with increased morbidity but not mortality.[10]

Pathophysiology of weaning

The 'mechanical' pivotal point in the weaning strategy is the ratio between respiratory pump load, that is to say WOB for tidal volume, and ventilatory capacity, the maximum capacity to generate the inspiratory pressure (Pimax). Then, several other points have to be taken into account: cardiac and neuromuscular function, nutrition, metabolic balance, and psychological aspects.

Ventilatory load

The ventilatory load depends on:

- Reduced thoracopulmonary compliance: that is to say any pulmonary disease causing diffuse pulmonary infiltrates, or any pleural or chest wall disease. These diseases can be acute and be at least in part responsible of the ARF (pneumonia, pulmonary oedema, abdominal distension, or ascites), or chronic (parenchymal diseases, such as pulmonary fibrosis/interstitial lung disease, chest wall diseases, such as kyphoscoliosis, or obesity) and be responsible for increased difficulties in weaning. Pneumonia can be either the cause of ARF or a complication of endotracheal intubation (VAP), just as pulmonary oedema can be the primary cause of ARF or a complication of the pulmonary-induced ARF which is responsible of an increased cardiac workload. Reducing the length of MV is crucial to reduce the incidence of VAP which worsens the prognosis of these patients.[11,12] Furthermore, reduced compliance is present in the hyperinflated COPD patients due to the severity of airflow limitation, inducing a pre-existing static hyperinflation which can be worsened by iatrogenic dynamic hyperinflation during MV. Patient/ventilator interaction may further increase the WOB in case of dyssynchrony
- An increase of airways resistance can be induced by bronchoconstriction in COPD and asthma, bronchial inflammation, and airways oedema, and this resistive workload may be partially reversible with medical therapy. Then, an additional resistive load is put on the respiratory pump during SBT by ETT resistance and, after extubation, by laryngeal oedema or excessive airways secretions.[13]

Ventilatory capacity

The ventilatory capacity needs a sufficient central drive and efficacious respiratory muscles activity to generate the negative inspiratory pressure which is necessary to deal with the WOB and maintain an alveolar ventilation sufficient to meet the metabolic demands. An inefficient central drive may ensue from neurologic diseases (encephalitis or brainstem dysfunction), metabolic alkalosis, or sedative drugs. A peripheral dysfunction may be caused by neuromuscular diseases such as Guillain–Barré syndrome and myasthenia gravis which are sometimes diagnosed in the evaluation of a difficult-to-wean patient; in other cases, weakness may be acquired during the ICU stay, as in the case of CIP or CIM.[14] One study showed that ICU-acquired paresis was an independent contributor to MV duration after awakening from the acute phase of critical illness.[15] Hypokalaemia, hypophosphataemia, hypomagnesaemia, anaemia,[16] and malnutrition may further impair the process of liberation from MV. Adrenal insufficiency may also play a role during weaning, and this should be suspected in the critically ill when random cortisol concentrations are lower than 25 g/dL and if cortisol increments are less than 9 g/dL with ACTH stimulation testing.[17]

Iatrogenic factors

Excessive sedation is related to prolonged weaning, and daily awakening is useful to carefully evaluate readiness to breathe spontaneously.[18] Indeed, this practice is safe, decreases the length of MV, and may be associated with reductions in PTSD.[19]

Concerns have been raised that MV may itself have harmful effects on the diaphragm. In animals, diaphragmatic inactivity associated with controlled MV leads to muscle fibre atrophy in the diaphragm and a reduction in its force-generating capacity,[20] a condition referred to as 'ventilator-induced diaphragmatic dysfunction' (VIDD).[21] Levine et al.[22] reported that diaphragmatic inactivity induced by MV in brain-dead organ donors is associated with preferential fibre atrophy and increase in markers of proteolysis within the diaphragm, thus supporting the existence of VIDD in these patients. A more recent study[23] demonstrates the rapid onset of diaphragmatic weakness and atrophy in mechanically ventilated humans and, in addition, showed that MV is associated with a structural injury to diaphragm muscle fibres and an upregulation of the calpain proteolytic system. Collectively, these data highlight the need to avoid, when possible, modes of MV aimed at a maximal reduction of the patient's inspiratory effort.

Acquired weakness in critically ill patients may be induced by drug-related neuromuscular junction defects, polyneuropathy, and myopathy.[24] Acute quadriplegic myopathy typically affects patients with status asthmaticus requiring MV and the administration of high-dose IV corticosteroids and/or non-depolarizing NMBAs.[25] Another observational study shows that one-third of the patients admitted to the ICU due to acute exacerbation of COPD and receiving high doses of corticosteroids developed acute quadriplegic myopathy.[26]

Cardiac load

During SBT, as the ventilator support is withdrawn, two major modifications of cardiovascular balance happen:

+ The increased metabolic demand, due to increased WOB, which must be met with a build-up of CO

+ The recurrence of negative intrathoracic inspiratory pressure which induces an increment of right heart filling, with increased preload, and an increased left ventricular afterload.

Weaning thus represents a stress test for the cardiovascular system which is either difficult to bear for patients with chronic heart disease or may unmask a latent cardiac dysfunction.[27,28] Cardiac ischaemia and/or pulmonary oedema may ensue, especially in those patients with a previous episode of MI.[29] The protective effect on cardiac function of the positive intrathoracic pressure induced by positive pressure MV is confirmed by the efficacy of NIV in the ARF caused by cardiogenic pulmonary oedema.[30]

Other factors

Psychological alterations, such as delirium,[31,32] anxiety, and depression, may increase the length of MV. In particular, depressive disorders were diagnosed in 42% of patients during weaning from prolonged ventilation, and these patients were more likely to experience weaning failure and death.[33]

Timing

According to the International Task Force,[1] there are six stages to consider during the weaning process, defined as follows: (1) treatment of ARF, (2) suspicion that weaning may be possible, (3) assessment of readiness to wean, (4) SBT, (5) extubation, and possibly (6) reintubation.

As the ARF improves, the chance to withdraw IMV as soon as possible must not be missed. Any unjustified delay increases the window for ICU-related complications to develop and complicate the process of liberation from MV. The outcome of self-extubated patients, both those in full mechanical support and those already in weaning,[2,34] and the readiness to wean of 'unweanable' subjects as soon as they change the caring staff[35] support the idea that often MV is unnecessarily prolonged.

Daily screening of the respiratory function of adults receiving MV, followed by trials of spontaneous breathing in appropriate patients and notification of their physicians when the trials were successful, can reduce the duration of MV and the cost of intensive care and is associated with fewer complications than usual care.[36] This strategy may also reduce the number of self-extubations, tracheostomies, and the incidence of VAP.[37]

Depressed mental status is usually viewed as an obstacle to successful extubation, but, in one study, a low reintubation rate was shown in brain-injured patients with a low GCS.[4] In a small study performed in neurocritical care of patients undergoing extubation trial, traditional weaning parameters do not predict extubation failure.[38]

In these patients with neurologic diseases, however, a systematic approach to weaning and extubation reduces the rate of reintubation secondary to extubation failure, without affecting the duration of MV, and is overall positively perceived by ICU professionals.[39] Daily spontaneous awakening trials (i.e. interruption of sedatives, coupled with SBTs) result in better outcomes for mechanically ventilated patients in intensive care than current standard approaches, and some authors have suggested that this should become routine practice.[40]

The assessment of readiness to wean is based on the confidence in clinical stability of the patient and on their capacity to bear the WOB. This assessment considers several points which do not necessarily all need to be fulfilled:[1]

- Significant and persistent improvement of the acute disease which caused ARF
- Ability to cooperate (which includes tolerating withdrawing of sedation)
- Satisfactory capacity to deal with tracheobronchial secretions (effective cough and manageable amount of secretions)[41]
- Adequate gas exchange ($PaO_2/FiO_2 > 150$ mmHg) with PEEP < 8 cmH$_2$O
- Tolerable ventilatory demand (minute ventilation < 10 L/min)
- Manageable respiratory acidosis
- Adequate ventilatory pump performance (vital capacity > 10 mL/kg, tidal volume > 5 mL/kg, maximal inspiratory pressure (MIP) < -20 cmH$_2$O, respiratory rate < 35 breaths/min, rapid shallow breathing index (RSBI) < 105).

An air leak test (presence of air flow around the ETT after having deflated the cuff) should be performed before extubation to evaluate the presence of a potential upper airways obstruction.[42,43]

Predictors of weaning failure

Besides the most common indices of weaning success or failure, the clinician must base her/his decision to extubate the patient on objective clinical criteria after a trial of weaning, irrespective of the strategy used. The presence of respiratory distress (like thoracoabdominal paradox, excessive use of accessory muscle), diaphoresis and anxiety, sensorium impairment, haemodynamic instability, and oxygen desaturation may be objective signs that the patient is unable to sustain unsupported breathing.

Several 'single' indices of weaning success were proposed in the literature like vital capacity, tidal volume, airway occlusion pressure (P0.1), minute ventilation, respiratory rate, MIP; however, in a general ICU, the areas under the curve showed that the tests do not accurately discriminate between successful and unsuccessful weaning.[44]

Composite indices, such as P0.1/Pimax (ratio of airway occlusion pressure 0.1 s after the onset of inspiratory effort to MIP) and CROP (integrative index of compliance, rate, oxygenation, and pressure),[45,46] were also proposed. The former is dependent on the quality of the measurement recorded directly from the ventilator that is not always reliable, and the latter is somewhat cumbersome to use in the clinical setting, as it requires measurements of many variables, with the potential risk of errors in the measurement techniques.

RSBI is the ratio between respiratory rate and tidal volume and is able to predict a successful SBT and is probably the mostly used predictor in clinical practice.[46] As a matter of fact, patients who cannot stand a spontaneous breathing tend to rapidly increase the breathing frequency, reducing at the same time tidal volume, so the RSBI increases. In a landmark study, an RSBI > 105 breaths/min/L was associated with weaning failure, while lower values predicted weaning success with good sensitivity and satisfactory specificity. Recent systematic reviews supported, however, the idea that the likelihood ratios are better measures than sensitivity and specificity, because they are independent of the pretest probability,[47,48] and that a negative likelihood ratio is better at identifying the patients who will fail than a positive likelihood ratio at depicting the patients who will be weaned successfully.

During an SBT, Wysocki et al.[49] showed that breathing variability is greater in patients successfully separated from the ventilator and the ETT and that variability indices are sufficient to separate success from failure cases.

SBT can be performed with low levels of inspiratory support (PS < +8 cmH$_2$O) or with continuous positive airway pressure (CPAP) without impairing its predictive power of successful extubation.[50–52] CPAP is helpful in COPD patients during SBT, as it helps to overcome the load imposed by intrinsic PEEP, but this 'assistance' has not yet been formally studied. The use of an automatic compensation of the resistive load imposed by ETT (ATC)[53] does not consider that, in real life, the patient has to get through the resistance of inflamed upper airways after extubation so that post-extubation WOB is simulated better without this ATC.[13,54] Some studies have shown that failure is evident within 20 minutes when a patient does not overcome an SBT[9,46] and that a 30-minute SBT is as successful as a 120-minute SBT in predicting extubation success.[9]

There are both objective measurements and subjective criteria (agitation, dyspnoea, diaphoresis, cyanosis, depressed mental status, use of accessory muscles, and facial signs of distress) for sentencing an SBT failure.[55] The objective indices are:

- Hypoxaemia ($PaO_2 < 50$–60 mmHg with $FiO_2 > 50\%$)
- Hypercapnia ($PaCO_2 > 50$ mmHg or increase > 8 mmHg during the SBT)
- Acidosis (pH < 7.32 or reduction of pH > 0.07 of pH units)
- RSBI > 105
- Tachypnoea (respiratory rate > 35 breaths/minute or increased by 50%)
- Tachycardia (heart rate > 140/min or increased $> 20\%$)
- Hypertension > 180 mmHg or increased $> 20\%$
- Hypotension < 90 mmHg
- Arrhythmias.

Only 13% of patients who successfully completed an SBT needs reintubation;[1] on the contrary, 40% of subjects extubated without an SBT have to be reintubated.[56] When a patient fails an SBT, he/she should be ventilated using a non fatiguing mode (A/C or PSV) to recover waiting for the next SBT.

Methods of weaning

According to an international survey, daily SBT is probably the most used weaning method, and it is performed in half of the cases using a T-tube (less used are low PS or CPAP).

Gradual reduction of inspiratory pressure support is the second most popular method, especially in those patients with difficult weaning, and it is based on the principle of progressively reducing the 'external' aid until a level < 7 cmH$_2$O is reached. This has been shown to simulate quite well the WOB of the patient, once she/he is extubated.

A recent physiological trial showed that PSV and PSV plus PEEP markedly modified the breathing pattern (with reduced respiratory rate and increased tidal volume) and reduced inspiratory muscle effort and cardiovascular response (reduced pulmonary artery pressure and LV HF), as compared to the T-piece, so that most subjects in this small group of difficult-to-wean patients failed the T-piece trial but succeeded the other two.[57]

Synchronized intermittent mandatory ventilation (SIMV) was much used in the past. It is a mode of MV which ensures minimal minute ventilation by deciding tidal volume and respiratory rate. The ventilator breaths are synchronized with the patient's inspiratory efforts. The patient can increase ventilation by pressure-supported breaths. Weaning is performed by decreasing respiratory rate; furthermore, the pressure support given to spontaneous breaths has to be withdrawn.

What is considered to be the best method of weaning among these three most popular ones? Several trials showed that intermittent use of spontaneous breathing via a T-tube was comparable to PSV as a weaning mode. Thus, after failed SBT, the use of progressively increased time on a T-piece is also an effective means of liberating patients from the ventilator. According to the International Task Force, the use of PSV may also be helpful in liberating patients from MV after several failed attempts at spontaneous breathing. Some studies, however, reported a different rate of weaning success using PSV or T-tube trial, but this may reflect the different attitude, training, and confidence of a specific team of clinicians with one method, rather than its superiority. Most of the studies comparing these three methods indicate that SIMV was inferior to PSV or T-piece in speeding-up the weaning process. Indeed, the literature does not support the use of SIMV alone as a weaning mode, and little data exist for the use of SIMV and PSV combined.[58,59] Besides these three most popular weaning approaches, some other ventilatory modes have been proposed in the literature.

Advanced closed-loop systems were proposed to simplify ventilator management by making the weaning process interactive, responsive, and adaptive. Despite some positive results,[60–62] the role of these automated modes in reducing weaning practice pattern variation and facilitating knowledge translation remains to be established. Indeed, automation during weaning does not yet supersede the need for close patient observation and monitoring. The most popular of these techniques include mandatory minute ventilation (MMV)[63] that combines features of controlled ventilation with mandatory breaths and PSV to augment spontaneous respiratory efforts. The ventilator adapts the mandatory breath rate to meet the predetermined minute ventilation by taking the patient's spontaneous respiratory rate into consideration. If a patient's spontaneous breathing meets or exceeds the preset minute volume, no mandatory breaths are provided in MMV. Adaptive support ventilation (ASV) automatically selects a target ventilatory pattern, based on clinicians' inputs (predicted body weight (PBW), minimum minute volume, and pressure limit) and respiratory mechanics data from the ventilator monitoring system (respiratory system expiratory time constant and dynamic compliance).[64] The algorithm is aimed to minimize total work of inspiration, and the ventilator continuously adapts to match changes in respiratory mechanics by using automatic controls for level of inspiratory pressure above PEEP, frequency, and inspiratory time of ventilator-initiated breaths. SmartCare®, also known as 'Neoganesh' or the automated weaning system, is the first commercially available automated system specifically designed to guide the weaning process. SmartCare®/PS monitors the patient's respiratory status every 2 or 5 minutes and periodically adapts pressure support to maintain the patient in a defined 'respiratory zone of comfort'. Once SmartCare® has successfully minimized the level of inspiratory support, an observation period occurs, which may be followed by a recommendation to 'consider separation' (proceed, if clinically indicated, to patient extubation).

PAV and neurally adjusted ventilatory assist (NAVA) are relatively newer weaning modes, and some authors have postulated a potential role of these two methods in weaning patients from MV, but there are actually no studies to verify this hypothesis.[65,66]

NIV to shorten the duration of intubation

As stand-alone technique, the use of NIV was proposed to shorten the duration of ventilation in a subset of patients, mostly those with persistent hypercapnia and chronic respiratory disorders. From a physiological point of view, NIV is similar to invasive MV; in fact, it reduces the breathing work and frequency, decreases the negative deflections of intrathoracic pressure, improves gas exchange, and decreases the effort of the respiratory muscles.[67] Indeed, both invasive and non-invasive pressure support are equally effective, and NIV may be used as a 'full alternative' for invasive ventilation.

Burns et al. in a meta-analysis and systematic review identified 12 RCTs enrolling 530 participants, mostly with COPD. Compared with invasive weaning, non-invasive weaning was significantly associated with reduced mortality (RR 0.55, 95% CI 0.38–0.79), VAP (RR 0.29, 95% CI 0.19–0.45), length of stay in ICU (weighted mean difference −6.27 days, −8.77 to −3.78) and hospital (−7.19 days, −10.80 to −3.58), total duration of ventilation, and duration of invasive ventilation. Non-invasive weaning had no effect on weaning failures or weaning time.[68]

More recently, Girault completed an RCT with a large number of patients in 17 centres in France in patients with chronic hypercapnic respiratory failure intubated for ARF.[69] Patients were randomized into three groups: to continue MV with conventional weaning, to start NIV, or to receive supplemental oxygen after extubation. Reintubation rates were 30%, 37%, and 32% for invasive weaning, oxygen therapy, and NIV group, respectively. Weaning failure rates, including

Table 39.1 Advantages and limitations associated with ventilator liberation strategies

Method of weaning	Advantages	Disadvantages
T-piece trial	– Simulates spontaneous breathing – The major diagnostic test to determine if patients can be successfully extubated	– Too 'brisk' for some patients, with a potential increase in anxiety
Gradual decrease in inspiratory support	– Simulates spontaneous breathing – To be used in the case of SBT failure	– Requires protocolized actions (i.e. number and amount of daily modifications of inspiratory support)
SIMV		Increases WOB vs T-piece ot PS Slows the process of weaning vs SBT and PS
Automatic tube compensation	– May be used for those patients with a narrow ETT	– Does not consider the resistances 'external' to the ETT – Lack of solid scientific evidences
Closed-loop systems	– May simplify ventilator management	– Still requiring the need for close patient observation and monitoring – Lack of solid scientific evidences
NIV	– Allows precox extubation, even in the case of SBT failure – Reduces the risk of VAP	– To be used only in COPD patients – Requires skilled team

post-extubation ARF, were 54%, 71%, and 33%, respectively, and this was statistically significant in favour of NIV. Rescue NIV success rates for invasive and oxygen therapy groups were 45% and 58%, respectively. Apart from a longer weaning time in NIV than in invasive group (2.5 vs 1.5 days; $P = 0.033$), no significant outcome difference was observed between groups. It was therefore concluded that NIV decreases the intubation duration and may improve the weaning results in difficult-to-wean patients with hypercapnic respiratory failure by reducing the risk of post-extubation ARF.

Some small, non-randomized trials have been performed using NIV to wean trauma patients with hypoxaemic respiratory failure[70] and non-COPD patients with persistent ARF after early extubation.[71,72] However, based on these studies, we cannot recommend NIV as a weaning strategy in severely hypoxic patients. The poor tolerance of facial interfaces and the possible difficulties in fitting masks have been considered as possible causes for failure of NIV in the weaning process.[73] Lately, the helmet has been considered as a potential alternative for NIV. In a case report, Klein et al.[74] described rapid liberation of a COPD patient intubated for an ARF by using the helmet during NIV. They showed good patient compliance, lower costs and nurse workload, and mostly fewer complications related to sedation and infections, compared to invasive ventilation.

The advantages and disadvantages of the various weaning methods are summarized in Table 39.1.

Post-extubation respiratory failure

Post-extubation respiratory failure is a major clinical problem in ICUs. It is usually defined when respiratory distress (i.e. increased breathing frequency and indirect signs of incipient fatigue such as massive activation of accessory muscles and/or inward movements of the lower rib cage), worsening of arterial blood gases (i.e. increase of $PaCO_2 > 10$ mmHg and decrease in pH > 0.10; $PaO_2 < 60$ mmHg or $SaO_2 < 90\%$ while receiving $FiO_2 > 0.50$), or inability to protect the airways because of upper airways obstruction or excessive secretions, occuring within the first 48 hours after extubation.[75]

Post-extubation failure requiring reintubation occurs, on average, in 13% of patients. The prognosis of these patients is very poor, because their hospital mortality exceeds 30–40%, with the cause of extubation failure and the time to reintubation being independent predictors of outcome.[75,76]

The most common reasons for reintubation are respiratory failure, CHF, aspiration or excess pulmonary secretions, and upper airway obstruction. Mortality is significantly higher for patients failing, because of non-airway aetiologies, compared with those who failed principally because of an airway problem (52.9% vs 17.4%).[76]

The mortality rate increases with increasing duration of time from extubation to reintubation and is significantly lower for patients reintubated within either 12 hours (24% vs 51%) or 24 hours (30.2% vs 58.1%) of extubation when compared with those reintubated after longer periods of time.[76]

Moreover, reintubation represents 'per-se' an independent risk factor for nosocomial pneumonia, as assessed by Torres in a case-control study.[77]

There is a certain subset of patients whose clinical characteristics at the time of extubation may predict reintubation, so that it was suggested that the application of NIV in this selected population of at-risk patients may avoid the occurrence of post-extubation failure and consequently the possibility of reintubation. Based on this hypothesis, two randomized trials[78,79] were therefore performed to assess whether NIV is effective in preventing the occurrence of post-extubation failure in patients at 'highest risk' when compared to standard medical treatment. The two trials adopted similar criteria to define the category of patients at potential risk (i.e. persistent weaning failure, post-extubation hypercapnia, age, weak cough reflex, or a pre-existing cardiac disease) and similar design (i.e. sequential use of NIV in the first 48 hours).

In the first study, the use of NIV was associate with a 16% reduction in the risk for reintubation, whereas the protective effect on ICU mortality was close to achieving a statistical significance. In the second randomized trial, differently from the previous study, NIV was also used as rescue therapy in patients from the two groups in case of respiratory failure after extubation without needing immediate reintubation. The authors found that NIV significantly reduced the incidence of respiratory failure after extubation, but the differences between the two groups in the reintubation rate failed to be significant. This was due to the efficacy of NIV as rescue therapy to avoid reintubation. The beneficial effects of NIV on survival appear restricted to patients with chronic respiratory disorders and hypercapnia during the SBT. To confirm the result found in this subgroup of patients, Ferrer and colleagues[80] performed a multicentre RCT specifically designed for patients who developed hypercapnia during an SBT. They found that respiratory failure was less frequent in the NIV arm than in the other one (standard treatment) (15% vs 25%). NIV was also independently associated with a lower risk of respiratory failure after extubation, and, in patients with respiratory failure, NIV as a rescue therapy avoided reintubation. The overall 90-day mortality was significantly lower in the group of NIV (11% vs 31%).

The use of NIV has also been suggested in an attempt to avoid reintubation in patients who show already signs of 'incipient', or even overt, respiratory failure following extubation.

In an RCT,[81] patients developing ARF within 48 hours after extubation were randomized to receive standard medical therapy alone or NIV. The authors did not find any difference in reintubation rate, hospital mortality rate, and ICU and hospital stay, despite a trend towards a shorter duration of hospital stay in the NIV group. Esteban et al.[82] conducted a large multicentre randomized trial to evaluate the effect of NIV on mortality of patients who had post-extubation respiratory failure. The study was stopped prematurely during an interim analysis, because the authors found a higher mortality rate in the NIV group, compared to the standard therapy (25% vs 14%, respectively). However, the dissimilarity appeared to be due to differences in the rate of death among the patients who required reintubation (38% in NIV group vs 22% in standard therapy group). This could correlate with the result of a longer interval between the onset of ARF and reintubation in the NIV group. This study was performed in an unselected group of patients; consequently, the authors concluded that there was the potential that selected patients (i.e. those with COPD) may still benefit from NIV, but the sample was too small to allow meaningful conclusions.

In general, NIV is not presently indicated for the treatment of patients showing respiratory distress or failure after extubation, but future studies are certainly needed in selected population of patients such as those with a chronic respiratory disorder or signs of respiratory pump failure.

Conclusion

Last, the word weaning means 'the act of taking from the breast and nourishing by other means',[83] and this may not be the best way to characterize an event, like liberation from a machine, which is associated with difficulty, pain, and disease. The individual who first coined the term weaning in this context made a perceptive choice to remind us that the disconnection from MV is not only a matter of numbers, strategies, protocols, ventilatory modes, and costs, but also care, dedication, and emotional support required by the patients who have to abandon the security of a ventilator and start breathing again by themselves. Selecting the optimal strategy for liberation from MV must consider evidence from individual experience and common sense approaches.[84] A rational approach to weaning is proposed in Figure 39.1. The recommendations from Task

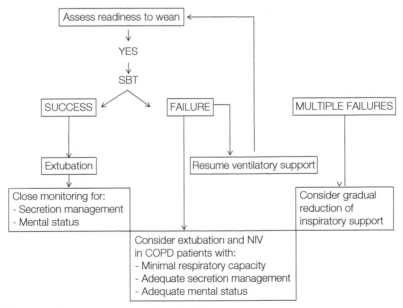

Fig. 39.1 Ventilator liberation strategy: flow chart for a rational approach.

Forces, the implementation of protocols, and the application of weaning strategies have improved the approach to the problem in the last few years; however, practice remains partly empirical and based on subjective impressions, including the patient's feeling about her/his possibility of being liberated from the ventilator.

References

1 Boles JM, Bion J, Connors A, et al. Weaning from mechanical Ventilation. *Eur Respir J* 2007;**29**: 1033–56.

2 Epstein SK, Nevins ML, Chung J. Effect of unplanned extubation on outcome of mechanical ventilation. *Am J Respir Crit Care Med* 2000;**161**:1912–16.

3 Esteban A, Alía I, Ibanez J, Benito S, Tobin MJ. Modes of mechanical ventilation and weaning: a national survey of Spanish hospitals. *Chest* 1994;**106**:1188–93.

4 Coplin WM, Pierson DJ, Cooley KD, Newell DW, Rubenfeld GD. Implications of extubation delay in brain injured patients meeting standard weaning criteria. *Am J Respir Crit Care Med* 2000;**161**: 1530–6.

5 Esteban A, Anzueto A, Frutos F, et al. Mechanical Ventilation International Study Group. Characteristics and outcomes in adult patients receiving mechanical ventilation: a 28 days international study. *JAMA* 2002;**287**:345–55.

6 Wunsch H, Linde-Zwirble WT, Angus DC, et al. The epidemiology of mechanical ventilation use in the United States. *Crit Care Med* 2010;**38**:1947–53.

7 Zilberberg MD, Shorr AF. Prolonged acute mechanical ventilation and hospital bed utilization in 2020 in the United States: implications for budgets, plant and personnel planning. *BMC Health Serv Res* 2008;**8**:242.

8 Vallverdu I, Calaf N, Subirana M, Net A, Benito S, Mancebo J. Clinical characteristics, respiratory functional parameters, and outcome of a two hours T-piece trial in patients weaning from mechanical ventilation. *Am J Respir Crit Care Med* 1998;**158**:1855–62.

9 Esteban A, Alia I, Tobin MJ, et al. Effect of spontaneous breathing trial duration on outcome of attempts to discontinue mechanical ventilation. *Am J Respir Crit Care Med* 1999;**159**:512–18.

10 Funk GC, Anders S, Breyer MK, et al. Incidence and outcome of weaning from mechanical ventilation according to new categories. *Eur Respir J* 2010;**35**:88–94.

11 Chastre J, Fagon JY. Ventilator-associated pneumonia. *Am J Respir Crit Care Med* 2002;**165**:867–903.

12 American Thoracic Society. Guidelines for the management of adults with hospital-acquired, ventilator-associated, and healthcare-associated pneumonia. *Am J Respir Crit Care Med* 2005;**171**: 388–416.

13 Straus C, Louis B, Isabey D, Lemaire F, Harf A, Brochard L. Contribution of the endotracheal tube and the upper airway to breathing workload. *Am J Respir Crit Care Med* 1998;**157**:23–30.

14 Garnacho-Montero J, Amaya Villar R, Garcia-Garmendia JL, Madrazo-Osuna J, Ortiz-Leyba C. Effect of critical illness polyneuropathy on the withdrawal from mechanical ventilation and the length of stay in septic patients. *Crit Care Med* 2005;**33**:349–54.

15 De Jonghe B, Bastuji-Garin S, Sharshar T, Outin H, Brochard L. Does ICU-acquired paresis lengthen weaning from mechanical ventilation? *Intensive Care Med* 2004;**30**:1117–21.

16 Shonhofer B, Wenzel M, Geibel M, Kohler D. Blood transfusion and lung function in chronically anemic patients with severe chronic obstructive pulmonary disease. *Crit Care Med* 1998;**26**:1824–8.

17 Huang CJ, Lin HC. Association between adrenal insufficiency and ventilator weaning. *Am J Respir Crit Care Med* 2006;**173**:276–80.

18 Kress JP, Pohlman AS, O'Connor MF, Hall JB. Daily interruption of sedative infusions in critically ill patients undergoing mechanical ventilation. *N Engl J Med* 2000;**342**:1471–7.

19 Kress JP, Gehlbach B, Lacy M, Pliskin N, Pohlman AS, Hall JB. The long-term psychological effects of daily sedative interruption on critically ill patients. *Am J Respir Crit Care Med* 2003;**168**: 1457–61.

20 Le Bourdelles G, Viires N, Boczkowski J, Seta N, Pavlovic D, Aubier M. Effects of mechanical ventilation on diaphragmatic contractile properties in rats. *Am J Respir Crit Care Med* 1994;**149**: 1539–44.

21 Vassilakopoulos T, Petrof BJ. Ventilator-induced diaphragmatic dysfunction. *Am J Respir Crit Care Med* 2004;**169**:336–41.

22 Levine S, Nguyen T, Taylor N, et al. Rapid disuse atrophy of diaphragm fibers in mechanically ventilated humans. *N Engl J Med* 2008;**358**:1327–35.

23 Jaber S, Petrof BJ, Jung B, et al. Progressive diaphragmatic weakness and injury during mechanical ventilation in humans. *Am J Respir Crit Care Med* 2011;**183**:364–71.

24 Stevens RD, Hart N, de Jonghe B, Sharshar T. Weakness in the ICU: a call to action. *Crit Care Med* 2009 ;**37**(Suppl):S299–308.

25 Leatherman JW, Fluegel WL, David WS, Davies SF, Iber C. Muscle weakness in mechanically ventilated patients with severe asthma. *Am J Respir Crit Care Med* 1996;**153**:1686–90.

26 Amaya-Villar R, Garnacho-Montero J, García-Garmendía JL, et al. Steroid-induced myopathy in patients intubated due to exacerbation of chronic obstructive pulmonary disease. *Intensive Care Med* 2005;**31**:157–61.

27 Lemaire F, Teboul JL, Cinotti L, et al. Acute left ventricular dysfunction during unsuccessful weaning from mechanical ventilation. *Anesthesiology* 1988;**69**:171–9.

28 Pinsky MR. Breathing as exercise: the cardiovascular response to weaning from mechanical ventilation. *Intensive Care Med* 2000;**26**:1164–6.

29 Srivastava S, Chatila W, Amoateng-Adjepong Y, et al. Myocardial ischemia and weaning failure in patients with coronary artery disease: an update. *Crit Care Med* 1999;**27**:2109–12.

30 Nava S, Carbone G, DiBattista N, et al. Noninvasive ventilation in cardiogenic pulmonary oedema: a multicentre trial. *Am J Respir Crit Care Med* 2003;**168**:1432–7.

31 Lin SM, Liu CY, Wang CH, et al. The impact of delirium on survival of mechanically ventilated patients. *Crit Care Med* 2004;**32**:2254–9.

32 Ely EW, Shintani A, Truman B, et al. Delirium as a predictor of mortality in mechanically ventilated patients in the intensive care unit. *JAMA* 2004;**291**:1753–62.

33 Jubran A, Lawm G, Kelly J, et al. Depressive disorders during weaning from prolonged mechanical ventilation. *Intensive Care Med* 2010;**36**:828–35.

34 Betbese AJ, Perez M, Bak E, Rialp G, Mancebo J. A prospective study of unplanned endotracheal extubation in intensive care unit patients. *Crit Care Med* 1998;**26**:1180–6.

35 Vitacca M, Vianello A, Colombo D, et al. Comparison of two methods for weaning patients with chronic obstructive pulmonary disease requiring mechanical ventilation for more than 15 days. *Am J Respir Crit Care Med* 2001;**164**:225–30.

36 Ely EW, Baker AM, Dunagan DP, et al. Effect on the duration of mechanical ventilation of identifying patients capable of breathing spontaneously. *N Engl J Med* 1996;**335**:1864–9.

37 Grap MJ, Strickland D, Tormey L, et al. Collaborative practice: development, implementation, and evaluation of a weaning protocol for patients receiving mechanical ventilation. *Am J Crit Care* 2003;**12**:454–60.

38 Ko R, Ramos L, Chalela JA. Conventional weaning parameters do not predict extubation failure in neurocritical care patients. *Neurocrit Care* 2009;**10**:269–73.

39 Navalesi P, Frigerio P, Moretti MP, et al. Rate of reintubation in mechanically ventilated neurosurgical and neurologic patients: evaluation of a systematic approach to weaning and extubation. *Crit Care Med* 2008;**36**:2986–892.

40 Girard TD, Kress JP, Fuchs BD, et al. Efficacy and safety of a paired sedation and ventilator weaning protocol for mechanically ventilated patients in intensive care (Awakening and Breathing Controlled trial): a randomised controlled trial. *Lancet* 2008;**371**:126–34.

41 Khamiees M, Raju P, DeGirolamo A, Amoateng-Adjepong Y, Manthous CA. Predictors of extubation outcome in patients who have successfully completed a spontaneous breathing trial. *Chest* 2001;**120**:1262–70.

42 De Bast Y, De Backer D, Moraine JJ, Lemaire M, Vandenborght C, Vincent JL. The cuff leak test to predict failure of tracheal extubation for laryngeal oedema. *Intensive Care Med* 2002;**28**:1267–72.

43 Jaber S, Chanques G, Matecki S, et al. Post extubation stridor in intensive care units patients. Risk factors evaluation and importance of the cuff leak test. *Intensive Care Med* 2003;**29**:69–74.

44 Conti G, Montini L, Pennisi MA, et al. A prospective, blinded evaluation of indexes proposed to predict weaning from mechanical ventilation. *Intensive Care Med* 2004;**30**:830–6.

45 Montgomery AB, Holle RH, Neagley SR, Pierson DJ, Schoene RB. Prediction of successful ventilator weaning using airway occlusion pressure and hypercapnic challenge. *Chest* 1987;**91**:496–9.

46 Yang KL, Tobin MJ. A prospective study of indexes predicting the outcome of trials of weaning from mechanical ventilation. *N Engl J Med* 1991;**324**:1445–50.

47 Meade M, Guyatt G, Cook D, et al. Predicting success in weaning from mechanical ventilation. *Chest* 2001;**120**(6 Suppl):400S–24S.

48 Tobin MJ, Jubran A. Variable performance of weaning-predictor tests: role of Bayes' theorem and spectrum and test-referral bias. *Intensive Care Med* 2006;**32**:2002–12.

49 Wysocki M, Cracco C, Teixeira A, et al. Reduced breathing variability as a predictor of unsuccessful patient separation from mechanical ventilation. *Crit Care Med* 2006;**34**:2076–83.

50 Kollef MH, Shapiro SD, Silver P, et al. A randomized, controlled trial of protocol-directed versus physician directed weaning from mechanical ventilation. *Crit Care Med* 1997;**25**:567–74.

51 Matic I, Majeric-Kogler V. Comparison of pressure support and T-tube weaning from mechanical ventilation: randomized prospective study. *Croat Med J* 2004;**45**:162–6.

52 Jones DP, Byrne P, Morgan C, Fraser I, Hyland R. Positive end-expiratory pressure versus T-piece. Extubation after mechanical ventilation. *Chest* 1991;**100**:1655–9.

53 Haberthur C, Mols G, Elsasser S, Bingisser R, Stocker R, Guttmann J. Extubation after breathing trials with automatic tube compensation, T-tube, or pressure support ventilation. *Acta Anaesthesiol Scand* 2002;**46**:973–9.

54 Mehta S, Nelson DL, Klinger JR, Buczko GB, Levy MM. Prediction of post-extubation work of breathing. *Crit Care Med* 2000;**28**:1341–6.

55 Perren A, Domenighetti G, Mauri S, Genini F, Vizzardi N. Protocol-directed weaning from mechanical ventilation: clinical outcome in patients randomized for a 30-min or 120-min trial with pressure support ventilation. *Intensive Care Med* 2002;**28**:1058–63.

56 Zeggwagh AA, Abouqal R, Madani N, Zekraoui A, Kerkeb O. Weaning from mechanical ventilation: a model for extubation. *Intensive Care Med* 1999;**25**:1077–83.

57 Cabello B, Thille AW, Roche-Campo F, Brochard L, Gómez FJ, Mancebo J. Physiological comparison of three spontaneous breathing trials in difficult-to-wean patients. *Intensive Care Med* 2010;**36**:1171–9.

58 Brochard L, Rauss A, Benito S, et al. Comparison of three methods of gradual withdrawal from ventilatory support during weaning from mechanical ventilation. *Am J Respir Crit Care Med* 1994;**150**: 896–903.

59 Esteban A, Frutos F, Tobin MJ, et al. A comparison of four methods of weaning patients from mechanical ventilation. Spanish Lung Failure Collaborative Group. *N Engl J Med* 1995;**332**:345–50.

60 Iotti GA, Polito A, Belliato M, et al. Adaptive support ventilation versus conventional ventilation for total ventilatory support in acute respiratory failure. *Intensive Care Med* 2010;**36**:1371–9.

61 Davis S, Potgieter PD, Linton DM. Mandatory minute volume weaning in patients with pulmonary pathology. *Anaesth Intensive Care* 1989;**17**:170–4.

62 Lellouche F, Mancebo J, Jolliet P, et al. A multicenter randomized trial of computer-driven protocol-ized weaning from mechanical ventilation. *Am J Respir Crit Care Med* 2006;**174**:894–900.

63 Hewlett AM, Platt AS, Terry VG. Mandatory minute volume. A new concept in weaning from mechan-ical ventilation. *Anaesthesia* 1977;**32**:163–9.

64 Brunner JX, Iotti GA. Adaptive Support Ventilation (ASV). *Minerva Anestesiol* 2002;**68**:365–8.

65 Georgopoulos D. Proportional assist ventilation: an alternative approach to wean the patient. *Eur J Anaesthesiol* 1998;**15**:756–60.

66 Sinderby C, Beck J. Proportional assist ventilation and neurally adjusted ventilatory assist-better approaches to patient ventilator synchrony? *Clin Chest Med* 2008;**29**:329–42.

67 Vitacca M, Ambrosino N, Clini E, et al. Physiological response to pressure support ventilation deliv-ered before and after extubation in patients not capable of totally spontaneous autonomous breathing. *Am J Respir Crit Care Med* 2001;**164**:638–41.

68 Burns KE, Adhikari NK, Keenan SP, Meade M. Use of non-invasive ventilation to wean critically ill adults off invasive ventilation: meta-analysis and systematic review. *BMJ* 2009;**338**:1574.

69 Girault C, Bubenheim B, Fekri Abroug Al; for the VENISE trial group. Noninvasive ventilation and weaning in patients with chronic hypercapnic respiratory failure. A randomized multicenter trial. *Am J Respir Crit Care Med* 2011;**184**:672–9.

70 Gregoretti C, Beltrame F, Lucangelo U, et al. Physiologic evaluation of non-invasive pressure support ventilation in trauma patients with acute respiratory failure. *Intensive Care Med* 1998;**24**:785–90.

71 Kilger E, Briegel J, Haller M, et al. Effects of noninvasive positive pressure ventilatory support in non-COPD patients with acute respiratory insufficiency after early extubation. *Intensive Care Med* 1999;**25**:1374–80.

72 Vaschetto R, Turucz E, Dellapiazza F, et al. Noninvasive ventilation after early extubation in patients recovering from hypoxemic acute respiratory failure: a single-centre feasibility study. *Intensive Care Med* 2012;**38**:1599–606.

73 Nava S, Hill N. Non-invasive ventilation in acute respiratory failure. *Lancet* 2009;**374**:250–9.

74 Klein M, Weksler N, Bartal C, Gurman GM. Helmet noninvasive ventilation for weaning from mechanical ventilation. *Respir Care* 2004;**49**:1035–7.

75 Epstein SK, Ciubotaru RL, Wong JB. Effect of failed extubation on the outcome of mechanical ventila-tion. *Chest* 1997;**112**:186–92.

76 Epstein SK, Ciubotaru RL. Independent effects of etiology of failure and time to reintubation on out-come for patients failing extubation. *Am J Respir Crit Care Med* 1998;**158**:489–93.

77 Torres A, Gatell JM, Aznar E, et al. Re-intubation increases the risk of nosocomial pneumonia in patients needing mechanical ventilation. *Am J Respir Crit Care Med* 1995;**152**:137–41.

78 Nava S, Gregoretti C, Fanfulla F, et al. Noninvasive ventilation to prevent respiratory failure after extu-bation in high-risk patients. *Crit Care Med* 2005;**33**:2465–70.

79 Ferrer M, Valencia M, Nicolas JM, Bernadich O, Badia JR, Torres A. Early noninvasive ventila-tion averts extubation failure in patients at risk: a randomized trial. *Am J Respir Crit Care Med* 2006;**173**:164–70.

80 Ferrer M, Sellarés J, Valencia M, et al. Non-invasive ventilation after extubation in hypercapnic patients with chronic respiratory disorders: randomised controlled trial. *Lancet* 2009;**374**:1082–8.

81 Keenan SP, Powers C, McCormack DG, Block G. Noninvasive positive-pressure ventilation for postex-tubation respiratory distress: a randomized controlled trial. *JAMA* 2002;**287**:3238–44.

82 Esteban A, Frutos-Vivar F, Ferguson ND, et al. Non-invasive positive pressure ventilation for respiratory failure after extubation. *N Engl J Med* 2004;**350**:2452–60.

83 **Williams and Wilkins Lippencott.** *Stedman's ilustrated medical dictionary.* 24th ed. Baltimore, MD: Lippencott, Williams and Wilkins; 1992. p. 1575.

84 Milic-Emili J. Is weaning an art or a science? *Am Rev Respir Dis* 1986;**134**:1107–8.

Chapter 40

Rethinking Sedation in the ICU

Sinead Galvin, Lisa Burry, and Sangeeta Mehta

Introduction

The seasonal polio epidemics of the 1940s and 1950s solidified the role of formal ICUs and also MV. The historical photographs of these ICUs show the negative pressure 'iron-lung' ventilators, with awake patients interacting with the health care staff. The following decades saw a well-intentioned trend towards the liberal use of opioids and sedatives as a compassionate means of limiting suffering for our mechanically ventilated patients. However, research in this area over the last two decades has led us to the clear understanding that excessive sedation is detrimental for both short-term and longer-term patient outcomes.

Sedation, as an umbrella term, encompasses many agents used in the ICU, disparate in terms of their mechanism of action, pharmacological profiles, and short- and longer-term side effect profiles. Arroliga and colleagues conducted an international, multicentre study (n = 5183 patients) highlighting the extent of sedative medication use, reporting sedative use in over two-thirds of patients at some point during their course of MV. This group found sedative use to be independently associated with longer durations of MV and ICU stay.[1] Analgesic and sedative medications are commonly used for the management of critically ill patients to provide analgesia, relieve anxiety, provide hypnosis when indicated, facilitate painful procedures, and promote tolerance of MV. Sedative medications may be beneficial when attempting to normalize sleep-wake patterns and may have a protective role in patients with intracranial hypertension. Table 40.1 presents the pharmacology and kinetics for commonly used analgesics and sedatives. There are many patient-specific factors that influence the selection of sedatives, including age, specific organ dysfunction, perceived pain threshold, predicted length of MV, clinical trajectory, alcohol or substance misuse history,[2] and prior psychiatric or chronic pain disorders. There may be tacit input from nursing, physicians, and other allied health care professionals, representing their personal beliefs that may also impact on the drug regimens chosen.

From work published in the last two decades, we have learned that the manner in which we administer, titrate, and monitor analgesia and sedation can impact not only ICU outcomes, but also other longer-term patient outcomes. The concept of sedation strategies that minimize drug doses is accepted and has been consolidated in subsequent trials. The overall objectives of sedation have changed, such that a calm, comfortable, awake, and interactive patient is the goal. This can be achieved using an individualized, restrictive, goal-directed, and protocolized approach to analgo-sedation. There are published interprofessional guidelines and decision support tools to guide sedation of ICU patients.[3]

Analgesia——treat pain first, all else after

Pain in the ICU

Pain is a subjective and individual sensation, and health care providers should resist from judging patients, based on preconceived notions of the severity. Studies suggest that many or most

Table 40.1 Comparison of sedative and analgesic agents[33,34]

Drug class	Agent/route	Therapeutic effect	Onset of action	Duration of effect	PK/PD	Common adverse effects
α2-adrenergic agonist	Dexmedetomidine (IV)	Activation of α_{2a}-adrenoceptor in brainstem which inhibits norepinephrine release Anaesthetic adjunct Sedation ↓ opioid needs	15–30 min	1–4 hours	M: hepatic (CYP2A6) PB: 94% $t_{1/2}$: 6 min E: renal	Hypotension Cardiac dysrhythmia (e.g. bradycardia, atrial fibrillation) Respiratory depression Nausea
Benzodiazepines	Lorazepam (PO, IM, IV)	Inhibit neuronal excitability of GABA Anxiolysis	IV 15 min	6–8 hours	M: 75% hepatic PB: 85% $t_{1/2}$: 12–18 hours E: renal	Respiratory depression/apnoea Hypotension Visual hallucinations Delirium
	Diazepam (PO, PR, IM, IV)	Sedation Amnesia Anti-convulsant Treatment of delirium tremens	IV <10 min	20–30 min	M: hepatic (CYP2C19/3A4) PB: 98% $t_{1/2}$: 20–90 hours E: renal	Paradoxical agitation Withdrawal syndrome Accumulation with prolonged use (>24 hours)
	Midazolam (PO, IM, IV)		IV <5 min	2 hours	M: hepatic (CYP3A4) PB: 95% $t_{1/2}$: 1–4 hours E: renal	High-dose lorazepam infusions may result in propylene glycol toxicity due to diluent accumulation.

Table 40.1 (continued) Comparison of sedative and analgesic agents

Drug class	Agent/route	Therapeutic effect	Onset of action	Duration of effect	PK/PD	Common adverse effects
General anaesthetics	Ketamine (IM, IV)	Non-barbiturate anaesthetic, analgesic; acts directly on cortex and limbic system to produce a cataleptic-like state by binding the NMDA and sigma opioid receptors	IV <1 min	5–10 min	M: hepatic (CYP450) PB: 50% $t_{1/2}$: 2–3 hours E: renal	Hypertension Tachycardia Hyperglycaemia Myoclonus Emergence reactions (e.g. vivid dreams, dissociative experiences)
	Propofol (IV)	Alkyl-phenoic compound Anaesthetic adjunct Anti-convulsant Treatment of delirium tremens	IV <1 min	3–10 min	M: hepatic PB: 99% $t_{1/2}$: 1.5–12 hours E: renal	Do NOT use if allergy to eggs/soy Hypotension Bradycardia Respiratory depression Hypertriglyceridaemia PRIS—acute bradycardia, with ≥1 of: metabolic acidosis, rhabdomyolysis, renal failure, hyperlipidaemia, enlarged or fatty liver

Table 40.1 (continued) Comparison of sedative and analgesic agents

Drug class	Agent/route	Therapeutic effect	Onset of action	Duration of effect	PK/PD	Common adverse effects
Opioids — Opium derivatives	Morphine (PO, EPI, IM, IV, SC, PR)	Bind to stereospecific opioid mu receptors in CNS to alter pain perception	PO 30 min IV 5–10 min	PO 4–5 hours IV 4 hours	M: hepatic (CYP2D6) PB: 30–35% $t_{1/2}$: 2–4 hours E: renal	Respiratory depression Hypotension Bradycardia Increased ICP
	Hydromorphone (PO, PR, IM, IV, SC)	Analgesia Anaesthetic adjunct Anxiolysis	PO 30 min IV 5–10 min	PO 4–5 hours IV 4 hours	M: hepatic (CYP2D6) PB: 30–35% $t_{1/2}$: 2–4 hours E: renal	Myoclonus Muscle rigidity Confusion Delirium
Opioids — Synthetic opioids	Fentanyl (Top, PO, EPI, IM, IV, SC)		IV <1 min	IM 1–2 hours IV 0.5–1 hour	M: hepatic (CYP3A4) PB: 80–85% $t_{1/2}$: 2–4 hours E: renal	Pruritus, urticaria Constipation, nausea, vomiting
	Alfentanil (IV, IM, EPI)		IV <1 min	IV 30–60 min	¼ fentanyl's potency M: hepatic (CYP3A) PB: 92% $t_{1/2}$: 80–100 min E: renal	
	Remifentanil (IV)		1–3 min	<10 min	M: esterases PB: 70% (not albumin) $t_{1/2}$: 3–10 min E: renal	
	Sufentanil (IV, EPI)		IV 1–3 min	IV 30 min	7–10x more potent than fentanyl M: hepatic PB: 91–93% $t_{1/2}$: 2.5–3 hours E: renal	

E, elimination; EPI, epidural; IV, intravenous; IM, intramuscular; M, metabolism; PB, protein binding; PD, pharmacodynamics; PK, pharmacokinetics; PO, oral; PR, rectal; SC, subcutaneous; Top, topical; t1/2, half-life.

critically ill patients experience pain, with one study reporting moderate to severe pain in 50% of patients surveyed.[4] It is estimated that as many as 70% of patients experience at least moderate intensity procedure-related or post-operative pain during their stay in the ICU.[5,6] Pain may be under-recognized and undertreated, and sources of pain may not be obvious to the care provider. Commonly reported causes of pain include tracheal suctioning, pressure areas, IV injection sites, inability to rotate weight distribution, and ETT and tracheostomy traction. Inadequately recognized and undertreated pain has detrimental effects, including patient distress, sympathetic overactivity, sleep disturbance, delayed mobilization, secretion retention/atelectasis, delirium, PTSD, and the development of chronic pain syndromes. There is individual variation in the response to pain, which is influenced by genetics, age, gender, and cultural background. Our approach should be patient-centred and focus on pre-emptive pain control, regular scheduled dosing, and minimizing the adverse effects of our interventions.

Systems approach

Recognition of the extent of pain in ICU patients has popularized an analgesia-first approach entitled 'analgosedation'. Breen and colleagues[7] demonstrated that analgesia-first-based sedation approach was well tolerated, consistently achieved the desired comfort goals, and was associated with a reduced duration of MV, compared to hypnotic-first-based sedation. Institutional clinical pathways or algorithms for pain management have been shown to be effective.[8,9] The use of a pain resource nurse programme[10] and of a referral source,[11] such as an acute pain service, have also shown good results. The American Pain Society regularly publishes concise, rigorous guidelines to address pain management in specific patient populations, and these are invaluable in the education, decision support, and the quality improvement process (available at: http://www. ampainsoc.org). Their most recent quality improvement recommendations are: (1) recognize and treat pain promptly, (2) involve patients and families in the pain management plan, (3) improve treatment patterns, (4) reassess and adjust the pain management plan as needed, and (5) monitor processes and outcomes of pain management.[12]

ICU staff should use validated methods and assess pain scores frequently. An assessment method that is suitable for the individual patient should be used. The validated numerical rating or VAS (see Table 40.2) may be ideal for an awake, alert patient, but a facial pain rating scale may be needed for a disorientated, uncooperative patient. It is also vitally important to clearly document the results and adverse effects of any pain intervention; as these will help the health care team to formulate future analgesia plans.

Pharmacological approach

Many pain interventions in the ICU involve the use of potent opioids, which are reliable and rapid in the management of moderate to severe pain. However, all opioids have the potential to cause deep sedation, reduced respiratory drive, and hypotension. The push towards awake and mobile ICU patients may necessitate a re-evaluation in the management of pain in ICU patients. A balanced, multi-modal, and holistic approach to pain may be useful. The non-pharmacological approaches will be addressed later in this review. A balanced, multi-modal approach to analgesia works on the premise that using two or more agents, with different mechanisms of actions, achieve superior analgesic effect while limiting adverse effects by avoiding increased doses of a single agent. Acetaminophen and NSAIDs are effective for low-intensity pain or as adjuncts or opioid-sparing agents in moderate to severe pain. Given the extent of organ dysfunction in ICU patients,

Table 40.2 Pain, delirium, and sedation assessment tools for use in mechanically ventilated patients

Assessment tool (year)	Scale design	Conditions measured					Validity and reliability testing
		Consciousness	Agitation	Ventilator synchrony	Pain	Delirium	
Pain BPS (2001)[58,99,100]	Sum score of the components: facial expression, movement of upper limbs, compliance with MV				◆		Reliability (r 0.5–0.71) Validated in medical-surgical ICU patients during painful and non-painful procedures Responsiveness decreases with deeper sedation
CPOT (2006)[101,102]	Sum score of four components: facial expression, body movements, muscle tension, compliance if intubated (vocalization if not intubated)				◆		Validated in cardiac surgery patients, using periods of rest, painful stimulation, and 20 minutes after stimulation Evaluations conducted while patients were conscious and unconscious
Ramsay (1974)[49]	6-level scale describes consciousness, agitation, and anxiety Only a single level to describe agitation or anxiousness (score = 1)	◆	◆				Reliability (κ 0.94) Validated in medical ICU patients vs RASS and BIS (r –0.4 to –0.78)
Sedation SAS (1994)[50,51]	7-level scale describes consciousness and agitation	◆	◆				Reliability (κ 0.85–0.93) Validated in medical and surgical ICU patients vs Ramsay, VAS, and BIS (r 0.43–0.90)
MAAS (1999)[52]	7-level scale describes consciousness and agitation	◆	◆				Reliability (κ 0.83) Validated in surgical ICU patients vs VAS, BP, HR, and agitation-related sequelae (P = 0.001)
VICS (2000)[53]	Two domains: interaction, calmness 5 questions per domain; each question has six responses from 'strongly agree' to 'strongly disagree'	◆	◆				Reliability (κ 0.89–0.90) Validated in medical and surgical ICU patients vs need for intervention (r –0.83) Responsive

Assessment tool (year)	Scale design	Conditions measured Consciousness	Agitation	Ventilator synchrony	Pain	Delirium	Validity and reliability testing
RASS (2002)[54,55]	10-level scale from −4 to +5 to describe consciousness, agitation, and cognition or comprehension. Used in step 1 of CAM-ICU delirium tool	◆	◆				Reliability (κ 0.64–0.96). Validated in medical and surgical MV patients vs Ramsay, VAS, SAS, BIS (r 0.78–0.91). Also extensively tested in other populations: neurological, cardiac, trauma. Responsive
ATICE (2003)[56]	5-item scale: awakeness and comprehension, calmness, ventilator synchrony, facial relaxation. Divided into two domains: consciousness, tolerance. Also tests cognition or comprehension	◆	◆	◆			Reliability (κ 0.82–0.99). Validated in adult medical ICU patients vs Ramsay, VAS, SAS, GCS (r 0.37–0.95). Responsive. Sum of multiple subscales adds to complexity scoring
MSAT (2004)[57]	Arousal domain. Awakeness domain (spontaneous, then response to auditory and physical stimuli). Motor activity domain	◆		◆			Reliability (κ 0.72–0.85). Validated in adult medical and surgical MV patients vs VICS (r −0.41 to 0.68)
CAM-ICU (2001)[70–72]	2-step approach: (A) If RASS >−4, → B) assess four features of delirium: acute onset or fluctuating course, inattention, disorganized thinking, altered level of consciousness. Yes/no questions for use with non-verbal patients	◆				◆	High inter-rater reliability (P <0.0001). Validated in medical and cardiac ICU patients. High sensitivity (0.9–1.0) and specificity (0.89–1.0), compared to psychiatric DSM-IV assessment
ICDSC (2001)[73]	2-step approach: (A) assessment of consciousness. If patient responsive, proceed to: (B) assess eight features: consciousness, inattention, disorientation, hallucinations, psychomotor agitation, mood speech, sleep-wake cycle disturbances, symptom fluctuation	◆				◆	Validated in medical and surgical patients. Sensitivity (0.99), specificity (0.64) vs psychiatric DSM-IV assessment

Delirium

ATICE, Adaptation to the Intensive Care Environment; BIS, Bispectral Index; BPS, Behaviour Pain Scale; MV, mechanical ventilation; GCS, Glasgow Coma Scale; K, κ statistic; MAAS, Motor Activity Assessment Scale; MSAT, Minnesota Sedation Assessment Tool; r, correlation; RASS, Richmond Agitation Sedation Scale; SAS, Sedation Agitation Scale; VICS, Vancouver Interactive and Calmness Scale; VAS, Visual Analogue Scale.

there may be a reticence to use these agents, particularly NSAIDs. Their use may be justified in more stable patients with normal renal and liver function. Gabapentin and pregabalin are related GABA analogues, anti-convulsant medications that have an established role in pain therapy; both drugs exert their effects by selectively binding presynaptic P/Q type voltage-dependent calcium channels. Pregabalin is a newer, lipophilic GABA analogue, substituted to enhance diffusion across the BBB.[13] Pregabalin has been used to good effect in both neuropathic-type pain and acute incisional post-procedural pain. Pregabalin has also been shown to have a favourable sleep-inducing profile, increasing slow-wave restorative sleep in healthy volunteers.[14] While both of these agents can cause dose-related sedation, this is less profound than seen with potent IV opioid administration. A recent study evaluated pregabalin use in elderly (>75 years) post-cardiac surgical patients. The treatment group received pregabalin preoperatively and twice daily for 5 post-operative days, and the control arm received placebo.[15] In the pregabalin group, cumulative consumption of parenteral oxycodone during 16 hours after extubation was reduced by 44%, and total oxycodone consumption from extubation to the end of the fifth post-operative day was reduced by 48%. These GABA analogue agents seem to have potential in the pain armamentarium in the ICU. Another option for analgesia in longer-term ICU patients are the weaker opioid agents such as tramadol and codeine. These agents may be useful for treating baseline, mild to moderate pain in certain patients. As with the GABA analogues, they can be sedating but usually to a lesser extent than the potent opioids. They can be dosed orally and regularly, and the dosing schedules could be timed to give analgesic coverage for physiotherapy and mobilization sessions. Other adjuvant agents listed in balanced approach ladders include ketamine and clonidine. Both agents are useful for treating moderate and severe pain, but they are associated with effects which may limit mobilization and DIS. These agents may represent a reasonable choice as targeted analgosedation for short, planned interventions such as dressing and line changes. Clonidine may have a particular role in the setting of sympathetic overactivity syndromes associated with alcohol and drug withdrawal and in the sedative weaning phase.[16]

Another aspect of a balanced approach to analgesia is regional anaesthesia. The use of regional anaesthesia techniques is common in surgical and trauma ICUs. A variety of techniques from wound infiltration to peripheral nerve or plexus blockade (single shot or catheter technique) to neuraxial blockade (epidural or subarachnoid blockade, via single shot, catheter technique, or patient-controlled system) are utilized. These modalities are often initiated in the operating room by anaesthesiology and managed in the ICU by a pain outreach service. There may be less familiarity initiating these techniques in general or medical ICUs. The staffing demographics of an ICU may also impact on user familiarity with regional techniques. Presumably, those with an anaesthesia or surgical background may be more familiar with the techniques. There are many potential contraindications to regional anaesthesia, including local or systemic infection,[17] coagulopathy, anticoagulant or antiplatelet medication,[18] or patient refusal. Nevertheless, these techniques certainly have a role in procedural pain in certain patients to offset the need or reduce the dose of sedating medication. Rigorous attention to adequate and generous local anaesthesia preparation of IV access sites, percutaneous tracheostomy sites, or thoracocentesis sites can reduce procedural pain. Repeated intercostal nerve blocks can be considered for ongoing thoracostomy discomfort. Epidural placement has been described to offset the pain of severe acute pancreatitis[19] and blunt chest trauma in the ICU.[20] Other indications for peripheral nerve blockade might include destructive cancer pain or painful ischaemic tissue loss. As with any approach to patient management, education, quality assurance, and decision support tools are invaluable. The European Society of Regional Anaesthesia (available at: http://www.ESRA.org)

and New York Society of Regional Anaesthesia (available at: http://www.NYSORA.com) have detailed education and resource websites.

Sedation administration strategies

Sedation minimization

DIS has many potential advantages, including the opportunity to cease drug infusions completely or to reduce dosage, the opportunity to perform a comprehensive neurological and delirium assessment, and to assess the patient for readiness for liberation from the ventilator. Two pivotal trials that focused on reducing sedation altered the way in which we apply analgesia and sedation for MV patients. Brook and colleagues compared the impact of a nursing-implemented sedation protocol vs usual sedation care on duration of MV and other important clinical outcomes.[21] Sedation was titrated to a Ramsay score of 2–3, and the protocol emphasized the reduction of continuous sedative infusions in favour of intermittent sedation. They demonstrated a significant reduction in the duration of MV (55 hours vs 117 hours, $P = 0.004$) for patients randomized to the nurse-directed sedation protocol, compared to the usual care group. The intervention group also had shorter durations of both ICU and hospital lengths of stay and lower tracheostomy rates. In another single-centre randomized trial, Kress and colleagues compared daily interruption of sedative/analgesic infusions with usual sedation management.[22] The median duration of MV in the DIS group was 4.9 days, compared to 7.3 days in the control group ($P = 0.004$), in whom infusions were interrupted only at the discretion of the clinician. After adjustment for baseline variables, the DIS group was discharged earlier from ICU. The DIS group required fewer tests to evaluate decreased level of consciousness (9% vs 27% in control group) and received approximately 50% of the midazolam doses as the control group. The DIS group had no increase in adverse events; in particular, self-extubation rates were similar in the two groups.

Following the work by Brook[21] and Kress,[22] subsequent trials have expanded upon the concept of sedation minimization strategies. Girard and colleagues[23] evaluated a paired approach of an SBT and DIS, compared with usual sedation care and an SBT. The treatment 'wake up and breathe' group had more days breathing without assistance (14.7 vs 11.6 days, $P = 0.02$), shorter hospital and ICU length of stays, but no differences in ICU or hospital mortality. The intervention group had a higher incidence of self-extubation (16 patients vs six patients in the control group). At 1 year, mortality was significantly, but inexplicably, lower in the intervention than the control group, with a number to treat (NNT) of 7, suggesting that, for every seven patients treated with the intervention, one life was saved.

Strom and colleagues[24] compared a protocol of no sedation, consisting of opioid analgesia boluses only, with a control sedation infusion group (using propofol and midazolam, DIS, and rescue opioid analgesia boluses) in 140 medical-surgical ICU patients. The no sedation group had significantly more VFDs (13.8 vs 9.6 days, $P = 0.019$) and shorter stays in both ICU and hospital. Criticisms of this study include the stringent exclusion criteria, such that only 140 of 428 patients were randomized; and the control group was sicker by SOFA (day 1) and SAPS II scoring methods. There was no demonstrable increase in adverse events, such as accidental extubation in the no sedation group, but delirium was recorded more frequently in the intervention group (20% vs 7%), necessitating more frequent use of haloperidol. However, speculatively, this could represent improved delirium recognition by staff in the awake patients or also a trend towards more hyperactive symptoms, rather than hypoactive symptomatology in the awake patients. An extra person was needed at the bedside in the intervention group to comfort and reassure patients. The economic implication of this increased manpower demand may potentially be offset by reduced pharmaceutical costs and reduced ICU stay, but this will require complex further economic analysis of both direct and indirect costing. However, this trial clearly shows that a limited sedation approach is feasible, may be associated with improved important outcomes, seems to be safe; and is certainly worthy of ongoing study. Clearly, a move towards no sedation in our ICU patients will demand further evidence to support improved outcomes, a major change in not only staff, but also patient and family attitudes and ongoing education. A renewed focus on other means of improving patient comfort will be imperative such as increased family and caregiver presence, bedside sitters, local anaesthesia techniques and regional blocks for invasive lines, and interactive ventilator modes to increase comfort.

More recently, a multicentre randomized trial compared protocolized sedation with combined protocolized sedation plus daily sedation interruption in 423 critically ill mechanically ventilated medical and surgical patients.[25] There was no difference in the primary outcome of duration of MV nor in ICU and hospital lengths of stay between the groups. Furthermore, patients in the daily interruption group received higher daily opioid and benzodiazepines doses, and nurses reported higher workload in this group. Thus, while daily sedation interruption appears to be safe, its effectiveness likely depends on the usual institutional sedation care; and, if patients are kept lightly sedated, daily interruption does not add further benefit.

Considering the earlier DIS data from over a decade ago, it had a startling impact in terms of outcome improvement and practice change. Subsequent studies have at times not demonstrated a benefit.[26,27] In contrast to the study by Brook et al.,[21] Bucknall et al.[26] did not find any clinical benefits to the use of a nurse-directed sedation protocol, compared with usual care in an Australian ICU. They proposed that the lack of observed benefit was due to a new era of more restrictive sedation practice where depth of sedation monitoring is enforced. They suggest that earlier trial benefits may have come from the relative reduction in cumulative dosing, and thus, in this current more restrictive dosing environment, DIS may not be as vital. Given also that protocolized sedation directs titration of therapy to prevent bioaccumulation, its use may not be advantageous or necessary when administering drugs with an ultrashort half-life such as propofol. In fact, in certain groups of patients, such as those with active myocardial ischaemia, raised intracranial pressure (ICP), or substance dependence, DIS may not be the most ideal model of approach. A study by DeWit and colleagues[28] raised concerns about the use of DIS in patients with a history of alcohol or substance misuse. Surveys have shown that ICU clinicians have concerns about DIS in certain patient groups.[29]

Choice of agent

A complex review of these agents is beyond the scope of this chapter; thus, we have briefly summarized the key individual characteristics in Table 40.1. Guidelines for sedation and analgesia in the ICU produced by a Task Force of the American College of Critical Care Medicine in 2002 recommended midazolam and propofol for short-term sedation (< 24 hours), and lorazepam for longer-term sedation (>24 hours).[3] However, these recommendations were based on a small number of RCTs. Trials published since 2002 have produced mixed results regarding the 'best' agent to use in various critically ill populations. Several RCTs have documented faster time to awakening and reduced duration of MV with propofol, compared to benzodiazepines, but no difference in ICU length of stay or mortality.[30–32] However, propofol is associated with a number of undesirable features such as hypotension, hypertriglyceridaemia, propofol infusion syndrome (PRIS), and high acquisition cost.[33–35] Surveys of North American clinicians document high use of lorazepam and midazolam, with a smaller proportion of respondents (<25%) citing propofol as their primary sedative of choice.[29,36,37] International surveys suggest morphine is still the favoured analgesic for most clinicians, but the use of fentanyl and newer short-acting fentanyl derivatives is increasing.[36-38]

Novel pharmacological agents

Dexmedetomidine, a centrally acting α2-adrenergic agonist with both sedative and analgesic properties, with little effect on respiratory drive, has been studied primarily in the post-operative setting.[39] Recent randomized trials have explored the use of this drug beyond 72 hours in medical and surgical mechanically ventilated ICU patients, with promising results.[40-42] In the MENDS trial, Pandharipande and colleagues[42] randomized 106 patients to dexmedetomidine or lorazepam for up to 120 hours and demonstrated an increased number of days alive without delirium or coma in the dexmedetomidine group (7 vs 3 days, $P = 0.01$), without any reductions in duration of MV or ICU length of stay. In the larger 375-patient multicentre SEDCOM trial, patients treated with dexmedetomidine for up to 30 days had shorter median times to extubation (3.7 vs 5.1 days, $P = 0.01$) and experienced significantly less delirium (54% vs 76.6% of patients, $P < 0.001$) than midazolam-treated patients.[40] The most notable adverse effect was bradycardia, occurring twice as often in the dexmedetomidine group (42.2% vs 18.9%, $P < 0.001$). A 20-patient pilot study of dexmedetomidine vs haloperidol use in already delirious intubated patients showed shorter median times to extubation and shorter ICU stays in the dexmedetomidine group.[43] At present, dexmedetomidine may not be available in all countries and is costly, and its utility in the general ICU population is not fully delineated, given that patients with significant organ dysfunction were excluded from some of the trials previously described, and the ideal dosing regimen is somewhat unclear. However, it shows promising results as an analgosedative agent in those at high risk of delirium or those who are already delirious.

Remifentanil is an ultrashort-acting synthetic opioid. The context-sensitive half-life is 3-5 minutes, even in prolonged infusion, as plasma clearance occurs rapidly by non-specific esterases.[33] Remifentanil has been shown in several RCTs to decrease the duration of MV and ICU length of stay when compared to morphine, fentanyl, or midazolam.[44-47] Other desirable effects may include decreased cerebral metabolism and ICP, with minimal cerebral perfusion pressure changes. The routine use of remifentanil in the ICU is limited by high cost, rapid emergence of pain upon drug discontinuation, unless carefully titrated or substituted with a longer-acting agent, and the paucity of data for prolonged use in varied ICU populations. Remifentanil may have a particular role in neuro ICU where blunting of central hyperventilation and resultant hypocarbia must be balanced with regular, sedation-interrupted neurological assessment.[44]

Sevoflurane is a halogenated, volatile inhalational agent, commonly used in the operating theatre for both induction and maintenance of anaesthesia. Sevoflurane has a short duration of action and a brief elimination delay. In a recent three-arm study, Mesnil et al. compared longer-term (> 24 hours) goal-directed sedation in 47 ICU patients, using either inhaled sevoflurane, IV midazolam, or propofol.[48] The sevoflurane intervention group had significantly shorter wake-up time and extubation delay times than either of the IV agent groups. The proportion of the study time spent at the desired Ramsay Sedation Scale level 3-4 was similar between the groups; there were fewer hallucinations reported in the sevoflurane group and a tendency towards less post-extubation opioid use, suggesting an antihyperalgesia effect from sevoflurane. This small study suggests that sevoflurane may be a valid agent for ICU sedation in the future, pending further data.

Sedation monitoring

Objective goal-directed sedation is now a recommended standard to avoid oversedation, to promote earlier liberation from MV, and to minimize ICU length of stay. Standardized sedation assessment tools are used to judge the depth of sedation through indicators such as movement and response to verbal or physical stimuli. A useful sedation assessment tool should have discrete criteria that are easy to recall, apply, and interpret when used by frontline care providers. There are numerous validated scales with good inter-rater reliability (see Table 40.2).[49–57] Several newer scales, such as the ATICE[56] and Motor Activity Assessment Scale (MAAS),[52] have the added advantage of evaluation of multiple domains such as consciousness, agitation, motor activity, sleep, or patient-ventilator synchrony. The RASS, ATICE, and the Vancouver Interaction and Calmness Scale (VICS) have also been shown to accurately reflect responsiveness (change in sedation status over time).[53,54,56] Several single-centre studies have shown a reduction in oversedation, duration of MV, and costs with the introduction of a sedation scale.[58–61] Whether the use of a particular scale, compared to another, results in superior clinical outcomes in not yet known. Table 40.2 presents a summary of pain, delirium, and sedation assessment tools for use in mechanically ventilated patients.

Patient-controlled sedation (PCS)

The concept of patient-controlled analgesia is not new in ICU, particularly in surgical or mixed units. The concept of patient-controlled analgesia accepts that health care providers are subjective and not the best judge of patients' pain or distress. Preselected patient groups can take control of both opioid and epidural analgesia regimes, with good effect. Studies suggest better patient satisfaction, less analgesic consumption overall, and better pain scores. The history and experience for patient-controlled analgesia comes predominantly from the acute pain literature. The concept of PCS is newer and, to date, has only been described outside the critical care setting for shorter invasive procedures. A proof of concept pilot study evaluated a select group of MV patients using dexmedetomidine PCS with strict lockout parameters (with a nurse-controlled basal infusion rate).[62] Staff and patients were satisfied with the resultant sedation in this study. There were some adverse physiological side effects, such as hypotension and bradycardia, which were likely agent-specific. This pilot study raises the feasibility of PCS in the ICU sphere and is certainly worthy of ongoing study.

Non-pharmacological approaches to analgosedation in the ICU

The ultimate goal is awake, alert, and mobile ICU patients, such that intensivists must limit the use of sedating medication, while recognizing that patients may experience pain, anxiety, disordered sleep patterns, and distress while in ICU. Other non-pharmacological approaches may be helpful, though, in truth, there are little compelling data from either the ICU or the pain literature. However, the popularity for these alternative approaches has grown rapidly, such that the NIH established the Office of Alternative Medicine in 1992 (now the National Centre for Complementary and Alternative Medicine). We describe several simple non-pharmacological interventions here.

Noise reduction and optimum lighting

ICU must deliver 24-hour care to the sickest patients, making it one of the noisier places in the hospital. The recommended noise levels are frequently exceeded.[63] Our patients are consistently exposed to harsh lighting, phones ringing, pagers, other devices, alarms, and staff conversations.

Patients report major concerns with the level of noise in intensive care.[64] Simple interventions, such as safely reducing alarm volumes, diverting phone calls to a central area at night, patient earplugs, and discouraging noisy discussion at the bedside, may be helpful. Natural light access is a priority in ICU design and planning nowadays, as this may help in normalizing the night-day rhythm cycles of our patients. Otherwise, dimming the overhead lights at night and avoiding harsh fluorescent lights, except for procedures, seems prudent. An interventional study to decrease noise in a neurocritical care unit showed significantly improved observed sleep with the introduction of twice-daily quiet-time and light-dimming protocol.[65]

Massage therapy

Massage therapy efficacy is established in sleep promotion and relaxation in ICU patients.[66] Massage can help to relieve muscle pain and tension from positioning, contractures, or exercise. It is a simple, cheap, and comforting approach to patient discomfort. Basic staff training and prior patient consent are imperative. Family members can also be instructed in simple techniques like hand and foot massage, and this may help empower the family. TENS machines are used for the relief of acute and chronic pain syndromes. The evidence for their efficacy is relatively conflicting, but certain patients report very good pain relief. The mechanism of action is thought to be via both mediation and closing of gated pain channels and via natural endorphin stimulation. TENS machines are not advised for patients who are pacemaker-dependent or who have a seizure disorder. Otherwise, it is a benign intervention; it is easy to apply the electrodes, either while in bed or mobile, and it may work for some patients. Other simple interventions worth trying include sequential hot packs and ice packs to tender muscle groups or joints. These packs should be avoided in insensate areas, given the risk of thermal injury. The relief from all these interventions may be small, but cumulative, and patients can feedback in terms of the perceived benefit.

Distraction therapy

This encompasses therapies such as music therapy, hypnosis, and imagery therapy. These methods all come under the umbrella term complementary or alternative therapy. For music therapy, the genre selection, audio volume, and timing should be dictated by the patient and can be relaxing and comforting. The same holds for imagery therapy where familiar photographs or familiar image projection may help relaxation and recall of pleasant memories.

Increased family presence

The extent of family presence allowed in ICUs varies greatly. 'Restricted' visiting practice allows a fixed number of visitors and very specific time allowances, usually preset by hospital policy. The rationale for such a practice includes undisturbed patient sleep, a less crowded ICU, and less interruption of nursing duties and medical procedures. 'Open' visiting allows families to visit any time during the 24-hour day, often for as long as they wish. The rationale for this approach includes improved patient mood and emotional well-being and the perception of the family as instrumental in the care and communication process. Gonzalez et al.[67] examined patients' preferences for family visiting in an ICU and a complex care medical unit. Patients participated in a structured interview that assessed their preferences for visiting, stressors and benefits of visiting, and their perceived satisfaction with hospital guidelines for visiting. This study clearly shows that patients in both units rated visiting as a non-stressful experience, because visitors offered reassurance, comfort, and calm. Patients in the ICU valued the fact that visitors could assist them in interpreting the information provided by health care providers and that visitors could provide information to help nurses understand a patient's personality and coping style. With increased awareness of acute delirium in ICU and of the dangers of excessive sedative medications, we may need to allow and facilitate more bedside family presence. This increased presence may help to orientate and calm the agitated patient. The family member can thus be more instrumental in the simpler care interventions for their loved ones. In neonatal and paediatric ICUs, extended-hours family presence and involvement in routines, such as dressing, bathing, and feeding, are often the norm. This may well be a model we need to borrow from in our adult practice.

Counselling and communication

Simple, frequent, and repeated communication is vital in helping the patient to adjust to the ICU environment. In busy ICUs, this aspect of direct communication with the patient may be overlooked. By explaining any medical updates and planned intervention to the patient and by staff taking the time to understand patient's discomfort, worries, and values, the patient may be comforted. Patients can gain a realistic view of the care limitations, such that we can promise pain relief but may not be able to guarantee 'pain-free status'.

Acupuncture

Acupuncture may have a role in anxiolysis, the reduction of nausea, and acute pain management in the ICU. Again, there are little robust data as yet to solidify its role. The need for informed patient consent and for trained staff and contraindications, such as bleeding disorders, will make acupuncture unfeasible in some cases. Some pilot studies in ICU[68] have shown promising results, and larger trials may be justified.

Other

There are many other means of potentially comforting and limiting the suffering of our critical care patients. These include animal-assisted therapy, accompanied trips outside the ICU, and alternative Eastern medicine approaches.

Delirium: prevention, assessment, and management

Delirium is an acute and fluctuating disturbance of consciousness and cognition that can be characterized as either hyperactive (increased psychomotor activity with agitated behaviour), hypoactive (decreased psychomotor behaviour, somnolence, and lethargy), or mixed. Delirium, or acute brain dysfunction, is common in ICU patients and may go unnoticed.[69] The reported prevalence of delirium in the ICU ranges between 20 and 80%, depending on patient severity of illness and the method of detection.[70–74] The Diagnostic and Statistical Manual of Mental Disorders, 4th edition (DSM-IV) provides the gold standard criteria for the diagnosis of delirium,[75] but the assessment requires a minimum of 30 minutes by a psychiatrist, which is usually impractical in the ICU. The DSM-IV defines delirium as the presence of: (1) a disturbance of consciousness with inattention, accompanied by (2) an acute change in cognition (i.e. disorientation, perceptual disturbances) not accounted for by pre-existing, established, or evolving dementia; (3) development over a short period of time (hours to days), with fluctuation over time; and (4) evidence that the disturbance is caused by the direct physiological consequences of a general medical condition.[75] The CAM-ICU and ICDSC are two delirium screening tools. These two ICU-specific assessment instruments have established validity and reliability for the diagnosis of delirium by a non-psychiatric physician (see Table 40.2).[70–73] Either of these tools can be used to detect hypo- or hyperactive delirium, as they assess clarity of thought, rather than focusing on level of consciousness. Recent data suggest that the ICDSC (see Table 40.2) may have potential benefits over the CAM-ICU. The ICDSC was specifically developed and validated for screening delirium in mechanically ventilated ICU patients and has been shown to have excellent validity, compared to psychiatrist assessment using DSM-IV criteria.

The link between exposure to benzodiazepines and opioids and a 2–3-fold risk of delirium in the ICU has been well documented, lending further support to the judicious use of these agents in ICU patients.[40,42,74,76–80] Ely et al.[81] evaluated delirium as a predictor of mortality in a prospective cohort of 275 MV adult patients. In this study, delirium, after covariate adjustment, was associated with longer ICU and hospital stay, fewer VFDs, and higher incidence of cognitive impairment at discharge. Not only was delirium a predictor of 6-month mortality (34% vs 15%), but also the number of days spent in a delirious state was predictive of mortality. Up to 11% of survivors had persistent delirium at hospital discharge. These investigators also found that delirious patients, compared to non-delirious patients, received higher daily and cumulative doses of lorazepam, propofol, morphine, and fentanyl and suggested a causal relationship.

Multi-component interventions aimed at preventing delirium have shown good results in geriatric and surgical hospitalized patients but have not been formally evaluated in the ICU population.[82–84] These interventions include (but are not limited to): review of medications for agents that may cause or exacerbate delirium, restoration of the sleep-wake cycle, frequent reorientation, removal of unnecessary catheters, reintroduction of eye glasses and hearing aids, and early mobilization. Evidence supporting the use of pharmacologic agents for delirium in the ICU is also lacking. While the SCCM guidelines recommended haloperidol as the drug of choice for ICU delirium, at the time of the publication, there were no published trials supporting its use.[3]

There still exist limited data evaluating the use of antipsychotics in the ICU. Only three small randomized trials have evaluated antipsychotics in critically ill patients.[85–87] In a randomized feasibility trial, Girard et al.[85] showed similar mean duration of days alive without delirium and coma for patients treated with haloperidol, ziprasidone, or placebo (14, 15, and 13.5 days, respectively, P = 0.66) and no difference in adverse drug events. In a pilot study (n = 36), quetiapine was compared to placebo in 36 patients diagnosed with delirium, based on ICDSC screening.[86] Quetiapine resulted in faster first resolution of delirium (median 1 day vs 4.5 days, P = 0.001), reduced duration of delirium (median 36 hours vs 120 hours, P = 0.006), and fewer hours of agitation (median 6 hours vs 36 hours, P = 0.002). A single–centre, unblinded trial comparing haloperidol to olanzapine found no difference in delirium severity nor the proportion of patients requiring benzodiazepines.[87] An Australian pilot study compared haloperidol vs dexmedetomidine in the treatment of established delirium,[43] with a suggestion of improved outcome variables in the dexmedetomidine group. It is important to note that the use of antipsychotic agents is not without complications (e.g. extrapyramidal effects, anticholinergic effects, malignant hyperthermia) and has been associated with increased mortality in elderly patients.[88,89]

Sleep disturbance in the ICU

Sleep disturbance is widespread in mechanically ventilated patients. On average, ICU patients sleep only 2 hours per day, and less than 10% of this is restorative or REM sleep.[90] A recent study suggested that noise and patient care activities account for less than 30% of arousals and awakenings and suggested that other elements contribute to this sleep disturbance such as underlying illness, medications, and disordered circadian rhythm.[91] Sleep in the ICU is difficult to reliably assess; polysomnography (PSG) is the objective gold standard but is challenging and expensive to undertake in ICU patients. Other objective sleep measurement tools, such as BIS and actigraphy, have not been validated for ICU patients. Subjective measurements of sleep include nursing and patient assessment, and, in clinical practice, they offer the only real means of assessing the efficacy of interventions in attempting to improve patients' sleep. There is a necessity for further research in the techniques for measuring sleep in the critical care patient. Concurrent assessment of sleep and delirium is especially important if we are to appropriately guide pharmacological and non-pharmacological therapies.

Early mobilization in the ICU

Early mobilization of ICU patients was commonplace in earlier decades. In more recent decades, deep sedation, prolonged bed rest, and generally sicker patients became the ICU norm. Many ICU patients receive little physiotherapy or mobilization, certainly until almost ready for ICU discharge.[92] Recent compelling evidence has shown us that early physiotherapy and OT interventions can improve long-term outcomes.[93,94] These favourable outcomes have included length of MV, length of ICU stay, ICUAW, delirium-free days, improved longer-term return to physical/cognitive baseline, and ultimate home discharge. It also appears that this drive towards early physical activity is acceptable to patients and is safe. When we consider the safety aspects of regularly mobilizing our ventilated patients, we need to ensure pain-free, awake, alert, and delirium-free patients. This will further necessitate regularly interrupting sedation, using boluses, rather than infusions, using agents with less accumulation potential, using strict protocols, and identifying unresolved pain. The goals of pain relief should be complete dynamic analgesia, which can be challenging. The involvement of acute pain services may guide us in addressing this need, as dynamic analgesia has been the goal of acute pain services for many years. The reward of seeing ambulatory, interactive patients on the ICU more than justifies the necessary attention to detail needed with our sedation practice.

Conclusion

While the field of sedation administration in the ICU has progressed over the last two decades, there remain many areas for further improvement and exploration. Standardization of ICU sedation practices, in line with best RCT-derived evidence and international guidelines, is enticing. However, as in many other areas of critical care practice, despite rigorous evidence-based recommendations, there is a delay or gap in their implementation. This gap between the evidence and actual practice has been highlighted in the various surveys on sedation practices, particularly in those carried out post-publication of the 2002 SCCM guidelines.[1,36,38,95–98]

We still need robust data on the safety and relative efficacy of the newer sedative agents, such as dexmedetomidine, on optimizing analgosedation for patients who are candidates for early mobilization, on alternative quantitative methods of measuring the depth of sedation, such as BIS, on the prevention of, and best pharmacologic management, of ICU delirium, and on the impact of drugs and titration strategies on sleep and long-term psychological morbidity.

References

1 **Arroliga A, Frutos-Vivar F, Hall J, et al.** Use of sedatives and neuromuscular blockers in a cohort of patients receiving mechanical ventilation. *Chest* 2005;**128**:496–506.

2 **de Wit M, Wan SY, Gill S, et al.** Prevalence and impact of alcohol and other drug use disorders on sedation and mechanical ventilation: a retrospective study. *BMC Anesthesiol* 2007;**7**:3.

3 **Jacobi J, Fraser GL, Coursin DB, et al.** Clinical practice guidelines for the sustained use of sedatives and analgesics in the critically ill adult. *Crit Care Med* 2002;**30**:119–41.

4 Desbiens NA, Wu AW, Broste SK, et al. Pain and satisfaction with pain control in seriously ill hospi-
talized adults: findings from the SUPPORT research investigations. For the SUPPORT investigators.
Study to Understand Prognoses and Preferences for Outcomes and Risks of Treatmentm. *Crit Care
Med* 1996;**24**:1953–61.

5 Gelinas C. Management of pain in cardiac surgery ICU patients: have we improved over time?
Intensive Crit Care Nurs 2007;**23**:298–303.

6 Puntillo KA, White C, Morris AB, et al. Patients' perceptions and responses to procedural pain: results
from Thunder Project II. *Am J Crit Care* 2001;**10**:238–51.

7 Breen D, Karabinis A, Malbrain M, et al. Decreased duration of mechanical ventilation when comparing analgesia-based sedation using remifentanil with standard hypnotic-based sedation for up to 10
days in intensive care unit patients: a randomised trial [ISRCTN47583497]. *Crit Care* 2005;**9**:R200–10.

8 Reimer-Kent J. From theory to practice: preventing pain after cardiac surgery. *Am J Crit Care*
2003;**12**:136–43.

9 Cullen L, Greiner J, Bombei C, Comried L. Excellence in evidence-based practice: organizational and
unit exemplars. *Crit Care Nurs Clin North Am* 2005;**17**:127–42.

10 Pasero C, Gordon D, McCaffrey M. Building institutional committment to improving pain management. In: McCaffrey M, Pasero C (eds.) *Pain: clinical manual.* 3rd ed. St Louis, MO: Mosby; 1999.
pp. 711–44.

11 Miaskowski C, Crews J, Ready LB, Paul SM, Ginsberg B. Anesthesia-based pain services improve the
quality of postoperative pain management. *Pain* 1999;**80**:23–9.

12 Gordon DB, Dahl JL, Miaskowski C, et al. American Pain Society recommendations for improving
the quality of acute and cancer pain management: American Pain Society Quality of Care Task Force.
Arch Intern Med 2005;**165**:1574–80.

13 Gajraj NM. Pregabalin: its pharmacology and use in pain management. *Anesth Analg* 2007;**105**:1805–15.

14 Hindmarch I, Dawson J, Stanley N. A double-blind study in healthy volunteers to assess the effects on
sleep of pregabalin compared with alprazolam and placebo. *Sleep* 2005;**28**:187–93.

15 Pesonen A, Suojaranta-Ylinen R, Hammaren E, et al. Pregabalin has an opioid-sparing effect in elderly patients after cardiac surgery: a randomized placebo-controlled trial. *Br J Anaesth* 2011;**106**:873–81.

16 Liatsi D, Tsapas B, Pampori S, et al. Respiratory, metabolic and hemodynamic effects of clonidine in
ventilated patients presenting with withdrawal syndrome. *Intensive Care Med* 2009;**35**:275–81.

17 Wedel DJ, Horlocker TT. Regional anesthesia in the febrile or infected patient. *Reg Anesth Pain Med*
2006;**31**:324–33.

18 Horlocker TT, Wedel DJ, Rowlingson JC, et al. Regional anesthesia in the patient receiving
antithrombotic or thrombolytic therapy: American Society of Regional Anesthesia and Pain Medicine
Evidence-Based Guidelines (Third Edition). *Reg Anesth Pain Med* 2010;**35**:64–101.

19 Bernhardt A, Kortgen A, Niesel H, Goertz A. [Using epidural anesthesia in patients with acute pan-
creatitis--prospective study of 121 patients]. *Anaesthesiol Reanim* 2002;**27**:16–22.

20 Wu CL, Jani ND, Perkins FM, Barquist E. Thoracic epidural analgesia versus intravenous patient-
controlled analgesia for the treatment of rib fracture pain after motor vehicle crash. *J Trauma* 1999;**47**:564–7.

21 Brook AD, Ahrens TS, Schaiff R, et al. Effect of a nursing-implemented sedation protocol on the
duration of mechanical ventilation. *Crit Care Med* 1999;**27**:2609–15.

22 Kress JP, Pohlman AS, O'Connor MF, Hall JB. Daily interruption of sedative infusions in critically ill
patients undergoing mechanical ventilation. *N Engl J Med* 2000;**342**:1471–7.

23 Girard TD, Kress JP, Fuchs BD, et al. Efficacy and safety of a paired sedation and ventilator weaning
protocol for mechanically ventilated patients in intensive care (Awakening and Breathing Controlled
trial): a randomised controlled trial. *Lancet* 2008;**371**:126–34.

24 Strom T, Martinussen T, Toft P. A protocol of no sedation for critically ill patients receiving mechanical ventilation: a randomised trial. *Lancet* 2010;**375**:475–80.

25 Mehta S, Burry L, Cook D, et al.; SLEAP Investigators; Canadian Critical Care Trials Group. Daily sedation interruption in mechanically ventilated critically ill patients cared for with a sedation protocol: a randomized controlled trial. *JAMA* 2012;**308**:1985–92.

26 Bucknall TK, Manias E, Presneill JJ. A randomized trial of protocol-directed sedation management for mechanical ventilation in an Australian intensive care unit. *Crit Care Med* 2008;**36**:1444–50.

27 Elliott R, McKinley S, Aitken LM, Hendrikz J. The effect of an algorithm-based sedation guideline on the duration of mechanical ventilation in an Australian intensive care unit. *Intensive Care Med* 2006;**32**:1506–14.

28 de Wit M, Gennings C, Jenvey WI, Epstein SK. Randomized trial comparing daily interruption of sedation and nursing-implemented sedation algorithm in medical intensive care unit patients. *Crit Care* 2008;**12**:R70.

29 Tanios MA, de Wit M, Epstein SK, Devlin JW. Perceived barriers to the use of sedation protocols and daily sedation interruption: a multidisciplinary survey. *J Crit Care* 2009;**24**:66–73.

30 McCollam JS, O'Neil MG, Norcross ED, Byrne TK, Reeves ST. Continuous infusions of lorazepam, midazolam, and propofol for sedation of the critically ill surgery trauma patient: a prospective, randomized comparison. *Crit Care Med* 1999;**27**:2454–8.

31 Hall RI, Sandham D, Cardinal P, et al. Propofol vs midazolam for ICU sedation : a Canadian multicenter randomized trial. *Chest* 2001;**119**:1151–9.

32 Carson SS, Kress JP, Rodgers JE, et al. A randomized trial of intermittent lorazepam versus propofol with daily interruption in mechanically ventilated patients. *Crit Care Med* 2006;**34**:1326–32.

33 McEvoy G (ed.). *AHFS drug information 2005*. Bethesda, MD: American Society of Health-System Pharmacists; 2005.

34 Repchinsky C (ed.). *Compendium of pharmaceuticals and specialties (CPS)*. Ottawa, ON: Canadian Pharmaceutical Association; 2009.

35 MacLaren R, Sullivan PW. Economic evaluation of sustained sedation/analgesia in the intensive care unit. *Expert Opin Pharmacother* 2006;**7**:2047–68.

36 Mehta S, Burry L, Fischer S, et al. Canadian survey of the use of sedatives, analgesics, and neuromuscular blocking agents in critically ill patients. *Crit Care Med* 2006;**34**:374–80.

37 Mehta S, McCullagh I, Burry L. Current sedation practices: lessons learned from international surveys. *Crit Care Clin* 2009;**25**:471–88, vii–viii.

38 Payen JF, Chanques G, Mantz J, et al. Current practices in sedation and analgesia for mechanically ventilated critically ill patients: a prospective multicenter patient-based study. *Anesthesiology* 2007;**106**:687–95; quiz 891–2.

39 Shehabi Y, Grant P, Wolfenden H, et al. Prevalence of delirium with dexmedetomidine compared with morphine based therapy after cardiac surgery: a randomized controlled trial (DEXmedetomidine COmpared to Morphine-DEXCOM Study). *Anesthesiology* 2009;**111**:1075–84.

40 Riker RR, Shehabi Y, Bokesch PM, et al. Dexmedetomidine vs midazolam for sedation of critically ill patients: a randomized trial. *JAMA* 2009;**301**:489–99.

41 Ruokonen E, Parviainen I, Jakob SM, et al. Dexmedetomidine versus propofol/midazolam for long-term sedation during mechanical ventilation. *Intensive Care Med* 2009;**35**:282–90.

42 Pandharipande PP, Pun BT, Herr DL, et al. Effect of sedation with dexmedetomidine vs lorazepam on acute brain dysfunction in mechanically ventilated patients: the MENDS randomized controlled trial. *JAMA* 2007;**298**:2644–53.

43 Reade MC, O'Sullivan K, Bates S, et al. Dexmedetomidine vs haloperidol in delirious, agitated, intubated patients: a randomised open-label trial. *Crit Care* 2009;**13**:R75.

44 Karabinis A, Mandragos K, Stergiopoulos S, et al. Safety and efficacy of analgesia-based sedation with remifentanil versus standard hypnotic-based regimens in intensive care unit patients with brain injuries: a randomised, controlled trial [ISRCTN50308308]. *Crit Care* 2004;**8**:R268–80.

45 Dahaba AA, Grabner T, Rehak PH, List WF, Metzler H. Remifentanil versus morphine analgesia and sedation for mechanically ventilated critically ill patients: a randomized double blind study. *Anesthesiology* 2004;**101**:640–6.

46 Richman PS, Baram D, Varela M, Glass PS. Sedation during mechanical ventilation: a trial of benzodiazepine and opiate in combination. *Crit Care Med* 2006;**34**:1395–401.

47 Muellejans B, Matthey T, Scholpp J, Schill M. Sedation in the intensive care unit with remifentanil/propofol versus midazolam/fentanyl: a randomised, open-label, pharmacoeconomic trial. *Crit Care* 2006;**10**:R91.

48 Mesnil M, Capdevila X, Bringuier S, et al. Long-term sedation in intensive care unit: a randomized comparison between inhaled sevoflurane and intravenous propofol or midazolam. *Intensive Care Med* 2011;**37**:933–41.

49 Ramsay MA, Savege TM, Simpson BR, Goodwin R. Controlled sedation with alphaxalone-alphadolone. *Br Med J* 1974;**2**:656–9.

50 Riker RR, Picard JT, Fraser GL. Prospective evaluation of the Sedation-Agitation Scale for adult critically ill patients. *Crit Care Med* 1999;**27**:1325–9.

51 Riker RR, Fraser GL, Simmons LE, Wilkins ML. Validating the Sedation-Agitation Scale with the Bispectral Index and Visual Analog Scale in adult ICU patients after cardiac surgery. *Intensive Care Med* 2001;**27**:853–8.

52 Devlin JW, Boleski G, Mlynarek M, et al. Motor Activity Assessment Scale: a valid and reliable sedation scale for use with mechanically ventilated patients in an adult surgical intensive care unit. *Crit Care Med* 1999;**27**:1271–5.

53 de Lemos J, Tweeddale M, Chittock D. Measuring quality of sedation in adult mechanically ventilated critically ill patients. the Vancouver Interaction and Calmness Scale. Sedation Focus Group. *J Clin Epidemiol* 2000;**53**:908–19.

54 Sessler CN, Gosnell MS, Grap MJ, et al. The Richmond Agitation-Sedation Scale: validity and reliability in adult intensive care unit patients. *Am J Respir Crit Care Med* 2002;**166**:1338–44.

55 Ely EW, Truman B, Shintani A, et al. Monitoring sedation status over time in ICU patients: reliability and validity of the Richmond Agitation-Sedation Scale (RASS). *JAMA* 2003;**289**:2983–91.

56 De Jonghe B, Cook D, Griffith L, et al. Adaptation to the Intensive Care Environment (ATICE): development and validation of a new sedation assessment instrument. *Crit Care Med* 2003;**31**:2344–54.

57 Weinert C, McFarland L. The state of intubated ICU patients: development of a two-dimensional sedation rating scale for critically ill adults. *Chest* 2004;**126**:1883–90.

58 Chanques G, Jaber S, Barbotte E, et al. Impact of systematic evaluation of pain and agitation in an intensive care unit. *Crit Care Med* 2006;**34**:1691–9.

59 Brattebo G, Hofoss D, Flaatten H, et al. Effect of a scoring system and protocol for sedation on duration of patients' need for ventilator support in a surgical intensive care unit. *Qual Saf Health Care* 2004;**13**:203–5.

60 De Jonghe B, Bastuji-Garin S, Fangio P, et al. Sedation algorithm in critically ill patients without acute brain injury. *Crit Care Med* 2005;**33**:120–7.

61 Botha JA, Mudholkar P. The effect of a sedation scale on ventilation hours, sedative, analgesic and inotropic use in an intensive care unit. *Crit Care Resusc* 2004;**6**:253–7.

62 Chlan LL, Weinert CR, Skaar DJ, Tracy MF. Patient-controlled sedation: a novel approach to sedation management for mechanically ventilated patients. *Chest* 2010;**138**:1045–53.

63 Freedman NS, Gazendam J, Levan L, Pack AI, Schwab RJ. Abnormal sleep/wake cycles and the effect of environmental noise on sleep disruption in the intensive care unit. *Am J Respir Crit Care Med* 2001;**163**:451–7.

64 Hofhuis JG, Spronk PE, van Stel HF, et al. Experiences of critically ill patients in the ICU. *Intensive Crit Care Nurs* 2008;**24**:300–13.

65 Olson DM, Borel CO, Laskowitz DT, Moore DT, McConnell ES. Quiet time: a nursing intervention to promote sleep in neurocritical care units. *Am J Crit Care* 2001;**10**:74–8.

66 Richards KC. Effect of a back massage and relaxation intervention on sleep in critically ill patients. *Am J Crit Care* 1998;**7**:288–99.

67 Gonzalez CE, Carroll DL, Elliott JS, Fitzgerald PA, Vallent HJ. Visiting preferences of patients in the intensive care unit and in a complex care medical unit. *Am J Crit Care* 2004;**13**:194–8.

68 Nayak S, Wenstone R, Jones A, et al. Surface electrostimulation of acupuncture points for sedation of critically ill patients in the intensive care unit--a pilot study. *Acupunct Med* 2008;**26**:1–7.

69 Ely EW, Stephens RK, Jackson JC, et al. Current opinions regarding the importance, diagnosis, and management of delirium in the intensive care unit: a survey of 912 healthcare professionals. *Crit Care Med* 2004;**32**:106–12.

70 Ely EW, Margolin R, Francis J, et al. Evaluation of delirium in critically ill patients: validation of the Confusion Assessment Method for the Intensive Care Unit (CAM-ICU). *Crit Care Med* 2001;**29**:1370–9.

71 Ely EW, Inouye SK, Bernard GR, et al. Delirium in mechanically ventilated patients: validity and reliability of the confusion assessment method for the intensive care unit (CAM-ICU). *JAMA* 2001;**286**:2703–10.

72 Lin SM, Liu CY, Wang CH, et al. The impact of delirium on the survival of mechanically ventilated patients. *Crit Care Med* 2004;**32**:2254–9.

73 Bergeron N, Dubois MJ, Dumont M, Dial S, Skrobik Y. Intensive Care Delirium Screening Checklist: evaluation of a new screening tool. *Intensive Care Med* 2001;**27**:859–64.

74 Ouimet S, Kavanagh BP, Gottfried SB, Skrobik Y. Incidence risk factors and consequences of ICU delirium. *Intensive Care Med* 2007;**33**:66–73.

75 American Psychiatric Association. *Diagnostic and statistical manual of mental disorders.* 4th ed. Washington, DC: American Psychiatric Association; 1994. pp. 124–33.

76 Dubois MJ, Bergeron N, Dumont M, Dial S, Skrobik Y. Delirium in an intensive care unit: a study of risk factors. *Intensive Care Med* 2001;**27**:1297–304.

77 Ely EW, Gautam S, Margolin R, et al. The impact of delirium in the intensive care unit on hospital length of stay. *Intensive Care Med* 2001;**27**:1892–900.

78 Marcantonio ER, Juarez G, Goldman L, et al. The relationship of postoperative delirium with psychoactive medications. *JAMA* 1994;**272**:1518–22.

79 Pandharipande P, Shintani A, Peterson J, et al. Lorazepam is an independent risk factor for transitioning to delirium in intensive care unit patients. *Anesthesiology* 2006;**104**:21–6.

80 Pandharipande P, Cotton BA, Shintani A, et al. Prevalence and risk factors for development of delirium in surgical and trauma intensive care unit patients. *J Trauma* 2008;**65**:34–41.

81 Ely EW, Shintani A, Truman B, et al. Delirium as a predictor of mortality in mechanically ventilated patients in the intensive care unit. *JAMA* 2004;**291**:1753–62.

82 Inouye SK, Bogardus ST, Jr, Charpentier PA, et al. A multicomponent intervention to prevent delirium in hospitalized older patients. *N Engl J Med* 1999;**340**:669–76.

83 Lundstrom M, Edlund A, Karlsson S, et al. A multifactorial intervention program reduces the duration of delirium, length of hospitalization, and mortality in delirious patients. *J Am Geriatr Soc* 2005;**53**:622–8.

84 Marcantonio ER, Flacker JM, Wright RJ, Resnick NM. Reducing delirium after hip fracture: a randomized trial. *J Am Geriatr Soc* 2001;**49**:516–22.

85 Girard TD, Pandharipande PP, Carson SS, et al. Feasibility, efficacy, and safety of antipsychotics for intensive care unit delirium: the MIND randomized, placebo-controlled trial. *Crit Care Med* 2010;**38**:428–37.

86 Devlin JW, Roberts RJ, Fong JJ, et al. Efficacy and safety of quetiapine in critically ill patients with delirium: a prospective, multicenter, randomized, double-blind, placebo-controlled pilot study. *Crit Care Med* 2010;**38**:419–27.

87 Skrobik YK, Bergeron N, Dumont M, Gottfried SB. Olanzapine vs haloperidol: treating delirium in a critical care setting. *Intensive Care Med* 2004;**30**:444–9.

88 Schneider LS, Dagerman KS, Insel P. Risk of death with atypical antipsychotic drug treatment for dementia: meta-analysis of randomized placebo-controlled trials. *JAMA* 2005;**294**:1934–43.

89 Wang PS, Schneeweiss S, Avorn J, et al. Risk of death in elderly users of conventional vs atypical antipsychotic medications. *N Engl J Med* 2005;**353**:2335–41.

90 Aurell J, Elmqvist D. Sleep in the surgical intensive care unit: continuous polygraphic recording of sleep in nine patients receiving postoperative care. *Br Med J* 1985;**290**:1029–32.

91 Gabor JY, Cooper AB, Crombach SA, et al. Contribution of the intensive care unit environment to sleep disruption in mechanically ventilated patients and healthy subjects. *Am J Respir Crit Care Med* 2003;**167**:708–15.

92 Needham DM. Mobilizing patients in the intensive care unit: improving neuromuscular weakness and physical function. *JAMA* 2008;**300**:1685–90.

93 Truong AD, Fan E, Brower RG, Needham DM. Bench-to-bedside review: mobilizing patients in the intensive care unit--from pathophysiology to clinical trials. *Crit Care* 2009;**13**:216.

94 Schweickert WD, Pohlman MC, Pohlman AS, et al. Early physical and occupational therapy in mechanically ventilated, critically ill patients: a randomised controlled trial. *Lancet* 2009;**373**:1874–82.

95 Rhoney DH, Murry KR. National survey of the use of sedating drugs, neuromuscular blocking agents, and reversal agents in the intensive care unit. *J Intensive Care Med* 2003;**18**:139–45.

96 Samuelson KA, Larsson S, Lundberg D, Fridlund B. Intensive care sedation of mechanically ventilated patients: a national Swedish survey. *Intensive Crit Care Nurs* 2003;**19**:350–62.

97 Guldbrand P, Berggren L, Brattebo G, et al. Survey of routines for sedation of patients on controlled ventilation in Nordic intensive care units. *Acta Anaesthesiol Scand* 2004;**48**:944–50.

98 Botha J, Le Blanc V. The state of sedation in the nation: results of an Australian survey. *Crit Care Resusc* 2005;**7**:92–6.

99 Payen JF, Bru O, Bosson JL, et al. Assessing pain in critically ill sedated patients by using a behavioral pain scale. *Crit Care Med* 2001;**29**:2258–63.

100 Young J, Siffleet J, Nikoletti S, Shaw T. Use of a Behavioural Pain Scale to assess pain in ventilated, unconscious and/or sedated patients. *Intensive Crit Care Nurs* 2006;**22**:32–9.

101 Gelinas C, Fillion L, Puntillo KA, Viens C, Fortier M. Validation of the critical-care pain observation tool in adult patients. *Am J Crit Care* 2006;**15**:420–7.

102 Gelinas C, Harel F, Fillion L, Puntillo KA, Johnston CC. Sensitivity and specificity of the critical-care pain observation tool for the detection of pain in intubated adults after cardiac surgery. *J Pain Symptom Manage* 2009;**37**:58–67.

Chapter 41

Sleep-Promoting Strategies

Vito Fanelli, Lucia Mirabella, Stefano Italiano,
Michele Dambrosio, and V. Marco Ranieri

Introduction

Severe disruption of sleep architecture, with respect to both quantity and quality, has been extensively demonstrated in critical ill patients.[1,2] The aetiology of sleep perturbation in ICU patients is multifactorial, and it is noteworthy that sleep disruption is associated with the derangement of several physiological regulatory processes that may impact clinical outcome of patients admitted to ICU.

The objectives of this chapter are to summarize the most important factors, which contribute to poor quality of sleep, and provide the rationale of strategies aiming to improve sleep quality in critically ill patients.

Normal sleep architecture

Normal sleep architecture is divided into two distinct states: NREM sleep and REM sleep. NREM is composed of three separate stages, based on EEG criteria. Stages 1 (N1) and 2 (N2) reflect light sleep and are followed by stages 3 (N3) and 4 (N4), which are characterized by slow-wave EEG activity and are considered the deep phase of sleep.[3]

REM sleep is characterized by basic parasympathetic (vagal) activity that is episodically interrupted by sympathetic bursts corresponding to the rapid eye movements,[4] irregular respiratory and cardiac rate, sudden increase in blood pressure, and paralysis of the major muscle groups (excluding the diaphragm and upper airway musculature).[5] During this stage, the EEG activity resembles wakefulness, and, for this reason, it is also called 'paradoxical' sleep.[6] Thus, REM sleep is a catabolic state,[3] useful for some stage of learning and memory consolidation.[6] SWS, on the other hand, is an anabolic state, and it is considered the most restorative stage of sleep,[7] during which physiologic repair of the organism occurs.[6]

Regulation of the sleep-wave cycle is a complex process, and it is controlled by two main processes: the sleep homeostasis (or S-process, or homeostatic drive for sleep), regulating the quantity and intensity of sleep, according to the time spent awake or asleep;[6,8] and the circadian rhythm (C-process), regulated by the internal pacemaker localized in the SCN that activates the pineal gland to secrete melatonin.[8,9]

The neurobiochemical transmission regulating sleep time and stages involves cholinergic, noradrenergic, and serotoninergic activities. During REM sleep, GABAergic pathways from the ventrolateral preoptic (VLPO) nucleus of the hypothalamus inhibit histaminergic activity of the tuberomammillary nucleus, and the orexinergic pathway from the perifornical nucleus is inactivated.[6] This explains why catecholamines, histamine, glutamate, orexin, and acetylcholine promote wakefulness, why acetylcholine promotes REM sleep, and why noradrenaline, and serotonin inhibit REM sleep. Meanwhile, GABA and serotonin are SWS-promoting. Melatonin is the most important biochemical regulator of the circadian rhythm that is involved in the modulation of the function of different systems and apparatuses of the organism (hypothalamic-pituitary-adrenal axis, immune function, coagulation, cardiovascular, pulmonary, hepatic, and renal apparatus).[10]

This complex molecular interaction is important in order to understand how severe clinical conditions and the ICU environment (medication, nursing, abnormal light and noise exposure, loss of physical activity and social interaction, sedation) can easily modify these biochemical pathways, with grave consequences on sleep patterns and architecture.

PSG and sleep alterations in the critically ill patients

Up to 60% of patients surviving ICU admission report poor sleep quality or deprivation,[11,12,13] which may negatively impact their QoL after ICU discharge.[14,15] Several studies using PSG objectively revealed a severe disruption of sleep architecture with respect to both quantity and quality.[4,5,15–20] In fact, in ICU patients, sleep is characterized by a longer onset and a poorer sleep efficacy, as demonstrated by the prevalence of N1 and N2 stages, a reduction or absence of N3 stage and REM sleep, and an increased sleep fragmentation.[5,18,21,22]

Various PSG studies have shown a 'normal' amount of TST through the 24-hour period, but this was the result of the combination of an abnormal daytime sleep with short periods of nocturnal sleep. This disrupted sleep (with daytime sleep that can represent up to the 40–50% of TST)[3,5,17,23] is clearly not beneficial as the nocturnal physiologic sleep.

PSG is the gold standard technique to study sleep.[18] However, there are several issues that limit its application in the ICU. First, PSG is a time-consuming and uncomfortable procedure, and nursing and medical activities may negatively interfere with PSG recordings. Second, the current Rechtschaffen and Kales methodology for sleep analysis is problematic to apply to critically ill patients who typically show a severe alteration in sleep pattern and architecture.[8,17,20] For instance, ICU patients may present N2 stage without spindles and k-complexes,[5,20] τ and δ EEG activity during wakefulness, REMs during N2 stage, and rapid fluctuations between wakefulness and REM stage.[17] Toward this end, Druot and colleagues described the PSG pattern of patients with an 'atypical sleep' and 'pathological wakefulness' as similar to the EEG pattern of delirious patients.[24]

Implications of sleep alteration in ICU

Sleep disturbances in critically ill patients have deleterious biological and neuropsychological consequences[17] (see Figure 41.1). Sleep restriction increases energy consumption and cortisol concentration and impairs the release of many hormones and neurotransmitters such as epinephrine, GH, and TSH.[4,22] Moreover, glucose metabolism may be deranged to similar levels of patients with type 2 diabetes.[23]

Sleep deprivation may increase sympathetic and decrease parasympathetic cardiac activity, respectively, resulting in an increased risk of MI.[23] Impaired sleep can also affect respiratory function, reducing the ventilatory response to hypercapnia and hypoxaemia; the inspiratory muscle endurance and maximal voluntary ventilation can be decreased without affecting the respiratory muscle strength.[17] In this context, the weaning process may be compromised. In patients with

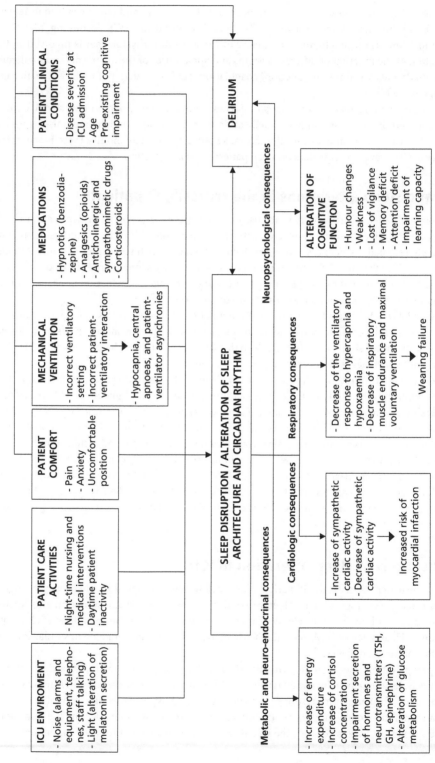

Fig. 41.1 Risk factors and biological and neuropsychological consequences of sleep disturbances in critically ill patients.

acute hypercapnic respiratory failure, Roche Campo et al. demonstrated that poor sleep quality was more frequently associated with late NIV failure.[25]

Neuropsychological involvement corresponds to the damage caused by sleep deprivation to cognitive functions. Typical findings include humour changes, weakness, loss of vigilance, memory deficit, attention and learning capacity up to delirium.[8,17,23,26]

Factors contributing to sleep disruption and strategies to improve sleep in ICU patients

In the following section, potential risk factors involved in sleep disruption, such as ICU environment, patient care activities, patient discomfort, MV, medications, and delirium strategies will be reviewed. Moreover, strategies aimed to minimize poor sleep quality in ICU will be pointed out (see Table 41.1).

ICU environment

The ICU environment is thought to be an important factor in sleep disruption.[27] One of the most studied stressors is the noise in ICU. Although the US Environmental Protection Agency recommends that hospital noise level should be less than 45 and 35 dB at daytime and night-time,[28]

Table 41.1 Principal factors contributing to poor sleep quality in ICU and strategies aiming to improve sleep quality in critically ill patients

Factors contributing to sleep disruption in ICU		Strategies to improve sleep in ICU
ICU enviroment	Noise Abnormal light exposure	Education of staff regarding noise (reduce conversation near the bedside, correct setting of non-critical alarms) Individual patient rooms Earplug, white noise, music therapy use Natural light at daytime Normal light/dark alternation
Patients care activities	Nursing interventions (i.e. bath, wound dressing, medication administration, monitoring)	Coordinate nursing activities to allow patient sleep periods
Patient comfort	Anxiety Pain MV	Inform exhaustively and reassure patient (i.e. before sleeping time, before procedures) Orientate patient with respect to daytime Prevent or treat pain by comfortable bed position, massage, or analgesic drugs Optimize patient-ventilator interaction
MV	Sleep deprivation and fragmentation (arousal and awakening) due to patient-ventilator asynchrony	Check ventilator setting in order to avoid overassistance (central apnoeas) or ineffective effort during MV
Medications	Sleep deprivation, alteration of sleep architecture, and EEG patterns (analgesics, sedatives/hypnotics, corticosteroids, antidepressants)	Use the minimum dose of sedative and analgesic to obtain pain control and patient comfort Adopt analgosedation protocols Interrupt daily sedative drug infusion Prevent and promptly treat delirium

this threshold is largely exceeded in ICU, with a daily ambient noise levels of 60–65 dB and a mean sound peak level of 83.6 ± 0.1 dB. Moreover, the longest has been reported to be only 22 minutes.[29] Nonetheless, among the sources of noise in the ICU environment, such as alarms, ventilator sounds, suctioning sounds, physician beepers, telephone, and television, staff talking accounted for 26% of the noise and had the highest peak decibel level; thus, it was perceived to be the most disruptive factor of sleep.[11,30,31]

Some authors[32] suggest that it is not the peak noise levels that create disruption, but rather the changes in noise levels. Recent emphasis has been on noise reduction, and studies have shown that implementing guidelines and education of staff regarding noise can effectively change staff behaviour and reduce peak noise levels.[29,31,33] Although many studies indicate that noise is one of the most important stressors in the ICU environment, its impact on sleep disruption is not clear. PSG studies in ICU patients show that only 10–30% of arousals/awakenings could be attributed to noise.[30,34] Many factors have been advocated to explain these conflicting results. First, the simultaneous presence of stressful factors at the same time may account for sleep disruption, such as disease severity, pain, and patient ventilator dyssynchrony. In fact, Gabor et al. showed that noise and patient care were responsible for only 30% of arousals and awakenings, whereas the cause of the remaining 70% of sleep disruptions was unknown.[30] Second, the effect of noise could be overestimated if concomitant stressors are not measured. In fact, some arousals may coincidentally occur after a noise peak but not be causally related.[35]

Abnormal light exposure is another contributing factor in poor quality of sleep, especially because it may interfere with circadian rhythms. Circadian melatonin secretion has been demonstrated to be severely impaired in ICU patients. Compared to patients in the ward, Shilo and colleagues demonstrated that 12 of 14 ICU patients had flattened melatonin concentration in the urine and this was associated with sporadic sleep.[36] Nocturnal melatonin secretion can be acutely suppressed by light, and 100 lx is sufficient to impact nocturnal melatonin secretion.[37] Reported nocturnal illumination in ICUs varies widely, with mean levels ranging between 5 and 1400 lx.[28,29] Attention to controlling the patients' environment is a reasonable strategy, aimed at improving sleep quality. Exposure to brighter light during the day (turn on the lights, open the curtains) and turning off the lights by 10.00 p.m. should be encouraged. Moreover, decreasing noise with earplugs and the use of eye masks has shown to improve sleep efficiency in normal subjects who were sleeping in a simulated ICU environment.[38–41] Finally, sound masking and absorption seems to be the most promising strategy to improve sleep and will require more collaborative work between acousticians and physicians.[35]

Patient care activities

ICU patients rate nursing interventions to be as disruptive to sleep as noise.[11] Studies from both medical and surgical ICUs show that 40–50 care interventions typically occur per patient per night shift[42,43] for activities such as wound dressings, medicine administration, and nightly baths. Approximately 10% of arousals and awakenings over a 24-hour period are due to patient care activities.[30] It could be argued that nurses have an around-the-clock presence and a coordinating function in the ICU and should be able to coordinate nursing care with other activities to allow for patient sleep periods.[44] Staff need to coordinate with the patient's nurse all activities of ICU care; this may require changing routine schedules to facilitate night-time sleep. For example, the frequency of overnight monitoring can be decreased. These can include finger sticks, blood drawing for laboratory testing, and checking for vital signs. Also, bathing, dressing changes, and room switches can be minimized during night hours.

Patient comfort

The inability to relax due to pain, anxiety, or uncomfortable positioning in bed[45] is reported to be an important cause of sleep deprivation in the ICU. Adjusting the patient's position in the bed, providing pain relief, and informing the patient when it is time to sleep seem to be valid interventions. Moreover, it is important to orient the patient with respect to daytime, also plan routine activities,[22] and reassure that he will be looked after when sleeping.[46] In addition, performing foot or hand massage, holding the patient's hand, sitting within visual distance if the patient is anxious, or offering television, radio, or music if the patient desires such entertainment before sleeping are adjunctive measures to apply.[44]

MV

The majority of ICU patients are mechanically ventilated, and several studies have been conducted to investigate how MV may affect sleep. Ventilation mode, ventilator settings, and patient-ventilator interaction are critical factors that may influence sleep quality. Currently, there are conflicting results from several studies addressing the hypothesis that ventilation mode itself may affect sleep. In a seminal study, Parthasarathy and colleagues compared two modes of MV—ACV and PSV—on the effect on sleep fragmentation. The authors showed that PSV was associated with a higher proportion of sleep fragmentation—the number of arousals and awakenings per hour of sleep—compared to ACV. However, this difference disappeared when a dead space was added to the ventilator circuit during PSV. This effect then seemed to be related to the central apnoea induced by hypocapnia during PSV mode. Additionally, more than half of the patient population suffered from CHF in this study, which may, in turn, cause hypocapnia and central apnoeas.[1] On the contrary, low levels of assistance during PSV, especially in patients with high resistive load, may be related to poor quality of sleep.[47] However, these results were not confirmed in a separate study that compared ACV mode to two different modalities of PSV, clinically and automatically adjusted. Sleep efficiency, as well as minute ventilation and levels of assistance, were similar across the three ventilation modes. Taken together, these results highlight the importance of ventilator setting, rather than the mode, in determining sleep quality. In fact, a stereotypical application of high levels of assistance at night-time seems to be the strongest factor that negatively affects sleep quality. A landmark study published by Meza and colleagues showed that the level of overassistance was associated with a poor quality of sleep in healthy subjects.[48] Moreover, in a cohort of patients with neuromuscular disease, Fanfulla and colleagues showed that optimizing ventilator settings, based on the patient's respiratory effort, improved sleep efficiency.[49] Patients were randomized to two NIV strategies: clinically adjusted PSV, in which the level of inspiratory pressure was set to reduce the awake $PaCO_2$ by more than 5% of that recorded during spontaneous breathing; and physiologically adjusted PSV, in which the level of inspiratory pressure was set to reduce transdiaphragmatic pressure (Pdi) swing by more than 40% and less than 80% and/or to avoid any positive deflection in oesophageal pressure (Poes) during expiration. Of note, patients in the physiologically adjusted PSV group had less ineffective efforts during sleep, and this condition positively correlated with a better sleep architecture.[49] Along with the idea that a more physiologic approach may improve sleep quality, Bosma and colleagues demonstrated that patient-ventilator dyssynchrony plays a pivotal role in sleep disruption.[50] In a randomized crossover clinical trial, ICU patients, who were ready for weaning, were randomized to receive PSV or PAV. In both groups, the ventilator setting was optimized to obtain a 50% reduction of inspiration work during an SBT. At night-time, PAV significantly improved sleep architecture and fragmentation. Interestingly, this better quality of sleep showed a good correlation with fewer patient-ventilator asynchronies per hour.[50] Recently, a new mode of ventilation NAVA has been shown to improve sleep quality probably through better neuromechanical coupling.[51] Fourteen patients were randomized to four periods—4 hours each—of PSV or NAVA ventilation, in which PSG was performed. PSV and NAVA levels of assistance were adjusted to obtain a tidal volume of 8 mL/kg and respiratory rate less than 35. Compared to PSV, NAVA increased REM and decreased sleep fragmentation. Moreover, NAVA improved patient-ventilator interaction, reducing inspiratory and expiratory trigger delay.[51]

In conclusion, hypocapnia- and central apnoea-induced high levels of assistance play a pivotal role in sleep disruption during MV. Optimizing ventilator settings to improve patient-ventilator synchrony seems to be the better strategy to ameliorate sleep quality. However, optimal adjustments of ventilator settings by the physician during sleep time is difficult to determine, whereas more physiological modalities of assisted ventilation, such as PAV and NAVA, seem to be promising for the overall improvement of sleep quality.

Medications

It is difficult to ascertain a single drug's effect on sleep architecture in critically ill patients. because many prescribed drugs may concomitantly affect sleep. Moreover, different volumes of distribution, renal and hepatic clearance/metabolism, and the confounding effect of sympathetic activation from acute stress may concomitantly affect sleep.[52,53]

Most ICU patients require administration of sedatives and analgesics to improve patient-ventilator interaction and avoid pain. There are two main classes of hypnotic drugs commonly used in ICU patients. First are those that act through GABA receptors, such as benzodiazepines and propofol, thus enhancing the signal of this neurotransmitter. Second are those that act on alpha 2 (α_2) receptors in the brainstem, resulting in inhibition of NE release.[2]

At low doses, benzodiazepines and propofol suppress SWS which is characteristic of stages 3 and 4 of NREM sleep. Moreover, they shorten sleep latency, decrease arousal, and increase duration of stage 2. At higher doses, they progressively slow the EEG until burst suppression. All of these EEG patterns correlate with a reduction of brain metabolism. In a small cohort of surgical patients, Treggiari-Venzi and colleagues showed that sleep quality tended to improve from day 1 to day 5 after ICU entry. Moreover, anxiety levels were similar in the two groups, and only depression tended to be higher in the midazolam group.[54] Benzodiazepine administration is associated with the development of delirium. For patients who need continuous sedation as those who are mechanically ventilated, the use of propofol is a reasonable alternative. In fact, animal studies have demonstrated that prolonged sedation with propofol does not result in sleep deprivation.[55] However, more studies are necessary to address if one drug is superior to the other.

Dexmedetomidine is an agonist of the α_2 receptor at the locus coeruleus, and it exerts its sedative effects through reducing NE release. EEG pattern is characterized by a decrease in the percentage of REM and an increase of NREM phases 2, 3, and 4. Sleep induced by dexmedetomidine resembles natural sleep, as shown by fMRI and some clinical observations such as easy arousal and preserved cognitive power. Despite the favourable profile of dexmedetomidine, it was shown not to be superior to propofol in promoting better sleep perception. Corbett and colleagues randomized patients who underwent coronary artery bypass surgery to propofol or dexmedetomidine sedation regimens during MV in the post-operative period.[56] Dosing adjustments were based on a standardized ICU nursing protocol to maintain a Ramsay score of 5 for the first 2 hours post-operatively, followed by a score of 3–4, until they were intubated. To investigate patient satisfaction, a modified Hewitt sedation questionnaire was administered within 24 hours of extubation. Patients were asked about comfort level, pain level, ability to interact with health care providers and family, agitation, anxiety, ability to sleep or rest, and satisfaction with ICU experience. There were no differences between the two groups in global perception of sleep in the post-operative period.[56] This study investigated sleep quality through a questionnaire that, despite being a valuable tool to understand patient's perception, does not object to other factors influencing sleep such as patient-ventilator dyssynchrony, noise environment, and disease severity.

Opioids are medications commonly used in ICU patients to control pain (i.e. after surgery) and to ameliorate patient-ventilator synchrony, in conjunction with hypnotics. At higher doses, they produce hypnotic effects acting on the pontothalamic arousal pathway, which is most involved in REM sleep. Opioids suppress REM, SWS stages 2 and 4 of NREM sleep that are overall EEG patterns associated with poor quality of sleep. However, in the post-operative period, pain represents the most important sleep disruptor. For this reason, a satisfactory analgesic greatly improves the overall perception of sleep quality. In fact, Cronin and colleagues showed that REM sleep was completely abolished in the first post-operative night in a cohort of 14 patients who underwent gynaecologic surgery. The percentage of deep sleep was significantly lower in the group of patients treated with opioids, compared to those treated with locoregional anaesthetics.[57] Despite a different PSG pattern, the molecule used for pain control did not affect patients' perception of sleep quality.[57]

Melatonin, a naturally occurring hormone, promotes sleep, without inducing daytime sedation or respiratory depression, and maintains normal sleep architecture.[52,58,59] Investigators reported that melatonin increased TST and decreased sleep fragmentation, and improved sleep efficiency in patients on MV.[60] Side effects of melatonin are uncommon; however, drug-drug interactions may occur, particularly with immunosuppressor agents, due to its pro-immunologic actions.[61,62] In animal models of sepsis, melatonin is known to have immunologic properties and is necessary for free radical scavenging, antioxidant properties, and survival from sepsis.[61,62] Mundliger demonstrated that the circadian secretion of melatonin is altered in septic vs non-septic ICU patients. Septic patients maintained a continuous secretion of melatonin, in contrast to normal cyclic variation in the non septic patients. The continuous excretion noted in septic patients supports the immunologic role of melatonin and suggest that increased sleep is necessary for recovery from illness.[63]

Delirium

Delirium is a clinical syndrome characterized by an impairment of consciousness and attention and cognitive dysfunction, and it may affect up to 80% of critically ill patients.[64,65] Moreover, it presents an independent risk factor for ICU poor outcome such as increased mortality and hospital length of stay and higher costs.[64-69] Many risk factors have been implicated in the development of delirium such as disease severity, advanced age, medication (benzodiazepines, opioids, anticholinergic and sympathomimetic drugs, corticosteroids), and electrolyte abnormalities. Recently, sleep deprivation or poor quality of sleep experienced by critically ill patients has been advocated as an important risk factor for delirium. To date, its causative effect is not completely demonstrated.[70] However, the reciprocal relation between delirium and poor quality of sleep lies in similarities shared by these two pathological conditions.[70] First, risk factors for the development of delirium coincide with those for sleep deprivation. In fact, pre-existing cognitive impairment, disease severity at ICU entry, patient-ventilator asynchrony, pain, and medications (benzodiazepines, opioids, anticholinergic and sympathomimetic drugs, corticosteroids) predispose to both conditions. Second, clinical features of hypoactive delirium (and not hyperactive) are recognized in sleep-deprived patients such as sleepiness, and attention and memory impairment. Third, PSG analysis of both conditions show a typical pattern characterized by a decrease of deep—stages 3 and 4 of NREM—sleep and of REM sleep, and an increase of wakefulness and light sleep—stages 1 and 2 of NREM sleep. Recently, Trompeo and colleagues demonstrated an association between REM sleep deprivation and delirium in mechanically ventilated ICU patients.[71] In this study, ready-to-wean patients not sedated for at least 24 hours were divided in two groups: severe or not deprived of REM sleep, based on PSG evidence of 6% reduction in REM sleep. Patients in the severe REM sleep deprivation group were more severe, as indicated by median SAPS II at ICU entry, and they were dependent on MV for a longer period of time. Of interest, a clear correlation was established between REM sleep reduction, delirium, and the use of lorazepam.[71] In light of these considerations, strategies aimed at improving both ICU sleep quality and the incidence of delirium may likely ameliorate short- and long-term outcomes of critically ill patients.

Conclusion

In conclusion, poor sleep quality and sleep deprivation in the ICU are associated with a profound change of physical homeostasis of the whole organism. A correlation between poor cardiovascular, respiratory, and cognitive function and disturbed sleep has been clearly shown. Sleep disturbances have been directly implicated as a driver of adverse outcome in the critically ill. Critical care physicians should seek to minimize risk factors for sleep disruption. Research is needed into viable strategies to ameliorate sleep in the ICU.

References

1 Puntillo KA, Arai S, Cohen NH, et al. Symptoms experienced by intensive care unit patients at high risk of dying. *Crit Care Med* 2010;**38**:2155–60.

2 Weinhouse GL, Watson PL. Sedation and sleep disturbances in the ICU. *Crit Care Clin* 2009;**25**: 539–49, ix.

3 Hardin KA. Sleep in the ICU: potential mechanisms and clinical implications. *Chest* 2009;**136**:284–94.

4 Bijwadia JS, Ejaz MS. Sleep and critical care. *Curr Opin Crit Care* 2009;**15**:25–9.

5 Parthasarathy S, Tobin MJ. Sleep in the intensive care unit. *Intensive Crit Care Nurs Med* 2004;**30**: 197–206.

6 Sanders RD, Maze M. Contribution of sedative-hypnotic agents to delirium via modulation of the sleep pathway. *Can J Anaesth* 2011;**58**:149–56.

7 Desbiens NA, Wu AW, Broste SK, et al. Pain and satisfaction with pain control in seriously ill hospitalized adults: findings from the SUPPORT research investigations. For the SUPPORT investigators. Study to Understand Prognoses and Preferences for Outcomes and Risks of Treatment. *Crit Care Med* 1996;**24**:1953–61.

8 Figueroa-Ramos MI, Arroyo-Novoa CM, Lee KA, Padilla G, Puntillo KA. Sleep and delirium in ICU patients: a review of mechanisms and manifestations. *Intensive Care Med* 2009;**35**:781–95.

9 Olofsson K, Alling C, Lundberg D, Malmros C. Abolished circadian rhythm of melatonin secretion in sedated and artificially ventilated intensive care patients. *Acta Anaesthesiol Scand* 2004;**48**:679–84.

10 Chan MC, Spieth PM, Quinn K, Parotto M, Zhang H, Slutsky AS. Circadian rhythms: from basic mechanisms to the intensive care unit. *Crit Care Med* 2012;**40**:246–53.

11 Freedman NS, Kotzer N, Schwab RJ. Patient perception of sleep quality and etiology of sleep disruption in the intensive care unit. *Am J Respir Crit Care Med* 1999;**159**:1155–62.

12 **Nelson JE, Meier DE, Oei EJ, et al.** Self-reported symptom experience of critically ill cancer patients receiving intensive care. *Crit Care Med* 2001;**29**:277–82.

13 **Simini B.** Patients' perceptions of intensive care. *Lancet* 1999;**354**:571–2.

14 **Granja C, Lopes A, Moreira S, Dias C, Costa-Pereira A, Carneiro A; JMIP Study Group.** Patients' recollections of experiences in the intensive care unit may affect their quality of life. *Crit Care* 2005; 9:R96–109.

15 **Watson P.** Sleep in the ICU: where dreams go to die. *Minerva Anestesiol* 2011;**77**:568–70.

16 **Cabello B, Mancebo J, Brochard L.** [Sleep quality in ventilated patients: is the ventilatory method important or its adjustment?]. *Med Intensiva* 2006;**30**:392–5.

17 **Drouot X, Cabello B, d'Ortho MP, Brochard L.** Sleep in the intensive care unit. *Sleep Med Rev* 2008;**12**:391–403.

18 **Mistraletti G, Carloni E, Cigada M, et al.** Sleep and delirium in the intensive care unit. *Minerva Anestesiol* 2008;**74**:329–33.

19 **Parthasarathy S.** Sleep during mechanical ventilation. *Curr Opin Pulm Med* 2004;**10**:489–94.

20 **Weinhouse GL.** Sleep in the critically ill: an epoch adventure. *Sleep Med* 2012;**13**:3–4.

21 **Friese RS, Diaz-Arrastia R, McBride D, Frankel H, Gentilello LM.** Quantity and quality of sleep in the surgical intensive care unit: are our patients sleeping? *J Trauma* 2007;**63**:1210–14.

22 **Friese RS.** Sleep and recovery from critical illness and injury: a review of theory, current practice, and future directions. *Crit Care Med* 2008;**36**:697–705.

23 **Salas RE, Gamaldo CE.** Adverse effects of sleep deprivation in the ICU. *Crit Care Clin* 2008;**24**:461–76, v–vi.

24 **Drouot X, Roche-Campo F, Thille AW, et al.** A new classification for sleep analysis in critically ill patients. *Sleep Med* 2012;**13**:7–14.

25 **Roche Campo F, Drouot X, Thille AW, et al.** Poor sleep quality is associated with late noninvasive ventilation failure in patients with acute hypercapnic respiratory failure. *Crit Care Med* 2010;**38**: 477–85.

26 **Matthews EE.** Sleep disturbances and fatigue in critically ill patients. *AACN Adv Crit Care* 2011;**22**: 204–24.

27 **Boyko Y, Ording H, Jennum P.** Sleep disturbances in critically ill patients in ICU: how much do we know? *Acta Anaesthesiol Scand* 2012;**56**:950–8.

28 **Meyer TJ, Eveloff SE, Bauer MS, Schwartz WA, Hill NS, Millman RP.** Adverse environmental conditions in the respiratory and medical ICU settings. *Chest* 1994;**105**:1211–16.

29 **Walder B, Francioli D, Meyer JJ, Lançon M, Romand JA.** Effects of guidelines implementation in a surgical intensive care unit to control nighttime light and noise levels. *Crit Care Med* 2000;**28**:2242–7.

30 **Gabor JY, Cooper AB, Crombach SA, et al.** Contribution of the intensive care unit environment to sleep disruption in mechanically ventilated patients and healthy subjects. *Am J Respir Crit Care Med* 2003;**167**:708–15.

31 **Kahn DM, Cook TE, Carlisle CC, Nelson DL, Kramer NR, Millman RP.** Identification and modification of environmental noise in an ICU setting. *Chest* 1998;**114**:535–40.

32 **Stanchina ML, Abu-Hijleh M, Chaudhry BK, Carlisle CC, Millman RP.** The influence of white noise on sleep in subjects exposed to ICU noise. *Sleep Med* 2005;**6**:423–8.

33 **Monsen MG, Edell-Gustafsson UM.** Noise and sleep disturbance factors before and after implementation of a behavioural modification programme. *Intensive Crit Care Nurs* 2005;**21**:208–19.

34 **Freedman NS, Gazendam J, Levan L, Pack AI, Schwab RJ.** Abnormal sleep/wake cycles and the effect of environmental noise on sleep disruption in the intensive care unit. *Am J Respir Crit Care Med* 2001;**163**:451–7.

35 **Bosma KJ, Ranieri VM.** Filtering out the noise: evaluating the impact of noise and sound reduction strategies on sleep quality for ICU patients. *Crit Care* 2009;**13**:151.

36 Shilo L, Dagan Y, Smorjik Y, et al. Patients in the intensive care unit suffer from severe lack of sleep associated with loss of normal melatonin secretion pattern. *Am J Med Sci* 1999;**317**:278–81.

37 Boivin DB, Duffy JF, Kronauer RE, Czeisler CA. Dose-response relationships for resetting of human circadian clock by light. *Nature* 1996;**379**:540–42.

38 Richardson A, Crow W, Coghill E, Turnock C. A comparison of sleep assessment tools by nurses and patients in critical care. *J Clin Nurs* 2007;**16**:1660–8.

39 Scotto CJ, McClusky C, Spillan S, Kimmel J. Earplugs improve patients' subjective experience of sleep in critical care. *Nurs Crit Care* 2009;**14**:180–4.

40 Topf M, Davis JE. Critical care unit noise and rapid eye movement (REM) sleep. *Heart Lung* 1993;**22**:252–8.

41 Wallace CJ, Robins J, Alvord LS, Walker JM. The effect of earplugs on sleep measures during exposure to simulated intensive care unit noise. *Am J Crit Care* 1999;**8**:210–19.

42 Celik S, Oztekin D, Akyolcu N, Işsever H. Sleep disturbance: the patient care activities applied at the night shift in the intensive care unit. *J Clin Nurs* 2005;**14**:102–6.

43 Tamburri LM, DiBrienza R, Zozula R, Redeker NS. Nocturnal care interactions with patients in critical care units. *Am J Crit Care* 2004;**13**:102–12; quiz 114–15.

44 Eliassen KM, Hopstock LA. Sleep promotion in the intensive care unit-a survey of nurses' interventions. *Intensive Crit Care Nurs* 2011;**27**:138–42.

45 Parker KP. Promoting sleep and rest in critically ill patients. *Crit Care Nurs Clin North Am* 1995;**7**:337–49.

46 Evans JC, French DG. Sleep and healing in intensive care settings. *Dimens Crit Care Nurs* 1995;**14**:189–99.

47 Toublanc B, Rose D, Glerant JC, et al. Assist-control ventilation vs. low levels of pressure support ventilation on sleep quality in intubated ICU patients. *Intensive Care Med* 2007;**33**:1148–54.

48 Meza S, Mendez M, Ostrowski M, Younes M. Susceptibility to periodic breathing with assisted ventilation during sleep in normal subjects. *J Applied Physiol* 1998;**85**:1929–40.

49 Fanfulla F, Delmastro M, Berardinelli A, Lupo ND, Nava S. Effects of different ventilator settings on sleep and inspiratory effort in patients with neuromuscular disease. *Am J Respir Crit Care Med* 2005;**172**:619–24.

50 Bosma K, Ferreyra G, Ambrogio C, et al. Patient-ventilator interaction and sleep in mechanically ventilated patients: pressure support versus proportional assist ventilation. *Crit Care Med* 2007;**35**:1048–54.

51 Delisle S, Ouellet P, Bellemare P, Tétrault JP, Arsenault P. Sleep quality in mechanically ventilated patients: comparison between NAVA and PSV modes. *Ann Intensive Care* 2011;**1**:42.

52 Bourne RS, Mills GH. Sleep disruption in critically ill patients--pharmacological considerations. *Anaesthesia* 2004;**59**:374–84.

53 Pandharipande P, Ely EW. Sedative and analgesic medications: risk factors for delirium and sleep disturbances in the critically ill. *Crit Care Clin* 2006;**22**:313–27, vii.

54 Treggiari-Venzi M, Borgeat A, Fuchs-Buder T, Gachoud JP, Suter PM. Overnight sedation with midazolam or propofol in the ICU: effects on sleep quality, anxiety and depression. *Intensive Care Med* 1996;**22**:1186–90.

55 Tung A, Bergmann BM, Herrera S, Cao D, Mendelson WB. Recovery from sleep deprivation occurs during propofol anesthesia. *Anesthesiology* 2004;**100**:1419–26.

56 Corbett SM, Rebuck JA, Green CM, et al. Dexmedetomidine does not improve patient satisfaction when compared with propofol during mechanical ventilation. *Crit Care Med* 2005;**33**:940–5.

57 Cronin AJ, Keifer JC, Davies MF, King TS, Bixler EO. Postoperative sleep disturbance: influences of opioids and pain in humans. *Sleep* 2001;**24**:39–44.

58 Ibrahim MG, Bellomo R, Hart GK, et al. A double-blind placebo-controlled randomised pilot study of nocturnal melatonin in tracheostomised patients. *Crit Care Resusc* 2006;**8**:187–91.

59 Zhdanova IV, Wurtman RJ, Morabito C, Piotrovska VR, Lynch HJ. Effects of low oral doses of melatonin, given 2–4 hours before habitual bedtime, on sleep in normal young humans. *Sleep* 1996;**19**:423–31.

60 Bellapart J, Boots R. Potential use of melatonin in sleep and delirium in the critically ill. *Br J Anaesthesia* 2012;**108**:572–80.

61 Escames G, Leon J, Macías M, Khaldy H, Acuña-Castroviejo D. Melatonin counteracts lipopoly-saccharide-induced expression and activity of mitochondrial nitric oxide synthase in rats. *FASEB J* 2003;**17**:932–4.

62 Sener G, Toklu H, Kapucu C, et al. Melatonin protects against oxidative organ injury in a rat model of sepsis. *Surg Today* 2005;**35**:52–9.

63 Mundigler G, Delle-Karth G, Koreny M, et al. Impaired circadian rhythm of melatonin secretion in sedated critically ill patients with severe sepsis. *Crit Care Med* 2002;**30**:536–40.

64 Ely EW, Shintani A, Truman B, et al. Delirium as a predictor of mortality in mechanically ventilated patients in the intensive care unit. *JAMA* 2004;**291**:1753–62.

65 Ouimet S, Kavanagh BP, Gottfried SB, Skrobik Y. Incidence, risk factors and consequences of ICU delirium. *Intensive Care Med* 2007;**33**:66–73.

66 Ely EW, Gautam S, Margolin R, et al. The impact of delirium in the intensive care unit on hospital length of stay. *Intensive Care Med* 2001;**27**:1892–900.

67 Lin SM, Liu CY, Wang CH, et al. The impact of delirium on the survival of mechanically ventilated patients. *Crit Care Med* 2004;**32**:2254–9.

68 Milbrandt EB, Deppen S, Harrison PL, et al. Costs associated with delirium in mechanically ventilated patients. *Crit Care Med* 2004;**32**:955–62.

69 Thomason JW, Shintani A, Peterson JF, Pun BT, Jackson JC, Ely EW. Intensive care unit delirium is an independent predictor of longer hospital stay: a prospective analysis of 261 non-ventilated patients. *Crit Care* 2005;**9**:R375–381.

70 Weinhouse GL, Schwab RJ, Watson PL, et al. Bench-to-bedside review: delirium in ICU patients - importance of sleep deprivation. *Crit Care* 2009;**13**:234.

71 Trompeo AC, Vidi Y, Locane MD, et al. Sleep disturbances in the critically ill patients: role of delirium and sedative agents. *Minerva Anestesiol* 2011;**77**:604–12.

Chapter 42

Effects of Insulin and Glycaemic Management on Neuromuscular Function

Greet Hermans

Introduction

Acute illness or injury induces insulin resistance and hyperglycaemia, labelled stress hyperglycaemia or 'diabetes of injury'. High glucose levels in critically ill patients are associated with poor outcome, as demonstrated by the J-shaped association of glucose levels with mortality.[1] Hyperglycaemia in this setting is also linked to morbidity. Over 20 years ago, hyperglycaemia was identified as one of the risk factors for the development of ICUAW.[2] This syndrome of muscle weakness, involving peripheral as well as respiratory muscles, is caused by CIP, CIM, or a combination of both (CIP/CIM). The problem of ICUAW is a frequent complication of ICU stays,[3] with major impact on short-[4] as well as long-term outcome[5] in ICU survivors, and is presumed to have major socio-economical impact. This chapter will focus on the data currently available on the neuromuscular effects of hyperglycaemia in critically ill patients and the neuromuscular effects of controlling glycaemia using insulin in this setting. We further elaborate on potential mechanisms of action and discuss the available literature on this topic.

Clinical data

Soon after the first description of CIP by Bolton in the eighties,[6] observational studies focused on the identification of risk factors for this problem. The first study to address this question was performed by Witt and co-workers.[2] They identified hyperglycaemia as one of the predisposing factors. Since then, several prospective trials have studied the relationship between various indicators of glucose control in critically ill patients and the presence of clinical muscle weakness or electrophysiological signs of CIP/CIM (see Table 42.1). In total, in four out of seven trials, hyperglycaemia was associated with an increased risk. In two of these trials, including the largest one, hyperglycaemia was also found to be independently related to CIP/CIM or ICUAW, using multivariate models. The absence of effect of glucose in some other trials[7–9] may be due to the differences in the sample size as well as to the use of different criteria to evaluate glucose control, the specific characteristics of the patient populations studied, and distinct definitions of CIP/CIM and ICUAW (see Table 42.1). In a retrospective trial of 50 ARDS patients, those with muscle weakness exhibited significantly higher mean daily peak glucose levels.[10] To examine whether hyperglycaemia actually contributed to morbidity and mortality, rather than just representing an adaptive response in the critically ill, the first randomized trials[11–13] of glycaemic control in the ICU were performed as single-centre studies. These trials evaluated overall outcome effects of controlling glycaemia to levels normal for age on morbidity and mortality vs a 'do not

Table 42.1 Studies evaluating the effect of glycaemia on CIP/CIM

	No. of patients included	Type of ICU	Type of patients studied	Diagnosis	Incidence of CIP/CIM	Glucose criteria studied	Univariate analysis of effect of glucose P value	Multivariate analysis of effect of glucose OR (95% CI)	P value
Retrospective studies									
Bercker (2005)[10]	50	Mixed	ARDS	MRC sum score	27/50 (60%)	Daily peak glucose, mean/28 days	**<0.001**	NA	NA
Hermans (2009)[26]	620	Mixed	Weakness/weaning failure receiving electrophysiology	Electrophysiology	220/452 (48.7%) vs 125/168 (74.4%)	Before vs after institution of IIT, aiming between 80 and 180 mg/dL	**<0.0001**	0.25 (0.14–0.43)[a]	**<0.0001**
Prospective studies									
Witt (1991)[2]	43	Mixed	ICU ≥5 days + sepsis + ≥2 organ failures	Electrophysiology	30/43 (70%)	Serum glucose level	**0.002**	NA	**<0.0001**
Campellone (1998)[44]	87	SICU	Liver transplant recipients hospitalized >14 days or MV >7 days	Quadriparesis	7/87 (8%)	Mean serum glucose	**0.007**	No effect	NA
Thiele (2000)[7]	19	SICU	MV >3 days, cardiac surgery	Electrophysiology	12/19 (63%)	Mean serum glucose	**NS**	NA	NA
Garnacho-Montero (2001)[9]	73	NA	Sepsis + ≥2 organ failures + MV >10 days	Electrophysiology	50/73 (68.5%)	Glycaemia >250 mg/dL for >24 hours	0.9	NA	NA
De Jonghe (2002)[45]	95	Mixed	MV ≥7 days	MRC sum score <48	24/95 (25.3%)	Highest blood glucose	**0.001**	No effect	NA
Bednarik (2005)[8]	61	Mixed	≥2 organ failures	Electrophysiology + MRC score (≤2)	17/61 (27.9%) 35/61 (57.4%)	NA	NS	NA	NA

Table 42.1 (continued) Studies evaluating the effect of glycaemia on CIP/CIM

	No. of patients included	Type of ICU	Type of patients studied	Diagnosis	Incidence of CIP/CIM	Glucose criteria studied	Univariate analysis of effect of glucose P value	Multivariate analysis of effect of glucose OR (95% CI)	P value
Nanas (2008)[46]	185	Mixed	In ICU >10 days	MRC sum score (<48)	44/185 (23.8%)	Mean morning glucose >150 mg/dL	0.006	2.862 (1.301–6.296)[b]	0.009
RCTs									
Van den Berghe (2005)[19]	405	SICU	In ICU ≥7 days	Electrophysiology	46/181 (25%) vs 109/224 (49%)		<0.0001	1.26 (1.09–1.46)[c]	0.002
Hermans (2007)[20]	420	MICU	In ICU ≥7 days	Electrophysiology	81/208% (39%) vs 107/212 (51%)		0.02	0.61 (0.40–0.92)[d]	0.02

NA, not available; IIT, intensive insulin therapy; CIT, conventional insulin therapy; SICU, surgical intensive care unit; MICU, medical intensive care unit; OR, odds ratio; CI, confidence interval.

[a] Odds ratio after IIT vs before IIT.

[b] Odds ratio for hyperglycaemia vs no hyperglycaemia.

[c] Odds ratio per mmol/L of morning blood glucose.

[d] Odds ratio for IIT vs CIT

touch' strategy, accepting hyperglycaemia up to the renal threshold. After the impressive beneficial results observed in these three Leuven trials, involving surgical,[11] medical,[12] and paediatric[13] populations, other randomized trials were performed.[14–16] These trials tempered some of the initial enthusiasm and called for caution and potential harm when implementing this strategy on a large scale,[16] albeit by using methods and protocols different from the original setting.[1] These included different glucose target ranges, insulin administration routes, types of infusion pumps, sampling sites, accuracies of glucometers, nutritional strategies, and varying levels of expertise. One of the main concerns when implementing the treatment is hypoglycaemia. Hypoglycaemia was associated with an increased risk of death, although a causal relationship cannot be proven.[17] On the other hand, when hypoglycaemia is detected early, using accurate devices, and quickly corrected, it did not affect intelligence 3 years after ICU stay in a paediatric population.[18]

Only two of these RCTs[11,12] specifically addressed the neuromuscular effects of tight glycaemic control. The studies were performed in the medical and surgical ICU, respectively. A total of 1548 surgical patients[11] and 1200 medical patients[12] were included. In both trials, all patients who stayed in the ICU for at least 7 days and had no prior neuromuscular disorders received weekly electrophysiological screening during their ICU stay. This consisted of NCS and needle EMG. The muscles analysed were the *m. extensor digitorum communis*, *m. biceps*, *m. quadriceps*, and *m. gastrocnemius*. When findings were equivocal, additional muscles were evaluated. Muscles susceptible to pressure palsies were avoided. The diagnosis of critical illness polyneuromyopathy (CIPNM) was solely based on the presence of abundant spontaneous electrical activity manifested as positive sharp waves or fibrillation potentials. Electrophysiological data were obtained in 420 medical and 405 surgical patients. Results showed that IIT significantly reduced the electrophysiological incidence of CIP/CIM from 49% to 25% in the surgical population[19] and from 51% to 39% in the medical population.[20] Multivariate logistic regression analysis, including baseline risk factors and other known risk factors for CIP/CIM, confirmed that IIT was an independent protective factor. Meta-analysis of these data resulted in a relative risk of 0.65 (95% CI 0.55–0.78) for the development of CIP/CIM for patients treated with IIT, compared to those treated with conventional insulin therapy (CIT).[21] The beneficial effects on electrophysiological parameters were related with glucose control, rather than insulin dose.[19] Pooled data from both trials also indicated that the beneficial effects on CIP/CIM were only present in the group of patients in which normoglycaemia was reached (80–110 mg/dL), in contrast with patients in whom mild hyperglycaemia (110–150 mg/dL) was still present.[22] These electrophysiological effects were accompanied by a significant reduction in the need for PMV, defined as MV for at least 7 days, from 47% to 35% in the medical and from 42% to 32% in the surgical population.

IIT could possibly also avert some of the negative neuromuscular effects that GCs may have in critically ill patients. The role of GCs in causing myopathy is well known, but the actual clinical impact of GC treatment in critically ill patients remains controversial.[23] GCs had protective electrophysiological effects only in the subgroup of patients that received IIT.[20] This observation elicited the hypothesis that counteracting the hyperglycaemia induced by GCs may permit its anti-inflammatory activity to prevail.[24] Increased spontaneous electrical activity may occur in axonopathy or muscle necrosis, but this finding is not seen with muscle membrane inexcitability, a feature of CIM which is identified by reduced CMAPs; hence, the use of spontaneous electrical activity as a diagnostic endpoint may overestimate the relative prevalence of axonopathy. Therefore, the benefit of GCs would involve neuroprotection, rather than muscle protection. Indeed, muscle atrophy appeared to be aggravated by GCs, as shown by markers of atrophy and proteolysis in muscle biopsies of critically ill patients.[25]

These observations were made in the controlled setting of a randomized trial, during which study nurses were continuously monitoring the quality of the glycaemic control. For this reason, it is not obvious to extrapolate these data into the setting of tight glycaemic control in daily care. Consequently, this particular question was evaluated, using a retrospective analysis of data from our centre, comparing electrophysiological outcome data obtained during the periods before the insulin trials, at which time the conventional regimen was the standard regimen, and after the trials when strict glycaemic control was implemented into routine clinical practice. This analysis included electrophysiological data obtained during routine clinical practice in 620 patients.[26] The same electrophysiological criteria were used to diagnose CIP/CIM, as used in the randomized trials. Results were also very similar and showed a significant reduction in the electrophysiological diagnosis of CIP/CIM in the screened long-stay patients from 74.4% to 48.7%. This benefit was observed in the medical as well as in the surgical patients, and multivariate analysis pointed to an independent effect of the introduction of IIT (OR 0.25, 95% CI 0.14–0.43). Notably, the absolute incidence of CIP/CIM, based on electrophysiological testing, in this retrospective cohort is higher than during the randomized trials for the IIT as well as CIT groups, as all electrophysiological tests were performed because of clinical weakness or weaning failure and at a later stage of the ICU stay, rather than being part of a routine and early screening. The institution of IIT was also independently related to a reduction in the need for PMV (OR 0.4, CI 0.22–0.72). Absolute and relative values of SNAPs, used as a surrogate marker for CIP, were improved after the institution of IIT, and the presence of a myopathic component in the tracings obtained during voluntary contraction was significantly lower (before IIT 30%, after institution of IIT 18%). The major limitation of these data is the retrospective nature of these results which was, however, inevitable, given the positive results on mortality obtained in the RCTs in our centre.

Neuromuscular effects of glycaemic control at the pathophysiological level

The pathophysiology of ICUAW is very complex and includes changes at the level of the muscles as well as the nerves (see Figure 42.1). The global effect is loss of muscle mass and function. Aspects involved include axonal degeneration and excitability changes at the nerve membrane, hormonal imbalances favouring a catabolic muscle state, with relative decrease in protein synthesis and increased proteolysis, changes in the excitation-contraction coupling, bioenergetic failure, and muscle membrane inexcitability. Several potential mechanisms may be invoked to explain the beneficial neuromuscular effects of strict glycaemic control in critically ill patients.

Insulin resistance is a key feature of critical illness. Insulin normally acts as an anabolic hormone, suppressing proteolysis and stimulating protein synthesis and cell proliferation. In prolonged critical illness, the insulin-independent GLUT-1 and GLUT-3 transporters are upregulated, which may put the muscle at risk for passive glucose uptake and overload, whereas the insulin-dependent GLUT-4 transporters are downregulated. Treatment with IIT reduces insulin resistance, reflected by the downregulation of GLUT-1 and GLUT-3 transporters and normalization of GLUT-4 expression in skeletal muscle.[27] This coincided with increased overall protein content in the muscle of a subgroup of surgical patients treated with IIT, compared to those treated with CIT.[28,29] In several other catabolic states, insulin has protein-sparing effects.[30–32] Muscle biopsies from critically ill patients receiving insulin therapy showed increased Akt-dependent signalling, suggesting activated protein synthesis. A positive correlation was found with the insulin dose administered and phosphorylated Akt (p-Akt).[33] These data are in accordance with significantly increased amounts of p-Akt in post-mortem biopsies of patients treated with IIT, compared to

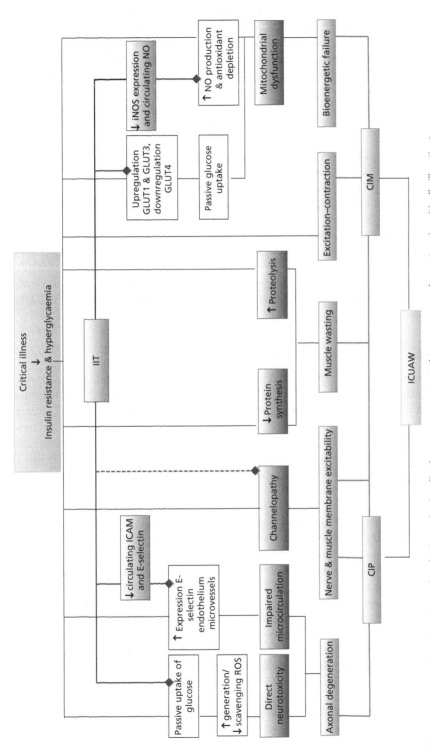

Fig. 42.1 Presumed mechanisms whereby intensive insulin therapy may protect the neuromuscular system in critically ill patients.

Reproduced from Hermans G, De Jonghe B, Bruyninckx F, Van den BG, 'Interventions for preventing critical illness polyneuropathy and critical illness myopathy', Cochrane Database Systematic Reviews, 2009, CD006832, with permission. Copyright © 2009 The Cochrane Collaboration. Published by John Wiley & Sons, Ltd.

those treated with CIT.[34] Further analysis of 208 muscle biopsies, either collected *in vivo* (n = 64, *m rectus femoris, vastus lateralis*) or post-mortem (n = 144, *m rectus abdominis*) during the insulin trials and compared to healthy controls, revealed that loss of fibre size during critical illness, however, was not affected by IIT.[25] No significant differences were noted in the myofibrillar protein synthesis capacity at the level of gene expression. Proteolytic activity was also not affected by IIT. In these samples, myosin/actin ratios were overall reduced, compared with controls, and multivariate logistic regression analysis identified IIT as an independent protective factor against severely reduced myosin/actin ratios in the post-mortem samples. However, in the *in vivo* biopsies, IIT did not affect myosin/actin ratio or the proportion of patients with a severely reduced myosin/actin ratio in the *in vivo* biopsies.

Another potential mechanism of action at the muscular level could be linked to the iNOS enzyme. Critically ill patients exhibit increased levels of circulating NO, which has pro-inflammatory capacities and may contribute to organ damage in I/R. Increased local production of NO, antioxidant depletion, and mitochondrial dysfunction are documented in the skeletal muscle of critically ill patients and are presumed to contribute to bioenergetic failure of the muscle.[35] Sepsis-induced expression and activation of iNOS coincided with a reduction of *in vitro* muscle force of the human rectus abdominus muscle.[36] In biopsies taken from the same muscle in critically ill patients, IIT reduced iNOS gene expression and also lowered circulating NO levels.[37] IIT further protected mitochondrial activity in the liver; however, no similar beneficial effects could be observed in the muscle.[28]

Integrating clinical data and bench work

The observational studies suggest a detrimental role of hyperglycaemia in the development of ICUAW, which is further confirmed by the significant reduction of electrophysiological incidence of CIP/CIM and associated reduction in the need for PMV in two RCTs normalizing glycaemia using insulin. Muscle biopsies from these patients show downregulation of protein synthesis at the level of gene expression and increased proteolytic activity, affecting myosin to a greater extent than actin, resulting in a decreased myosin/actin ratio. IIT overall did not substantially alter this response at the level of the skeletal muscle, and no mitochondrial protection could be confirmed. There may be several explanations for this apparently contradictory finding.

Beneficial effects could be largely situated at the level of the nerve, rather than in the muscle. The myosin/actin ratio indeed is not affected in axonal neuropathy.[38] The electrophysiological criteria used in the RCTs consisted solely of the presence of spontaneous electrical activity. The syndrome of muscle membrane inexcitability therefore may have been overlooked, and the electrophysiological diagnosis may have favoured the identification of axonal neuropathy, rather than myopathy. This is supported by the observation that markers of denervation or neuronal inactivity were increased in patients with positive electrophysiological findings but not in patients with reduced myosin/actin ratio.[25] Human nervous tissue samples from critically ill patients are not often collected, as this is an invasive procedure, and are therefore not available for these randomized trials. The pathophysiology of the neuropathic component of ICUAW is thus even more obscure than the muscle component. Endothelial cells in the microvessels in the endoneurium of the peripheral nerves from critically ill patients with neuromuscular disorders are activated, as shown by increased expression of E-selectin.[39] This is presumed to be involved in the development of axonopathy in these patients. IIT protects the endothelium, as evidenced by reduced circulating ICAM and E selectin,[37] and could therefore have a neuroprotective effect; however, this has not been demonstrated.

The peripheral nervous system depends on the extracellular concentration of glucose for its uptake, which occurs passively. Hyperglycaemia could potentially cause direct neurotoxicity by increased passive uptake, causing increased generation and decreased scavenging of ROS, compromising mitochondrial function.[40] This is one of the mechanisms responsible for glucose neurotoxicity in diabetes, in addition to the accumulation of sorbitol, protein glycation, and altered intracellular signalling.[41] The clinical scenario of diabetic neuropathy differs in many aspects from the situation of critically ill patients developing hyperglycaemia. Nevertheless, some of the pathways involved could be similar but remain currently unexplored in CIP.

Finally, nerve membrane inexcitability is considered to be involved in the pathogenesis of CIP, as part of a generalized inexcitability phenomenon, also affecting the muscle and the heart. Rich et al. described a rapidly reversible neuropathy in critically ill patients, suggesting that this mechanism may be more important than nerve degeneration or is possibly preceding actual neuronal damage in CIP.[42] Animal data confirm that inactivation of sodium channels contributes to reduced nerve excitability. In diabetic polyneuropathy, nerve excitability changes have been documented.[43] The potential role of hyperglycaemia on nerve excitability in critically ill patients has not been studied yet.

It is nevertheless too simplistic to state that the beneficial effects observed in the randomized trials are purely neuroprotective. The first reason to support this statement is that no difference was found in the markers of denervation/neuronal inactivity between the IIT and CIT groups.[25] Secondly, spontaneous electrical activity can also be present in patients with myopathy, and not solely in neuropathy. It may be, however, that the electrophysiological findings preceded the changes in myosin/actin levels, and, therefore, the latter appeared rather unaffected by IIT in the currently available data. Finally, we need to consider that no large series yet have studied the relationship between the electrophysiological presence of spontaneous electrical activity and muscle weakness and that muscle strength was not formally evaluated in the randomized studies. Abundant spontaneous electrical activity may occur in axonopathy or muscle necrosis. This criterion may miss the entity of muscle membrane inexcitability, which is a feature of myopathy that is identified with reduced CMAPs. Early signs of neuromyopathy may also remain unrecognized as spontaneous electrical activity only appears later in the process compared with the very early reduction in CMAPs. Clinical data from both studies in the surgical and medical ICU in our centre do suggest that these electrophysiological criteria used are indeed clinically relevant. IIT significantly reduced the need for PMV. Whether this benefit results from overall benefit of treatment on morbidity or is specifically caused by improved muscle function cannot be distinguished. The observation that the electrophysiological diagnosis as such was found to be independently associated with PMV, however, supports the latter hypothesis.

Conclusion

Several observational studies identified hyperglycaemia as a risk factor for CIP/CIM. Additionally, two large randomized interventional trials, comparing strict glycaemic control with a strategy of tolerating hyperglycaemia, showed that this intervention reduced the electrophysiological incidence of CIP/CIM, which was accompanied by a reduction in the need for PMV, in addition to decreased mortality. These results were confirmed in a retrospective analysis evaluating the effects of implementation of strict glycaemic control in a daily care setting. Mechanisms of action remain unclear. Although, at the level of the muscle, potential anabolic effects and mitochondrial protection have been suggested, this could not be clearly confirmed on human skeletal muscle tissue from critically ill patients treated to normoglycaemia. This may be explained by a time lag in certain pathological changes or may suggest that the benefits largely consist of neuroprotection. Several conceptual benefits at the level of the nerve can be identified. Due to invasiveness of nerve biopsy, human data, however, are currently lacking.

Controversy exists on the optimal level of glucose control in critically ill patients, as multicentre trials could not replicate the overall beneficial effects on mortality and even pointed to potential harm. Several methodological issues may explain the divergent study results. It is not recommended to embark on strict normalization of glycaemia if the methodological prerequisites from the Leuven trials are not met.

References

1 Van den Berghe G, Schetz M, Vlasselaers D, et al. Clinical review: intensive insulin therapy in critically ill patients: NICE-SUGAR or Leuven blood glucose target? *J Clin Endocrinol Metab* 2009;**94**:3163–70.

2 Witt NJ, Zochodne DW, Bolton CF, et al. Peripheral nerve function in sepsis and multiple organ failure. *Chest*. 1991;**99**:176–84.

3 Stevens RD, Dowdy DW, Michaels RK, Mendez-Tellez PA, Pronovost PJ, Needham DM. Neuromuscular dysfunction acquired in critical illness: a systematic review. *Intensive Care Med* 2007;**33**:1876–91.

4 De Jonghe B, Bastuji-Garin S, Durand MC, et al. Respiratory weakness is associated with limb weakness and delayed weaning in critical illness. *Crit Care Med* 2007;**35**:2007–15.

5 Herridge MS, Cheung AM, Tansey CM, et al. One-year outcomes in survivors of the acute respiratory distress syndrome. *N Engl J Med* 2003;**348**:683–93.

6 Bolton CF, Gilbert JJ, Hahn AF, Sibbald WJ. Polyneuropathy in critically ill patients. *J Neurol Neurosurg Psychiatry* 1984;**47**:1223–31.

7 Thiele RI, Jakob H, Hund E, et al. Sepsis and catecholamine support are the major risk factors for critical illness polyneuropathy after open heart surgery'. *Thorac Cardiovasc Surg* 2000;**48**:145–50.

8 Bednarik J, Vondracek P, Dusek L, Moravcova E, Cundrle I. Risk factors for critical illness polyneuromyopathy. *J Neurol* 2005;**252**:343–51.

9 Garnacho-Montero J, Madrazo-Osuna J, Garcia-Garmendia JL, et al. Critical illness polyneuropathy: risk factors and clinical consequences. A cohort study in septic patients. *Intensive Care Med* 2001;**27**:1288–96.

10 Bercker S, Weber-Carstens S, Deja M, et al. Critical illness polyneuropathy and myopathy in patients with acute respiratory distress syndrome. *Crit Care Med* 2005;**33**:711–15.

11 Van den Berghe G, Wouters P, Weekers F, et al. Intensive insulin therapy in the critically ill patients. *N Engl J Med* 2001;**345**:1359–67.

12 Van den Berghe G, Wilmer A, Hermans G, et al. Intensive insulin therapy in the medical ICU. *N Engl J Med* 2006;**354**:449–61.

13 Vlasselaers D, Milants I, Desmet L, et al. Intensive insulin therapy for patients in paediatric intensive care: a prospective, randomised controlled study. *Lancet* 2009;**373**:547–56.

14 Brunkhorst FM, Engel C, Bloos F, et al. Intensive insulin therapy and pentastarch resuscitation in severe sepsis. *N Engl J Med* 2008;**358**:125–39.

15 Preiser JC, Devos P, Ruiz-Santana S, et al. A prospective randomised multi-centre controlled trial on tight glucose control by intensive insulin therapy in adult intensive care units: the Glucontrol study. *Intensive Care Med* 2009;**35**:1738–48.

16 Finfer S, Chittock DR, Su SY, et al. Intensive versus conventional glucose control in critically ill patients. *N Engl J Med* 2009;**360**:1283–97.

17 Finfer S, Liu B, Chittock DR, et al. Hypoglycemia and risk of death in critically ill patients. *N Engl J Med* 2012;**367**:1108–18.

18 Mesotten D, Gielen M, Sterken C, et al. Neurocognitive development of children 4 years after critical illness and treatment with tight glucose control: a randomized controlled trial. *JAMA* 2012;**308**:1641–50.

19 Van den Berghe G, Schoonheydt K, Becx P, Bruyninckx F, Wouters PJ. Insulin therapy protects the central and peripheral nervous system of intensive care patients. *Neurology*. 2005;**64**:1348–53.

20 Hermans G, Wilmer A, Meersseman W, et al. Impact of Intensive Insulin Therapy on Neuromuscular Complications and Ventilator-dependency in MICU. *Am J Respir Crit Care Med* 2007;**175**:480–9.

21 Hermans G, De Jonghe B, Bruyninckx F, Van den Berghe G. Interventions for preventing critical illness polyneuropathy and critical illness myopathy. *Cochrane Database Syst Rev* 2009;**1**:CD006832.

22 Van den Berghe G , Wilmer A, Milants I, et al. Intensive insulin therapy in mixed medical/surgical intensive care units: benefit versus harm. *Diabetes*. 2006;**55**:3151–9.

23 De Jonghe B, Lacherade JC, Sharshar T, Outin H. Intensive care unit-acquired weakness: risk factors and prevention. *Crit Care Med* 2009;**37**:S309–15.

24 Bloch S, Polkey MI, Griffiths M, Kemp P. Molecular mechanisms of intensive care unit acquired weakness. *Eur Respir J* 2011;**39**:1000–11.

25 Derde S, Hermans G, Derese I, et al. Muscle atrophy and preferential loss of myosin in prolonged critically ill patients. *Crit Care Med* 2012;**40**:79–89.

26 Hermans G, Schrooten M, Van Damme P, et al. Benefits of intensive insulin therapy on neuromuscular complications in routine daily critical care practice: a retrospective study. *Crit Care* 2009;**13**:R5.

27 Langouche L, Van den Berghe G. Glucose metabolism and insulin therapy. *Crit Care Clin* 2006;**22**: 119–29, vii.

28 Vanhorebeek I, De VR, Mesotten D, Wouters PJ, De Wolf-Peeters C, Van den Berghe G. Protection of hepatocyte mitochondrial ultrastructure and function by strict blood glucose control with insulin in critically ill patients. *Lancet* 2005;**365**:53–9.

29 Langouche L, Vander Perre S, Wouters P, and Van den Berghe G. Expression of glucose transporters in critical illness. *Crit Care* **2006;10**(Suppl 1):P252.

30 Gore DC, Wolf SE, Sanford AP, Herndon DN, Wolfe RR. Extremity hyperinsulinemia stimulates muscle protein synthesis in severely injured patients. *Am J Physiol Endocrinol Metab* 2004;**286**:E529–34.

31 Thomas SJ, Morimoto K, Herndon DN, et al. The effect of prolonged euglycemic hyperinsulinemia on lean body mass after severe burn. *Surgery* 2002;**132**:341–7.

32 Biolo G, De Cicco M, Lorenzon S, et al. Treating hyperglycemia improves skeletal muscle protein metabolism in cancer patients after major surgery. *Crit Care Med* 2008;**36**:1768–75.

33 Jespersen JG, Nedergaard A, Reitelseder S, et al. Activated protein synthesis and suppressed protein breakdown signaling in skeletal muscle of critically ill patients. *PLoS One* 2011;**6**:e18090.

34 Langouche L, Vander Perre S, Wouters PJ, D'Hoore A, Hansen TK, Van den Berghe G. Effect of intensive insulin therapy on insulin sensitivity in the critically ill. *J Clin Endocrinol Metab* 2007;**92**:3890–7.

35 Brealey D, Brand M, Hargreaves I, et al. Association between mitochondrial dysfunction and severity and outcome of septic shock. *Lancet* 2002;**360**:219–23.

36 Lanone S, Mebazaa A, Heymes C, et al. Muscular contractile failure in septic patients: role of the inducible nitric oxide synthase pathway. *Am J Respir Crit Care Med* 2000;**162**:2308–15.

37 Langouche L, Vanhorebeek I, Vlasselaers D, et al. Intensive insulin therapy protects the endothelium of critically ill patients. *J Clin Invest* 2005;**115**:2277–86.

38 Stibler H, Edstrom L, Ahlbeck K, Remahl S, Ansved T. Electrophoretic determination of the myosin/actin ratio in the diagnosis of critical illness myopathy. *Intensive Care Med* 2003;**29**:1515–27.

39 Fenzi F, Latronico N, Refatti N, Rizzuto N. Enhanced expression of E-selectin on the vascular endothelium of peripheral nerve in critically ill patients with neuromuscular disorders. *Acta Neuropathol (Berl)* 2003;**106**:75–82.

40 Van den Berghe G. How does blood glucose control with insulin save lives in intensive care? *J Clin Invest* 2004;**114**:1187–95.

41 Tomlinson DR, Gardiner NJ. Glucose neurotoxicity. *Nat Rev Neurosci* 2008;**9**:36–45.

42 Novak KR, Nardelli P, Cope TC, et al. Inactivation of sodium channels underlies reversible neuropathy during critical illness in rats. *J Clin Invest* 2009;**119**:1150–8.

43 Krishnan AV, Lin CS, Kiernan MC. Activity-dependent excitability changes suggest Na +/K + pump dysfunction in diabetic neuropathy. *Brain* 2008;**131**:1209–16.

44 Campellone JV, Lacomis D, Kramer DJ, Van Cott AC, Giuliani MJ. Acute myopathy after liver transplantation. *Neurology* 1998;**50**:46–53.

45 De Jonghe B, Sharshar T, Lefaucheur JP, et al. Paresis acquired in the intensive care unit: a prospective multicenter study. *JAMA* 2002;**288**:2859–67.

46 Nanas S, Kritikos K, Angelopoulos E, et al. Predisposing factors for critical illness polyneuromyopathy in a multidisciplinary intensive care unit. *Acta Neurol Scand* 2008;**118**:175–81.

Chapter 43

Physical and Occupational Therapy in the ICU

William D. Schweickert and John P. Kress

Introduction

Survival from critical illness is improving substantially. The groundswell of improvements stemming from recent advances in evidence-based patient care strategies is quite encouraging.[1-6] The survival of such extremely sick people, previously destined to die, brings novel modes of recovery, with a rehabilitation process that is long, arduous, and often incomplete. A substantial burden on the recovering ICU patient is the deconditioning and neuromuscular weakness so commonly noted. This is particularly common in those suffering from ARDS, sepsis, and/or SIRS.[7,8] The reasons and mechanisms underpinning the final pathway of weakness and functional debilitation are poorly understood; this is likely, in part, due to the fact that numerous disease processes and pathophysiologies may culminate in the end result of physical weakness in ICU survivors.

Over previous decades, as intensive care advanced, bed rest—a state of suspended physical and mental animation—became commonplace.[9] The use of potent sedative and analgesic drugs was a major reason for this immobilized state, though growing abilities to care for patients with extremely high severity of illness was an additional contributor. It is interesting that awareness of the harmful effects of complete bed rest have been recognized for over 60 years,[10,11] but modern intensive care has seemed to attend more to remarkable advances in ways to maintain homeostasis by artificial means; until recent times, such artificial life support strategies have failed to consider the cost of 'taking over' for natural body functions. Yet the philosophy of 'fully taking over' for failing organ systems (i.e. a failing body) is not without cost. Recent evidence suggests that an ICU care strategy which calls upon dysfunctional organ systems to 'do some of the work' may be better than complete normalization of physiology by artificial means (e.g. MV, permissive hypercapnia,[12] reduced reliance on full MV support,[13,14] less aggressive RRT[15,16]). Running parallel with this shift of care philosophy has been reconsideration—in all patients—of the wisdom and necessity of complete bed rest.

Long-term effects of critical illness

Awareness of the long-term issues which confront ICU survivors recently has grown in both medical and lay communities alike. Likewise, long-term problems in ICU survivors with respiratory failure have become a major focus of recent clinical investigations. As ICU outcome research has proliferated, awareness has grown regarding extreme and long-standing **physical** impairments.[17-19] One of the earliest reports came from work by Herridge et al. This group followed survivors of ARDS for 1 year after hospital discharge. ARDS is a common condition, with data published in 2005 suggesting that there were nearly 200 000 annual cases of ALI in the US, with 74 500 deaths and 3.6 million hospital days reported in such patients.[20] It is likely that these numbers are currently even higher. The above landmark study by Herridge et al. interviewed and tested ARDS survivors for physical as well as mental functional problems. The evaluation was quite extensive, with the investigators even travelling long distances to perform home visits to ensure the accuracy and completeness of their data. Despite a very young median age of 45 years, **all** of the 109 patients evaluated noted loss of muscle bulk, proximal muscle weakness, and fatigue; half of this relatively young group of patients were unemployed 1 year after their ICU experience.[21] A recent report of the same cohort, now 5 years out from hospital discharge, noted persistent (permanent?) physical limitations in the 64 remaining survivors, with 6-minute walk tests and physical component scores on the SF-36 Health Survey that were noted to be far below normal.[17] It is remarkable that the majority (94%) of survivors were able to return to work in spite of the refractory nature of their physical limitations. Nevertheless, these important studies signal that physical debilitation in ICU survivors has major public health implications.

While it may seem self-evident that the prolonged physical immobilization that is so common in mechanically ventilated ICU patients leads to neuromuscular weakness, the science supporting this notion was relatively limited until very recently. In an elegant study reported more than 15 years ago, Griffiths and colleagues compared the effects of CPM of one leg in critically ill patients with respiratory failure during neuromuscular blockade;[22] the patients' contralateral leg served as a control. Muscle fibre atrophy was prevented, and muscle DNA to protein ratios (an established index of wasting) and muscle protein content were reduced less profoundly in the leg receiving passive range of motion. The authors concluded that, in critically ill patients, an intervention as simple as passive muscle stretching could preserve the architecture of muscle fibres.

Studies of early physical therapy in the ICU

In the last few years, several investigators have begun reporting on a novel strategy of ICU patient care where the traditional model of deep sedation and prolonged bed rest is substituted by a strategy of early mobilization. Teams of specialists, including physical and occupational therapists, nurses, respiratory therapists, and patient care technicians, are coming to the ICU and working with patients to get them out of bed. This intervention is occurring very early, even while patients are still requiring MV through an ETT. Table 43.1 summarizes the published literature on early mobilization in the ICU.

In order to undergo any mobilization strategy, patients must be awake and able to interact with their environment. Accordingly, ICU care strategies that rationalize and limit sedation are necessary. It seems self-evident that deep sedation and immobility go hand in hand, yet the detrimental effects on neuromuscular function have only recently been reported. De Jonghe and colleagues described the results of a sedation algorithm designed to allow patients to be more alert.[23] This algorithm was designed around the ATICE instrument. This instrument, which targets consciousness (with awakeness and consciousness subdomains) and tolerance (with calmness, ventilatory synchrony, and face relaxation subdomains), was used to direct a nursing sedation algorithm. In this 'before-after' trial, transitioning from usual care to the algorithm reduced time to awakening, ventilator time, and ICU length of stay. It is interesting that it also reduced pressure sores by 50%, presumably due to reductions in a drug-induced state of immobility.

Bailey and colleagues reported a significant advance with the first publication of early mobilization in mechanically ventilated ICU patients.[24] The study was a descriptive prospective cohort

Table 43.1 Summary of studies of ICU mobilization

	Intervention	Outcomes	Adverse events reported
De Jonghe et al. (2005)[23]	Before-after trial—nursing sedation algorithm	50% reduction in bed sores	None
Bailey et al. (2007)[24]	Mobilization with physical and respiratory therapist, nurse critical care technician	103 patients had ~1500 activities; ~40% intubated patients performed physical therapy activities	Falls, oxygen desaturation, blood pressure changes, medical device removal—all <1%
Thomsen et al. (2008)[25]	Mobilization with physical and respiratory therapist, nurse, critical care technician	Patients in an ICU that targeted early mobility were more than twice as likely to receive it	None
Morris et al. (2011)[26]	Block assignment— mobilization with physical therapist, nurse, nursing assistant	Improved time to getting out of bed; reduced hospital length of stay	None
Burtin et al. (2009)[27]	Randomized trial—bedside bicycle ergometer exercises	Improved 6-minute walk test; improved SF-36 physical function scores; improved quadriceps force	Oxygen desaturation, blood pressure changes <4%
Bourdin et al. (2010)[28]	Observational trial—bedside mobilization team	Chair sitting in more than half of patients, walking in 11%	Drops in muscle tone without falls, oxygen desaturation, orthostatic hypotension, medical device removal 3%
Needham et al. (2010)[29]	Before-after trial—physical and occupational therapist	Reduced sedative use, reduced ICU delirium, ICU and hospital length of stay	None
Schweickert et al. (2009)[30]	Randomized, blinded trial— physical and occupational therapist	Improved functional independence, reduced delirium, reduced ventilator days, improved discharge to home	Falls, oxygen desaturation, blood pressure changes, medical device removal—all <4%

report of patients with respiratory failure admitted to a special ICU at LDS Hospital in Salt Lake City, Utah. In this 'respiratory ICU', a culture of minimal sedation and early mobilization was embraced. These patients were transferred from another ICU where they had been residing an average of 10 days. Mobilization in the respiratory ICU commenced as soon as patients were responsive to verbal stimulation and had respiratory and cardiovascular 'stability', defined as ventilator settings of $FiO_2 \leq 0.6$ and $PEEP \leq 10\ cmH_2O$, and absence of orthostatic hypotension and catecholamine infusions, respectively. The protocol of mobilization used a team approach that included a physical and respiratory therapist, a nurse, and a critical care technician. The mobilization algorithm targeted a sequential strategy where activities progressed from lesser to greater complexity, according to the patient's level of tolerance. Specifically, the sequence of activities started with sitting on the edge of the bed, with progression to sitting in a chair after bed transfer and ultimately to ambulation. Such a sequential approach to mobilization is utilized routinely by physical therapists caring for patients in less acute settings. In this trial, nearly 1500 activity events were recorded in 103 patients. Ambulation was quite common, even in patients with high illness acuities. Indeed, greater than 40% of activity events occurred in patients who were still intubated and mechanically ventilated. The authors reported a very low incidence of adverse events such as falls to knees (n = 5), notable blood pressure changes (n = 5), severe oxyhaemoglobin desaturations (n = 3), and medical device removal (n = 1). It is important to remember that adverse events, such as desaturation, blood pressure changes, and unplanned device removal (e.g. self-extubation), occur in patients during routine standard care. Accordingly, these occurrences cannot be viewed as 'never events' in ICU patients. This publication was the first to systematically describe the safety and feasibility of mobilization in mechanically ventilated ICU patients. A follow-up study by this same group reported the importance of a culture and philosophy of ICU care that embraced patient mobility.[25] In this study, patients transferred to the LDS respiratory ICU from another ICU were 2.5 times more likely to receive a care plan that included mobilization.

In 2008, Morris and colleagues published the first prospective trial of mobilization in mechanically ventilated medical ICU patients at Wake Forest University. The mobility team in this study consisted of a physical therapist, a critical care nurse, and a nursing assistant. The strategy of mobilization was again sequential and based upon patient cognitive awareness, tolerance, and capability with regard to performing mobilization procedures. This group likewise utilized a minimalist approach to sedation during MV, utilizing a strategy of daily interruption of sedative infusions. A total of 330 patients were enrolled in a non-randomized block allocation manner. Eighty per cent of patients in the group assigned to mobilization had at least one PT session, compared to only 47% in the usual care group. The mobilization group was able to move out of bed 5 days faster than the control group and had 2 fewer hospital days; both of these findings were statistically significant. Importantly, the authors reported no adverse events or unintentional removal of medical devices during **any** of the mobilization sessions. This group recently reported the results of a 1-year follow-up of this cohort. Eighty-five per cent of the 330 patients had survived the original hospitalization. Those not subjected to early mobilization had a nearly twofold higher likelihood of death or hospital readmission within a year after discharge (OR, 1.77, 95% CI 1.04–3.01).[26]

In 2009, Burtin and colleagues reported the results of an RCT of early exercise, using a bedside bicycle ergometer, in patients with expected prolonged stays in medical and surgical ICUs. The majority of patients in this trial came from surgical ICUs.[27] The bicycle ergometer intervention was delayed from the time of ICU admission by approximately 2 weeks. Patients randomized to the intervention group used a bedside cycle ergometer that was attached to the foot of the bed. For 5 of 7 days each week, patients underwent a cycling exercise session. In patients who were not awake enough to actively participate, the feet could be strapped to the pedals of the cycle so that passive range-of-motion exercises could occur. Once awake enough to participate, active cycling exercise began. Eighty-four per cent of the patients in this trial were intubated and mechanically ventilated for at least a portion of their ICU stay. Strength and functional assessments were measured as the outcomes of interest. The 6-minute walk distance at hospital discharge was higher in the intervention patients (196 vs 143 m, $P < 0.05$). Likewise, the SF-36 physical function score at hospital discharge was higher (21 vs 15, $P < 0.05$), and the quadriceps force at hospital discharge was better in the intervention group (2.37 vs 2.03 N/kg, $P < 0.05$). The cycling sessions were well tolerated in this group of ICU patients. There was a total of 425 cycling sessions in the study, with no serious adverse events. Adverse events of any sort occurred rarely, with only 4% of sessions unable to be completed. Reasons for rare premature stoppage included oxyhaemoglobin desaturation and unexpected changes in blood pressure during the cycling sessions.

Bourdin and colleagues recently reported an observational study of 20 patients.[28] This cohort began mobilization after a median of 5 ICU days, with one-third of interventions occurring during MV. The investigators utilized a conservative approach to initiating mobilization by excluding all patients with conditions such as shock, sedation, and ongoing renal support. Accordingly, a contraindication to mobilization was noted on nearly half of the days, with sedation (15%), shock (11%), and renal support (9%) being the most frequent reasons that mobilization was contraindication. The mobilization included chair sitting (56%), tilting up with arms unsupported (25%), walking (11%), and tilting up with arms supported (8%). Adverse events were rare, occurring in 3% of the total of 424 interventions. The reported adverse events included drops in muscle tone without falls (n = 7), hypoxaemia (SpO_2 <88% for >1 min), one unscheduled extubation, and one orthostatic arterial hypotensive event. There were no deaths, MIs, dysrhythmias, or pulmonary emboli noted. This report utilized a very conservative approach to beginning mobilization therapy. The fact that 15% of patients did not undergo mobilization, because of ongoing sedation, underscores the importance of minimization of this impediment if mobilization is to be successful.

A report by Needham and colleagues[29] described a before/after quality improvement project, focused on increasing mobilization in ICU patients. The investigators recognized the need to reduce deep sedation and delirium in order to permit mobilization in ICU patients and improve patients' functional mobility. This quality improvement project utilized a multidisciplinary team that provided increased ICU staffing to include full-time physical and occupational therapists. This effort included a change in the ICU from traditional deep sedation and bed rest to systematic mobilization throughout the ICU. As a result of this quality improvement project, sedative and opiate use decreased and ICU delirium improved. These changes were associated with patients receiving more rehabilitation treatments and accomplishing a higher level of functional mobility. ICU length of stay decreased by an average of 2.1 days (95% CI 0.4–3.8); hospital length of stay decreased by 3.1 days (95% CI 0.3–5.9). Both clinicians and hospital administrative professionals noted the remarkable improvements in patient outcomes in this 'before-after' analysis. The result of this intervention was a full supportive endeavour by the hospital administration to provide ongoing financial support of this novel intervention. In addition to the obvious importance of the clinical findings of this trial, the message to administrative professionals is quite important. Hospital administrative personnel must embrace novel interventions that improve patient outcomes in order to be successful with regard to widespread implementation. The work by Needham and colleagues nicely demonstrates the importance of a patient care plan that moves beyond the bedside care providers. It is only by utilizing such a strategy of communication between clinicians and administrators that implementation of novel care strategies can gain widespread acceptance.

In 2009, Schweickert and colleagues reported findings from a prospective randomized blinded trial of very early PT and OT therapy from the **inception** of respiratory failure requiring MV.[30] This project was novel in that it was the first randomized and blinded project evaluating early mobilization in mechanically ventilated ICU patients. The investigators began the mobilization protocol immediately, rather than waiting for several days. The intent of this trial was to initiate mobilization before deconditioning had occurred. The two-centre study enrolled patients from medical ICUs undergoing MV for less than 72 hours who were functionally independent prior to their ICU admission. They were randomized to an intervention group that underwent a progressive PT and OT therapy regimen, focused on mobilization and achievement of occupational tasks (i.e. ADLs), compared to a control group who did not receive early mobilization while intubated. Patients in both groups received the following established therapies: daily sedative interruption,[31] daily SBTs,[32] early EN, and tight glucose control.[33] After awakening from sedation, a team consisting of a physical and an occupational therapist worked with patients in a progressive, step-wise manner. This mobilization team led patients through exercises such as sitting at the edge to the bed, engaging in simulated ADLs, transfer training, and ambulation. Progression of the mobilization protocol was dependent on patient tolerance and stability. Control patients also received PT and OT, but this was done under the direction of the primary care team. Therapy in this group was typically initiated once patients were extubated.[24,25,34–37] A group of therapists who were blinded to patient randomization assignment performed evaluations of functional outcomes. The primary endpoint of the trial was the return to 'functional independence' at hospital discharge. Functional independence was defined a priori as the ability to perform ADLs (bathing, dressing, eating, grooming, transfer from bed to chair, toileting) and walk independently.

Compared to the previous studies, where therapy was typically initiated more than 5 days after ICU admission, patients in this trial began therapy an average of 1.5 days after intubation. Patients in this trial were able to accomplish impressive milestones, even while still requiring MV through an ETT. A total of 244 therapy sessions occurred in 49 patients who were intubated. Bed mobility was accomplished in 76%, a median of 1.7 days after intubation; standing was accomplished in 33% (median 3.2 days after intubation); chair sitting was accomplished in 33% (median 3.1 days after intubation); ambulation was accomplished in 15% (median 3.8 days after intubation; median ambulation distance 15 ft).[38]

As noted previously, the intent of immediate mobilization, limited only by the time required for consent, was anchored on the notion that neuromuscular deconditioning occurs rapidly in mechanically ventilated patients. Indeed, recent evidence has reported the loss of structural and functional integrity of the diaphragm that occurs in a matter of **hours** after initiation of full ventilatory support.[13,39] These data suggest that neuromuscular integrity is in peril in ICU patients, even in the earliest stages of critical illness. This problem, while not as transparent to the bedside clinician as circulatory or respiratory compromise, brings a substantial burden to the survivor of critical illness.

The protocol of an extremely early mobilization strategy led to a 1.7-fold increase in patients who were functionally independent when they left the hospital (59 vs 35%, $P = 0.02$). More patients in the early mobilization group went directly home after hospitalization than in the control group (43 vs 24%, $P = 0.06$). The duration of MV was reduced (3.4 vs 6.1 days, $P = 0.02$) and VFDs increased (23.5 vs 21.1, $P = 0.05$). ICU delirium days were reduced by 50% (2.0 vs 4.0 days, $P = 0.03$) in spite of no differences in sedatives administered. The early mobilization patients had better maximal walking distances (33.4 vs 0 m, $P = 0.004$), greater numbers of ADLs performed at hospital discharge (6 vs 4, $P = 0.06$), and more VFDs (23.5 vs 21.1, $P = 0.05$).[30] Adverse events were rare and included oxyhaemoglobin desaturation >5% in 6% of sessions, heart rate increase >20% in 4% of sessions, ventilator asynchrony in 4% of sessions, agitation in 2% of sessions, and device removal in 0.8% of sessions. Premature stoppage of a therapy session occurred in only 4% of sessions. The intervention in this trial embraced a philosophy where virtually all patients were approached and considered for early mobilization. Patients considered 'unstable' by traditional criteria were mobilized without adverse events. These patients included those with ALI (58% of all mobilization sessions), morbid obesity (41% of all mobilization sessions), shock requiring vasoactive infusions (17% of all mobilization sessions), and RRT (9% of all mobilization sessions).

Conclusion

ICU survivors recovering from respiratory failure requiring MV often have neuromuscular weakness and functional impairment. It is clear that the burden of acute illness carries a phase of long, and often incomplete, recovery in those fortunate enough to survive their illnesses. The notion of a multidisciplinary care plan for ICU patients is slowly moving into the mainstream of critical care. While PT and OT have not traditionally played a role in the management of mechanically ventilated patients, the potential for such disciplines to provide unique benefits to such patients is indisputable. It is clear from recent literature that mobilization of mechanically ventilated patients is feasible and safe. In order for widespread utilization of such a care model, continued focus on minimization of sedation must occur. The critical care community must move away from the traditional hierarchical model of care and embrace this philosophy of a multidisciplinary model; the benefits are substantial, and the potential for future beneficial outcomes is great. More research is needed to identify whether there are specific groups of patients that stand to benefit from early mobilization more than others. Continued emphasis on the problems associated with deep sedation and prolonged immobility is needed in order to change ICU culture to one of more mental and physical animation in this group of high-risk patients.

References

1 Lilly CM, Cody S, Zhao H, et al. Hospital mortality, length of stay, and preventable complications among critically ill patients before and after tele-ICU reengineering of critical care processes. *JAMA* 2011;**305**:2175–83.

2 Brochard L, Mancebo J, Wysocki M, et al. Noninvasive ventilation for acute exacerbations of chronic obstructive pulmonary disease. *N Engl J Med* 1995;**333**:817–22.

3 Papazian L, Forel JM, Gacouin A, et al. Neuromuscular blockers in early acute respiratory distress syndrome. *N Engl J Med* 2010;**363**:1107–16.

4 Rivers E, Nguyen B, Havstad S, et al. Early goal-directed therapy in the treatment of severe sepsis and septic shock. *N Engl J Med* 2001;**345**:1368–77.

5 The National Heart L, and Blood Institute Acute Respiratory Distress Syndrome (ARDS) Clinical Trials Network. Ventilation with lower tidal volumes as compared with traditional tidal volumes for acute lung injury and the acute respiratory distress syndrome. The Acute Respiratory Distress Syndrome Network. *N Engl J Med* 2000;**342**:1301–8.

6 Briel M, Meade M, Mercat A, et al. Higher vs lower positive end-expiratory pressure in patients with acute lung injury and acute respiratory distress syndrome: systematic review and meta-analysis. *JAMA* 2010;**303**:865–73.

7 de Letter MA, Schmitz PI, Visser LH, et al. Risk factors for the development of polyneuropathy and myopathy in critically ill patients. *Crit Care Med* 2001;**29**:2281–6.

8 Latronico N. Neuromuscular alterations in the critically ill patient: critical illness myopathy, critical illness neuropathy, or both? *Intensive Care Med* 2003;**29**:1411–13.

9 Petty TL. Suspended life or extending death? *Chest* 1998;**114**:360–1.

10 Dock W. The evil sequelae of complete bed rest. *JAMA* 1944;**125**:1083–5.

11 Asher RA. The dangers of going to bed. *Br Med J* 1947;**2**:967.

12 Ijland MM, Heunks LM, van der Hoeven JG. Bench-to-bedside review: hypercapnic acidosis in lung injury—from 'permissive' to 'therapeutic'. *Crit Care* 2010;**14**:237.

13 Hussain SN, Mofarrahi M, Sigala I, et al. Mechanical ventilation-induced diaphragm disuse in humans triggers autophagy. *Am J Respir Crit Care Med* 2010;**182**:1377–86.

14 Futier E, Constantin JM, Combaret L, et al. Pressure support ventilation attenuates ventilator-induced protein modifications in the diaphragm. *Crit Care* 2008;**12**:R116.

15 Palevsky PM, Zhang JH, O'Connor TZ, et al. Intensity of renal support in critically ill patients with acute kidney injury. *N Engl J Med* 2008;**359**:7–20.

16 Bonventre JV. Dialysis in acute kidney injury—more is not better. *N Engl J Med* 2008;**359**:82–4.

17 Herridge MS, Tansey CM, Matte A, et al. Functional disability 5 years after acute respiratory distress syndrome. *N Engl J Med* 2011;**364**:1293–304.

18 Misak CJ. The critical care experience: a patient's view. *Am J Respir Crit Care Med* 2004;**170**:357–9.

19 Misak C. ICU psychosis and patient autonomy: some thoughts from the inside. *J Med Philos* 2005;**30**:411–30.

20 Rubenfeld GD, Caldwell E, Peabody E, et al. Incidence and outcomes of acute lung injury. *N Engl J Med* 2005;**353**:1685–93.

21 Herridge MS, Cheung AM, Tansey CM, et al. One-year outcomes in survivors of the acute respiratory distress syndrome. *N Engl J Med* 2003;**348**:683–93.

22 Griffiths RD, Palmer TE, Helliwell T, MacLennan P, MacMillan RR. Effect of passive stretching on the wasting of muscle in the critically ill. *Nutrition* 1995;**11**:428–32.

23 De Jonghe B, Bastuji-Garin S, Fangio P, et al. Sedation algorithm in critically ill patients without acute brain injury. *Crit Care Med* 2005;**33**:120–7.

24 Bailey P, Thomsen GE, Spuhler VJ, et al. Early activity is feasible and safe in respiratory failure patients. *Crit Care Med* 2007;**35**:139–45.

25 Thomsen GE, Snow GL, Rodriguez L, Hopkins RO. Patients with respiratory failure increase ambulation after transfer to an intensive care unit where early activity is a priority. *Crit Care Med* 2008;**36**:1119–24.

26 Morris PE, Griffin L, Berry M, et al. Receiving early mobility during an intensive care unit admission is a predictor of improved outcomes in acute respiratory failure. *Am J Med Sci* 2011;**341**:373–7.

27 Burtin C, Clerckx B, Robbeets C, et al. Early exercise in critically ill patients enhances short-term functional recovery. *Crit Care Med* 2009;**37**:2499–505.

28 Bourdin G, Barbier J, Burle JF, et al. The feasibility of early physical activity in intensive care unit patients: a prospective observational one-center study. *Respir Care* 2010;**55**:400–7.

29 Needham DM, Korupolu R, Zanni JM, et al. Early physical medicine and rehabilitation for patients with acute respiratory failure: a quality improvement project. *Arch Phys Med Rehabil* 2010;**91**:536–42.

30 Schweickert WD, Pohlman MC, Pohlman AS, et al. Early physical and occupational therapy in mechanically ventilated, critically ill patients: a randomised controlled trial. *Lancet* 2009;**373**:1874–82.

31 Kress JP, Pohlman AS, O'Connor MF, Hall JB. Daily interruption of sedative infusions in critically ill patients undergoing mechanical ventilation. *N Engl J Med* 2000;**342**:1471–7.

32 Ely EW, Baker AM, Dunagan DP, et al. Effect on the duration of mechanical ventilation of identifying patients capable of breathing spontaneously. *N Engl J Med* 1996;**335**:1864–9.

33 van den Berghe G, Wouters P, Weekers F, et al. Intensive insulin therapy in the critically ill patients. *N Engl J Med* 2001;**345**:1359–67.

34 Gosselink R, Bott J, Johnson M, et al. Physiotherapy for adult patients with critical illness: recommendations of the European Respiratory Society and European Society of Intensive Care Medicine Task Force on Physiotherapy for Critically Ill Patients. *Intensive Care Med* 2008;**34**:1188–99.

35 Hodgin KE, Nordon-Craft A, McFann KK, Mealer ML, Moss M. Physical therapy utilization in intensive care units: Results from a national survey. *Crit Care Med* 2009;**37**:561–6.

36 Martin UJ, Hincapie L, Nimchuk M, Gaughan J, Criner GJ. Impact of whole-body rehabilitation in patients receiving chronic mechanical ventilation. *Crit Care Med* 2005;**33**:2259–65.

37 Morris PE, Goad A, Thompson C, et al. Early intensive care unit mobility therapy in the treatment of acute respiratory failure. *Crit Care Med* 2008;**36**:2238–43.

38 Pohlman MC, Schweickert WD, Pohlman AS, et al. Feasibility of physical and occupational therapy beginning from initiation of mechanical ventilation. *Crit Care Med* 2010;**38**:2089–94.

39 Levine S, Nguyen T, Taylor N, et al. Rapid disuse atrophy of diaphragm fibers in mechanically ventilated humans. *N Engl J Med* 2008;**358**:1327–35.

Chapter 44

Neuromuscular Electrical Stimulation: A New Therapeutic and Rehabilitation Strategy in the ICU

Vasiliki Gerovasili and Serafim N. Nanas

Introduction

Medical and technological advances contribute to a constantly increasing number of ICU survivors.[1] However, survival after critical illness is associated with important costs both to society and the individuals that are involved. Survivors of critical illness suffer from impaired physical function and QoL that may persist for years after discharge from the ICU.[2] In a landmark study of functional ability in survivors of ARDS 5 years after ICU discharge, the majority of previously healthy individuals did not return to premorbid functional status.[2] The burden to society can be considerable. Five years after ARDS survival, 23% of patients could not return to work, and there are data indicating increased utilization of health care services and consequent increased health care costs.[2,3]

ICUAW is the most common neuromuscular complication of critical illness, presenting with generalized muscle weakness, diminished tendon reflexes, difficult weaning from MV,[4,5] and is associated with prolonged ICU and hospital stay.[6] ICUAW is reported to have an incidence ranging from 23% to more than 50%, depending on the criteria used for diagnosis—clinical or electrophysiological—and the patient population evaluated.[4,5] In patients with ICUAW, muscle weakness may persist for months, and a percentage may never fully recover.[7] In view of this, the need for a preventive tool for ICUAW is highly desirable.

Several risk factors have been proposed for the development of ICUAW. Sepsis—especially Gram-negative bacteraemia[5]—and SIRS cause microcirculatory alterations which compromise the supply of oxygen and nutrients to peripheral nerves and skeletal muscles, causing functional and structural damage. Medications that have neuromuscular toxicity (such as NMBAs and aminoglycosides) and immobilization may also be important contributors.[4,8,9]

Critical illness is commonly viewed as a condition that requires bed rest and deep sedation, as the emphasis is placed on treatment of acute illness and failing organ systems. Patients are often considered 'too sick' to be mobilized, and the neuromuscular system tends to be overlooked during the acute phase of critical illness. Attention to it is drawn after the interruption of sedation when severe muscle weakness has already occurred.

The effect of bed rest and immobilization on skeletal muscle of the critically ill

The effect of immobilization on peripheral skeletal muscle is detrimental. In healthy subjects, immobilization results in profound loss of muscle mass. In a recent study,[10] 5 weeks of immobilization resulted in a loss of up to 12% of muscle mass, as assessed with CT, and up to 20% of muscle strength.

The effect of immobilization on skeletal muscle is more pronounced in critically ill, septic patients. Severe illness and sepsis induce a catabolic state for the muscle tissue, accelerating the effect of immobilization on the loss of muscle tissue. In an earlier study, 21 days of immobilization of critically ill patients resulted in the loss of approximately 1 kg of skeletal muscle mass, as assessed with DEXA.[11] Interestingly, two-thirds of the loss of skeletal muscle mass occurred during the first 5 days of immobilization. In a recent case report, a 33-day ICU stay resulted in the loss of 11.2 kg, of which 33% was skeletal muscle.[12] In a recent study by our group, we showed that 1 week of immobilization resulted in approximately 13% loss of the cross-sectional diameter of rectus femoris muscle, as assessed with ultrasonography.[13] Electrophysiological studies assessing the incidence of ICUAW have shown evidence of neurophysiological abnormalities present during the first week of critical illness; changes are also apparent on muscle biopsy, indicating structural muscular damage within the first 15 days of illness onset.[14] These data imply that any intervention aimed at preventing the development of ICUAW needs to be applied very early after ICU admission—probably immediately after initial stabilization—in order for it to be effective.

Early mobilization protocols in the critically ill

Recently, there has been growing interest in implementing early rehabilitation for the prevention of critical illness-related muscle weakness.[15] Actually, the concept of early mobilization is not novel. Studies dating back to the Second World War reported on the benefits of early mobilization,[16] even in mechanically ventilated patients.[17]

A number of studies have reported on the feasibility and effectiveness of early rehabilitation in the critically ill. Early mobilization has been shown to be safe,[15] and there are data showing that patients who receive early mobilization ambulate further at ICU discharge[15] and have a shorter ICU and hospital stay.[18] Moreover, lack of early mobilization is associated with readmissions or death during the first year after ICU discharge.[19] Early PT and OT during ICU stay results in increased return to independent functional status.[20] Finally, bedside bicycle therapy, in addition to standard PT in respiratory patients, contributed to improved ambulation at hospital discharge and better QoL.[21] Early rehabilitation therefore appears to be feasible and safe in critically ill patients and, despite the use of different outcome measures, beneficial for the critically ill.

Neuromuscular electrical stimulation (NMES)—basic principles

NMES is an alternative form of exercise that can be used in combination with other rehabilitation tools for the early mobilization of the critically ill. NMES is especially advantageous during the acute phase of critical illness, because it is during this time period that a considerable number of critically ill patients cannot participate in physical rehabilitation due to sedation or cognitive impairment. NMES overcomes this problem, since it does not rely on patient cooperation and can be implemented even in sedated patients. It is therefore an alternative to early mobilization in the ICU setting.

NMES is an alternative form of exercise that has been used extensively in healthy subjects[22] and in patient populations.[23,24] NMES uses electrical impulses to elicit muscle contraction. Low-voltage electrical impulses are delivered through electrodes, placed on the skin surface, to the respective muscle. These electrical impulses elicit non-volitional muscle contractions that have similar characteristics with volitional, repetitive muscle contractions during mild exercise.

The main NMES characteristics that need to be determined for NMES application are the type of electrical current, pulse duration, pulse frequency, pulse intensity, and duty cycle. The type of electrical current most widely used is pulse biphasic current that may have different shapes (e.g. rectangular, trapezoid). Pulse duration determines the duration of each current impulse. It usually ranges between 0.2 and 0.5 ms, although longer durations are not uncommon. The pulse frequency refers to the number of current impulses delivered during a specific time, measured in Hz. In patient populations, pulse frequencies between 10 and 50 Hz are most common. Low-frequency currents (between 10 and 20 Hz) are thought to mainly stimulate type I muscle fibres (aerobic) and are preferred in NMES programmes targeted at enhancing muscle endurance, whereas higher frequencies are thought to mainly stimulate type II muscle fibres (anaerobic) that are responsible for muscle strength. Pulse intensity is an NMES characteristic that determines the number of fibres that will be stimulated with each muscle contraction. It usually depends on patient tolerance. Finally, duty cycle refers to the amount of time that electrical current is delivered to the muscle. Usually, electrical current is delivered for a few seconds (in impulses of

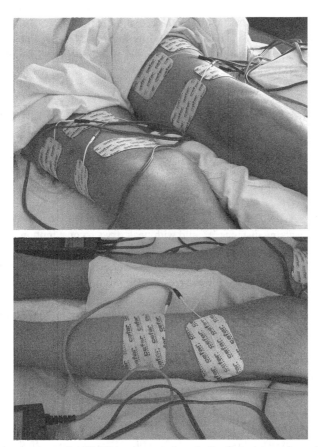

Fig. 44.1 Electrode placement for NMES implementation. In the first picture, four electrodes are placed on the quadriceps muscle after appropriate skin preparation, including shaving, and, in the second picture, the electrodes are placed on peroneus longus.

predefined duration, frequency, and intensity), followed by a few seconds of complete muscle rest, to avoid muscle damage.

NMES is easily applicable, and, in home-based rehabilitation programmes, patients have been trained to apply NMES themselves.[24] After appropriate skin preparation (shaving may be required), electrodes are placed on the skin surface, according to the selected muscle, and electrical current is delivered through the electrodes from the stimulator device (see Figure 44.1). The duration of each session ranges from 30 minutes[25] to 4 hours.[26] Local skin irritation and pain during the session are the most important side effects. Pain is generally well managed by decreasing the current intensity to the highest tolerable level. As patients get accustomed to NMES, they can usually tolerate higher current intensities, so the current intensity should be regularly revisited.

NMES is currently contraindicated in patients with implanted defibrillators and pacemakers, although preliminary data indicate that it may be safe.[27]

NMES in healthy subjects

NMES has been used in healthy subjects and athletes and has been shown to improve muscle strength.[22] A recent meta-analysis in healthy subjects showed that NMES is effective in increasing the muscle strength of quadriceps muscle. In healthy subjects, NMES, combined with volitional exercise, has been shown to be more effective than exercise alone. However, physical exercise is more effective than NMES alone in healthy subjects.[22]

NMES in patients with chronic heart failure (CHF) and COPD

During the last decade, NMES has been increasingly used in patients with CHF and COPD, alone or combined with volitional exercise, as part of a rehabilitation programme.[23–26] These patients, who are unable to participate in physical exercise due to cardiac or pulmonary impairment, benefit from NMES in terms of exercise capacity,[26] muscle strength,[23,25] and QoL.[24]

In patients with severe COPD and CHF, NMES improves aerobic exercise capacity, as assessed with the 6-minute walking distance[26,28] and with peak oxygen consumption during incremental maximum exercise testing.[26,28]

NMES also results in improvement of muscle strength and endurance in patients with COPD[23,25] and CHF.[24,26,28] In COPD patients, NMES results in significant increase of muscle strength[23,25] and endurance,[29] and similar changes have been noted in patients with CHF.[24,26,28] Structural changes in skeletal muscle, following an NMES programme, have been shown with an increase in type I muscle fibres and citrate synthase enzyme activity.[26]

QoL also seems to improve, following an NMES rehabilitation programme. Patients with severe COPD have reported decreased sense of dyspnoea,[23] following an NMES rehabilitation programme. In patients with severe CHF, improvement has been shown in ADLs, which reflect improved functionality.[24] Finally, in a study with refractory CHF, improvement in NYHA status has been reported, following an NMES programme.[24]

These data indicate that NMES can be safely used in patients with severe cardiac or pulmonary insufficiency as an alternative rehabilitation tool or as part of a structured rehabilitation programme. In these patients, NMES is beneficial in terms of exercise capacity, muscle strength and endurance, and QoL.

NMES in the critically ill

Nine studies[30–37] have assessed the effect of NMES on critically ill patients, and also a protocol concerning an ongoing clinical trial utilizing NMES in a medical ICU has been published[38] (see Table 44.1). Of these, nine clinical trials were conducted in the ICU during the acute phase of critical illness, and one trial[25] was conducted in a high dependency unit with patients receiving chronic MV. Six trials were conducted in a multidisciplinary ICU,[30–34,37] and three trials in a medical ICU.[35,36,38] Seven studies were RCTs,[25,31–33,37,38] one study was not randomized,[30] and, in the remaining two studies, one side (left or right) was randomly selected for NMES application, with the other serving as a control.[34,35]

Patient population characteristics

In these studies, different patient populations were enrolled; however, some patient characteristics were consistent in all of the studies. Patients were severely ill, as assessed with severity scores; they were mechanically ventilated, and the majority was sedated and treated during the acute phase of their critical illness. In one study, patients were in a high dependency unit, following 30 days of ICU study, receiving long-term MV.[25] Six studies enrolled a mixed population of critically ill patients that included medical and surgical diagnoses at ICU admission as well as trauma,[30–33,36,37] two studies required septic shock as inclusion criteria for the study,[34,35] one study included only patients with COPD,[25] and one ongoing clinical trial is enrolling mechanically ventilated patients in a medical ICU.[38] However, it should be noted that in all studies conducted in the ICU setting, severe sepsis and/or septic shock occurred in the majority of patients at some point during their ICU stay.

All studies to date have included a relatively small number of critically ill patients. The largest trial has randomized 140 patients, of which 52 patients were analysed with an intention-to-treat analysis, according to the primary outcome measure.[32] The rest of the trials have included smaller numbers of patients, ranging from 8 to 49 randomized critically ill patients. Eight studies have used a control group that received routine care or sham NMES,[25,30–33,36–38] and two studies stimulated one part of the body (left or right), with the other part serving as control.[34,35]

Despite the differences in patient population characteristics and the relatively small sample size, it can be argued that, in all trials, severely ill patients—most of them with sepsis and/or septic shock, sedated, and mechanically ventilated—were included. These patients are representative of a typical critically ill population, which facilitates generalization of the results.

Muscle groups stimulated

The muscle groups that have primarily been used for NMES in critically ill patients include large muscle groups in the lower extremities. Three studies[33,34,36] have used the quadriceps muscle only; six studies have stimulated the quadriceps, together with other muscle groups in the lower extremities (peroneus longus, vastus glutei, tibialis anterior, and gastrocnemius),[25,30–32,37,38] and one study has used the quadriceps and the brachial biceps muscle[35] (see Table 44.1).

The choice of muscle groups to be stimulated is dictated by the need to stimulate the largest possible muscle mass. Stimulation of the largest possible muscle mass is more important than the choice of specific muscle groups, because, as it has been shown,[30] the systemic effect of exercise with NMES implies that beneficial results can be delivered in muscle groups not directly stimulated. Limitations to the choice of muscle groups are accessibility of the desired muscle group, especially in non-cooperative, sedated patients, and the fear of interference with monitoring

Table 44.1 Studies of NMES in critically ill patients, showing study design, NMES characteristics chosen for each study, and muscle groups stimulated

Author	ICU type	Study design	Population	Number (enrolled/analysed)	Control	Muscle group	Control	Hz	Pulse duration (micro second)	Intensity	Duty cycle	Session (week)	Duration (min)
Zanotti (2003)[25]	HDU	Randomized	COPD	24	12	Quadriceps + vastus glutei	ALM	35	350	Maximum tolerance	NR	5	30
Gerovasili (2009)[30]	Multidisciplinary	Not randomized	Mixed	34	6	Quadriceps + peroneus longus	Usual care	45	400	Visible contractions	12 on/6 off	NA	45
Gerovasili (2009)[31]	Multidisciplinary	Randomized	Mixed	49/26	13	Quadriceps + peroneus longus	Usual care	45	400	Visible contractions	12 on/6 off	7	45
Routsi (2010)[32]	Multidisciplinary	Randomized	Mixed	140/52	28	Quadriceps + peroneus longus	Usual care	45	400	Visible contractions	12 on/6 off	7	45
Gruther (2010)[33]	Multidisciplinary	Randomized	Mixed	46/33	18	Quadriceps	Sham	50	350	Maximum tolerance	8 on/24 off	5	30–60
Meesen (2010)[36]	Medical	Randomized	Mixed	25/19	12	Quadriceps	Usual care	5–100	250–330	Visible contractions	Variable	7	30
Rodriquez (2011)[35]	Medical	Randomized (side)	Septic shock	16/14	NA	Quadriceps + brachial biceps	NA	100	300	Visible contractions	2 on/4 off	7	30 x 2
Poulsen (2011)[34]	Multidisciplinary	Randomized (side)	Septic shock	8/8	NA	Quadriceps	NA	35	300	50% above threshold	4 on/6 off	7	60
Karatzanos (2012)[37]	Multidisciplinary	Randomized (subgroup analysis)	Mixed	140/52	28	Quadriceps + peroneus longus	Usual care	45	400	Visible contractions	12 on/6 off	7	45
Kho (2012)[38]	Medical	Randomized	Medical	NA	NA	Quadriceps + tibialis anterior + gastrocnemius	Sham	50	250	Visible contractions	5 on/10 off	7	60

ICU, intensive care unit; ALM, active limb mobilization; NA, non-applicable; NR, not reported.

devices when stimulating muscles of the upper extremities or the thorax. Stimulation of lower extremities seems to be the most beneficial, because it includes large, easily accessible muscle groups and is away from monitoring devices. In the only study where a muscle group in upper extremities (brachial biceps) was used, the authors reported no interference with monitoring devices.[35] However, the muscle mass of the upper extremities is considerably less than that of lower extremities, and therefore they are not expected to contribute considerably to the systemic effect of exercise with NMES.

NMES characteristics

The choice of NMES characteristics is relatively heterogeneous. In most studies, daily NMES sessions were delivered;[30–32,34–38] however, in two studies, sessions were delivered 5 days per week.[25,33] The duration of each session is also variable, ranging from 30 minutes to 1 hour, usually once daily, although, in one study, twice-daily 30-minute sessions were preferred.[35]

Similar heterogeneity is notable in the rest of the NMES characteristics. Stimulation frequency ranges between 35 and 100 Hz, with one study even using a frequency range between 5 and 100 Hz during one NMES session.[36] However, most studies have used stimulation frequencies between 35 and 50 Hz. The pulse duration chosen is usually between 300 and 400 microseconds, and the duty cycle is widely different between the studies, with the most intense programme being 12 s on, followed by 6 s off. The level of intensity was chosen according to maximum tolerance in cooperative patients,[25,33] and, in the rest of the studies, the intensity was increased until visible contractions could be seen. In one study,[34] the authors used an intensity 50% higher than the 'threshold intensity', with the threshold intensity being defined as the intensity level at which visible contractions could be seen. In critically ill patients with tissue oedema, combined with electrolyte and metabolic changes, tissue conductivity might be impaired, requiring higher intensities than those needed for healthy subjects or even other patient groups (see Table 44.1).

Acute systemic effects of NMES in the critically ill

In the earliest study conducted in the ICU setting, the acute effect of NMES on cardiovascular and microcirculatory parameters of critically ill patients was assessed.[30] The authors evaluated 35 critically ill patients, of whom 86% were mechanically ventilated, half were sedated, and one-third (33%) were in need of continuous vasopressor support. A total of 29 patients received NMES of both lower extremities (quadriceps and peroneus longus), and six critically ill patients served as controls. The microcirculation was assessed with near-infrared spectroscopy (NIRS) in the thenar muscle of the hand, which did not receive any stimulation. Basic cardiovascular parameters, such as heart rate and blood pressure, were recorded.

In this study, a statistically significant, but clinically insignificant, increase of heart rate by 5 beats/min and of systolic blood pressure by 10 mmHg was reported in the NMES group, as compared to no change in the control group. This finding of a minimal increase in heart rate and blood pressure has been reported previously in healthy subjects[39] and in patients with CHF.[40] The marginal increase in systolic blood pressure and heart rate observed in critically ill patients implies a cardiovascular response. The respiratory rate increased by 1 breath/min during the NMES session, suggesting a mild increase in minute ventilation. The authors noted no change in arterial blood gases, lactate levels, and central venous oxygen saturation during the session.

The most important finding of this study was that one NMES session of the lower extremities caused a microcirculatory response in the thenar muscle of the hand, which did not receive any contractions. A statistically significant increase in the oxygen consumption rate and the reperfusion rate of the thenar, as assessed with NIRS vascular occlusion, occurred after the NMES session. This finding is indicative of the presence of factors induced by NMES that act in a systemic way. These factors could include the release of molecules, such as cytokines, at the loci of NMES that act in a systemic way, or the activation of metabo- and ergoreflex or activation of central command.[41] Regardless of the involved mechanisms, the systemic effect of NMES implies that beneficial results of an NMES-based early rehabilitation programme could be anticipated in muscle groups other than those directly stimulated.

Outcome measures

So far, all studies have focused on outcome measures related to muscle properties and function, and some of them reported on the development of ICUAW.[32,35,37] One study has reported data on the ICU length of stay of these patients. No data have been reported yet on the long-term outcomes of these patients such as the functional status after ICU discharge or their QoL.

Assessment of muscle properties

Several muscle properties have been assessed so far in critically ill patients undergoing NMES sessions, rendering mixed results. Muscle thickness of the quadriceps or biceps muscle has been reported in three studies;[31,33,35] muscle volume, with the use of CT, was used in one study,[34] and two studies have shown data on muscle circumference.[35,36] Differences in study design, including patient characteristics, type and duration of NMES sessions, timing of assessment of outcome measures, and the presence or not of a control group, make comparison between studies and generalization of results difficult.

As far as the assessment of muscle thickness via ultrasound is concerned, in one randomized study of critically ill patients during the first days of critical illness, daily NMES sessions of both lower extremities resulted in attenuated loss of muscle thickness, as compared to the control group which received usual care.[31] In a pilot randomized study including a mixed population of critically ill patients—long-term and acute care group—NMES sessions resulted in an increase of muscle thickness in the long-term group, whereas, in the acute care group, NMES contributed to less, though not significant, decrease in muscle thickness.[33] Both studies assessed the cross-sectional diameter of the quadriceps muscle, and discrepancies between them could be attributed to the small number of patients evaluated, the differences in stimulation characteristics, and the time of inclusion in the study. It has been shown that the most profound loss of muscle mass occurs within the first 5–7 days of critical illness,[11] and, therefore, even minor delay of the onset of NMES sessions could be significant. In the first study, all patients were randomized on the second day after admission, whereas, in the second study of acute care, critically ill patients, the onset of NMES sessions was delayed until the third or fourth day in the stimulated and control group, respectively.

The third study assessed the muscle thickness of the biceps muscle and found no significant difference between the stimulated and control side, although, after awakening, differences in muscle strength in favour of the NMES side were reported by the authors.[35] The authors stimulated one side of the body, with the other serving as control. Taking into account the systemic effect of NMES and the fact that, contrary to other studies, no loss of muscle thickness was reported in the control side, it could be speculated that the systemic effect of NMES may have contributed to preservation of muscle thickness both on the stimulated and control side.

The loss of muscle volume, as assessed with CT, was evaluated in a small, but well-designed, randomized study of septic shock patients.[34] No differences were found between the stimulated and non-stimulated side, and severe loss of quadriceps muscle volume were reported by the authors. As already mentioned, the differences in stimulation characteristics, the specific patient characteristics, as well as the delay of onset of NMES sessions—patients could be included even after 5 days of septic shock—could account for the lack of benefit of NMES in this study.

Finally, the arm and leg circumference, a crude measure of muscle mass, was assessed in two studies showing preserved[35] or increased[36] circumference of the stimulated side.

Muscle function

Assessment of muscle function requires patient cooperation and is therefore often impossible in critically ill patients or has to be reserved until interruption of sedation and patient awakening. Two studies have reported data on muscle strength after awakening in critically ill patients,[32,35] and similarly one study which was conducted in a high dependency unit in COPD mechanically ventilated patients after ICU stay for COPD exacerbation.[25] All three studies have used manual muscle testing, with the MRC scale for muscle strength (scores 0–5). One study[37] has reported data on handgrip dynamometry.

The first study, an RCT, showed that daily NMES sessions of lower extremities resulted in significantly increased muscle strength, as assessed with the MRC scale for muscle strength, in the intervention group, as compared to the control group.[32] In the second study,[35] septic shock patients received daily NMES sessions of one part of the body (left or right), with the other serving as control. At awakening, the side that was stimulated had higher muscle strength, as assessed clinically with the MRC scale, than the control side.

The fourth study has a different patient population than the rest of the studies:[25] COPD patients, mechanically ventilated and after a 30-day ICU stay for COPD exacerbation, were included. All patients were awake and cooperative in a high dependency unit and were extremely weak at randomization, with a mean MRC score of less than 2; namely, they had visible muscle contraction and could partially move their limbs against gravity. As opposed to the other studies, in which NMES was used to prevent the loss of muscle mass and/or strength, this study aimed to assess whether NMES could restore the muscle weakness. Patients randomized to the NMES group had a higher MRC score than the control group and were able to move from the bed to chair 4 days earlier than patients in the control group. No data as to the treatment of ICUAW and the long-term outcome of patients were reported.

Handgrip dynamometry was assessed in a subgroup analysis[37] of previously published data.[32] No differences were noted between patients assigned to the NMES group and control group in handgrip strength, whether expressed in absolute values or percentage predicted. However, the study was underpowered.

ICUAW

In one study, the effect of daily NMES sessions on the prevention of ICUAW was assessed.[32] Critically ill patients were randomly assigned to the NMES group or the control group, and patients were assessed at awakening for the development of ICUAW by non-blinded examiners. Patients assigned to the NMES group received daily NMES sessions of both lower extremities from the second day after admission until ICU discharge. A total of 140 critically ill patients were randomly assigned to one of two groups, and, of those, 52 could be clinically evaluated for the development of ICUAW—the rest of the patients either died or were non-cooperative and could not be assessed with the MRC scale. The authors found that daily NMES sessions of both lower extremities resulted in significantly lower incidence of ICUAW, 13% in the intervention group, as compared to 39% in the control group. It is the first study to show that daily NMES sessions of lower extremities in critically ill patients could prevent the development of ICUAW. The results of this study are expected to be confirmed by other studies.

Weaning from MV and ICU length of stay

Weaning from MV and ICU length of stay were also assessed as secondary outcomes in the latter study.[32] Interestingly, patients assigned to the NMES group had a shorter duration of weaning, which is indication of the presence of a relationship between limb and respiratory muscle weakness. As has been mentioned, an acute systemic effect has been reported after one NMES session which could act as an anabolic stimulus to the respiratory muscles. The shorter duration of weaning in patients assigned to the NMES group implies a beneficial effect of NMES on respiratory muscle function and reinforces the clinical significance of this study. No difference in the ICU length of stay could be documented between the NMES group and control group; however, it tended to be lower in the intervention group.

Conclusion

NMES is a rehabilitation tool that can be used in critically ill, sedated patients, it does not require patient cooperation and is therefore a promising tool for early mobilization in the critically ill. Data in critically ill patients show that NMES sessions can preserve the muscle properties and prevent the development of ICUAW and even contribute to shorter duration of weaning from MV. NMES seems therefore to have a clinical role for critically ill ICU patients. Further studies are needed to evaluate the long-term effect of NMES and to explore the NMES characteristics most appropriate for each group of critically ill patients.

References

1 Zilberberg MD, de Wit M, Shorr AF. Accuracy of previous estimates for adult prolonged acute mechanical ventilation volume in 2020: Update using 2000–8 data. *Crit Care Med* 2012;**40**:18–20.

2 Herridge MS, Tansey CM, Matte A, et al. Functional disability 5 years after acute respiratory distress syndrome. *N Engl J Med* 2011;**364**:1293.

3 Unroe M, Kahn JM, Carson SS, et al. One-year trajectories of care and resource utilization for recipients of prolonged mechanical ventilation: a cohort study. *Ann Intern Med* 2010;**153**:167–75.

4 Garnacho-Montero J, Madrazo-Osuna J, García-Garmendia JL, et al. Critical illness polyneuropathy: risk factors and clinical consequences. A cohort study in septic patients. *Intensive Care Med* 2001;**27**:1288–96.

5 Nanas S, Kritikos K, Angelopoulos E, et al. Predisposing factors for critical illness polyneuromyopathy in a multidisciplinary intensive care unit. *Acta Neurol Scand* 2008;**118**:175–81.

6 De Jonghe B, Sharshar T, Lefaucheur JP, et al. Paresis acquired in the intensive care unit: a prospective multicenter study. *JAMA* 2002;**288**:2859–67.

7 Fletcher SN, Kennedy DD, Ghosh IR, et al. Persistent neuromuscular and neurophysiologic abnormalities in long-term survivors of prolonged critical illness. *Crit Care Med* 2003;**31**:1012–16.

8 de Letter MA, Schmitz PI, Visser LH, et al. Risk factors for the development of polyneuropathy and myopathy in critically ill patients. *Crit Care Med* 2001;**29**:2281–6.

9 Gruther W, Benesch T, Zorn C, et al. Muscle wasting in intensive care patients: ultrasound observation of the M. quadriceps femoris muscle layer. *J Rehabil Med* 2008;**40**:185–9.

10 Berg HE, Eiken O, Miklavcic L, Mekjavic IB. Hip, thigh and calf muscle atrophy and bone loss after 5-week bedrest inactivity. *Eur J Appl Physiol* 2007;**99**:283–9.

11 Monk DN, Plank LD, Franch-Arcas G, Finn PJ, Streat SJ, Hill GL. Sequential changes in the metabolic response in critically injured patients during the first 25 days after blunt trauma. *Ann Surg* 1996;**223**:395–405.

12 Reid CL, Murgatroyd PR, Wright A, Menon DK. Quantification of lean and fat tissue repletion following critical illness: a case report. *Crit Care* 2008;**12**:R79.

13 Gerovasili V, Stefanidis K, Vitzilaios K, et al. Electrical muscle stimulation preserves the muscle mass of critically ill patients. A randomized study. *Crit Care* 2009;**13**:R161.

14 Ahlbeck K, Fredriksson K, Rooyackers O, et al. Signs of critical illness polyneuropathy and myopathy can be seen early in the ICU course. *Acta Anaesthesiol Scand* 2009;**53**:717–23.

15 Bailey P, Thomsen GE, Spuhler VJ, et al. Early activity is feasible and safe in respiratory failure patients. *Crit Care Med* 2007;**35**:139–45.

16   No authors listed. Editorial. Early rising after operation. *BMJ* 1948;**2**:1026–7.

17 Burns JR, Jones FL. Letter: Early ambulation of patients requiring ventilatory assistance. *Chest* 1975;**68**:608.

18 Morris PE, Goad A, Thompson C, et al. Early intensive care unit mobility therapy in the treatment of acute respiratory failure. *Crit Care Med* 2008;**36**:2238–43.

19 Morris PE, Griffin L, Berry M, et al. Receiving early mobility during an intensive care unit admission is a predictor of improved outcomes in acute respiratory failure. *Am J Med Sci* 2011;**341**:373–7.

20 Schweickert WD, Pohlman MC, Pohlman AS, et al. Early physical and occupational therapy in mechanically ventilated, critically ill patients: a randomised controlled trial. *Lancet* 2009;**373**:1874–82.

21 Burtin C, Clerckx B, Robbeets C, et al. Early exercise in critically ill patients enhances short-term functional recovery. *Crit Care Med* 2009;**37**:2499–505.

22 Bax L, Staes F, Verhagen A. Does neuromuscular electrical stimulation strengthen the quadriceps femoris? A systematic review of randomised controlled trials. *Sports Med* 2005;**35**:191–212.

23 Vivodtzev I, Pepin JL, Vottero G, et al. Improvement in quadriceps strength and dyspnea in daily tasks after 1 month of electrical stimulation in severely deconditioned and malnourished COPD. *Chest* 2006;**129**:1540–8.

24 Quittan M, Wiesinger GF, Sturm B, et al. Improvement of thigh muscles by neuromuscular electrical stimulation in patients with refractory heart failure: a single- blinded, randomized, controlled trial. *Am J Phys Med Rehabil* 2001;**80**:206–14.

25 Zanotti E, Felicetti C, Maini M, Fracchia C. Peripheral muscle strength training in bed-bound patients with COPD receiving mechanical ventilation: effect of electrical stimulation. *Chest* 2003;**142**:292–6.

26 Nuhr MJ, Pette D, Berger R, et al. Beneficial effects of chronic low- frequency stimulation of thigh muscles in patients with advanced chronic heart failure. *Eur Heart J* 2004;**25**:136–43.

27 Wiesinger GF, Crevenna R, Nuhr M, Huelsmann M, Fialka-Moser V, Quittan M. Neuromuscular electric stimulation in heart tranplantation candidates with cardiac pacemakers. *Arch Phys Med Rehabil* 2001;**82**:1476–7.

28 Maillefert JF, Eicher JC, Walker P, et al. Effects of low- frequency electrical stimulation of quadriceps and calf muscles in patients with chronic heart failure. *J Cardiopul Rehabil* 1998;**18**:277–82.

29 Bourjeily-Habr G, Rochester CL, Palermo F, Snyder P, Mohsenin V. Randomised controlled trial of transcutaneous electrical muscle stimulation of the lower extremities in patients with chronic obstructive pulmonary disease. *Thorax* 2002;**57**:1045–9.

30 Gerovasili V, Tripodaki E, Karatzanos E, et al. Short-term systemic effect of electrical muscle stimulation in critically ill patients. *Chest* 2009;**136**:1249–56.

31 Gerovasili V, Stefanidis K, Vitzilaios K, et al. Electrical muscle stimulation preserves the muscle mass of critically ill patients: a randomized study. *Crit Care* 2009;**13**:R161.

32 Routsi C, Gerovasili V, Vasileiadis I, et al. Electrical muscle stimulation prevents critical illness poly-neuromyopathy: a randomized parallel intervention trial. *Crit Care* 2010;**14**:R74.

33 Gruther W, Kainberger F, Fialka-Moser V, et al. Effects of neuromuscular electrical stimulation on muscle layer thickness of knee extensor muscles in intensive care unit patients: a pilot study. *J Rehabil Med.* 2010;**42**:593–7.

34 Poulsen JB, Moller K, Jensen CV, Weisdorf S, Kehlet H, Perner A. Effect of transcutaneous electrical muscle stimulation on muscle volume in patients with septic shock. *Crit Care Med* 2011;**39**:456–61.

35 Rodriguez PO, Setten M, Maskin LP, et al. Muscle weakness in septic patients requiring mechanical ventilation: Protective effect of transcutaneous neuromuscular electrical stimulation. *J Crit Care* 2012;**27**:319.e1–8.

36 Meesen RL, Dendale P, Cuypers K, et al. Neuromuscular Electrical Stimulation as a possible means to prevent muscle tissue wasting in artificially ventilated and sedated patients in the intensive care unit: a pilot study. *Neuromodulation* 2010;**13**:315–21.

37 Karatzanos E, Gerovasili V, Zervakis D, et al. Electrical muscle stimulation: an effective form of exercise and early mobilization to preserve muscle strength in critically ill patients. *Crit Care Res Pract* 2012;**2012**:432752.

38 Kho ME, Truong AD, Brower RG, et al. Neuromuscular Electrical Stimulation for Intensive Care Unit-Acquired Weakness: Protocol and Methodological Implications for a Randomized, Sham-Controlled, Phase II Trial. *Phys Ther* 2012;**92**:1564–79.

39 Banerjee P, Clark A, Witte K, Crowe L, Caulfield B. Electrical stimulation of unloaded muscles causes cardiovascular exercise by increasing oxygen demand. *Eur J Cardiovasc Prev Rehabil* 2005;**12**:503–8.

40 Quittan M, Sochor A, Wiesinger GF, et al. Strength improvement of knee extensor muscles in patients with chronic heart failure by neuromuscular electrical stimulation. *Artif Organs* 1999;**23**:432–5.

41 Tsuchimochi H, Hayes SG, McCord JL, Kaufman MP. Both central command and exercise pressor reflex activate cardiac sympathetic nerve activity in decerebrate cats. *Am J Physiol Heart Circ Physiol* 2009;**296**:H1157–63.

Chapter 45

Exercise and Early Rehabilitation in the Intensive Care Unit

Rik Gosselink

Introduction

The progress of intensive care medicine has dramatically improved survival of critically ill patients, especially in patients with ARDS.[1] This improved survival is, however, oftentimes associated with general deconditioning, muscle weakness,[2] and reduced functional status[3] at ICU discharge and with long-term disability in survivors of critical illness.[4–6] Deconditioning and specifically muscle weakness are suggested to have an important role in the impaired functional status.[6,7] Bed rest and immobility during critical illness may result in profound physical deconditioning. These effects can be exacerbated by inflammation, lack of glycaemic control, and pharmacological agents.[8] Skeletal muscle weakness in patients admitted to the ICU is observed in about 25% of patients that were ventilated for more than 7 days[9] and contributes to weaning failure[10] and mortality.[11] Although most patients under MV are extubated in less than 3 days, still approximately 20% require prolonged ventilatory support.[12] This prolonged ventilator dependence is not only a major medical problem but is also an extremely uncomfortable and potentially harmful state for the patient, carrying important psychosocial implications and affecting severely the functional performance in the short and long run.

Reductions in functional performance, exercise capacity, and QoL in ICU survivors indicate the need for rehabilitation **following** ICU stay[4] but specifically underscore the need for early assessment and treatment to prevent or attenuate deconditioning and loss of physical function **during** ICU stay. Recent evidence supports the safety and efficacy of an approach that emphasizes early physical activity and mobilization in critically ill patients.[13–20]

Assessment

The indications, safety, regimen, and implementation of early physical activity, exercise, and rehabilitation of patients in the ICU have only recently become a shared focus of interest to interdisciplinary teams practising in the ICU.[13–15,21,22] Rehabilitation focuses on deficiencies in the broader scope of health problems, as defined in the ICF.[23] This classification helps to identify problems and the prescription of interventions at the level of impairments of 'body structure and body function', 'activity' limitations, and 'participation' restrictions. Physical activity and exercise should be targeted at the appropriate intensity and with the appropriate exercise modality. The risk of moving a critically ill patient is weighed against the risk of immobility and recumbency and, when employed, requires stringent monitoring to ensure the mobilization is instituted appropriately and safely. Several algorithms to guide early mobilization and physical activity were developed over the last years.[14,24–26] All

Table 45.1 'Start to move' protocol University Hospitals Leuven: step-up approach of progressive mobilization and physical activity programme

	LEVEL 1	LEVEL 2	LEVEL 3	LEVEL 4	LEVEL 5
LEVEL 0					
NO COOPERATION S5Q[1] = 0	NO-LOW COOPERATION S5Q[1] < 3	MODERATE COOPERATION S5Q[1] ≥ 3	CLOSE TO FULL COOPERATION S5Q[1] ≥ 4/5	FULL COOPERATION S5Q[1] = 5	FULL COOPERATION S5Q[1] = 5
FAIL BASIC ASSESSMENT[2]	PASSES BASIC ASSESSMENT[3] +	PASSES BASIC ASSESSMENT[3] +	PASSES BASIC ASSESSMENT[3] +	PASSES BASIC ASSESSMENT[3] +	PASSES BASIC ASSESSMENT[3] +
BASIC ASSESSMENT = - Cardiorespiratory unstable: MAP < 60mmHg or FiO$_2$ > 60% or PaO$_2$/FiO$_2$ < 200 or RR > 30 bpm - Neurologically unstable - Acute surgery - Temp > 40°C	Neurological or surgical or trauma condition does not allow transfer to chair	Obesity or neurological or surgical or trauma condition does not allow active transfer to chair (even if MRCsum ≥ 36)	MRCsum ≥ 36 + BBS Sit to stand = 0 + BBS Standing = 0 + BBS Sitting ≥ 1	MRCsum ≥ 48 + BBS Sit to stand ≥ 0 + BBS Standing ≥ 0 + BBS Sitting ≥ 2	MRCsum ≥ 48 + BBS Sit to stand ≥ 1 + BBS Standing ≥ 2 + BBS Sitting ≥ 3
BODY POSITIONING[4] 2hr turning	BODY POSITIONING[4] 2hr turning Fowler's position Splinting	BODY POSITIONING[4] 2hr turning Splinting Upright sitting position in bed Passive transfer bed to chair	BODY POSITIONING[4] 2hr turning Passive transfer bed to chair Sitting out of bed Standing with assist (2 ≥ pers)	BODY POSITIONING[4] Active transfer bed to chair Sitting out of bed Standing with assist (≥ 1 pers)	BODY POSITIONING[4] Active transfer bed to chair Sitting out of bed Standing

Table 45.1 (continued) 'Start to move' protocol University Hospitals Leuven: step-up approach of progressive mobilization and physical activity programme

LEVEL 0	LEVEL 1	LEVEL 2	LEVEL 3	LEVEL 4	LEVEL 5
PHYSIOTHERAPY: No treatment	**PHYSIOTHERAPY**[4] Passive range of motion Passive bed cyclying NMES	**PHYSIOTHERAPY**[4] Passive/Active range of motion Resistance training arms and legs Passive/Active leg and/or cyclying in bed or chair NMES	**PHYSIOTHERAPY**[4] Passive/Active range of motion Resistance training arms and legs Active leg and/or arm cycling in bed or chair NMES ADL	**PHYSIOTHERAPY**[4] Passive/Active range of motion Resistance training arms and legs Active leg and/or arm cycling in chair or bed Walking (with assistance/frame) NMES ADL	**PHYSIOTHERAPY**[4] Passive/Active range of motion Resistance training arms and legs Active leg and arm cycling in chair Walking (with assistance) NMES ADL

[1] SSQ: response to five standardized questions for cooperation.

[2] FAILS = at least one risk factor present.

[3] If basic assessment failed, decrease to level 0.

[4] Safety: each activity should be deferred if severe adverse events (cardiovascular, respiratory, and subject's intolerance) occur during the intervention.

MRC, Medical Research Council muscle strength sum scale (0–60); BBS, Berg Balance score.

Adapted from Morris PE, Goad A, Thompson C, Taylor K, Harry B, Passmore L, et al. 'Early intensive care unit mobility therapy in the treatment of acute respiratory failure', *Critical Care Medicine*, 36, 8, pp. 2238–2243, copyright 2008, with permission from Wolters Kluwer and the Society of Critical Care Medicine.

address the issue of safety and clinical assessment of the medical condition (cardiorespiratory and neurological status), level of cooperation, and functional status (muscle strength, level of mobility). This provides information for the steps to gradually increase physical activity and mobilization in the critically ill.[14,24–26] Some of the algorithms limit the start to early rehabilitation to the time point where patients start be conscious,[14,24,27,28] while others initiate treatment in the phase where patients are unconscious or uncooperative due the acuteness of the critical illness.[25,26] The flow chart 'Start to Move' was developed in our centre (see Table 45.1), inspired from the one by Morris et al.,[14] and is an example of a multidisciplinary step-up approach. Six levels are identified, and each level defines, guided by assessment of the medical condition: cardiorespiratory and neurological status, level of cooperation and functional status (muscle strength, level of mobility), the modality of body positioning (mobilization), and physiotherapy. Each day, the ICU team defines the appropriate level of the 'Start to Move' protocol in every patient, especially in those facing an extended ICU stay.

Accurate assessment of level of cooperation and cardiorespiratory reserve, and rigorous screening for other factors that could preclude early mobilization is of paramount importance.[24] In addition to assessment of the safety and readiness of the patient for exercise and physical activity, specific measures of function (e.g. muscle strength, joint mobility), functional status (e.g. outcomes for functional performance such as the Functional Independence Measure (FIM), Berg Balance scale, Functional Ambulation Categories) must be considered.[29]

Basic assessment

This assessment includes the evaluation of the cardiorespiratory, neurological, and surgical status of the patient to judge the appropriateness of early physical activity and rehabilitation of the critically ill patient. In general, only global indications can be given to decide on the safety of early physical activity and mobilization. In addition, some unstable conditions will exclude mobilization but will allow cycling in bed. Therefore, decisions on the appropriateness of modalities for mobilization or physical activity should be made by the multidisciplinary team. As an example, in our 'Start to Move' protocol, we suggested, as contraindication for **any** physical activity, the following: MAP <60 mmHg or FiO_2 >60% or PaO_2/FiO_2 <200 or respiratory rate >30 breaths/min, neurologically unstable (e.g. intracranial bleeding), acute surgery, and body temperature >40°C. Stiller established a more detailed scheme of safety issues to be considered for **mobilization** of the critically ill patient.[21]

Level of cooperation

The level of cooperation is important to judge the ability to cooperate with assessment (muscle testing) and treatment (active vs passive modalities) and can be assessed with the GCS or with five standardized questions: (1) open and close your eyes, (2) look at me, (3) open your mouth and stick out your tongue, (4) nod your head, (5) I will count to 5, frown your eyebrows afterwards.[9] A score of 5 indicates an adequate level of cooperation.

Joint mobility

Knowledge on the epidemiology of major joint contractures in critically ill patients is limited. A recent systematic review reported a high prevalence of joint contractures in patient populations frequently admitted to ICU (spinal cord injuries, burns, brain injuries, and stroke).[30] Functionally significant contractures of major joints occurred in more than 30% of patients with prolonged ICU stay.[31] Elbows and ankles were the mostly affected joints both at ICU discharge as well as hospital discharge. This underscores the need for both assessment and treatment of (passive) range of motion in ICU patients. Frequent assessment of joint mobility and causes of limitation of range of motion (muscle tone, muscle length, capsule, skin, and oedema) is requested. Detailed assessment of joint mobility by physiotherapists can reveal undetected injuries.[32]

Limb muscle strength

Muscle strength, or more precisely the maximum muscle force or tension generated by a muscle or (more commonly) a group of muscles, can be measured in several ways and with a range of different equipment. Manual muscle testing with the 0–5 MRC scale is often used in clinical practice. The MRC sum score combines the strength scores of six upper and lower muscle groups bilaterally and originates from patients with Guillain–Barré syndrome.[33] De Jonghe et al. have proposed that a sum score of less than 48 reflects significant muscle weakness, suggestive for ICUAW. Assessment of muscle strength is specifically becoming important to guide the progression of ambulation[14] and to predict outcome.[11] Muscle strength in ICU patients can be reliably measured in cooperative patients with the MRC score,[34] handgrip dynamometer,[34] and handheld dynamometry (HHD).[35]

Respiratory muscle strength

Weaning failure is an important clinical feature in a minority of ventilated patients. There is accumulating evidence that weaning problems are associated with failure of the respiratory muscles to resume ventilation.[36–38] Respiratory muscle weakness might be treated with respiratory muscle training. In clinical practice, respiratory muscle strength is measured as maximal inspiratory and expiratory mouth pressures (Pimax and Pemax, respectively). In ventilated patients, inspiratory muscle strength is estimated from temporary occlusion of the airway.[39] The procedure involves a unidirectional expiratory valve to allow the patient to expire while inspiration is blocked. Optimal length of occlusion time is considered to be 25–30 s in adults[39] and 15 s in children.

Functional status

The assessment of functional status may seem to be inapplicable for acutely ill ICU patients but can be implemented in patients with protracted critical illness. Functional assessment tools are also successfully used to monitor progress of patients in several studies.[17,18,40,41] Furthermore, they can play a role in reconstructing the patient's functionality before ICU admission. The Barthel Index,[42] FIM,[43] and Katz ADL Scale[44] are commonly used valid tools to score the patient's ability to independently perform a range of activities, mostly related to mobility (e.g. transfers from bed to chair, walking, stair climbing) and self-care (e.g. bathing, grooming, toileting, dressing, feeding). Functional status, such as the ability to sit on a chair, to transfer from sitting to standing, and to stand, can be quantified on a 0 to 4 ordinal scale with components of the Berg Balance scale[45] (see Box 45.1). Walking ability can also be simply assessed, using the Functional Ambulation Categories[46] (see Box 45.2). In patients that are able to walk, the 6-minute walking test can be used to evaluate functional exercise capacity.[47]

Physical activity and exercise in the unconscious patient

To simulate the normal perturbations that the human body experiences in health, the patient who is critically ill needs to be positioned upright (well supported), and rotated when recumbent. These perturbations need to be scheduled frequently to avoid the adverse effects of prolonged static positioning on respiratory, cardiac, and circulatory function.[48] Other indications for positioning include the management of soft tissue contracture, protection of flaccid limbs and lax

Box 45.1 Three components of the Berg Balance score to assess components of functional status in ICU patients

Sitting to standing

4 Able to stand without using hands and stabilize independently

3 Able to stand independently using hands

2 Able to stand using hands after several tries

1 Needs minimal aid to stand or stabilize

0 Needs moderate or maximal assist to stand

Standing unsupported

4 Able to stand safely for 2 min

3 Able to stand 2 min with supervision

2 Able to stand 30 s unsupported

1 Needs several tries to stand 30 s unsupported

0 Unable to stand 30 s unsupported

Sitting with back unsupported but feet supported on floor or on a stool

4 Able to sit safely and securely for 2 min

3 Able to sit for 2 min under supervision

2 Able to able to sit for 30 s

1 Able to sit for 10 s

0 Unable to sit without support for 10 s

Reproduced with permission of the Canadian Public Health Association. Berg KO, Wood-Dauphinee SL, Williams JI, Maki B, 'Measuring balance in the elderly: validation of an instrument', *Canadian Journal of Public Health*, 1992, 83, Suppl 2, pp. S7–S11.

joints, nerve impingement, and skin breakdown. The efficacy of 2-hourly patient rotation, which is common in clinical practice, has not been verified scientifically. Bed design features in critical care should include hip and knee breaks so the patient can approximate upright sitting as much as can be tolerated. Heavy-care patients, such as those who are sedated, overweight, or obese, may need chairs with greater support such as stretcher chairs. Lifts may be needed to change a patient's position safely. Early rehabilitation beyond body positioning in ICU patients was considered as contraindicated, mainly due to shock, sedation, and renal replacement, in more than 40% of the ICU days of critically ill patients.[28,49] However, this practice is incorrect, since other treatment modalities, such as passive cycling, joint mobility, muscle stretching, and NMES do not require patient cooperation and are not interfering with renal replacement or sedation of the patient. Passive stretching or range-of-motion exercise may have a particularly important role in the management of patients who are unable to move spontaneously. Studies in healthy subjects have shown that passive stretching decreases stiffness and increases extensibility of the muscle.[50,51] In an RCT of critically ill patients, three times per day for 3 hours of CPM per day revealed an attenuation of fibre atrophy and protein loss of the tibialis anterior muscle, compared with passive stretching for 5 minutes, twice daily.[52] Recently, positive effects

Box 45.2 Functional Ambulation Categories (FAC)

FAC of '0' (non-functional ambulatory) indicates a patient who is not able to walk at all or needs the help of two therapists.

FAC of '1' (ambulatory, dependent on physical assistance (level II)) indicates a patient who requires continuous manual contact to support body weight as well as to maintain balance or to assist coordination.

FAC of '2' (ambulatory, dependent on physical assistance (level I)) indicates a patient who requires intermittent, continuous light touch to assist balance or coordination.

FAC of '3' (ambulatory, dependent on supervision) indicates a patient who can ambulate on level surface, without manual contact of another person, but requires standby guarding of one person either for safety or for verbal cueing.

FAC of '4' (ambulatory, independent, level surface only) indicates a patient who can ambulate independently on level surface but requires supervision to negotiate (e.g. stairs, inclines, non-level surfaces).

FAC of '5' (ambulatory, independent) indicates a patient who can walk everywhere independently, including stairs.

Reprinted from *Physical Therapy*, Holden MK et al., 'Clinical gait assessment in the neurologically impaired. Reliability and meaningfulness', 1984, 64, 1, pp. 35–40, with permission of the American Physical Therapy Association. Copyright © 1984 American Physical Therapy Association.

of four times of 2.5 hours of daily passive loading on muscle-specific force, but not of muscle mass, were observed.[53] For patients who cannot be actively mobilized and have high risk of soft tissue contracture, such as following severe burns, trauma, and some neurological conditions, splinting may be indicated.

The application of (low-intensity) exercise training in the early phase of ICU admission is often more complicated due to unconsciousness, lack of cooperation, and the clinical status of the patient. Recent technological development resulted in a bedside cycle ergometer for (active or passive) leg cycling (see Figure 45.1) during bed rest to perform prolonged continuous mobilization, allowing rigorous control of exercise intensity and duration. Furthermore, training intensity can be continuously adjusted to the patient's health status and the physiological responses to exercise. An RCT of early application of daily bedside (initially passive) leg cycling in critically ill patients showed improved functional status, muscle function, and exercise performance at hospital discharge, compared to patients receiving standard physiotherapy without leg cycling.[18] Of interest is also their finding that neither passive nor active cycling induced significant cardiorespiratory responses and thus does not stress the vital systems during this phase of critical illness.

However, about 30% of the patients were not eligible to participate in the study because of the inability to cycle due to obesity, surgery, catheters and drains, or body height.[18] In these patients, EMS might be an alternative therapy to exercise local muscle groups. The application of EMS in patients during the **acute phase** of critical illness is a very interesting treatment option, since, specifically in the early phase, selective type II atrophy is reported.[54] EMS has the unique feature that it activates fast motor units and thus specifically stimulates contraction of fast (type II) fibres. In patients with **protracted** critical illness, EMS of the quadriceps, in addition to active limb mobilization, enhanced muscle strength[55] or reduced loss of muscle mass[56] and hastened independent transfer from bed to chair.[55] In patients after major

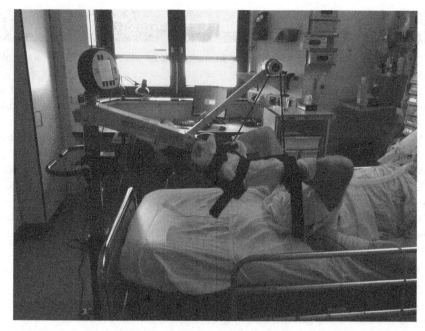

Fig. 45.1 Device for active and passive cycling in a bedridden patient in the intensive care.

abdominal surgery, a slower muscle protein catabolism and an increase in total RNA content were seen after EMS.[57] In **acute** critically ill patients in the ICU not able to move actively, the effectiveness of NMES is still controversial. Application of EMS in patients from the second day after admission to the ICU attenuated cross-sectional diameter loss of the quadriceps, compared to the non-stimulated leg,[58] while others were unable to revert muscle wasting in the early acute phase.[56,59] Although the application of EMS in the acute phase of critical illness seems a potential effective treatment to prevent or counteract muscle atrophy, several important issues remain to be resolved. The ability to stimulate the muscle might be hampered due to neuropathy, myopathy, sepsis, peripheral oedema, 'non-excitable membrane',[60] or medication.

Physical activity and exercise in the alert and cooperative patient

Mobilization refers to physical activity and exercise sufficient to elicit acute physiological effects that enhance ventilation, central and peripheral perfusion, circulation, muscle metabolism, and alertness. Strategies of mobilization—in order of intensity—include transferring in bed, sitting over the edge of the bed, moving from bed to chair, standing, stepping in place, and walking with or without support. Standing and walking frames enable the patient to mobilize safely with attachments for bags, lines, and leads that cannot be disconnected. Active rehabilitation and PT were applied safely (less than 1% adverse events) and effectively in ventilated patients,[13] even during extracorporeal membrane oxygenation in patients awaiting lung transplantation.[61] Walking and standing aids, and tilt tables enhance physiological responses[62] and promote early mobilization of critically ill patients. The frame either needs to be able to accommodate a portable O_2 tank, or a portable mechanical ventilator and seat, or a suitable trolley so equipment can

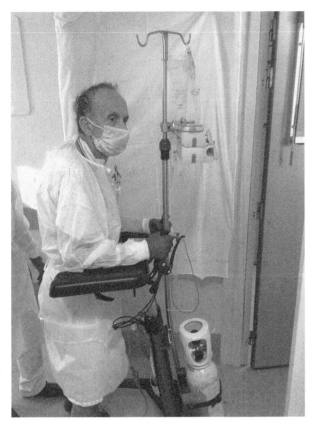

Fig. 45.2 Walking frame to assist a ventilator-dependent patient.

be used (see Figure 45.2). Transfer belts facilitate heavy lifts and protect both the patient and the nurse or physiotherapist. In ventilated patients, the ventilator settings may require adjustment to the patients' needs (i.e. increased minute ventilation). Although the approach of early mobilization has face validity and has been practised in Europe and Australia for many years, its effectiveness was only recently evaluated in formal clinical studies.[14,17] Morris et al. demonstrated in a prospective cohort study that patients receiving early mobility therapy by physical therapists had reduced ICU stay and hospital stay, with no differences in weaning time. No differences were observed in discharge location or in hospital costs of the usual care and early mobility patients. Schweickert et al. observed in an RCT that early PT and OT improved functional status at hospital discharge, shortened the duration of delirium, and increased VFDs. These findings did not result in differences in the length of ICU or hospital stay.[17]

Aerobic training and muscle strengthening, in addition to routine mobilization, improved walking distance more than mobilization alone in ventilated patients with CCI.[63] An RCT showed that a 6-week upper and lower limb training programme improved limb muscle strength, ventilator-free time, and functional outcomes in patients requiring long-term MV, compared to a control group.[40] These results are in line with a retrospective analysis of patients on long-term MV who participated in whole-body training and respiratory muscle training.[41] In patients recently weaned from MV,[64] the addition of upper limb exercise enhanced the effects of general mobilization on exercise endurance performance and dyspnoea.

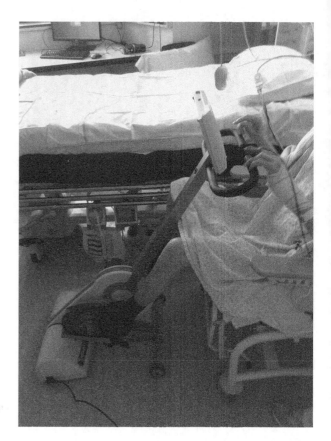

Fig. 45.3 Device for active and passive cycling in a patient in the intensive care.

Low-resistance multiple repetitions of resistive muscle training can augment muscle mass, force generation, and oxidative enzymes in the muscle. Sets of repetitions of muscle contractions within the patient's tolerance can be scheduled daily. Resistive muscle training can include the use of pulleys, elastic bands, and weight belts. The chair cycle (see Figure 45.3) and the bed cycle mentioned earlier allow patients to perform an individualized exercise training programme. The intensity of cycling can be adjusted to the individual patient's capacity, ranging from passive cycling, via assisted cycling, to cycling against increasing resistance.

Role for early rehabilitation in weaning failure

Only a small proportion of patients fail to wean from MV, but they require a disproportionate amount of resources. Several factors, including inadequate ventilatory drive, respiratory muscle weakness, respiratory muscle fatigue, increased WOB, or cardiac failure, are likely to contribute to weaning failure. There is accumulating evidence that weaning problems are associated with failure of the respiratory muscles to resume ventilation.[36–38] Respiratory muscle weakness is often observed in patients with weaning failure, and these patients are at risk of developing respiratory muscle fatigue.[38] Indeed, a high ratio of respiratory muscle workload and muscle capacity (Pi/Pimax) is a major cause of ventilator dependency and predicts the outcome of successful weaning.[36] 'Ventilator-induced diaphragm dysfunction' is suggested as an important cause of respiratory muscle failure, and intermittent loading of the respiratory muscles has been shown to attenuate respiratory muscle deconditioning.[65] Therefore, (intermittent) inspiratory muscle training (IMT) might be beneficial in patients with weaning failure. Some investigators might argue against the application of loaded breathing in the treatment of weaning failure, based on studies showing subcellular diaphragm muscle damage after loaded breathing.[66] However, these changes were observed after **continuous** loading, instead of **intermittent** loading, as applied during IMT (6–8 contractions, repeated in 3–4 series). A recent RCT, comparing IMT at moderate intensity (~50% of the Pimax) vs sham training in patients with weaning failure, showed that a statistically significant larger improvement in Pimax. In addition, a significantly higher proportion of the training group (76%) could be weaned, compared to the sham group (35%).[67] The addition of IMT in acute critically ill patients from the beginning of MV has shown contrasting findings. Caruso et al. submitted their patients in an RCT to IMT for 30 minutes per day and found that IMT neither improved Pimax or abbreviated the weaning duration nor decreased the reintubation rate.[68] In contrast, Cader et al. observed in an RCT that twice-daily IMT sessions at 30% Pimax for 5 minutes improved Pimax and reduced the weaning period (3.6 vs 5.3 days in comparison to the control group).[69]

From theory to clinical practice

Despite the evidence, the amount of rehabilitation performed in ICUs is often inadequate, and, as a rule, rehabilitation is better organized in weaning centres or respiratory ICUs.[22,63] Members of the rehabilitation team in the ICU (physicians, physiotherapists, nurses, and occupational therapists) should be able to prioritize and identify aims and parameters of treatment modalities of early mobilization and physical activity, ensuring that these treatment modalities are both therapeutic and safe by appropriate monitoring of vital functions.[24] The early intervention approach, although not easy, especially in patients still in need of supportive devices (MV, cardiac assists)[61] or unable to stand without support of personnel or standing aids, is a worthwhile endeavour.[16] The clinical consequences of a difference in the mentality of the team towards 'ambulation of the patient' were elegantly demonstrated in the study of Thomsen et al.[22] Transferring a patient from the acute intensive care to the respiratory intensive care increased the number of patients ambulating threefold, compared with pre-transfer rates. These improvements in ambulation rates were assigned to the differences in the team approach towards ambulating patients.[22] Garzon-Serrano et al. observed that physical therapists mobilize critically ill patients to higher levels of mobilization than nursing staff.[70] Based on their competence in exercise and physical activity, physiotherapists should be responsible for implementing mobilization plans and exercise prescription and should make recommendation for progression of the rehabilitation strategy jointly with medical and nursing staff.[15]

Conclusion

Exercise and early rehabilitation have an important role in the management of patients with critical illness. The assessment and treatment of critically ill patients concentrate on deconditioning (limb and respiratory muscle weakness, joint stiffness, impaired functional exercise capacity, physical inactivity) and weaning failure as targets for rehabilitation. A variety of modalities for exercise training and early mobility have been tested in clinical studies and can be implemented, depending on the stage of critical illness, comorbid conditions, and alertness and cooperation of the patient. Mobilization plans and exercise prescription for the patient is a team responsibility of physiotherapist, occupational therapist, intensivist, and nursing staff.

References

1 Eisner MD, Thompson T, Hudson LD, et al. Efficacy of low tidal volume ventilation in patients with different clinical risk factors for acute lung injury and the acute respiratory distress syndrome. *Am J Respir Crit Care Med* 2001;**164**:231–6.

2 Koch S, Spuler S, Deja M, et al. Critical illness myopathy is frequent: accompanying neuropathy protracts ICU discharge. *J Neurol Neurosurg Psychiatry* 2011;**82**:287–93.

3 van der Schaaf M, Dettling DS, Beelen A, Lucas C, Dongelmans DA, Nollet F. Poor functional status immediately after discharge from an intensive care unit. *Disabil Rehabil* 2008;**30**:1812–18.

4 Herridge MS, Tansey CM, Matte A, et al. Functional disability 5 years after acute respiratory distress syndrome. *N Engl J Med* 2011;**364**:1293–304.

5 Unroe M, Kahn JM, Carson SS, et al. One-year trajectories of care and resource utilization for recipients of prolonged mechanical ventilation: a cohort study. *Ann Intern Med* 2010;**153**:167–75.

6 Poulsen JB, Moller K, Kehlet H, Perner A. Long-term physical outcome in patients with septic shock. *Acta Anaesthesiol Scand* 2009;**53**:724–30.

7 Herridge MS, Cheung AM, Tansey CM, et al. One-year outcomes in survivors of the acute respiratory distress syndrome. *N Engl J Med* 2003;**348**:683–93.

8 Schefold JC, Bierbrauer J, Weber-Carstens S. Intensive care unit-acquired weakness (ICUAW) and muscle wasting in critically ill patients with severe sepsis and septic shock. *J Cachex Sarcopenia Muscle* 2010;**1**:147–57.

9 De Jonghe B, Sharshar T, Lefaucheur JP, et al. Paresis acquired in the intensive care unit: a prospective multicenter study. *JAMA* 2002;**288**:2859–67.

10 Hund EF. Neuromuscular complications in the ICU: the spectrum of critical illness-related conditions causing muscular weakness and weaning failure. *J Neurol Sci* 1996;**136**:10–16.

11 Ali NA, O'Brien JM, Jr, Hoffmann SP, et al. Acquired weakness, handgrip strength, and mortality in critically ill patients. *Am J Respir Crit Care Med* 2008;**178**:261–8.

12 Esteban A, Frutos F, Tobin MJ, et al. A comparison of four methods of weaning patients from mechanical ventilation. *N Engl J Med* 1995;**332**:345–50.

13 Bailey P, Thomsen GE, Spuhler VJ, et al. Early activity is feasible and safe in respiratory failure patients. *Crit Care Med* 2007;**35**:139–45.

14 Morris PE, Goad A, Thompson C, et al. Early intensive care unit mobility therapy in the treatment of acute respiratory failure. *Crit Care Med* 2008;**36**:2238–43.

15 Gosselink R, Bott J, Johnson M, et al. Physiotherapy for adult patients with critical illness: recommendations of the European Respiratory Society and European Society of Intensive Care Medicine Task Force on Physiotherapy for Critically Ill Patients. *Intensive Care Med* 2008;**34**:1188–99.

16 Needham DM. Mobilizing patients in the intensive care unit: improving neuromuscular weakness and physical function. *JAMA* 2008;**300**:1685–90.

17 Schweickert WD, Pohlman MC, Pohlman AS, et al. Early physical and occupational therapy in mechanically ventilated, critically ill patients: a randomised controlled trial. *Lancet* 2009;**373**:1874–82.

18 Burtin C, Clerckx B, Robbeets C, et al. Early exercise in critically ill patients enhances short-term functional recovery. *Crit Care Med* 2009;**37**:2499–505.

19 Morris PE, Griffin L, Berry M, et al. Receiving early mobility during an intensive care unit admission is a predictor of improved outcomes in acute respiratory failure. *Am J Med Sci* 2011;**341**:373–7.

20 Kasotakis G, Schmidt U, Perry D, et al. The surgical intensive care unit optimal mobility score predicts mortality and length of stay. *Crit Care Med* 2012;**40**:1122–8.

21 Stiller K. Safety issues that should be considered when mobilizing critically ill patients. *Crit Care Clin* 2007;**23**:35–53.

22 Thomsen GE, Snow GL, Rodriguez L, Hopkins RO. Patients with respiratory failure increase ambulation after transfer to an intensive care unit where early activity is a priority. *Crit Care Med* 2008;**36**:1119–24.

23 **World Health Organization.** *International Classification of Functioning, Disability and Health (ICF).* (2010). Available at: http://www.who.int/classifications/icf/en/.

24 **Stiller K, Philips A.** Safety aspects of mobilising acutely ill patients. *Physioth Theory and Pract* 2003;**19**:239–57.

25 **Hanekom S, Gosselink R, Dean E, et al.** The development of a clinical management algorithm for early physical activity and mobilization of critically ill patients: synthesis of evidence and expert opinion and its translation into practice. *Clin Rehabil* 2011;**25**:771–87.

26 **Gosselink R, Clerckx B, Robbeets C, Vanhullebusch T, Vanpee G, Segers J.** Physiotherapy in the intensive care unit. *Neth J Crit Care* 2011;**15**:66–75.

27 **Korupolu R, Gifford J, Needham DM.** Early mobilisation of critically ill patients: reducing neuromuscular complications. *Contemp Crit Care* 2009;**6**:1–12.

28 **Bourdin G, Barbier J, Burle JF, et al.** The feasibility of early physical activity in intensive care unit patients: a prospective observational one-center study. *Respir Care* 2010;**55**:400–7.

29 **Gosselink R, Needham D, Hermans G.** ICU-based rehabilitation and its appropriate metrics. *Curr Opin Crit Care* 2012;**18**:533–9.

30 **Fergusson D, Hutton B, Drodge A.** The epidemiology of major joint contractures: a systematic review of the literature. *Clin Orthop Relat Res* 2007;**456**:22–9.

31 **Clavet H, Hebert PC, Fergusson D, Doucette S, Trudel G.** Joint contracture following prolonged stay in the intensive care unit. *CMAJ* 2008;**178**:691–7.

32 **Schwartz Cowley R, Swanson B, Chapman P, Mackay LE.** The role of rehabilitation in the intensive care unit. *J Head Trauma Rehabil* 1994;**9**:32–42.

33 **Kleyweg RP, van der Meche FG, Schmitz PI.** Interobserver agreement in the assessment of muscle strength and functional abilities in Guillain-Barre syndrome. *Muscle Nerve* 1991;**14**:1103–9.

34 **Hermans G, Clerckx B, Van Hullebusch T, et al.** Inter-observer agreement of MRC-sum score and handgrip strength in the intensive care unit. *Muscle Nerve* 2012;**45**:18–25.

35 **Vanpee G, Segers J, Van MH, et al.** The interobserver agreement of handheld dynamometry for muscle strength assessment in critically ill patients. *Crit Care Med* 2011;**39**:1929–34.

36 **Vassilakopoulos T, Zakynthinos S, Roussos C.** The tension-time index and the frequency/tidal volume ratio are the major pathophysiologic determinants of weaning failure and success. *Am J Respir Crit Care Med* 1998;**158**:378–85.

37 **Zakynthinos SG, Vassilakopoulos T, Roussos C.** The load of inspiratory muscles in patients needing mechanical ventilation. *Am J Respir Crit Care Med* 1995;**152**:1248–55.

38 **Chang AT, Boots RJ, Brown MG, Paratz J, Hodges PW.** Reduced inspiratory muscle endurance following successful weaning from prolonged mechanical ventilation. *Chest* 2005;**128**:553–9.

39 **Marini JJ, Smith TC, Lamb V.** Estimation of inspiratory muscle strength in mechanically ventilated patients: the measurement of maximal inspiratory pressure. *J Crit Care* 1986;**1**:32–8.

40 **Chiang LL, Wang LY, Wu CP, Wu HD, Wu YT.** Effects of physical training on functional status in patients with prolonged mechanical ventilation. *Phys Ther* 2006;**86**:1271–81.

41 **Martin UJ, Hincapie L, Nimchuk M, Gaughan J, Criner GJ.** Impact of whole-body rehabilitation in patients receiving chronic mechanical ventilation. *Crit Care Med* 2005;**33**:2259–65.

42 **Mahoney FI, Barthel DW.** Functional evaluation: the Barthel index. *Md State Med J* 1965;**14**:61–5.

43 **Keith RA, Granger CV, Hamilton BB, Sherwin FS.** The functional independence measure: a new tool for rehabilitation. *Adv Clin Rehabil* 1987;**1**:6–18.

44 **Katz S, Ford AB, Moskowitz RW, Jackson BA, Jaffe MW.** Studies of illness in the aged. The index of ADL: a standardized measure of biological measure of biological and psychosocial function. *JAMA* 1963;**185**:914–19.

45 **Berg KO, Wood-Dauphinee SL, Williams JI, Maki B.** Measuring balance in the elderly: validation of an instrument. *Can J Public Health* 1992;**83**(Suppl 2):S7–11.

46 Holden MK, Gill KM, Magliozzi MR, Nathan J, Piehl-Baker L. Clinical gait assessment in the neurologically impaired. Reliability and meaningfulness. *Phys Ther* 1984;**64**:35–40.

47 American Thoracic Society. ATS Statement: Guidelines for the six-minute walking test. *Am J Respir Crit Care Med* 2002;**166**:111–17.

48 Convertino VA. Value of orthostatic stress in maintaining functional status soon after myocardial infarction or cardiac artery bypass grafting. *J Cardiovasc Nurs* 2003;**18**:124–30.

49 Needham DM, Korupolu R. Rehabilitation quality improvement in an intensive care unit setting: implementation of a quality improvement model. *Top Stroke Rehabil* 2010;**17**:271–81.

50 McNair PJ, Dombroski EW, Hewson DJ, Stanley SN. Stretching at the ankle joint: viscoelastic responses to holds and continuous passive motion. *Med Sci Sports Exerc* 2001;**33**:354–8.

51 Reid DA, McNair PJ. Passive force, angle, and stiffness changes after stretching of hamstring muscles. *Med Sci Sports Exerc* 2004;**36**:1944–8.

52 Griffiths RD, Palmer A, Helliwell T, Maclennan P, Macmillan RR. Effect of passive stretching on the wasting of muscle in the critically ill. *Nutrition* 1995;**11**:428–32.

53 Llano-Diez M, Renaud G, Andersson M, et al. Mechanisms underlying intensive care unit muscle wasting and effects of passive mechanical loading. *Crit Care* 2012;**16**:R209.

54 Bierbrauer J, Koch S, Olbricht C, et al. Early type II fiber atrophy in intensive care unit patients with nonexcitable muscle membrane. *Crit Care Med* 2012;**40**:647–50.

55 Zanotti E, Felicetti G, Maini M, Fracchia C. Peripheral muscle strength training in bed-bound patients with COPD receiving mechanical ventilation. Effect of electrical stimulation. *Chest* 2003;**124**: 292–6.

56 Gruther W, Kainberger F, Fialka-Moser V, et al. Effects of neuromuscular electrical stimulation on muscle layer thickness of knee extensor muscles in intensive care unit patients: a pilot study. *J Rehabil Med* 2010;**42**:593–7.

57 Strasser EM, Stattner S, Karner J, et al. Neuromuscular electrical stimulation reduces skeletal muscle protein degradation and stimulates insulin-like growth factors in an age- and current-dependent manner: a randomized, controlled clinical trial in major abdominal surgical patients. *Ann Surg* 2009;**249**:738–43.

58 Gerovasili V, Stefanidis K, Vitzilaios K, et al. Electrical muscle stimulation preserves the muscle mass of critically ill patients: a randomized study. *Crit Care* 2009;**13**:R161.

59 Poulsen JB, Moller K, Jensen CV, Weisdorf S, Kehlet H, Perner A. Effect of transcutaneous electrical muscle stimulation on muscle volume in patients with septic shock. *Crit Care Med* 2011;**39**: 456–61.

60 Weber-Carstens S, Koch S, Spuler S, et al. Nonexcitable muscle membrane predicts intensive care unit-acquired paresis in mechanically ventilated, sedated patients. *Crit Care Med* 2009;**37**: 2632–7.

61 Turner DA, Cheifetz IM, Rehder KJ, et al. Active rehabilitation and physical therapy during extracorporeal membrane oxygenation while awaiting lung transplantation-a practical approach. *Crit Care Med* 2011;**39**:2593–8.

62 Zafiropoulos B, Alison JA, McCarren B. Physiological responses to the early mobilisation of the intubated, ventilated abdominal surgery patient. *Aust J Physiother* 2004;**50**:95–100.

63 Nava S. Rehabilitation of patients admitted to a respiratory intensive care unit. *Arch Phys Med Rehabil* 1998;**79**:849–54.

64 Porta R, Vitacca M, Gile LS, et al. Supported arm training in patients recently weaned from mechanical ventilation. *Chest* 2005;**128**:2511–20.

65 Gayan-Ramirez G, Testelmans D, Maes K, et al. Intermittent spontaneous breathing protects the rat diaphragm from mechanical ventilation effects. *Crit Care Med* 2005;**33**:2804–9.

66 Orozco-Levi M, Lloreta J, Minguella J, Serrano S, Broquetas JM, Gea J. Injury of the human diaphragm associated with exertion and chronic obstructive pulmonary disease. *Am J Respir Crit Care Med* 2001;**164**:1734–9.

67 Martin AD, Smith BK, Davenport PD, et al. Inspiratory muscle strength training improves weaning outcome in failure to wean patients: a randomized trial. *Crit Care* 2011;**15**:R84.

68 Caruso P, Denari SD, Ruiz SA, et al. Inspiratory muscle training is ineffective in mechanically venti-lated critically ill patients. *Clinics* 2005;**60**:479–84.

69 Cader SA, Vale RG, Castro JC, et al. Inspiratory muscle training improves maximal inspiratory pressure and may assist weaning in older intubated patients: a randomised trial. *J Physiother* 2010;**56**: 171–7.

70 Garzon-Serrano J, Ryan C, Waak K, et al. Early mobilization in critically ill patients: patients' mobiliza-tion level depends on health care provider's profession. *PM R* 2011;**3**:307–13.

Part 7

Therapeutic and Rehabilitation Strategies in the Post-ICU Period

Chapter 46

Introduction: Therapeutic and Rehabilitation Strategies in the Post-ICU Period

Richard D. Griffiths

'The conflict in care': patients' and relatives' experience

To develop a robust rehabilitation strategy, the clinician must first appreciate that the goal of such a treatment is to facilitate the physical and psychological recovery of the patient towards a level similar to that experienced prior to admission to critical care.[1] This means involving the family and carers early in the stay in the ICU, since the effects of a critical illness are not merely experienced by the patient, but they have a deep impact on the family and the environment to which they will return. It is important to stress that rehabilitation is NOT follow-up, a later inclusive, but passive, observational process of information gathering that informs outcome. Experience shows that to 'recover lives' needs a distinct early active and selective decision-making process, with a therapeutic strategy starting within the ICU, to optimize the recovery of the patient and the family following what most likely has been their most challenging life experience.[2]

As we have learned more about the psychological problems after ICU, it is apparent psychological disturbances and behaviours start to become entrenched and, as such, established behaviour becomes hard to change in patients and relatives if not anticipated or prevented. If not addressed early, misunderstanding and misinterpretation will have been allowed to develop in patients and relatives that lead to what we have termed a **conflict in care** that reflects the often different experiences of patients vs their relative. Rehabilitation therefore starts early within ICU and is necessary to create a culture of recovery in both the deliverers and recipients of care and support.

To appreciate the importance of involving relatives and carers in rehabilitation, it is helpful to reflect on the different experiences encountered by patients and relatives and where these can create divergent perspectives on the same events. (see Table 46.1)

Conflict of care arises because of the very different expectations and anxieties and a failure to promote the right mix of incentives and support. For instance, a patient may be significantly motivated to drive their recovery forward, despite being weak, whilst their closest relative is so terrified of further mishap they overprotect and prevent the patient from mobilizing. These levels of anxiety in relatives must not be underestimated. Relatives have been known to lie awake at night, watching their newly returned partner, to check they are still breathing!

'Changing the culture': rehabilitations starts within ICU

The culture of rehabilitation therapy must start within ICU, but it is important to recognize who needs support and effort, and where resource should be focused. As important as it is to identify those patients who will need rehabilitation, it is equally important not to involve patients who will recover very well under their own steam where the short ICU stay is but a small part in their

Table 46.1 Conflict of care: the differences between patient and relative experiences

Patient	Relative
Amnesia for ICU	Vivid experiences of conflict with patients
➤ No true experience, gap in autobiography	➤ Overprotective and fearful
➤ Lack reality check and feelings of safety	➤ Unable to support and talk through with patient
➤ Distorted perspective on illness and recovery	
Delusions	Highly stressed
➤ Strongly held and frightening	➤ Risk of PTSD
➤ Risk of PTSD	➤ Exceeds personal and social coping
➤ Only experience of ICU if amnesic	

illness. Here, the recovery pathway, including their own, and their relatives' coping strategies are not exceeded, and unnecessary intervention and overmedicalization is avoided.

The culture of recovery and rehabilitation therapy

Clinically, during the ICU stay, it is not difficult to identify those who will have a longer recovery and specific rehabilitation needs. Simple clinical assessment integrates factors such as older age (>60 years), longer ICU stays (>10 days), severe sepsis, trauma or burn injury, extensive confusion and delirium, extensive drug use and withdrawal issues, or specific debility or dysfunction (e.g. swallowing). ICUAW[3] is a major challenge, but these clinical features help to define the likely degree of functional peripheral skeletal muscle (and often respiratory muscle) impairment. Including a more specific assessment during and on discharge of peripheral muscle function, cough function, swallow and mobility is part of risk assessment. Combining these factors with an assessment of the social framework and relatives' grasp of the illness allow the clinical team to focus on those patients and relatives most in need of support.

Creating a positive culture of rehabilitation therapy that is considered 'the treatment' is as important within ICU as it is afterwards. Several components are required, but central to this is the prevention of misunderstanding. This involves the nurse support of relatives so that realistic expectations are established that discuss progress and timescales. This sets the benchmark and, as the patient becomes more aware, allows achievable targets to be set and manageable and realistic milestones established. The cognitive impairment present in many patients negatively affects memory retention during the ICU admission. It is therefore essential that relatives are intimately involved early so that, when the patient becomes able to understand the timescales, the relative is in a position to facilitate conflict limitation. However, involving relatives adds the responsibility to the clinician in order to identify those that are not coping (e.g. not sleeping, discussion avoidance, extreme anxiety) so as to prevent establishment of more chronic anxiety states.

For some patients and relatives, the early mobility and healthy lifestyle approach is challenging, but it is important to stress that bed rest and immobility are counterproductive and that they have a role in helping to stimulate the mind and body during recovery. The clinician must stress to the patient and their relatives that active mobilization and physical rehabilitation are hard work and not easy. Frequent positive reinforcement, rewarding small achievements, and helping to reset expectation are necessary.

Managing the 'conflict in care'

Central to resolving the conflict in care that may arise after ICU is to provide a tool by which patients and relatives may realign their experiences so that they become shared and consistent. As will be discussed in Chapter 52, a patient and relative diary developed with nurses during the ICU stay, in partnership with the relatives, provides a framework to use during recovery.[4] It enables a shared understanding of the experience between the patient and their relatives, an appreciation from both sides of what each other has experienced that results in a coherent dialogue. Evidence suggests that it can reduce anxiety and significantly reduce the development of PTSD, which is a major limitation to recovery.

'Recovering lives': aftercare after ICU

In patients who were very sick during their ICU admission, there may be little, or no, recall of intensive care, and hence they start rehabilitation in a strange ward unconnected practically or emotionally with their illness. In addition, they are managed by clinicians who may not fully appreciate the details of their illness. It is therefore important that the processes and practices commenced in ICU, including risk assessment, are carried forward, including the involvement of relatives and carers. A clinical review process must inform and manage important issues such as drug withdrawal, cessation of unwanted medication, optimization of cardiorespiratory function, and screening for the associated physical problems of immobility.

Recognizing that cognitive impairment, especially in those who have sustained significant periods of delirium or confusion, may persist, even when no longer delirious, requires an approach to repeatedly provide information and advice. Screening for anxiety, depression, and PTSD is much easier, as simple tools have been developed. As within ICU, the approach is supportive, using a 'watch and wait' approach, to allow those who are coping well to recover whilst addressing physical, psychological, and social problems as they arise.

Timescales of recovery, in the light of progress, need to be re-addressed and involve the relatives to allow an assessment of their understanding and coping strategy to be made. This is summarized in UK NICE guidelines, suggesting that a clinical risk assessment and screening process should be performed during an ICU stay, with a formalized action plan documented on leaving ICU.[5]

Physical recovery

The physical functional impairment associated with critical illness includes abnormalities in central brain function as well as peripheral nerve and skeletal muscle problems. After ICU, the recovery of muscle wasting includes the provision of an adequate protein intake, combined with physical activity, and, where appropriate, adequate glycaemic control. Dietary management should focus on healthy eating, a reasonably spaced protein intake, and the avoidance of excess carbohydrates or fat to prevent excessive weight gain. Due to fluid loss after mobilization, it is not unusual to see body weight loss initially, following ICU discharge.

To maintain activity, the mobilization physiotherapy started in the ICU needs to continue on the general ward. For many, it is helpful to use a self-help effort-related exercise programme, with a diary record such as the 'The ICU recovery manual' that provides practical advice. This approach has been shown to improve physical well-being at 6 months in patients with a median ICU stay of 14 days.[6] In addition, patients may benefit from outpatient training sessions, and encouraging results are appearing.[7] These programmes are dependent on developing a culture of rehabilitation, including early exercise therapy, to enhance recovery. Starting after the patient has been discharged to the ward or after they have returned home may be too late to change behaviour to engage in rehabilitation. Furthermore, limited benefit may be observed in patients whose length of ICU stay is less than 1 week, and hence their correctable morbidity may be modest.[8,9]

Psychological recovery

Although the potential for some problems will be obvious, such as handling drug withdrawal or the very confused patient and/or anxious patient, for many patients, a process of normalization with a 'watch and wait' approach is necessary. Explanation and reassurance during recovery should focus on general well-being and enquiry into common distressing elements such as night-mares, delusions, persistent pain, unpleasant experiences, and non-refreshing sleep. Because of persistent cognitive impairment-associated amnesia and memory handling, it is often necessary to assume that this discussion needs repeating. A patient and relative diary then becomes a central aspect of support. A direct consequence of amnesia is the loss of the patient's own autobiography to place the changes that have occurred to them, e.g. generalized weakness, into context.[10] This impacts their comprehension of events as well as their perception of recovery. A diary allows the patient and their relatives both time and opportunity to discuss and contextualize their experi-ence. Although screening for PTSD risk is possible at 2 weeks[11] and can identify those patients who may need more specific therapy, the diary has other benefits, including assisting the relatives cope with their own distress.[12]

Cognitive dysfunction and social challenges

As discussed earlier, the recognition of acute brain dysfunction, e.g. delirium, is important as it can lead to longer-term cognitive impairment. From a practical perspective, explanation and reas-surance are required, as most patients will recover over several months. From experience, patients show considerable behavioural adaptation, and, as long as the patient and relative are forewarned, steps can be taken to ameliorate the consequences. The use of a diary, making lists as an 'aide-memoire', and seeking guidance with decisions are important supportive approaches.

'Recovering lives' requires the re-establishment of a social existence, including the social and emotional aspects of relationships incorporated into work and play. Hence, an approach of total rehabilitation ensures maximal recovery of the patient and permits those that support them to address these aspects where relevant. An understanding of nutritional importance[13] and strate-gies to overcome sexual dysfunction[14] should not be forgotten.

Outpatient review, e.g. at 3 months after hospital discharge, allows the progress in rehabilitation to be assessed. Furthermore, persistent non-resolving problems, such as joints problems, nerve and muscle damage, and post-tracheostomy airway issues, leading to exercise intolerance need to be managed. Finally, an assessment for ongoing psychosocial issues needs to be explored. For many patients, where the process of rehabilitation has been addressed early, this provides a use-ful milestone and reinforcement of the timescales of recovery. It is essential, however, that this appointment is for both the patient **and** the relative. In keeping with our understanding of the severity of muscle wasting and recovery time, a simple rule of thumb for the clinician, in order to understand the timescale of recovery, is that, for a young patient, each day in ICU requires 1 week of recovery and, for an older patient, this is extended to 2 weeks of recovery for each day in the ICU.

Conclusion

The heterogeneity of our ICU population in diagnosis, severity, and biological age means that recovery pathways and timescales are highly individual and varied. While there are some com-mon aspects to recovery, such as physical and behavioural, there is no unique post-ICU pattern of pathology, so the approach needs to be measured, selective, and appropriate to each patient, and hence it is a mistake to treat everyone the same and expect the same trajectory of recovery. Over the last few decades, we have learned much by listening to patients and relatives, and a clinician failing to include both of them in the recovery process is a serious mistake. Remember, we are merely the interim guardians; ultimate recovery involves rejoining their family and friends and reintegrating into their existing social networks.

References

1 Griffiths RD, Jones C. Recovering lives: the follow-up of ICU survivors. *Am J Respir Crit Care Med.* 2011;**183**:833–44.

2 Griffiths RD, Jones C. Seven lessons from 20 years of follow up of intensive care unit survivors. *Curr Opin Crit Care* 2007;**13**:508–13.

3 Griffiths RD, Hall J. Intensive care unit-acquired weakness. *Crit Care Med* 2010;**38**:779–87.

4 Jones C, Bäckman C, Capuzzo M, et al., and RACHEL group. Intensive care diaries reduce new onset PTSD following critical illness: a randomised, controlled trial. *Crit Care* 2010;**14**:R168.

5 National Institute for Health and Care Excellence. *Rehabilitation after critical illness: NICE clinical guideline 83.* 2009. Available at: http://www.nice.org.uk/CG83.

6 Jones C, Skirrow P, Griffiths RD, et al. Rehabilitation after critical illness: a randomised, controlled trial. *Crit Care Med* 2003;**31**:2456–61.

7 McWilliams DJ, Atkinson D, Carter A, Foe BA, Benington S, Conway DH. Feasibility and impact of a structured, exercise-based rehabilitation programme for intensive care survivors *Physiother Theory Pract* 2009;**25**:566–71.

8 Cuthbertson BH, Rattray J, Campbell MK, et al. The PRaCTICaL study of nurse led, intensive care follow-up programmes for improving long term outcomes from critical illness: a pragmatic randomised controlled trial. *BMJ* 2009;**339**:b3723–31.

9 Elliott D, McKinley S, Alison J, et al. Health-related quality of life and physical recovery after a critical illness: a multi-centre randomised controlled trial of a home-based physical rehabilitation program. *Crit Care* 2011;**15**:R142–52.

10 Griffiths RD, Jones C. Filling the intensive care memory gap? *Intensive Care Med* 2001;**27**:344–6.

11 Twigg E, Humphris G, Jones C, Bramwell R, Griffiths RD. Use of a screening questionnaire for post-traumatic stress disorder (PTSD) on a sample of UK ICU patients. *Acta Anaesthesiol Scand* 2008;**52**:202–8.

12 Jones C, Bäckman C, Griffiths RD. Intensive care diaries and relatives' symptoms of posttraumatic stress disorder after critical illness: a pilot study. *Am J Crit Care* 2012;**21**:172–6.

13 Griffiths RD. Nutrition after intensive care. In: Griffiths RD, Jones C (eds.) *Intensive care aftercare.* Oxford: Butterworth & Heinemann; 2002. pp. 48–52.

14 Waldmann C. Sexual problems and their treatment. In: Griffiths RD, Jones C (eds.) *Intensive care aftercare.* Oxford: Butterworth & Heinemann; 2002. pp. 39–47.

Chapter 47

Assessment of Peripheral and Respiratory Muscle Strength in ICU

Gerrard Rafferty and John Moxham

In critical care patients, skeletal muscle weakness affecting the respiratory and peripheral muscles is common[1-3] and can lead to difficulties in weaning from MV, prolonged ICU admission,[3] increased mortality,[4,5] and significant morbidity in survivors.[6,7] Neuromuscular diseases, endocrine and metabolic disorders, as well as medications, including aminoglycosides, corticosteroids, and NMBAS, can potentially impair muscle function. Malnutrition and chronic illnesses also detrimentally affect peripheral and respiratory muscle function. Phrenic nerve injury, with resultant diaphragm dysfunction, can occur as a complication of cardiac surgery,[8] heart-lung transplantation,[9] liver transplantation,[10,11] and traumatic spine injury involving the upper cervical roots.[12] In addition, skeletal muscle weakness can be caused by CIP, CIM, immobilization, or a combination of all three.

The structural changes in CIP and CIM include axonal nerve degeneration, muscle myosin loss, and muscle necrosis, while functional changes can lead to electrical inexcitability of nerves and muscles with reversible muscle weakness. Immobility in itself has marked effects on skeletal muscle strength, but, despite significant weakness and wasting, there is normal motor and sensory nerve conduction and EMGs. Muscle dysfunction can occur soon after admission to the ICU within hours of initiating MV,[13] and sequelae can last up to 5 years post-ICU discharge,[4,7,14] with many patients complaining of weakness for months to years after discharge and persistent exercise limitation.

Muscle biopsy and electrophysiological techniques, in combination with clinical examination, are used to assess neuromuscular dysfunction in patients on ICU, but accurate diagnosis is difficult. There may be pre-existing disorders, and testing is both time-consuming and requires skilled personnel.[15] Although electrophysiological and histological abnormalities are common in ICU patients, it can be difficult to determine whether such abnormalities have significant clinical impact.[16,17] Patients with sepsis and MOF can have decreased muscle strength without electrophysiological abnormalities,[17] and respiratory and peripheral muscle EMG findings do not predict the duration of MV or length of ICU stay in patients with CIP or SIRS.[18]

Volitional assessment of peripheral skeletal muscle strength

Routine quantitative assessment of peripheral skeletal muscle strength is commonly performed, using the MRC scale, a 6-point, categorized scale originally developed by Hughes et al.[19] to assess neuromuscular function in patients with Guillain–Barré syndrome. A modified score, the MRC sumscore,[20] was later introduced to provide a summation of the strength of six muscle groups bilaterally. The MRC sumscore ranges from 0 (paralysis) to 60 (normal strength), and both proximal and distal muscle groups are represented. The MRC sumscore has been proposed as a diagnostic criterion for ICUAW,[21] with a 'cut-off' value of less than 48 out of 60. The MRC scale provides a useful assessment tool, as each change in category is of clinical importance and steps between categories are well defined. The scale also has satisfactory reproducibility and intraclass correlation coefficient, indicating excellent inter-observer agreement,[22,23] albeit this has not been shown in patients in the earlier stage of critical illness. Furthermore, the MRC sumscore has previously been demonstrated to have correlations with respiratory muscle function, weaning, and mortality,[3,16,24] and, unlike other more complex, non-volitional tests, it is easy to perform and inexpensive, leading to more widespread availability. The MRC sumscore is, however, restricted in its application to conscious and cooperative patients and is therefore of limited value in ICU.[16,24,25] The volitional nature of the test limits its ability to distinguish poor motivation and impaired cognition from true loss of muscle function. In addition, the MRC sumscore is a crude means of assessing muscle strength, and each muscle group is scored on a non-linear ordinal scale. Grade 4 strength encompasses a large range of muscle strength, and, as the degree of active movement against gravity and some resistance is not quantified, it makes the discriminant ability poor above grade 3 strength.[26,27] The MRC scale does not make clear whether muscle tests should be performed through a range of motion or as an isometric contraction, potentially leading to discrepancies between measurements. The relative insensitivity of the MRC sumscore means that subtle changes in muscle strength may go undetected, despite marked electrophysiological changes.[28]

HHD provides a technique to objectively assess muscle strength by measuring maximal voluntary contraction (MVC) force. The operator resists movement by holding the dynamometer in an appropriate position, while the patient is encouraged to perform a maximal contraction of the muscle group of interest. The patient's posture and the point of measurement in the range of motion should be standardized[29] for test validity and reproducibility. HHD has good intra- and inter-rater reliability for knee extension, ankle dorsiflexion, and shoulder abduction.[30–32] In order to obtain valid measurements of muscle strength with HHD, the operator should be strong enough to counter the force produced by the muscle group during assessment to avoid underestimation of strength.[33–35]

Measurement of grip strength with a HHD provides a quick and simple alternative to comprehensive manual muscle testing,[24] and normative data are available.[36–38] Although providing an objective measure of muscle strength, dynamometry has similar limitations to the MRC sumscore, in that accuracy relies on the magnitude of the volitional effort which may be compromised by pain, sedation, delirium, or coma. Even in alert cooperative patients, volitional strength measurements can only rule out weakness if a subject can achieve values within the normal range; low values can be difficult to interpret, as they can reflect true weakness or submaximal effort.

Non-volitional assessment of peripheral skeletal muscle strength

Non-volitional assessment techniques that stimulate the motor nerve supply of the muscle, and hence remove the influence of patient cooperation and volition, provide reliable measures of muscle force in non-cooperative patients. A number of techniques are available, including measurement of adductor pollicis force following ulnar nerve stimulation,[17,39,40] quadriceps force elicited by femoral nerve stimulation[41,42] and ankle dorsiflexor force evoked by peroneal nerve stimulation.[43–45]

Ulnar nerve stimulation and adductor pollicis muscle strength

Eikermann[17] demonstrated a reduction in adductor pollicis force in 13 patients with sepsis and MOF, compared to healthy subjects, after limb immobilization. They were able to characterize muscle function by examining force generation at different stimulus frequencies (10–80 Hz), muscle contraction and half relaxation times, as well as the influence of fatigue using low-frequency stimulation.

Although tetanic motor nerve stimulation provides a non-volitional technique to assess muscle force production, stimulation at high frequencies can be painful and hence poorly tolerated by patients.[40] Rather than performing high-frequency nerve stimulation to measure force production during a tetanic contraction, it is possible to assess muscle contractility by measuring the force response to 1 Hz of supramaximal nerve stimulation. Harris et al.[39] demonstrated a reduction in adductor pollicis twitch tension (TwAP) in 12 ICU patients with a mean length of stay of 18.5 days, using electrical and also supramaximal magnetic ulnar nerve stimulation. The technique requires the use of a hand board[39,46] to immobilize the hand and forearm during stimulation (see Figure 47.1). Adductor pollicis force is measured using a strain gauge connected to a metal loop around the proximal phalanx of the thumb, and the ulnar nerve is stimulated between the flexor carpi ulnaris tendon and the ulnar artery. In a larger series using the same technique, Pickles et al. demonstrated a significant reduction in mean (SD) TwAP in 23 ICU patients (5.2 (2.1) N), compared to 29 healthy controls (8.0 (2.1) N).[47]

The use of isometric twitch tension as a measure of strength assumes a constant relationship between the force produced by the single twitch and the force produced by high-frequency stimulation and the resulting tetanic contraction (or a truly MVC). This relationship is known for a wide variety of animal and human skeletal muscles,[48] and the range of TwAP/MVC ratios in normal subjects is narrow (0.08–0.12), suggesting that this relationship is valid.[39] The TwAP technique causes minimal disruption to patient position or treatment and is well tolerated, even by the sickest of patients. Using magnetic, rather than electrical, ulnar nerve stimulation has the advantage that the stimulating coil requires less precise positioning and less surface pressure, and the presence of vascular catheters does not prevent measurements being performed. Also, as the firing threshold for motor fibres is much lower than for sensory fibres with magnetic stimulation,[49] the technique is painless. ES techniques require relatively high stimulating currents to overcome skin resistance. As

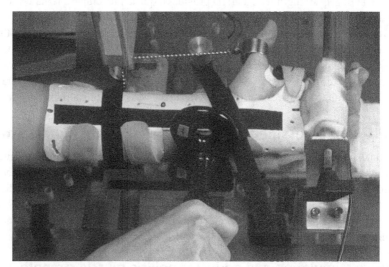

Fig. 47.1 Quadriceps twitch response following supramaximal femoral nerve stimulation in a healthy subject (left) and an ICU patient (right). TwQ is 12 kg in the healthy subject and 6.5 kg in the patient who had been in ICU for 13 days.

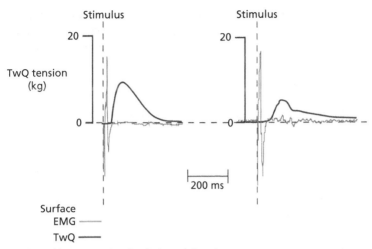

Fig. 47.2 TwAP elicited by magnetic stimulation of the ulnar nerve.

Reproduced with permission from Harris ML, Moxham J, 'Measuring respiratory and limb muscle strength using magnetic stimulation', *British Journal of Intensive Care*, 8, pp. 21–28, copyright 1998, Greycoat Publishing Ltd.

the stimulating currents are produced *in situ* during magnetic stimulation, their intensities can be very low which possibly explains the absence of pain.[50]

Femoral nerve stimulation and quadriceps muscle strength

Supramaximal magnetic stimulation of the femoral nerve allows quadriceps muscle contractility to be assessed.[41,42] The quadriceps is a primary locomotor muscle and of significant functional importance. Measurement in the ICU is, however, difficult, requiring the patient to be moved onto a modified strength-testing trolley[42,51] where they are positioned supine with the legs flexed at 90°. Quadriceps force is measured at the ankle using an inextensible strap attached to a strain gauge. Supramaximal electrical femoral nerve stimulation is possible, but it is technically difficult, and reproducibility is poor.[52] Transcutaneous ES of peripheral femoral nerve branches can be performed using skin surface electrodes placed over the muscle, but the technique is submaximal, as only a fraction of the muscle is activated.[52] Supramaximal magnetic stimulation of the femoral nerve is relatively easy to perform, painless, and reproducible.[41,42] A 70 mm figure-of-eight stimulating coil is placed high in the femoral triangle, lateral to the femoral artery, over the femoral nerve. The quadriceps twitch response (TwQ) can then be recorded, following supramaximal stimulation, to obtain a measure of muscle contractility. Harris et al.[42] demonstrated that mean (SD) TwQ was significantly reduced in 25 ICU patients (3.6 (1.7) kg), compared to 46 healthy control subjects (11.0 (3.1) kg) (see Figure 47.2).

Peroneal nerve stimulation and ankle dorsiflexor muscle strength

Peroneal nerve stimulation allows non-volitional assessment of ankle dorsiflexor muscle strength.[43,44] Ginz et al.[43] demonstrated a reduction in ankle dorsiflexor muscle strength in 19 ICU patients, compared to healthy control subjects, after 7 days of MV. The patients demonstrated reduced torque, shorter contraction time, and prolonged relaxation time, compared to the controls. Peroneal nerve stimulation may be preferable to ulnar nerve stimulation, as access to the site of assessment is generally less restricted than for the adductor pollicis. Seymour et al.[45] have demonstrated that 100 Hz ES of the peroneal nerve is tolerable both in healthy subjects and patients with COPD and that the evoked tetanic contraction force is equal to that obtained during an MVC.[53]

Technical considerations

Supramaximal stimulation, contact area, and temperature

Although providing valuable non-volitional techniques to assess skeletal muscle strength in non-cooperative critical care patients, a standardized approach to nerve stimulation is important to ensure valid measurements are obtained. Stimulation intensity should be supramaximal, ensuring the motor nerve is fully depolarized, leading to complete depolarization and contraction of the entire muscle. During ES, the intensity is increased to a level between 5% and 20% greater than that required to produce a maximal response as indicated by a plateau in the amplitude of the CMAP or in the force response. Stimulus intensity depends both on the current applied and the duration of the pulse (commonly 200 microseconds). Good skin preparation over the site of stimulation is required to optimize electrical contact, and appropriately sized stimulating electrodes that provide the optimal current density for nerve stimulation should be used. The electrode contact area should ideally be 7 mm to 11 mm, with an inter-electrode distance of 3–6 cm and the negative electrode placed distally.[54] Muscle preload should be standardized, as it directly affects force production. When measuring adductor pollicis strength, either a fixed thumb adduction angle (50°)[55] or a predetermined preload (3 g/kg body weight)[56] should be maintained throughout the protocol. Skeletal muscle function is markedly influenced by muscle temperature.[57] Critically ill patients can have impaired peripheral circulation, resulting in low skin and muscle temperature. The adductor pollicis is a small peripheral muscle with little thermal insulation from overlying subcutaneous fat. It is essential therefore to standardize muscle temperature during testing to prevent influences of changing temperature on the mechanical properties of muscle.[55,58] Maximal force production, shortening velocity, and the rate of tension development are reduced and relaxation rate slowed on cooling.[58] Harris et al.[39] immersed the hand and forearm in a water bath at 44°C for 10 min prior to assessment to enable muscle temperature to reach 35°C,[59] and the hand was subsequently kept warm by radiant heat provided by a lamp.

Muscle potentiation

Prior muscle contraction enhances the mechanical response to stimulation, leading to greater force generation, termed potentiation. Potentiation can occur as a result of either prior volitional muscle contraction[60] or non-volitional motor nerve stimulation.[61] The enhancement of the force response is particularly marked at low stimulation frequencies such as the single twitch response. When measuring the 1 Hz twitch response, completely resting the muscle for 20 min prior to measurement produces stable, reproducible, unpotentiated twitch responses, while twitch-on-twitch potentiation can be avoided by using a standardized stimulation protocol with 30 s between twitches.[39] When examining the forces produced over a range of stimulation frequencies, repeated single twitch stimulations, performed until a plateau is reached, is useful to establish a baseline level of potentiation.[62-64] Also, the duration of, and the interval between, trains of stimuli should be considered, so that such stimulation patterns do not, in themselves, induce muscle fatigue. Also, because prolonged stimulation at high frequencies can be painful, stimulating for 1–2 s, with a rest period of 60 s between trains, can be used for the generation of force-frequency curves.

Conclusion

A number of techniques can be used to assess peripheral skeletal muscle strength in ICU patients. Volitional techniques, using scoring systems or portable hand dynamometers, are relatively simple and quick to use and require little or no specialist equipment but can only be applied to conscious and cooperative patients. Such limitations prevent the assessment of muscle weakness early in admission to ICU. Non-volitional techniques remove the volitional component of testing and can provide measures of muscle force production but require specialist equipment. Normative data for comparative purposes are also limited. It is not clear which peripheral muscle best reflects generalized muscle weakness and the strength of the respiratory muscles, including the diaphragm.

Assessment of respiratory muscle strength

Respiratory muscle weakness can lead to difficulties in weaning from MV and prolonged ICU stay. As well as being affected directly by disease, trauma, and CIPNM, respiratory muscle function, in particular, the diaphragm as the principal muscle of inspiration, is also affected indirectly by the consequences of lung disease and the application of positive pressure ventilation on lung volume. Diaphragm length is reduced by hyperinflation,[65] and, as a consequence, its pressure-generating capacity is decreased.[66–70] This loss in pressure-generating capacity is principally due to a reduction in the ability of the diaphragm to lower intrathoracic pressure.[71]

Technical considerations for measuring pressure generation

Direct assessment of respiratory muscle strength is difficult because of the anatomical location of the muscles. Force production is assessed indirectly by measurement of pressure at the airway opening, which reflects global respiratory muscle function, or by invasive measurements of intrathoracic and intra-abdominal pressure which can provide assessment specific to the diaphragm, the transdiaphragmatic pressure. Contraction of the diaphragm results in a fall in intrathoracic pressure, which can be reliably estimated by measuring the pressure in the lower third of the oesophagus (Poes),[72] and an increase in abdominal pressure commonly assessed by measuring pressure in the stomach, gastric pressure (Pgas).[73] Transdiaphragmatic pressure is the difference between Poes and Pgas and is regarded as the 'gold standard' measurement of diaphragm function. A range of pressure catheters have been used to record Poes and Pgas, including air-filled pressure balloons,[74,75] fluid-filled,[76] and solid-state.[77,78] Regardless of the technique, it is important to determine the operating characteristics of the pressure-recording system and ensure that the frequency response is adequate. This is of particular importance when recording the diaphragm pressure (Pdi) responses evoked by phrenic nerve stimulation or during the sniff manoeuvre. In addition, the volume of air used to fill balloon catheters may need to be adjusted when making measurements in supine ICU patients.[79] Correct placement of the pressure catheters is important to ensure accurate measurement of Pdi.[75,80] A positive deflection of Pgas on palpation of the abdomen or during an inspiratory effort indicates placement of the catheter in the stomach. Agreement of Poes and mouth pressures within 10% during an inspiratory effort against an occluded airway[82] indicates correct positioning of the oesophageal catheter. Placement of catheters can also be difficult when a tracheostomy or an ETT is in place, and, under such circumstances, sedation of the patient may be required. Sedative drugs can affect diaphragm contractility, and the investigator can either accept this as a limitation of the data or wait for the effects of the drugs to wear off before assessment is undertaken. Placement under direct vision, using a bronchoscope positioned in the pharynx, can be helpful in some patients.

Non-invasive volitional testing

There are a range of non-invasive and invasive, volitional and non-volitional tests available to assess diaphragm and global inspiratory and expiratory muscle strength. Simple non-invasive, volitional measures of strength can be obtained by recording the pressure generated at the mouth or ETT during a maximal sustained inspiratory (Pimax) or expiratory (Pemax) effort[81] or in the nostril during a maximal sniff—sniff nasal inspiratory pressure (SNIP).[82–84] The inspiratory manoeuvres can be combined with invasive measurements of nasopharyngeal,[82] oesophageal (Sniff Poes),[85] or transdiaphragmatic (Sniff Pdi)[83,86] pressures. In addition to performing a maximal effort, a number of alternative inspiratory manoeuvres have been used.[86–88] A unidirectional valve attached to the ETT which allows expiration, but not inspiration, has been used to improve the assessment of inspiratory muscle strength.[89–91]

Invasive non-volitional testing

Invasive measures overcome the problems associated with impaired pressure transmission in obstructive lung disease or upper airway congestion by measuring pressure *in situ*; however, all volitional tests require the patient to make a maximal effort. Volitional tests are therefore of limited value in the ICU, unless the results are unequivocally normal. Standardized procedures and normal values are available[92] (see Table 47.1). By contrast, non-volitional techniques

Table 47.1 Normal values and cut-offs for inspiratory and expiratory muscle strength, as calculated by Steier et al. (2007)[115]

Test	Sex	Normal (mean (SD)) (cmH$_2$O)	Cut-off (cmH$_2$O)	Reference
Pimax	M	106 (31)	45	Wilson et al. (1984)[126]
	F	73 (21)	30	
Pemax	M	147 (34)	80	Wilson et al. (1984)[126]
	F	92 (16)	60	
Sniff Poes	M	105 (26)	55	Laroche et al. (1988)[85]
	F	92 (22)	50	
SNIP	M	96	50[†]	Heritier et al. (1994)[125]
	F	84	45[†]	
Sniff Pdi	M	148	100	Miller et al. (1985)[83]
	F	121	70	
TwPdi	M and F	28 (5)	18	Luo et al. (2002)[114]
TwT10	M and F	39.4 (26.6)[*]	16	Steier et al. (2007)[115]

M, male; F, female.

[*]Median and interquartile range.

[†]Lower limit of normal cut-off derived using the values from the Sniff Poes, multiplied by 0.91; the ratio of Sniff Pnasal/Sniff Poes determined by Heritier et al.[125]

are independent of patient cooperation and motivation, and, in addition to the assessment of diaphragm strength,[75,93,94] techniques are available to assess expiratory[95–98] and accessory muscle[99,100] strength, although the latter techniques have limited normative data and their applicability in critically ill patients remains untested.

Recording the Pdi response evoked by phrenic nerve stimulation provides a robust effort-independent technique to assess diaphragm strength. Ideally, the Pdi response would be recorded for a range of stimulus frequencies to enable the force-frequency curve to be constructed, thereby providing a comprehensive assessment of diaphragm function. Such stimulation, however, is uncomfortable and not tolerated by patients. As for peripheral skeletal muscles, it is possible to assess diaphragm contractility by measuring the twitch response to 1 Hz of supramaximal nerve stimulation (twitch Pdi (TwPdi)), the amplitude of which is proportional to maximal tetanic tension, the true diaphragm strength.

The phrenic nerves can be stimulated bilaterally to assess overall diaphragm strength or unilaterally to assess individual hemidiaphragm/phrenic nerve function. Transcutaneous ES is the classical technique used for phrenic nerve stimulation and provides a supramaximal stimulus which can be localized to the phrenic nerve.[101,102] The stimulating electrodes are positioned over the phrenic nerve behind the sternocleidomastoid over scalenous muscles.[103] Accurate, reproducible measurements, using bilateral ES, have proved difficult in the ICU, as the technique requires the precise location of the phrenic nerve to be identified with the stimulating electrode and subsequently maintained to achieve repeated supramaximal stimulations. Obesity, anatomic deformity, and indwelling vascular catheters can obstruct access to the point of stimulation. Reduced or absent TwPdi may result therefore from abnormal muscle or nerve function or failure to locate and stimulate the nerve. This can lead to diagnostic uncertainty and repeated attempts to locate and stimulate the phrenic nerves, which may be painful and lead to twitch potentiation.[104] Because of these limitations, the technique is sufficiently imprecise that the lower limit of normal overlaps with diaphragm weakness of both mild and moderate severity.[102]

Many of the problems associated with ES can be overcome using magnetic phrenic nerve stimulation.[11,93,94,105,106] The relatively less tightly focused nature of the magnetic field during magnetic stimulation allows easier location of the phrenic nerves, making the technique less technically demanding. Also, because the stimulating currents are produced *in situ* by the magnetic field, they are much lower than with ES, and hence the technique is relatively painless. The original technique involved bilateral stimulation of the cervical nerve roots by placing a coil over the cervical spine and has been used clinically to assess diaphragm strength.[71,107,108] As cervical magnetic stimulation (CMS) requires the placement of the coil over the cervical spine, it can be difficult in supine ICU patients. In addition, it may not always be possible to achieve supramaximal phrenic nerve stimulation,[105] and the technique may also recruit extradiaphragmatic muscles.[105,108] Similowski et al.[105] demonstrated activation of the deltoid, trapezius, and rhomboid muscles, following CMS. Current practice is bilateral, anterolateral magnetic phrenic nerve stimulation (BAMPS), using two 43 mm figure-of-eight coils placed over the phrenic nerves on the anterolateral aspects of the neck at the level of the cricoid cartilage.[93] Such an approach allows supramaximal phrenic nerve stimulation to be performed in supine ICU patients,[47,75,110] and all studies have reported significant reductions in diaphragm contractility in the critically ill (see Table 47.2). Both bilateral and unilateral phrenic nerve stimulation can be performed (see Figure 47.3). Bilateral TwPdi is thought to provide a better indication of overall diaphragm strength than unilateral TwPdi. Bilateral TwPdi is 25–30% greater than the sum of TwPdi when the left and right phrenic nerves are stimulated separately.[111] During unilateral phrenic nerve stimulation, the stimulated hemidiaphragm contracts and descends, while the contralateral hemidiaphragm ascends, the resulting

Table 47.2 Summary of studies using bilateral magnetic phrenic nerve stimulation to non-volitionally assess diaphragm strength in ICU patients

	Number of patients studied	Bilateral TwPdi (cmH$_2$O)	Duration of ICU stay (days)	Percentage of patients with TwPdi <18 cmH$_2$O*
Watson et al. (2001)[75]	25	10.8	25	88%
Laghi et al. (2003)[110]	19	9.6	23	89%
Cattapan et al. (2003)[127]	13	10.4	13	92%
Pickles et al. (2005)[47]	23	11.9	18	91%
Total/mean	72	10.7	19.8	90%

*Lower limit of normal TwPdi 18 cmH$_2$O (Luo et al. 2002).[114]

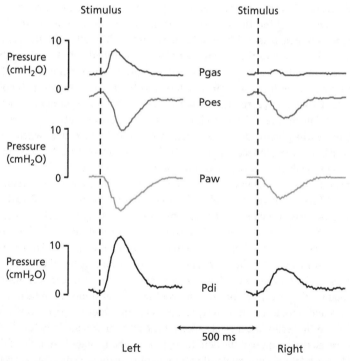

Fig. 47.3 Representative traces of diaphragm force responses following left and right unilateral ante-rolateral magnetic phrenic nerve stimulation in a critically ill 15-year-old patient. The difference in TwPdi after left and right phrenic nerve stimulation was >50%. *Pgas*, gastric pressure; *Paw*, airway pressure; *Poes*, oesophageal pressure; *Pdi*, transdiaphragmatic pressure.

TwPdi being dependent upon the compliance of the unstimulated hemidiaphragm and of the abdominal wall.[111,112] Patients are generally studied supine or semi-recumbent after 20 min of relaxed breathing to minimize the effect of potentiation.[104] Stimulations are performed at end-expiration to control for the effect of lung volume on diaphragm contractility,[113] and the values reported for unilateral and bilateral stimulation are the average of at least five stimulations. Normal values for unilateral and bilateral TwPdi in healthy subjects are available[114,115] (see Table 47.1). Values are reported for the seated posture, but the supine posture makes little difference to TwPdi values.[116] In addition, a recent meal can influence the TwPdi, probably due to a change in abdominal compliance,[117] hence studies in intensive care are best performed at least 1–2 hours after nasogastric feeding has been stopped. A manual or automated occlusion valve can be inserted into the ventilator circuit between the ETT or tracheostomy and ventilator manifold.[118] Occluding the airway during phrenic nerve stimulation ensures a quasi-isometric contraction of the diaphragm. Although BAMPS at 100% stimulator output has been shown to be supramaximal, it is good practice to demonstrate supramaximality by administering a series of stimulations at 95% and 90% as well as 100% of stimulator output. There should be no appreciable difference (<5%) in the TwPdi response across these stimulus intensities.

Non-invasive, non-volitional testing

The insertion of pressure catheters to measure Pdi is not always possible in intubated/tracheostomized patients or may be contraindicated. A non-invasive alternative is the measurement of twitch airway pressure (TwPaw)[75,119] during a brief occlusion. Unlike in spontaneously breathing subjects, where glottic closure can adversely affect the transmission of pressure to the airway opening, intubation/ tracheostomy removes the influence of the upper airway on pressure transmission, and hence reliable TwPaw measurements can be obtained. TwPaw reflects TwPoes, rather than TwPdi [75,120] (see Figure 47.3), and this can make interpretation of the TwPaw response more difficult. TwPoes is usually 50–60% of the overall TwPdi. Hence, if TwPdi is reduced by disease, trauma, or ICUAW, TwPaw may be small and difficult to measure. In addition, increases in lung volume, as a result of elevated end-expiratory pressure, can disproportionately diminish TwPoes and hence TwPaw.[70]

Expiratory muscle function

As with the inspiratory muscles, it is possible to assess expiratory muscle function non-volitionally. The principal expiratory muscles are those of the abdominal wall, hence measuring Pgas during abdominal muscle contraction provides a measure of expiratory muscle strength. Unlike ES,[95] magnetic stimulation of the thoracic nerve roots, using a 90 mm double, circular coil placed approximately over the tenth thoracic vertebra, is relatively painless and activates a substantially greater proportion of the abdominal musculature, some supramaximally.[121] Stimulation is performed at end-expiration, and, although there are few normative data,[115] the technique is well tolerated by patients and has been used to demonstrate weakness in amyotrophic lateral sclerosis[122] and tetraplegia.[123] There are no data available for ICU patients.

Conclusion

Measurement of Pimax and Pemax are the most widely used techniques to assess respiratory muscle strength in ICU patients and are applicable to patients who can make some respiratory effort. As with all volitional techniques, however, reliability is limited, as many ICU patients cannot perform maximal manoeuvres. Phrenic nerve stimulation allows diaphragm and phrenic nerve function to be assessed directly, without patient cooperation, and normative values for comparative purposes are available. Magnetic phrenic nerve stimulation is well tolerated by ICU patients, can be performed in the presence of vascular catheters, and can be used to document respiratory muscle weakness and track progression in critically ill patients.

References

1 Berek K, Margreiter J, Willeit J, Berek A, Schmutzhard E, Mutz NJ. Polyneuropathies in critically ill patients: a prospective evaluation. *Intensive Care Med* 1996;**22**:849–55.

2 Herridge MS, Cheung AM, Tansey CM, et al. One-year outcomes in survivors of the acute respiratory distress syndrome. *N Engl J Med* 2003;**348**:683–93.

3 De Jonghe B, Bastuji-Garin S, Durand MC, et al. Respiratory weakness is associated with limb weakness and delayed weaning in critical illness. *Crit Care Med* 2007;**35**:2007–15.

4 Leijten FS, Harinck-de Weerd JE, Poortvliet DC, de Weerd AW. The role of polyneuropathy in motor convalescence after prolonged mechanical ventilation. *JAMA* 1995;**274**:1221–5.

5 Garnacho-Montero J, Madrazo-Osuna J, Garcia-Garmendia JL, et al. Critical illness polyneuropathy: risk factors and clinical consequences. A cohort study in septic patients. *Intensive Care Med* 2001;**27**:1288–96.

6 Coakley JH, Nagendran K, Yarwood GD, Honavar M, Hinds CJ. Patterns of neurophysiological abnormality in prolonged critical illness. *Intensive Care Med* 1998;**24**:801–7.

7 Fletcher SN, Kennedy DD, Ghosh IR, et al. Persistent neuromuscular and neurophysiologic abnormalities in long-term survivors of prolonged critical illness. *Crit Care Med* 2003;**31**:1012–16.

8 Diehl JL, Lofaso F, Deleuze P, Similowski T, Lemaire F, Brochard L. Clinically relevant diaphragmatic dysfunction after cardiac operations. *J Thorac Cardiovasc Surg* 1994;**107**:487–98.

9 Ferdinande P, Bruyninckx F, Van Raemdonck D, Daenen W, Verleden G. Phrenic nerve dysfunction after heart-lung and lung transplantation. *J Heart Lung Transplant* 2004;**23**:105–9.

10 McAlister VC, Grant DR, Roy A, et al. Right phrenic nerve injury in orthotopic liver transplantation. *Transplantation* 1993;**55**:826–30.

11 Rafferty GF, Greenough A, Manczur TI, et al. Magnetic phrenic nerve stimulation to assess diaphragm function in children following liver transplantation. *Pediatr Crit Care Med* 2001;**2**:122–6.

12 Glenn WW, Holcomb WG, Shaw RK, Hogan JF, Holschuh KR. Long-term ventilatory support by diaphragm pacing in quadriplegia. *Ann Surg* 1976;**183**:566–77.

13 Levine S, Nguyen T, Taylor N, et al. Rapid disuse atrophy of diaphragm fibers in mechanically ventilated humans. *N Engl J Med* 2008;**358**:1327–35.

14 Herridge MS, Tansey CM, Matte A, et al. Functional disability 5 years after acute respiratory distress syndrome. *N Engl J Med* 2011;**364**:1293–304.

15 Latronico N, Bolton CF. Critical illness polyneuropathy and myopathy: a major cause of muscle weakness and paralysis. *Lancet Neurol* 2011;**10**:931–41.

16 De Jonghe B, Sharshar T, Lefaucheur JP, et al. Paresis acquired in the intensive care unit: A prospective multicenter study. *JAMA* 2002;**288**:2859–67.

17 Eikermann M, Koch G, Gerwig M, et al. Muscle force and fatigue in patients with sepsis and multiorgan failure. *Intensive Care Med* 2006;**32**:251–9.

18 Zifko UA, Zipko HT, Bolton CF. Clinical and electrophysiological findings in critical illness polyneuropathy. *J Neurol Sci* 1998;**159**:186–93.

19 Hughes RA, Newsom-Davis JM, Perkin GD, Pierce JM. Controlled trial prednisolone in acute polyneuropathy. *Lancet* 1978;**2**:750–3.

20 Kleyweg RP, van der Meche FG, Meulstee J. Treatment of guillain-barre syndrome with high-dose gammaglobulin. *Neurology* 1988;**38**:1639–41.

21 Stevens RD, Marshall SA, Cornblath DR, et al. A framework for diagnosing and classifying intensive care unit-acquired weakness. *Crit Care Med* 2009;**37**:S299–308.

22 Fan E, Ciesla ND, Truong AD, Bhoopathi V, Zeger SL, Needham DM. Inter-rater reliability of manual muscle strength testing in icu survivors and simulated patients. *Intensive Care Med* 2010;**36**:1038–43.

23 Kleyweg RP, van der Meche FG, Schmitz PI. Interobserver agreement in the assessment of muscle strength and functional abilities in Guillain–Barré syndrome. *Muscle Nerve* 1991;**14**:1103–9.

24 Ali NA, O'Brien JM, Jr, Hoffmann SP, et al. Acquired weakness, handgrip strength, and mortality in critically ill patients. *Am J Respir Crit Care Med* 2008;**178**:261–8.

25 Hough CL, Herridge MS. Long-term outcome after acute lung injury. *Curr Opin Crit Care* 2012;**18**:8–15.

26 Bohannon RW. Measuring knee extensor muscle strength. *Am J Phys Med Rehabil* 2001;**80**:13–18.

27 Hough CL, Lieu BK, Caldwell ES. Manual muscle strength testing of critically ill patients: feasibility and interobserver agreement. *Crit Care* 2011;**15**:R43.

28 Mills KR. Wasting, weakness, and the MRC scale in the first dorsal interosseous muscle. *J Neurol Neurosurg Psychiatry* 1997;**62**:541–2.

29 Bohannon RW. Reference values for extremity muscle strength obtained by hand-held dynamometry from adults aged 20 to 79 years. *Arch Phys Med Rehabil* 1997;**78**:26–32.

30 Vanpee G, Segers J, Van Mechelen H, et al. The interobserver agreement of handheld dynamometry for muscle strength assessment in critically ill patients. *Crit Care Med* 2011;**39**:1929–34.

31 Hayes K, Callanan M, Walton J, Paxinos A, Murrell GA. Shoulder instability: management and rehabilitation. *J Orthop Sports Phys Ther* 2002;**32**:497–509.

32 O'Shea SD, Taylor NF, Paratz JD. Measuring muscle strength for people with chronic obstructive pulmonary disease: Retest reliability of hand-held dynamometry. *Arch Phys Med Rehabil* 2007;**88**:32–6.

33 Beck M, Giess R, Wurffel W, Magnus T, Ochs G, Toyka KV. Comparison of maximal voluntary isometric contraction and drachman's hand-held dynamometry in evaluating patients with amyotrophic lateral sclerosis. *Muscle Nerve* 1999;**22**:1265–70.

34 Visser J, Mans E, de Visser M, et al. Comparison of maximal voluntary isometric contraction and hand-held dynamometry in measuring muscle strength of patients with progressive lower motor neuron syndrome. *Neuromuscul Disord* 2003;**13**:744–50.

35 Martin HJ, Yule V, Syddall HE, Dennison EM, Cooper C, Aihie Sayer A. Is hand-held dynamometry useful for the measurement of quadriceps strength in older people? A comparison with the gold standard bodex dynamometry. *Gerontology* 2006;**52**:154–9.

36 Mathiowetz V, Kashman N, Volland G, Weber K, Dowe M, Rogers S. Grip and pinch strength: normative data for adults. *Arch Phys Med Rehabil* 1985;**66**:69–74.

37 Mathiowetz V, Wiemer DM, Federman SM. Grip and pinch strength: norms for 6- to 19-year-olds. *Am J Occup Ther* 1986;**40**:705–11.

38 Puh U. Age-related and sex-related differences in hand and pinch grip strength in adults. *Int J Rehabil Res* 2010;**33**:4–11.

39 Harris ML, Luo YM, Watson AC, et al. Adductor pollicis twitch tension assessed by magnetic stimulation of the ulnar nerve. *Am J Respir Crit Care Med* 2000;**162**:240–5.

40 Finn PJ, Plank LD, Clark MA, Connolly AB, Hill GL. Assessment of involuntary muscle function in patients after critical injury or severe sepsis. *JPEN J Parenter Enteral Nutr* 1996;**20**:332–7.

41 Polkey MI, Kyroussis D, Hamnegard CH, Mills GH, Green M, Moxham J. Quadriceps strength and fatigue assessed by magnetic stimulation of the femoral nerve in man. *Muscle Nerve* 1996;**19**:549–55.

42 Harris ML. *Magnetic nerve stimulation for the assessment of limb and respiratory muscle contractility in normal subjects and patients.* London: Department of Respiratory Medicine and Allergy, University of London; 2002. p. 229.

43 Ginz HF, Iaizzo PA, Girard T, Urwyler A, Pargger H. Decreased isometric skeletal muscle force in critically ill patients. *Swiss Med Wkly* 2005;**135**:555–61.

44 Ginz HF, Iaizzo PA, Urwyler A, Pargger H. Use of non-invasive-stimulated muscle force assessment in long-term critically ill patients: a future standard in the intensive care unit? *Acta Anaesthesiol Scand* 2008;**52**:20–7.

45 Seymour JM, Ward K, Raffique A, et al. Quadriceps and ankle dorsiflexor strength in chronic obstructive pulmonary disease. *Muscle Nerve* 2012;**46**:548–54.

46 Merton PA. Voluntary strength and fatigue. *J Physiol* 1954;**123**:553–64.

47 Pickles J, Kondili E, Harikumar G, et al. Respiratory and limb muscle strength following critical illness. *Am J Respir Crit Care Med* 2005;**171**:A787.

48 Close RI. Dynamic properties of mammalian skeletal muscles. *Physiol Rev* 1972;**52**:129–97.

49 Panizza M, Nilsson J, Roth BJ, Basser PJ, Hallett M. Relevance of stimulus duration for activation of motor and sensory fibers: implications for the study of h-reflexes and magnetic stimulation. *Electroencephalogr Clin Neurophysiol* 1992;**85**:22–9.

50 Barker AT, Freeston IL, Jalinous R, Jarratt JA. Magnetic stimulation of the human brain and peripheral nervous system: an introduction and the results of an initial clinical evaluation. *Neurosurgery* 1987;**20**:100–9.

51 Harris ML, Watson AC, Moxham J. Assessment of respiratory and limb muscle function in the intensive care. In: Vincent JL (ed.) *Yearbook of intensive care and emergency medicine*. Berlin, Heidelberg GmbH: Springer-Verlag; 1999. pp. 309–21.

52 Edwards RH, Young A, Hosking GP, Jones DA. Human skeletal muscle function: description of tests and normal values. *Clin Sci Mol Med* 1977;**52**:283–90.

53 Bigland-Ritchie B, Jones DA, Woods JJ. Excitation frequency and muscle fatigue: electrical responses during human voluntary and stimulated contractions. *Exp Neurol* 1979;**64**:414–27.

54 Fuchs-Buder T, Claudius C, Skovgaard LT, Eriksson LI, Mirakhur RK, Viby-Mogensen J. Good clinical research practice in pharmacodynamic studies of neuromuscular blocking agents II: the Stockholm Revision. *Acta Anaesthesiol Scand* 2007;**51**:789–808.

55 De Ruiter CJ, De Haan A. Temperature effect on the force/velocity relationship of the fresh and fatigued human adductor pollicis muscle. *Pflugers Arch* 2000;**440**:163–70.

56 Bittner EA, Martyn JA, George E, Frontera WR, Eikermann M. Measurement of muscle strength in the intensive care unit. *Crit Care Med* 2009;**37**:S321–30.

57 Wiles CM, Edwards RH. The effect of temperature, ischaemia and contractile activity on the relaxation rate of human muscle. *Clin Physiol* 1982;**2**:485–97.

58 de Ruiter CJ, Jones DA, Sargeant AJ, de Haan A. Temperature effect on the rates of isometric force development and relaxation in the fresh and fatigued human adductor pollicis muscle. *Exp Physiol* 1999;**84**:1137–50.

59 Edwards RH, Hill DK, Jones DA, Merton PA. Fatigue of long duration in human skeletal muscle after exercise. *J Physiol* 1977;**272**:769–78.

60 Vandervoort AA, Quinlan J, McComas AJ. Twitch potentiation after voluntary contraction. *Exp Neurol* 1983;**81**:141–52.

61 O'Leary DD, Hope K, Sale DG. Posttetanic potentiation of human dorsiflexors. *J Appl Physiol* 1997;**83**:2131–8.

62 Krarup C. Enhancement and diminution of mechanical tension evoked by staircase and by tetanus in rat muscle. *J Physiol* 1981;**311**:355–72.

63 Binder-Macleod SA, Dean JC, Ding J. Electrical stimulation factors in potentiation of human quadriceps femoris. *Muscle Nerve* 2002;**25**:271–9.

64 Kopman AF, Kumar S, Klewicka MM, Neuman GG. The staircase phenomenon: Implications for monitoring of neuromuscular transmission. *Anesthesiology* 2001;**95**:403–7.

65 Cassart M, Pettiaux N, Gevenois PA, Paiva M, Estenne M. Effect of chronic hyperinflation on diaphragm length and surface area. *Am J Respir Crit Care Med* 1997;**156**:504–8.

66 Rahn H, Otis AB, et al. The pressure-volume diagram of the thorax and lung. *Am J Physiol* 1946;**146**: 161–78.

67 Wanke T, Schenz G, Zwick H, Popp W, Ritschka L, Flicker M. Dependence of maximal sniff generated mouth and transdiaphragmatic pressures on lung volume. *Thorax* 1990;**45**:352–5.

68 Smith J, Bellemare F. Effect of lung volume on in vivo contraction characteristics of human diaphragm. *J Appl Physiol* 1987;**62**:1893–900.

69 Hamnegard CH, Wragg S, Mills G, et al. The effect of lung volume on transdiaphragmatic pressure. *Eur Respir J* 1995;**8**:1532–6.

70 Polkey MI, Hamnegard CH, Hughes PD, Rafferty GF, Green M, Moxham J. Influence of acute lung volume change on contractile properties of human diaphragm. *J Appl Physiol* 1998;**85**:1322–8.

71 Polkey MI, Kyroussis D, Hamnegard CH, Mills GH, Green M, Moxham J. Diaphragm strength in chronic obstructive pulmonary disease. *Am J Respir Crit Care Med* 1996;**154**:1310–17.

72 Cherniack RM, Farhi LE, Armstrong BW, Proctor DF. A comparison of esophageal and intrapleural pressure in man. *J Appl Physiol* 1955;**8**:203–11.

73 Tzelepis GE, Nasiff L, McCool FD, Hammond J. Transmission of pressure within the abdomen. *J Appl Physiol* 1996;**81**:1111–14.

74 Milic-Emili J, Mead J, Turner JM, Glauser EM. Improved technique for estimating pleural pressure from esophageal balloons. *J Appl Physiol* 1964;**19**:1101–6.

75 Watson AC, Hughes PD, Harris ML, et al. Measurement of twitch transdiaphragmatic, esophageal, and endotracheal tube pressure with bilateral anterolateral magnetic phrenic nerve stimulation in patients in the intensive care unit. *Crit Care Med* 2001;**29**:1325–31.

76 Wanke T, Formanek D, Schenz G, Popp W, Gatol H, Zwick H. Mechanical load on the ventilatory muscles during an incremental cycle ergometer test. *Eur Respir J* 1991;**4**:385–92.

77 Evans SA, Watson L, Cowley AJ, Johnston ID, Kinnear WJ. Normal range for transdiaphragmatic pressures during sniffs with catheter mounted transducers. *Thorax* 1993;**48**:750–3.

78 Stell IM, Tompkins S, Lovell AT, Goldstone JC, Moxham J. An in vivo comparison of a catheter mounted pressure transducer system with conventional balloon catheters. *Eur Respir J* 1999;**13**:1158–63.

79 Knowles JH, Hong SK, Rahn H. Possible errors using esophageal balloon in determination of pressure-volume characteristics of the lung and thoracic cage. *J Appl Physiol* 1959;**14**:525–30.

80 Baydur A, Behrakis PK, Zin WA, Jaeger M, Milic Emili J. A simple method for assessing the validity of the esophageal balloon technique. *Am Rev Respir Dis* 1982;**126**:788–91.

81 Black LF, Hyatt RE. Maximal respiratory pressures: normal values and relationship to age and sex. *Am Rev Respir Dis* 1969;**99**:696–702.

82 Koulouris N, Mulvey DA, Laroche CM, Sawicka EH, Green M, Moxham J. The measurement of inspiratory muscle strength by sniff esophageal, nasopharyngeal, and mouth pressures. *Am Rev Respir Dis* 1989;**139**:641–6.

83 Miller JM, Moxham J, Green M. The maximal sniff in the assessment of diaphragm function in man. *Clin-Sci* 1985;**69**:91–6.

84 Uldry C, Fitting JW. Maximal values of sniff nasal inspiratory pressure in healthy subjects. *Thorax* 1995;**50**:371–5.

85 Laroche CM, Mier AK, Moxham J, Green M. The value of sniff esophageal pressures in the assessment of global inspiratory muscle strength. *Am Rev Respir Dis* 1988;**138**:598–603.

86 Nava S, Ambrosino N, Crotti P, Fracchia C, Rampulla C. Recruitment of some respiratory muscles during three maximal inspiratory manoeuvres. *Thorax* 1993;**48**:702–7.

87 Laporta D, Grassino A. Assessment of transdiaphragmatic pressure in humans. *J Appl Physiol* 1985; **58**:1469–76.

88 Gandevia SC, Gorman RB, McKenzie DK, Southon FC. Dynamic changes in human diaphragm length: maximal inspiratory and expulsive efforts studied with sequential radiography. *J Physiol* 1992;**457**:167–76.

89 Marini JJ, Smith TC, Lamb V. Estimation of inspiratory muscle strength in mechanically ventilated patients: the measurement of maximal inspiration pressure. *J Crit Care* 1986;**1**:32–8.

90 Caruso P, Friedrich C, Denari SD, Ruiz SA, Deheinzelin D. The unidirectional valve is the best method to determine maximal inspiratory pressure during weaning. *Chest* 1999;**115**:1096–101.

91 Harikumar G, Moxham J, Greenough A, Rafferty GF. Measurement of maximal inspiratory pressure in ventilated children. *Pediatric Pulmonology* 2008;**43**:1085–91.

92 American Thoracic Society/European Respiratory Society. ATS/ERS Statement on respiratory muscle testing. *Am J Respir Crit Care Med* 2002;**166**:518–624.

93 Mills GH, Kyroussis D, Hamnegard CH, Polkey MI, Green M, Moxham J. Bilateral magnetic stimulation of the phrenic nerves from an anterolateral approach. *Am J Respir Crit Care Med* 1996;**154**:1099–105.

94 Mills GH, Kyroussis D, Hamnegard CH, Wragg S, Moxham J, Green M. Unilateral magnetic stimulation of the phrenic nerve. *Thorax* 1995;**50**:1162–72.

95 Mier A, Brophy C, Estenne M, Moxham J, Green M, De Troyer A. Action of abdominal muscles on rib cage in humans. *J Appl Physiol* 1985;**58**:1438–43.

96 Kyroussis D, Polkey MI, Mills GH, Hughes PD, Moxham J, Green M. Simulation of cough in man by magnetic stimulation of the thoracic nerve roots. *Am J Respir Crit Care Med* 1997;**156**:1696–9.

97 Polkey MI, Luo Y, Guleria R, Hamnegard CH, Green M, Moxham J. Functional magnetic stimulation of the abdominal muscles in humans. *Am J Respir Crit Care Med* 1999;**160**:513–22.

98 Suzuki J, Tanaka R, Yan S, Chen R, Macklem PT, Kayser B. Assessment of abdominal muscle contractility, strength, and fatigue. *Am J Respir Crit Care Med* 1999;**159**:1052–60.

99 Moxham J, Wiles CM, Newham D, Edwards RH. Sternomastoid muscle function and fatigue in man. *Clin Sci (Lond)* 1980;**59**:463–8.

100 Peche R, Estenne M, Gevenois PA, Brassinne E, Yernault JC, De Troyer A. Sternomastoid muscle size and strength in patients with severe chronic obstructive pulmonary disease. *Am J Respir Crit Care Med* 1996;**153**:422–5.

101 Bellemare F, Biglandritchie B. Assessment of human diaphragm strength and activation using phrenic-nerve stimulation. *Respir Physiol* 1984;**58**:263–77.

102 Mier A, Brophy C, Moxham J, Green M. Twitch pressures in the assessment of diaphragm weakness. *Thorax* 1989;**44**:990–6.

103 Sarnoff SJ, Sarnoff LC, Wittenberger JL. Electrophrenic respiration. VII. The motor point of the phrenic nerve in relation to external stimulation. *Surg Gynecol Obstet* 1951;**93**:190–6.

104 Wragg S, Hamnegard C, Road J, et al. Potentiation of diaphragmatic twitch after voluntary contraction in normal subjects. *Thorax* 1994;**49**:1234–7.

105 Similowski T, Fleury B, Launois S, Cathala HP, Bouche P, Derenne JP. Cervical magnetic stimulation: a new painless method for bilateral phrenic nerve stimulation in conscious humans. *J Appl Physiol* 1989;**67**:1311–18.

106 Rafferty GF, Greenough A, Dimitriou G, et al. Assessment of neonatal diaphragm function using magnetic stimulation of the phrenic nerves. *Am J Respir Crit Care Med* 2000;**162**:2337–40.

107 Hamnegard CH, Wragg SD, Mills GH, et al. Clinical assessment of diaphragm strength by cervical magnetic stimulation of the phrenic nerves. *Thorax* 1996;**51**:1239–42.

108 Hughes PD, Polkey MI, Harrus ML, Coats AJ, Moxham J, Green M. Diaphragm strength in chronic heart failure. *Am J Respir Crit Care Med* 1999;**160**:529–34.

109 Laghi F, Harrison MJ, Tobin MJ. Comparison of magnetic and electrical phrenic nerve stimulation in assessment of diaphragmatic contractility. *J Appl Physiol* 1996;**80**:1731–42.

110 Laghi F, Cattapan SE, Jubran A, et al. Is weaning failure caused by low-frequency fatigue of the diaphragm? *Am J Respir Crit Care Med* 2003;**167**:120–7.

111 Bellemare F, Bigland Ritchie B, Woods JJ. Contractile properties of the human diaphragm in vivo. *J Appl Physiol* 1986;**61**:1153–61.

112 **Merton PA.** Voluntary strength and fatique. *J Physiol (Lond)* 1954;**123**:553–64.

113 **Grassino A, Goldman MD, Mead J, Sears TA.** Mechanics of the human diaphragm during voluntary contraction: Statics. *J Appl Physiol* 1978;**44**:829–39.

114 **Luo YM, Hart N, Mustfa N, et al.** Reproducibility of twitch and sniff transdiaphragmatic pressures. *Respir Physiol Neurobiol* 2002;**132**:301–6.

115 **Steier J, Kaul S, Seymour J, et al.** The value of multiple tests of respiratory muscle strength. *Thorax* 2007;**62**:975–80.

116 **Mier A, Brophy C, Moxham J, Green M.** Influence of lung volume and rib cage configuration on transdiaphragmatic pressure during phrenic nerve stimulation in man. *Respir Physiol* 1990;**80**:193–202.

117 **Man WD, Luo YM, Mustfa N, et al.** Postprandial effects on twitch transdiaphragmatic pressure. *Eur Respir J* 2002;**20**:577–80.

118 **Spicer M, Hughes P, Green M.** A non-invasive system to evaluate diaphragmatic strength in ventilated patients. *Physiol Meas* 1997;**18**:355–61.

119 **Rafferty GF, Mustfa N, Man WD, et al.** Twitch airway pressure elicited by magnetic phrenic nerve stimulation in anesthetized healthy children. *Pediatr Pulmonol* 2005;**40**:141–7.

120 **Hamnegaard CH, Wragg S, Kyroussis D, et al.** Mouth pressure in response to magnetic stimulation of the phrenic nerves. *Thorax* 1995;**50**:620–4.

121 **Taylor BJ, How SC, Romer LM.** Exercise-induced abdominal muscle fatigue in healthy humans. *J Appl Physiol* 2006;**100**:1554–62.

122 **Polkey MI, Lyall RA, Green M, Nigel Leigh P, Moxham J.** Expiratory muscle function in amyotrophic lateral sclerosis. *Am J Respir Crit Care Med* 1998;**158**:734–41.

123 **Estenne M, Pinet C, De Troyer A.** Abdominal muscle strength in patients with tetraplegia. *Am J Respir Crit Care Med* 2000;**161**:707–12.

124 **Harris ML, Moxham J.** Measuring respiratory and limb muscle strength using magnetic stimulation. *Brit J Intens Care* 1998;**8**:21–8.

125 **Heritier F, Rahm F, Pasche P, Fitting JW.** Sniff nasal inspiratory pressure. A noninvasive assessment of inspiratory muscle strength. *Am J Respir Crit Care Med* 1994;**150**:1678–83.

126 **Wilson SH, Cooke NT, Edwards RHT, Spiro SG.** Predicted normal values for maximal respiratory pressures in caucasian adults and children. *Thorax* 1984;**39**:535–8.

127 **Cattapan SE, Laghi F, Tobin MJ.** Can diaphragmatic contractility be assessed by airway twitch pressure in mechanically ventilated patients? *Thorax* 2003;**58**:58–62.

Chapter 48

Clinical Pathways for the Continuum of Rehabilitation

Karen Hoffman, Amanda Thomas, and Stephen Brett

Introduction

Changing the focus of the critical care clinician

Until recently, critical care clinicians were content to discharge surviving patients entirely to the care of their primary medical or surgical team within the hospital with subsequent follow-up, following discharge from the acute care setting being provided by the community GP.[1] Other than mortality statistics from clinical studies, critical care practitioners had limited opportunity of understanding the full impact of critical illness on a patient, their family, and the wider economy. An increased recognition of broader patient-centred outcomes after intensive care and the post-discharge burden on patient and family has led to the development of a variety of different services for patients, following discharge from critical care. Multidisciplinary intensive care follow-up clinics were established to evaluate the physical and psychological outcome as well as QoL of patients and families.[2–4] Further details are provided in Chapter 53. This, in turn, highlighted the need to address acute psychological and physiological consequences earlier during inpatient stay,[5] with detailed description provided in Chapter 20 and Chapter 52. There is agreement across Europe, Australasia, and North America that early intervention will positively impact on recovery, length of stay, and cost of caring for these patients.[6] This chapter will discuss the clinical pathways for the continuum of rehabilitation and highlight the important issues with patient case histories to allow the clinician to reflect on their own current practice.

Clinical pathways

The physical and psychological consequences of critical illness have been discussed in previous chapters. Although our understanding of critical illness and post-critical illness recovery has increased over a relatively short period, a standardized, structured approach for the rehabilitation of physical and psychological (non-physical) consequences following critical care admission remains elusive. Clinical and critical pathways have been used in a multitude of other conditions and diagnostic groups to improve patient care and outcome. A variety of care pathways have been developed to guide clinical practice and acute care in the critical care setting, although no pathway for rehabilitation exists.[7] Clinical pathways can assist in focusing clinical staff on the clinical care they are providing and, more importantly, the constant process on how this could be improved. It can also highlight areas for concern, in particular, in the area of pathway documentation and communication.[8,9]

A recent Cochrane review[10] assessed the effect of clinical pathways on professional practice, patient outcomes, length of stay, and hospital costs. Results from 27 studies, involving 11 398 participants, indicated that clinical pathways are associated with reduced in-hospital complications

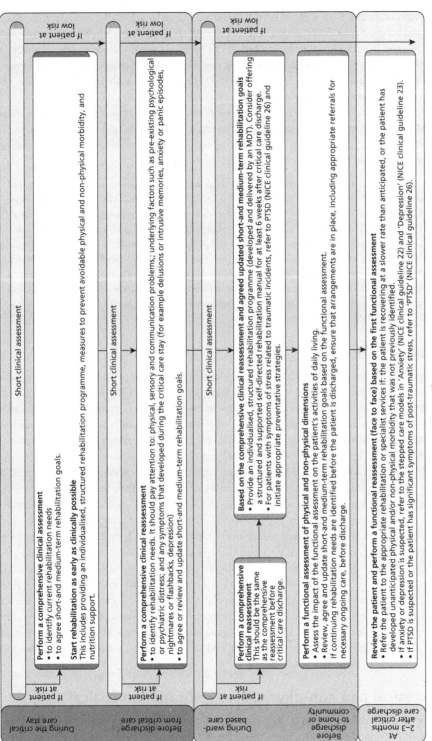

Fig. 48.1 NICE critical care rehabilitation care pathway (Tan et al., 2009).[12]
National Institute for Health and Clinical Excellence (2009) Adapted from 'CG 83: Rehabilitation after critical illness: quick reference guide'. London: NICE. Available from http://guidance.nice.org.uk/CG83. Reproduced with permission.

and improved documentation, without negatively impacting on length of stay and hospital costs.[10] Another Cochrane review concluded that early multidisciplinary rehabilitation can improve outcomes at the level of activity and participation.[11] The optimal intensity, frequency, and effects of rehabilitation over a longer period and associated social costs need further study. These reviews and several other research papers demonstrate the benefit of a rehabilitation care pathway to improve patient outcome and cost effectiveness.

In recognition of the complex rehabilitation needs of critical care patients and the benefit of clinical pathways, national clinical guidelines for critical illness rehabilitation were developed in the UK (NICE 2009).[12] The guidelines recognize the complex physical and non-physical rehabilitation issues during and following critical care and recommend that:

> Assessments and interventions should start as early as possible and continue throughout the patients' care pathway. All patients should be evaluated during and after their critical care stay to identify those who might benefit. Healthcare professionals from the multidisciplinary team e.g. rehabilitation medicine specialists, occupational therapists, speech and language therapists, physiotherapists, psychologists and other relevant specialists from secondary and primary care, should be involved in assessing the patient's physical and non-physical morbidity and their potential for rehabilitation at different stages during the recovery process. Careful coordination is crucial to ensure each patient has access to assessment and treatment by the relevant specialists to ensure they meet their rehabilitation potential. We believe that rehabilitation medicine specialists are particularly well-placed to fulfil this coordination role (see Figure 48.1).

Changing the culture

It is recognized that implementation of these guidelines may not be possible in all settings due to the varied patient case load or financial restrictions. Small-scale quality improvement projects may, however, assist in improving care and rehabilitation of patients. Examples of these include Needham et al.[13] who demonstrated the benefit of a critical care quality improvement project. ICU delirium, physical rehabilitation, and functional mobility were markedly improved and associated with decreased length of stay in the months following implementation of a multidisciplinary rehabilitation improvement project. Process changes included the development of mobility guidelines and guidelines for therapy. The availability of therapy within the unit was increased, and a change in sedation practice from continuous to bolus dose was encouraged. Project implementation elicited lower proportions of patients receiving sedatives during the critical care stay. Intervention subjects were more frequently alert and not delirious, compared to the control period. Consequently, more patients received therapy post-implementation (93%), compared to pre-implementation (70%). A total of 244 more physical treatments were delivered following project implementation, and functional mobility levels of sitting or higher occurred with greater frequency (56% pre and 78% post). The critical care length of stay was decreased from 7.0 days to 4.9 days, following project implementation. Similarly, the hospital length of stay decreased from 17.2 days to 14.1 days despite a 20% increase in admissions across the two time periods. Physical outcomes are clearly enhanced by well-organized and structured critical care environments that encourage a culture of early mobilization.[14]

Early physical and non-physical rehabilitation in critical care

The recommendations developed by NICE in 2009 were based on the best available evidence at the time of publication and the expert consensus of the guideline development group. Since that time, further publications have emerged which reinforce the guideline recommendations.

For example, the recommendation that rehabilitation should 'start as early as possible' within the critical care stay is now firmly accepted as best practice within most critical care communities.[15]

Early initiation of rehabilitation in patients with critical illness may have significant impact on physical and functional outcomes, in addition to decreasing length of ICU stay and its associated resource implications. Published accounts of critical care rehabilitation report low frequencies of adverse events, suggesting that early physical activity is both safe and feasible in this patient group, following either protocol-driven or individualized recruitment procedures.[14,16] The potential for initiation of rehabilitation activity should therefore be assessed immediately upon critical care admission in all patients and continue at regular intervals throughout the acute admission.[12]

Rehabilitation interventions in critically ill patients, often labelled 'mobilization', refer to movements, physical or functional tasks. Stiller and Phillips[17] defined mobilization as 'a hierarchy of patient activities ranging from moving around the bed to standing and walking'. Rehabilitation for critically ill patients has been defined by a task force on physiotherapy for adult patients with critical illness from the European Respiratory Society (ERS) and European Society of Intensive Care Medicine.[18] Activities, such as positioning, stretching, range-of-motion exercise, splinting, functional mobilization, aerobic training, and resistive exercise, have been recommended to both prevent and manage physical deconditioning and its related complications in the patient with critical illness. Clinical management algorithms for early physical activity and mobilization in critically ill patients have recently been published[19] which differentiate pathways for critically ill patients who are unconscious, conscious and physiologically stable, and those who are deconditioned. These algorithms reinforce the concepts of immediate initiation of early physical activity and clear documentation of specific functional goals in consultation with the patient or family member.

Differences in international critical care practice provide unique insights into the effects of early rehabilitation. They allow comparisons to be drawn between rehabilitation, which commences upon admission to critical care, and rehabilitation which begins at a later point in the critical care stay. Bailey et al.[14] and Thomsen et al.[20] demonstrated the benefit of early mobilization in critical care. An early mobility regime was implemented in a respiratory critical care unit (RICU), and the time to achieve four activities was recorded.[14] The activities included days to sit on the edge of the bed, days to chair sitting, days to walk, and days to walk greater than 100 ft. Results indicated that most of these tasks were achieved while in RICU, with only sitting on the edge of the bed achieved in a small group of patients prior to reaching the RICU. Ambulation was facilitated by the RICU early activity regime. The promotion of intense activity following transfer to a unit which prioritized early mobility was further demonstrated by Thomsen et al.[20] They investigated the difference in activity events occurring before and after transfer to an RICU. In the 24 hours preceding RICU transfer, only 11% of the patients had achieved ambulation. In contrast, 28% of patients were ambulating after 24 hours in the RICU, and 41% were ambulating 48 hours after transfer. Regression analysis revealed that RICU transfer was the strongest single predictor of ambulation. The authors attributed their findings to a culture where early mobility is a key component of patient care.

While research in early rehabilitation is ongoing, a standard rehabilitation protocol remains to be established. Several other research studies describe a variety of mobility protocols that demonstrate the effectiveness of early rehabilitation. Morris et al.[21] demonstrated that an immediate mobility protocol, compared to usual care, increased the amount of physical rehabilitation patients received during their hospital stay (80% vs 47.4%). The intervention group had fewer days in bed (8.5 days vs 13.7 days), fewer ICU days (5.5 days vs 6.9 days), and shorter adjusted overall hospital length of stay (11.2 days vs 14.5 days). The protocol intervention was immediately initiated on critical care admission, with treatments provided at a level determined by the patient's ability to interact and limb strength. Subjects in the usual care group received daily passive range of motion and second hourly repositioning.

Similarly, Schweickert et al.[22] reported a randomized trial comparing early exercise and mobilization (PT and OT), with physician-ordered PT and OT, in two medical centres which did not routinely provide PT for patients requiring MV for less than 2 weeks. Intervention subjects received therapy appropriate to their level of interaction during periods of sedation interruption. Unresponsive patients received passive range-of-motion exercises for all limbs, while responsive patients were progressed from active assisted exercises to bed mobility, sitting, transferring, and walking as tolerance increased. Not surprisingly, therapy began 1.5 days after intubation in the intervention subjects and 7.4 days in the control group. Time to functional milestones was significantly improved for intervention subjects, compared to controls. Standing occurred 3.2 (range 1.5–5.6) days following intubation in intervention subjects, compared to 6.0 (4.5–8.9) days in controls. Similarly, transferring to a chair occurred at 3.1 (1.8–4.5) days in the intervention group and 6.2 (4.5–8.4) days in controls. Subjects in the intervention group had significantly higher functional ability scores and greater walking distances (33 m vs 0 m), compared to controls, at hospital discharge. Return to independent function at hospital discharge occurred in 59% of intervention subjects, compared to 35% of controls.

Despite the fact that these trials excluded many patients from their research design, it remains clear that the achievement of functional milestones and improved functional ability at hospital discharge is enhanced by the initiation of early mobility paradigms. In clinical settings where early mobilization is standard practice, outcomes may be further enhanced by the implementation of a well coordinated rehabilitation care model (see Box 48.1).

Box 48.1 Addressing the physical and non-physical problems (case history 1)

A 69-year-old female was admitted to critical care with a pneumonia on a background of COPD requiring MV. The critical care admission was preceded by a 5-day inpatient stay, during which the patient remained bedbound due to shortness of breath. Prior to hospital admission, the patient was living independently but had limited community mobility. Within 2 days of her critical care admission, the nursing and physiotherapy staff identified the patient has significant pre-existing comorbities. Therefore, short-term physical rehabilitation goals were immediately established, and the patient was provided with twice-daily physical interventions. Active assisted strength training, functional activities, such as sitting, weight bearing, and walking, appropriate to her level of cooperation and ability at baseline physical assessments, were completed. Within 5 days of critical care admission, the patient was reviewed by the weekly multidisciplinary 'longer term' ward round. This ward round facilitated discussion within the multidisciplinary team regarding any limitations to her rehabilitation progression such as use of sedation, poor motivation, symptoms of delirium, and mood instability. As a result of the proactive approach, the medication chart was reviewed; referrals were made for OT; delirium screening tools were utilized, and her rehabilitation goals were updated. A member of the multidisciplinary team was assigned to coordinate her rehabilitation programme, facilitate ongoing referrals, update any assessments, and report progress to the weekly ward round while she remained within the critical care unit.

Specific critical care interventions

Specific interventions which may preserve muscular performance, such as NMES, should be also be considered in critically ill patients who are otherwise unable to perform active exercise for prolonged periods. This is discussed in greater detail in Chapter 44. Although the clinical use of ES in critically ill patients is limited, pilot evidence is emerging that the daily application of ES in selected patients early in critical illness reduces skeletal muscle.[23] In addition, there are data that support the use of ES in selected critically ill populations to prevent the development of CIPNM. Routsi et al.[24] describe a randomized parallel intervention in mechanically ventilated patients to investigate the effects of daily sessions of ES to the thigh muscles within 48 hours of critical care admission until ICU discharge. Intervention subjects demonstrated a lower incidence of CIPMN (12.5%), compared to controls (39%), and higher strength scores, as assessed by the MRC sum score.[25] Despite the recommendation by the ERS and the European Society of Intensive Care Medicine,[18] further research is required to both validate the clinical usefulness of neuromuscular ES and also to define the mechanisms of action of this therapy.

Inpatient and community rehabilitation following ICU discharge

The effects of specific rehabilitation interventions in the immediate post-critical care period remain largely unexplored. It is appreciated that this stage of the critical care patient journey is representative of the rehabilitation efforts of a wide multidisciplinary team, and a goal-oriented, coordinated approach to rehabilitation is urgently required. A pilot investigation from the UK[26] reported that enhancing standard physiotherapy with interventions delivered by a rehabilitation assistant increased physiotherapy frequency from 2.6 to 8.2 sessions per week, allowing a greater incidence of mobility treatments (3.3 to 14.6 per week). Disappointingly, at the 3-month follow-up, there were no differences observed between the standard and enhanced service in a battery of physical function tests, albeit that the numbers reviewed were small (n = 8).

The NICE (2009)[12] guideline recommends that patients receiving ward-based care may benefit from a self-help rehabilitation manual. This recommendation is based on an RCT that aimed to evaluate the impact of a 6-week rehabilitation programme on the physical and psychological recovery of critical care patients.[27] The control group received ward visits, three telephone calls on discharge, and outpatient follow-up. The intervention group received a self-help rehabilitation manual as well as a weekly telephone call and an outpatient clinic appointment. The intervention group demonstrated significantly better physical function scores on the SF-36 at 8 weeks and 6 months.

By contrast, a recent study has examined the effect of an 8-week home-based exercise programme that commenced 1 week following discharge from hospital.[28] Intervention participants received written instruction for an 8-week home-based graded physical rehabilitation programme which included strength and endurance components. This programme was reinforced by three home visits from a qualified physical trainer who also contacted the participant by phone during the study period. There were no differences in the rate of physical recovery, measured by 6-minute walk test or SF-36 physical function assessments, following 8 and 26 weeks between the control group and intervention group, although both groups of critical care survivors significantly improved their physical function over the study period. It remains unclear what the optimum time for the introduction of a post-critical care rehabilitation programme might be; however, comparison of these studies might suggest that the introduction of an individualized strength and endurance programme during ward-based care may enhance the recovery trajectory for critical care survivors. Further details on the models of rehabilitative care, post-ICU rehabilitation, and post-ICU follow-up clinic can be found in Chapter 50, Chapter 51, and Chapter 53, respectively.

Key workers and clinical pathway coordinators

Case managers and key workers are an essential component to the effective delivery of clinical pathways. They facilitate clear and concise information during transition between multiple levels of care during a single stay.[29] The NICE guidelines emphasize the importance of a key worker able to coordinate rehabilitation and communication along the rehabilitation pathway (see Figure 48.1). Other studies have demonstrated the effectiveness of case managers in conditions, such as acute MI,[30] and the management of older people post-acute discharge.[31] Furthermore, examples of successful rehabilitation coordinators are found in stroke and neurological rehabilitation.

The British Society for Rehabilitation Medicine's clinical standards for inpatient specialist rehabilitation services recommend the use of key workers or rehabilitation coordinators along the rehabilitation pathway.[32] It is not essential for a rehabilitation coordinator to have a medical qualification, but training in one of the therapy disciplines or nursing is an advantage, since close cooperation with the whole of the team as well as the patient and relatives is essential.[33] The rationale for the use of a rehabilitation coordinator is that one person, in the acute hospital, assumes responsibility for the continued interest in the patient, even though he or she may be in some other geographical location (see Box 48.2). This ensures continuity of care and improves the communication and delivery of important clinical information as the patient progresses through different health care services (see Table 48.1).

Box 48.2 Requirement for a rehabilitation pathway coordinator (case history 2)

A 66-year-old multi-trauma patient was discharged from the critical care unit following a 36-day stay. Her injuries included a fractured pelvis, spinal fractures, rib fractures, and bilateral upper limb fractures. While under the overall care of the 'trauma team', she was receiving input from an orthopaedic trauma team who were managing her pelvic and upper limb fractures and the neurosurgical trauma team who were conservatively managing her spinal fractures. A spinal brace had been provided, but the patient remained on both pelvic and spinal restrictions requiring logrolling. Therapy intervention was provided outside the critical care unit by specialist teams, although there was confusion regarding the extent of her movement restrictions with and without her brace, since the restrictions imposed by the orthopaedic team contradicted those imposed by the neurosurgical team. Therapy was suspended until clarification of these discrepancies could occur, and suspension of therapy occurred each time a change in restriction was documented, leading to many days on which no therapy could be delivered. Similar poor communication and therapy suspension occurred when the patient changed wards during her acute hospital stay, and consequently her rehabilitation was significantly delayed. A pathway coordinator would have responsibility for clarification of the opposing orthopaedic and neurosurgical management plans to facilitate communication between both surgical and therapy teams, enabling a seamless transition between environments and allowing rehabilitation to be maximized.

Table 48.1 Key components of a rehabilitation pathway coordinator

In the acute hospital and ICU	On discharge	Follow-up
◆ Improve the present uncoordinated referral system for the therapy services ◆ Coordinate therapy in the acute bed by good communication systems, regular meetings, handovers, and sharing of information ◆ Develop and implement rehabilitation policies for the hospital ◆ Establish a designated multidisciplinary team for injury patients ◆ Perform and monitor regular use of outcome assessment ◆ Plan treatment with agreed goals in the acute hospital with patients and therapists	◆ Find the appropriate setting for transfer or discharge from the acute hospital ◆ Perform an assessment and arrange treatment plans prior to discharge for the patient to take with him on transfer to his next hospital or centre without delay ◆ Coordinate timing and content of discharge reports—medical, nursing, therapists, and planned rehabilitation ◆ Establish a database of all available specialist centres for rehabilitation in the district where the patient comes from	◆ Improve referral systems to rehabilitation centres or community care ◆ Establish and maintain continuing care by GP or community ◆ Continue 3- and 6-monthly outcome assessments for research purposes as well as practical care ◆ Establish a central point where patients and their carers can refer to if they experience problems after discharge from the acute hospital ◆ Maintain a follow-up service to remedy problems after discharge due to inadequacies of provision in the community

Patient-centred outcome measures

Outcome research is important, as it drives the development of clinical practice guidelines, provides a structure for the assessment of the quality of medical care, and informs health policy decisions.[34] In turn, health outcome research is dependent on the appropriate use of valid, reliable, and appropriate patient rating scales. Rating scales are therefore one of the main dependent variables on which decisions are made that influence patient care and guide future research; the adequacy of these decisions depends directly on the scientific quality of the rating scales.[35]

Critical illness is not a disease with specific symptoms and functional impairments, which limits the development of a critical care disease-specific instrument. Nonetheless, the unique features of critical illness make it important that generic health status instruments are validated in this setting before they are used in clinical studies. Previous reviews emphasize the lack of consensus on which generic or disease-specific rating scales should be used in critical care outcome studies.[12,34,36] Moreover, this hinders the ability to carry out a systematic review or meta-analysis on critical care outcome studies. Table 48.2 summarizes the generic and disease-specific measures of impairment, functional status, and HRQoL that have been used in adult critical care (intensive care and high dependency).[36] Patient and family satisfaction with care represents another important domain of patient-centred outcomes.

Intensive care diaries

Many patients have limited memories of their stay in the ICU; others remember a mixture of real events and delusions, whilst a group remembers only delusions. It seems that people tend to hold onto delusions while failing to remember real events,[37] such that those patients with only delusional memories may have worse long-term psychological outcomes. In an effort to help 'fill in the gap',

Table 48.2 Summary of generic and disease-specific measures of impairment, functional status, and HRQoL that have been used in adult critical care (intensive care and high dependency) survivors

Measures of impairment	Measures of physical functional status	Measures of mental functional status	Measures of neuropsychological functioning	Measures of recovery	Measures of HRQoL
Respiratory volumes	Katz's ADL index	POMS	Trailmaking Tests A and B	GOS	SIP
Respiratory flow	Karnofsky Index	CES-D scale	WCST	Return to work	PQOL
Carbon monoxide	Barthel Index	HADS	Weschler Memory Scale	Residence	NHP
diffusing capacity	Activity levels	BDI	Benton's test for visual	Degree of recovery	SF-36
Visualization of the	Functional state	IES	retention	Productivity	Rosser's disability and
upper airway	measures		MMSE		distress categories
Hepatic, renal, and	NYHA functional		PASAT		Spitzer's QoL index and
haematological	class		Communication level		uniscale
measures	ATS respiratory				PGWB
	disease questionnaire				Fernandez's questionnaire
	Walk test				

ADL, activities of daily living; NYHA, New York Heart Association; ATS, American Thoracic Society; POMS, profile of mood states; CES-D, Center for Epidemiology Studies Depression Scale; HADS, Hospital Anxiety and Depression Scale; BDI, Beck Depression Inventory; IES, Impact of Event Scale; WCST, Wisconsin Card Sorting Test; MMSE, Mini-mental State Examination; PASAT, Paced Auditory Serial Addition Test; GOS, Glasgow Outcome Scale; SIP, Sickness Impact Profile; PQOL, Percieved Quality of Life Scale; NHP, Nottingham Health Profile; SF-36, Short-form 36; PGWB, Psychological General Well-Being Index.

Data from Hayes, J.A., Black, N.A., Jenkinson, C. et al (2000). Outcome measures for adult critical care: a systematic review. *Health Technol Assess.* 4(24):1–111.

which many patients describe as distressing, it was proposed that detailed illustrated diaries be kept which could be offered to patients during recovery.[38] Clearly, the creation of the diary must be contemporaneous, but evidence for benefit and the optimum model remained unclear. A recent RCT has demonstrated a reduced incidence of PTSD-related symptoms at 3 months post-discharge in patients with high symptom scores at 1 month;[39] all patients were reported as being positive about the diary, which appeared to be widely read by friends, family, and colleagues. Any critical care pathway must include the use of diary in order to maximize the non-physical support provided to the patient. This is covered in greater detail in Chapter 52.

Follow-up clinics

In an effort to improve continuity of care after discharge from hospitals, many institutions have established intensive care follow-up clinics,[4] although robust evidence for benefit from this approach is lacking. Cuthbertson and colleagues tested the concept of a nurse-led follow-up service in a three-centre randomized trial (The PRaCTICaL Trial).[40] The outcome measures were HRQoL and the incidences of depression, anxiety, and PTS. There was no benefit demonstrated in the intervention group at 12 months. As the existence of follow-up clinics has been pivotal to the development of our understanding of the consequences of critical illness, it is disappointing not to have proof of benefit. However, there were some complex methodological issues that may have reduced the chances of the study proving a benefit for particular patients, and these are discussed in Chapter 53. Anecdotally, many patients have been assisted by the management provided at the post-ICU clinic. It must be highlighted that the PRaCTICaL study was based on a nurse-led approach in an unselected post-critical care group of patients and therefore lacked the multidisciplinary approach to delivery rehabilitation to the groups most likely to benefit as is the approach in pulmonary, cardiac, and stroke rehabilitation.

Communication

The gap between discharge from the hospital and arrival in the community is substantial, and it is the responsibility of the hospital multidisciplinary team to ensure that clinical and other

---

Box 48.3 Clear communication required between hospital and community teams (case history 3)

A 72-year-old man required an extensive ICU admission following total resection of his pancreas, resulting in insulin dependency to manage his subsequent diabetes mellitus. He was reviewed routinely in the ICU follow-up clinic 3 months after discharge. The patient was questioned about his diabetes mellitus, in particular, his insulin requirements and glucose control. Surprisingly, the patient replied with the comment 'what diabetes?' On further questioning, it became apparent that the patient's wife was managing her husband's diabetic control by using her own insulin and equipment, as she was an also an insulin-dependent diabetic herself. The breakdown in communication between the hospital and community team is wholly evident and underlines the requirement for clear documentation, including copies issued to the patient and their carers.

information passes seamlessly to the GP and community teams (see Box 48.3). The NICE guideline[12] recommends that intensive care discharge summaries are transmitted to primary care, along with a rehabilitation plan. It is also recommended that the patient is issued with a copy of the discharge summary and rehabilitation plan. Whilst it may be difficult to demonstrate benefit, it would be hard to argue such an approach would be harmful, provided information was handled sensitively. In fact, in the UK, all hospital correspondence sent to the community GPs are routinely copied to the patient and or their carer to maximize communication with the patient.

Conclusion

Thus, the rehabilitation of complex critically ill patients needs to start early and subsequently will require continued focus and frequently multidisciplinary input. Many patients do not require this specialized approach, but, for those that do, this therapeutic approach is likely to have a better chance of success if all involved are clear about their responsibilities and communication duties. Arguably, a well-established and frequently used formal pathway can deliver this; it is currently unclear how widespread this organizational approach is.

References

1 **Broomhead LR, Brett SJ.** Clinical review: intensive care follow-up—what has it told us? *Crit Care* 2002;**6**:411–17.

2 **Department of Health.** *Critical care outreach: progress in developing services.* (2003). Available at: http://www.dh.gov.uk/en/Publicationsandstatistics/Publications/PublicationsPolicyAndGuidance/DH_4091873 (accessed 18 November 2012).

3 **Croker C.** A multidisciplinary follow-up clinic after patients' discharge from ITU. *Br J Nurs* 2003;**12**:910–14.

4 **Griffiths JA, Barber VS, Cuthbertson BH, et al.** A national survey of intensive care follow-up clinics. *Anaesthesia* 2006;**61**:950–5.

5 **Jones C, Griffiths RD.** Physical and psychological recovery. In: **Griffiths RD, Jones C** (eds.) *Intensive care aftercare.* Oxford: Butterworth-Heinemann; 2002. pp. 53–65.

6 **Kress JP.** Clinical trials of early mobilization of critically ill patients. *Crit Care Med* 2009;**37**(10 Suppl): S442–7.

7 **Wigfield A, Boon E.** Critical care pathway development: the way forward. *Br J Nurs* 1996;**5**:732–5.

8 **De Luk K.** Care pathways: an evaluation of their effectiveness. *J Adv Nurs* 2000;**32**:485–96.

9 **Gendron KM, Lai SY, Weinstein GS, et al.** Clinical care pathway for had and neck cancer. A valuable tool for decreasing resource. *Utilization Arch Otolaryngol Head Neck Surg* 2002;**128**:258–62.

10 **Rotter T, Kinsman L, James EL, et al.** Clinical pathways: effects on professional practice, patient outcomes, length of stay and hospital costs. *Cochrane Database Syst Rev* 2010;3:CD006632.

11 **Khan F, Ng L, Gonzalez S, et al.** (2008). Multidisciplinary rehabilitation programmes following joint replacement at the hip and knee in chronic arthropathy. *Cochrane Database Syst Rev* 2:CD004957.

12 **Tan T, Brett SJ, Stokes T, et al.** Rehabilitation after critical illness: summary of NICE guidance. *BMJ* 2009;**338**:822.

13 **Needham DM, Korupolu R, Kanni JM, et al.** Early physical medicine and rehabilitation for patients with acute respiratory failure: a quality improvement project. *Arch Phys Med Rehabil* 2010;**91**:536–42.

14 **Bailey PR, Thompsen GEM, Spuhler VJR, et al.** Early activity is feasible and safe in respiratory failure patients. *Crit Care Med* 2007;**35**:139–45.

15 **Stuki G, Stier-Jarmer M, Grill E, et al.** Rationale and principles of early rehabilitation care after an acute injury or illness. *Disabil Rehabil* 2005;**27**:353–9.

16 **Zeppos L, Patman S, Berney S, et al.** Physiotherapy intervention in intensive care is safe: an observational study. *Aust J Physiother* 2007;**53**:279–83.

17 **Stiller K, Phillips A.** Safety aspects of mobilising acutely ill inpatients. *Physiother Theory Pract* 2003;**19**: 239–57.

18 **Gosselink R, Bott J, Johnson M, et al.** Physiotherapy for adult patients with critical illness: recommendations of the European respiratory society and European society of intensive care medicine task force on physiotherapy for critically ill patients. *Intensive Care Med* 2008;**34**:1188–99.

19 **Hanekom S, Gosselink R, Dean E, et al.** The development of a clinical management algorithm for early physical activity and mobilization of critically ill patients: synthesis of evidence and expert opinion and its translation into practice. *Clin Rehabil* 2011;**25**:771–87.

20 **Thomsen GE, Snow GL, Rodriguez L, et al.** Patients with respiratory failure increase ambulation after transfer to an intensive care unit where early activity is a priority. *Crit Care Med* 2008;**36**:1119–24.

21 **Morris PE, Goad A, Thompson C, et al.** Early intensive care unit mobility therapy in the treatment of acute respiratory failure. *Crit Care Med* 2008;**36**:2238–43.

22 **Schweickert WD, Pohlman MC, Pohlman AS, et al.** Early physical and occupational therapy in mechanically ventilated, critically ill patients: a randomised controlled trial. *Lancet* 2009;**373**:1874–82.

23 **Gerovasili V, Stefanidis K, Vitzilaios K, et al.** Electrical muscle stimulation preserves the muscle mass of critically ill patients: a randomized study. *Crit Care* 2009;**13**:R161.

24 **Routsi C, Gerovasili V, Vasileiadis I, et al.** Electrical muscle stimulation prevents critical illness polyneuromyopathy: a randomized parallel intervention trial. *Crit Care* 2010;**14**:R74.

25 **Kleyweg RP, van der Meche FG, Schmitz PJ.** Intraobserver agreement in the assessment of muscle strength and functional abilities in Guillain-Barre syndrome. *Muscle Nerve* 1991;**14**:1103–9.

26 **Salisbury L, Merriweather JL, Walsh TS.** The development and feasibility of a ward based physiotherapy and nutritional rehabilitation package for people experiencing critical illness. *Clin Rehabil* 2010;**24**:489–500.

27 **Jones C, Skirrow P, Griffiths R, et al.** Rehabilitation after critical illness: a randomized, controlled trial. *Crit Care Med* 2003;**31**:2456–61.

28 **Elliott D, McKinley S, Alison J, et al.** Health related quality of life and physical recovery after critical illness: a multi-centre randomised controlled trial of home based physical rehabilitation program. *Crit Care* 2011;**15**:R142.

29 **Carr DD.** Case managers optimize patient safety by facilitating effective care transitions. *Prof Case Manag* 2007;**12**:70–80.

30 **DeBusk RF, Miller NH, Superko HR, et al.** A case-management system for coronary risk factor modification after acute myocardial infarction. *Ann Intern Med* 1994;**120**:721–9.

31 **Lim WK, Lambert SF, Gray LC.** Effectiveness of case management and post-acute services in older people after hospital discharge. *Med J Aust* 2003;**178**:262–6.

32 **Turner-Stokes L.** Clinical standards for inpatient specialist rehabilitation services in the UK. *Clin Rehabil* 2000;**14**:468–80.

33 **Hetherington H, Earlam RJ.** Rehabilitation after injury and the need for coordination. *Injury* 1994;**25**:527–31.

34 **Rubenfeld GD, Angus DC, Pinsky MR, et al.** Outcomes research. In critical care results of the American Thoracic Society Critical Care Assembly Workshop on Outcomes Research. *Am J Respir Crit Care Med* 1999;**160**:358–367.

35 **Hobart JC, Cano SJ, Zajicek JP, et al.** Rating scales as outcome measures for clinical trials in neurology: problems, solutions, and recommendations. *Lancet Neurol* 2007;**6**:1094–105.

36 **Hayes JA, Black NA, Jenkinson C, et al.** Outcome measures for adult critical care: a systematic review. *Health Technol Assess* 2000;**4**:1–111.

37 **Jones C, Griffiths RD, Humphris G, et al.** Memory, delusions, and the development of acute posttraumatic stress disorder-related symptoms after intensive care. *Crit Care Medicine* 2001;**29**:573–80.

38 Bäckman C, Walther SM. Use of personal diaries written on the ICU during critical illness. *Intensive Care Med* 2001;**27**:426–9.

39 Jones C, Bäckman C, Capuzzo M, et al. Intensive care diaries reduce new onset post traumatic stress disorder following critical illness: a randomised, controlled trial. *Crit Care* 2010;**14**:R168.

40 Cuthbertson BH, Rattray J, Campbell MK, et al. The PRaCTICaL study of nurse led, intensive care follow-up programmes for improving long term outcomes from critical illness: a pragmatic randomised controlled trial. *BMJ* 2009;**339**:3723.

Chapter 49

Prolonged Weaning

Benedict Creagh-Brown, Joerg Steier,
and Nicholas Hart

Introduction

Prolonged weaning from MV is the slow process of withdrawal of ventilatory support and gradual removal of the artificial airway and upper airways secretion management, which aims to liberate the patient from IMV and remove the tracheostomy. This requires adequate recovery of the neurorespiratory pathway as well as sufficient return of bulbar function. Another commonly employed strategy in the patient with prolonged weaning is the use of NIV as a bridge to decannulation. This may be particularly useful in patients who are considered at high risk of respiratory insufficiency, especially overnight during sleep, such as patients with pre-existing chronic lung disease, chest wall disease, spinal cord injury, obesity related respiratory failure, and inherited and acquired neuromuscular disease.

There has been a range of definitions for weaning, including the UK Department of Health Guidelines[1] (see Table 49.1a) and American Thoracic Society, ERS, European Society of Intensive Care Medicine, SCCM, and the Société de Réanimation de Langue Française International Consensus Guidelines[2] (see Table 49.1b). Due to the few data available, these guidelines have sparse detail on the patient with prolonged weaning and provide limited guidance on the use of NIV. Unless otherwise stated, the international consensus definition on prolonged weaning will be referred to throughout this chapter,[2] and we will focus on the management of the prolonged weaning patient with an overview, as provided in Figure 49.1. Complementary discussions about simple and difficult weaning are provided in Chapters 14 and 39.

Definition of prolonged weaning and weaning failure

Trial data report that around 75% of patients who require invasive ventilatory support can be liberated in less than 10 days from initiation of weaning.[3-5] However, in the remaining 25% of patients, weaning is more challenging, with 5–10% of patients still requiring ventilatory support at 30 days.[6] These data are supported by data from large observational cohort studies that have shown that 60% of patients receive IMV for less than 4 days.[7,8]

Using the UK Department of Health definition for **weaning failure**, defined as the need for ventilatory support for greater than **3** weeks in the absence of any non-respiratory factor preventing weaning,[1] the point prevalence of weaning failure has been reported at 7%.[1] Using the more recent international consensus definition of **prolonged weaning**, defined as a patient who undergoes more than three SBTs or greater than 7 days of weaning after the first SBT,[2] a large international observational cohort study showed that 6% of patients undergoing MV were classified as prolonged weaning. The similarity between the UK and European data highlights the overlap

Table 49.1a UK Department of Health Guidelines[1]

◆ Simple wean: patient who weans from IMV within 14 days
◆ Difficult wean: patient who weans from IMV between 14 and 21 days ('weaning delay')
◆ Very difficult wean: patient who weans from IMV in over 21 days ('weaning failure')

IMV, invasive mechanical ventilation.

United Kingdom Department of Health Guidelines (NHS Modernisation Agency Report, 2002). Public sector information licensed under the Open Government Licence v2.0. http://www.nationalarchives.gov.uk/doc/open-government-licence/version/2/

Table 49.1b International Consensus Definition[2]

◆ Simple wean: patient who proceeds from initiation of weaning to successful extubation on the first attempt
◆ Difficult wean: patient who fails initial weaning and requires up to three SBTs or up to 7 days from the first SBT to achieve successful weaning
◆ Prolonged wean: patient who fails at least three weaning attempts or requires greater than 7 days of weaning after the first SBT

SBT, spontaneous breathing trial.

International Consensus Definition (Boles et al., 2007).

Adapted and reproduced with permission of the European Respiratory Society: J-M. Boles, et al., 'Weaning from mechanical ventilation', *Eur Respir J* May 2007 29:1033-1056; doi:10.1183/09031936.00010206

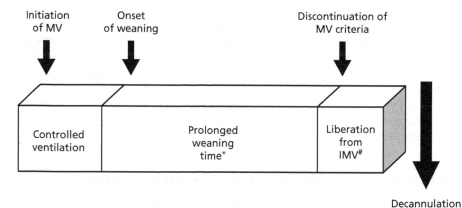

Fig. 49.1 Stages in prolonged weaning.

IMV, invasive mechanical ventilation. * Prolonged weaning time managed with a personalized management plan, including a combination of self-ventilation trials, CPAP, support and controlled modes of ventilatory support, tracheostomy cuff down trials, secretion clearance and exercise therapy, and mobilization. # Liberation from IMV is a process that can be facilitated in patients with chronic respiratory insufficiency, with the use on NIV as a bridge to decannulation and as part of a long-term management strategy in patients with sleep-disordered breathing and nocturnal hypoventilation, e.g. patients with chronic lung disease, chest wall disease, obesity-related respiratory failure, and inherited and acquired neuromuscular disease.

between these definitions.[1,2] We can consider the terms prolonged weaning and weaning failure, according to these definitions, as describing similar patient groups.

The prolonged weaning group has been shown, after adjustment for other variables, to be associated with a higher ICU mortality, compared with the simple weaning group, reported as 13% and 7%, respectively.[9] A similar study also observed an increased hospital mortality in the prolonged weaning group, compared with the simple weaning group.[10] Contributing to the excess mortality during the ICU admission is the increased risk of VAP[11,12] and chronic respiratory disease such as COPD.[13] Although the ICU and hospital mortality differed between the weaning groups, the 1-year mortality was similar, indicating that weaning failure patients who survive an episode of prolonged weaning are likely to be alive at 1 year and require ongoing nursing, therapy, and medical support.[14]

Physiological approach to weaning

CO_2 homeostasis is maintained by adequate alveolar ventilation, which is determined by the difference between minute and dead space ventilation. By focusing on the factors that influence respiratory frequency and tidal volume, the factors that impact on weaning failure can be understood. Neural respiratory drive, neuromuscular transmission, respiratory muscle action, and respiratory system impedance are all important, and impairment at one or more levels can result in weaning problems (see Figure 49.2). Weaning failure is recognized as an imbalance between neural respiratory drive, respiratory muscle load, and respiratory muscle capacity[15] (see Figure 49.3). A systematic approach can be applied in the prolonged weaning patient, and the clinical conditions implicated in failure of neural respiratory drive and neurotransmission, reduced respiratory muscle performance, and increased impedance is a rational approach that can be employed[15] (see Figure 49.4).

More recently, studies have investigated the effect of pulmonary mechanics, respiratory muscle strength, and fatigue on weaning outcome.[16,17] Whilst it has been shown that COPD patients who successfully wean from MV have lower airways resistance, intrinsic PEEP, and elastic load at the end of an SBT, compared with those who fail, the elastic, resistive, and threshold loads at the start of the trial are similar in both groups.[16] Furthermore, diaphragm strength is similar in patients that successfully wean from MV, compared with those who fail, and there is, in fact, no evidence of diaphragm fatigue in the weaning failure group.[16] Also, weaning time has been not

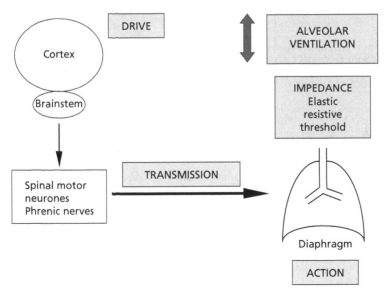

Fig. 49.2 Physiological factors determining alveolar ventilation.

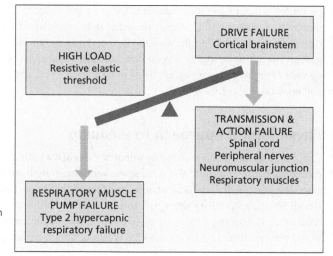

Fig. 49.3 Causes of weaning failure: imbalance between respiratory muscle drive, load, and capacity.

Reprinted from *Medicine*, 40, 6, Suh ES, and Hart N, 'Respiratory Failure', pp. 293–297, copyright 2012, with permission from Elsevier.

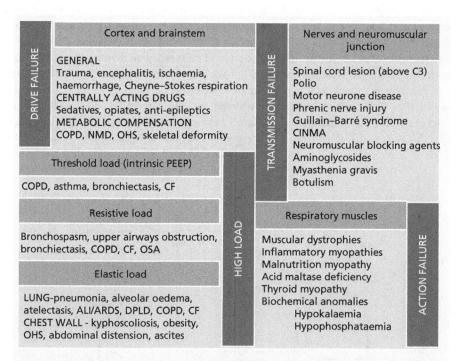

COPD, chronic obstructive pulmonary disease; NMD, neuromuscular disease; OHS, occipital hom syndrome; PEEP. positive end-expiratory pressure; CF, cystic fibrosis; OSA, obstructive sleep apnoea: ALI/ARDS. acute lung injury/acute respiratory distress syndrome; DPLD, diffuse parenchymal lung disease; CINMA, critical illness neuromuscular abnormalities.

Fig. 49.4 Causes of weaning failure: drive failure, transmission failure, action failure, and high impedance.

Reprinted from *Medicine*, 40, 6, Suh ES, and Hart N, 'Respiratory Failure', pp. 293–297, copyright 2012, with permission from Elsevier.

been shown to be associated with diaphragm strength.[17] All these data indicate that deterioration in pulmonary mechanics during a trial of spontaneous ventilation is one of the most important determinants of weaning outcome.

Contemporary approaches to weaning from MV

Mode of ventilation

Although synchronized IMV was originally designed as a weaning mode, it has been shown in two seminal studies[3,4] to be the inferior mode for weaning, which has resulted in a gradual decline in its clinical use, with the preference shifting toward supported ventilation modes from controlled modes of ventilation for weaning.[18] Furthermore, the increased awareness of the deleterious effects of continuous sedation,[19] data reporting that diaphragmatic inactivity causes diaphragm atrophy,[20,21] and the change in culture towards exercise therapy and mobilization early in the course of critical illness[22,23] have facilitated this movement away from controlled to support modes. This approach with the adoption of DIS strategy, as a component of international standard ventilator care bundles,[24,25] has led to an overall reduction in sedative use.[26] Furthermore, recent data have demonstrated that the use of protocolized sedation is as effective as protocolized sedation with daily sedation interruption in weaning patients from MV.[27]

Predictors and outcomes of prolonged weaning

A **Weaning Task Force** identified 462 weaning predictors in 65 observational studies and evaluated the ability of each variable to predict the outcome of an SBT.[28] The pooled likelihood ratios of the predictors were shown to have a low predictive power, indicating that weaning predictors should be disregarded. Although various definitions of weaning success have been proposed, these definitions are less than satisfactory for patients with prolonged weaning. A framework for outcomes for prolonged weaning patients, rather than an arbitrary time limit of self-ventilation, should be considered, including: (1) ventilator independence prior to discharge from ICU, weaning and rehabilitation centre, or LTAC hospital, (2) nocturnal NIV dependent prior to discharge from ICU, weaning and rehabilitation centre, or long-term acute care hospital, (3) invasively ventilator-dependent prior to discharge from ICU, weaning and rehabilitation centre, or LTAC hospital, and (4) within ICU, weaning and rehabilitation centre, or LTAC hospital death.

Protocolized weaning

This is a controversial issue in patients with prolonged weaning. The seminal study by Ely et al., similar to most of the other weaning studies, compared daily screening and a weaning protocol with physician-led care.[6] IMV time was reduced from 6 days to 4 days in the intervention group, but there was no difference in ICU length of stay, hospital length of stay, and overall cost of treatment. Although this trial supported the clinical benefit of protocolized weaning, it must be highlighted that 76% of the control group were weaned using synchronized intermittent mandatory ventilation, the least preferred mode of weaning from MV.[29,30] Furthermore, close inspection of the data[6] showed that, in patients with prolonged weaning, there was no difference between the protocolized weaning and physician-led weaning groups. Prolonged weaning should therefore be regarded as a complex task that requires an in-depth understanding and application of clinical and physiological principles. A recent meta-analysis reported that, if the organizational culture of the ICU included an optimum number of trained staff, there is no additional benefit from the use of weaning protocols,[31] which is reflected by the lack of widespread implementation of weaning protocols.[31]

Timing of tracheostomy insertion

Patients with prolonged weaning, in general, receive tracheostomy ventilation, with recent data guiding the clinician in terms of the timing of tracheostomy tube insertion. A single-centre RCT and a subsequent multicentre RCT demonstrated the beneficial effects of early, rather than late, placement of the tracheostomy tube.[32,33] In patients expected to require prolonged ventilation, tracheostomy insertion in the first week resulted in a shorter duration of IMV, a reduced ICU length of stay, a reduced pneumonia incidence, with more successful weaning and lower mortality, compared to patients who received tracheostomy insertion at the beginning of the third week.[32,33] These data advocate the early insertion of tracheostomy if prolonged weaning is expected.

Practical approach to the prolonged weaning patient

Patient cohorts

Prolonged weaning differs from simple and difficult weaning, albeit with similar fundamental goals. Such patients are in a relatively stable stage of CCI, with single organ respiratory failure, and therefore require less invasive monitoring and less support in terms of intensive nursing management. These patients have similar diagnoses, including COPD, neuromuscular disease, chest wall disease, spinal cord injury, and obesity,[34] all of which require differing levels of nursing care support and experience, depending on the physical and psychological needs of the patient during recovery from their critical illness.

Weaning strategy during prolonged weaning

The relatively small numbers of prolonged weaning patients has resulted in few evidence-based data to guide weaning. Regional weaning and rehabilitation centres have developed in Europe to specifically manage such patients, and these centres have reported their outcomes in observational cohort studies.[34–38] It has to be acknowledged that unit preference will determine the method of ventilatory support during prolonged weaning, but it has been shown that, in COPD patients, there was no difference in weaning outcome, duration of MV, hospital length of stay, and mortality between gradual reduction of inspiratory pressure support and increased periods of self-ventilation.[39] Specialist units develop personalized weaning and rehabilitation plans that combine self-ventilation trials, CPAP, support and controlled modes of ventilation, tracheostomy cuff down trials, exercise therapy, and mobilization. A practical clinical approach to these patients is provided in Box 49.1. The psychosocial needs of both the patient and their relatives are not discussed in detail, as this is dealt with in Chapters 10 and 11.

Secretion management

A secretion management plan is required to control both upper airway salivary secretions and lower airway bronchial secretions, in particular, in those patients with bulbar dysfunction and neuromuscular disease. Upper airway secretions can be controlled with carefully scheduled and timed use of tracheostomy cuff down trials, initially during wakefulness, and the transdermal application of hyoscine hydrobromide to reduce salivary gland secretion production. It is usually caused by an inability to swallow, rather than a real increase in the production of saliva. Bronchial

Box 49.1 Practical approach to the prolonged weaning patient

- Initial short daytime tracheostomy cuff down trials, with introduction of speaking valve in ventilator circuit, extended to 24-hour tracheostomy cuff down trials, with subsequent change to cuffless tracheostomy tube
  - ➤ Promotes airflow of vocal cords and soft palate to enhances bulbar function
  - ➤ Promotes phonation which is psychologically rewarding for patient
  - ➤ Reduces inspiratory pressure delivered to facilitate weaning
- Downsize nasogastric tube
  - ➤ Enhances limited swallow function
  - ➤ Improves patient comfort
- Downsize tracheostomy tube
  - ➤ 7.0–8.0 mm internal diameter tracheostomy tube is satisfactory for prolonged weaning
  - ➤ With a 7.0–8.0 mm internal diameter tracheostomy tube, with the cuff deflated, airflow is able to pass the vocal cords and soft palate which enhances bulbar function
- Check arterial blood gas
  - ➤ Drive down $PaCO_2$ if HCO_3^- level > 40 mmol/L, e.g. $PaCO_2$ 7.0–7.5 kPa
  - ➤ Maintain PaO_2 at a modified level in chronic respiratory disease, e.g. PaO_2 7.5–8.0 kPa
- Perform short self-ventilation trial
  - ➤ Up to 5 min, depending on physiological response
  - ➤ Inspiratory muscle function, e.g. assess thoraco-abdominal movement
  - ➤ Expiratory muscle function, e.g. cough and clear secretions
  - ➤ Lower airway secretion load, e.g. 'acquired' bronchiectasis with *Pseudomonas* colonization
  - ➤ Upper airways secretion load, e.g. poor bulbar function
  - ➤ Reduce WOB during cuff down trials, e.g. change reinforced extended length tracheostomy tube to shorter length tracheostomy tube (caution in the obese patient)
- Cough and secretion management
  - ➤ Nebulized antibiotics to reduce *Pseudomonas* colonization
  - ➤ Transdermal tropane alkaloid with anti-muscarinic properties to control upper airways secretion (e.g. hyoscine hydrobromide patch)
  - ➤ Assisted chest physiotherapy and mechanical insufflation-exsufflation cough assist device in neuromuscular and spinal cord injury patients
- Neurological assessment
  - ➤ Assess severity of ICUAW
  - ➤ Assess for neurological signs inconsistent with ICUAW, e.g. tongue and generalized muscle fasciculation, muscle wasting with brisk reflexes
  - ➤ EMG, NCS, and spinal cord MRI to exclude occult neurology if neurological signs inconsistent with ICUAW, e.g. amyotrophic lateral sclerosis

Box 49.1 Practical approach to the prolonged weaning patient *(continued)*

- ◆ Assessment and optimization of cardiorespiratory status
  - ➢ Manage fluid overload, and maintain a neutral fluid balance
  - ➢ ECHO for occult cardiac insufficiency, e.g. inherited neuromuscular patient group such as Duchenne muscular dystrophy, Becker's muscular dystrophy, limb girdle muscle dystrophy
  - ➢ High-resolution cross-sectional imaging of the thorax, e.g. chronic lung disease
  - ➢ Nocturnal monitoring, with full montage PSG or limited respiratory polygraphy, to adjust ventilator settings and optimize synchronization
- ◆ Nutrition assessment
  - ➢ 24-hour feed to 20-hour feed to overnight feed as clinical condition improves
  - ➢ Oral intake if tracheostomy cuff down trials successful and bulbar function preserved
- ◆ Rehabilitation assessment
- ◆ Mental health status assessment
- ◆ Assessment of pre-admission medical condition, level of function, and social care requirement

$PaCO_2$, arterial partial pressure of carbon dioxide; PaO_2, arterial partial pressure of oxygen; HCO_3^-, bicarbonate; ICUAW, intensive care unit-acquired weakness

secretion management requires regular assisted respiratory physiotherapy clearance techniques, including tracheobronchial suctioning, percussion and vibration therapy, positioning and postural drainage, lung volume recruitment with the use of a manual inflation, and, more recently, the use of the mechanical insufflation-exsufflation devices. The ability to generate a peak cough flow rate greater than 160 L/min has been shown to predict successful tracheostomy tube decannulation in patients with poor expiratory muscle function as a consequence of neuromuscular disease.[40] In addition, mechanical insufflation-exsufflation has been demonstrated to produce a greater increase in peak cough flow than other standard cough augmentation techniques in adults with neuromuscular disease.[41] Furthermore, in another small short-term physiological study of ventilator-dependent patients with amyotrophic lateral sclerosis, mechanical insufflation-exsufflation via a tracheostomy tube proved more effective in eliminating airway secretions than conventional tracheal suctioning.[42] Although there are no trials reporting the effectiveness of mechanical insufflation-exsufflation in patients with prolonged weaning, a recent trial in an unselected ICU patient group, excluding patients with neuromuscular disease, showed that the addition of mechanical insufflation-exsufflation three times a day to standard care reduced the early reintubation rate.[43] However, the trial included only simple weaning patients, as all the patients enrolled had fewer than three SBT attempts. The effectiveness of this technology in prolonged weaning patients needs to be further evaluated.

NIV as a bridge to decannulation

Although it has been shown in three trials that NIV is an effective tool to facilitate extubation in patients with chronic respiratory disease and persistent weaning failure,[44–46] there are limited published data on the use on NIV as a bridge to decannulation in prolonged weaning patients with sleep-disordered breathing and nocturnal hypoventilation. However, the lack of controlled trial data in the prolonged weaning and tracheostomy-ventilated groups is not surprising. Specifically, many of these patients have undiagnosed chronic respiratory failure, such as patients with chronic lung disease, chest wall disease, obesity-related respiratory failure, and inherited and acquired neuromuscular disease, prior to their acute crisis requiring critical care admission. There would therefore be ethical issues to withholding long-term NIV, as this is established as standard clinical care in these patients.[47–52] Effective titration of settings and establishment of nocturnal NIV require clinical expertise with interpretation of detailed overnight monitoring to maximize nocturnal ventilatory control and optimize the ventilator support.[53,54,55,56] This is outside the usual scope of a general medical and surgical ICU or LTAC hospital, and transfer to a specialist weaning and rehabilitation unit is recommended.

Cost and clinical effectiveness of long-term acute care hospitals and weaning centres

The number of LTAC hospitals in the US, which accommodate patients with prolonged weaning, have increased from 192 in 1997 to 408 in 2006.[57] The proportion of patients receiving MV in these facilities has increased from 16.4% in 1997–2000 to 29.8% in 2004–2006.[57] Of more concern is that the 1-year mortality of patients receiving MV transferred to these facilities was recently reported at 69.1%.[57] This is in contrast to the specialist weaning and rehabilitation centres that have been developed in Europe. Despite the variance in the reported clinical outcomes from these centres,[34–38] which is a reflection of the varying diagnoses amongst the different cohorts and the length of IMV prior to admission to the weaning unit, the overall mortality ranges between 15% and 25%. Furthermore, up to 45% of patients are completely weaned from MV, with up to 25% of patients requiring home nocturnal NIV and only 15% dependent on long-term IMV. The 1-year and 3-year survival ranges between 65–80% and 45–60%, respectively. There are obvious caveats to the direct comparison of data from a large epidemiological cohort of long-term general acute care hospitals and the relatively small data set from specialist weaning and rehabilitation centres. Despite this, these data highlight the clinical complexities of managing such patients in less specialist facilities, including the home setting.[58] This is important, as recent data have shown that lung-protective MV is associated with a substantial long-term survival benefit in patients with ALI.[59] The management of such patients is no longer the exclusive concern of critical care clinicians but now involves multiple health care professionals, including respiratory and rehabilitation specialists, to provide long-term management after the acute critical illness has resolved.[60]

Driving the expansion of LTAC hospitals in the US is a financial incentive with cost savings that favour the transfer out of the short-stay acute hospital. It was estimated in 1995 that there were over 11 000 ventilator-dependent patients with CCI in short-stay hospitals, costing over $9 million per day.[61] In addition to the relatively high margins from which the LTAC hospitals operate, short-stay hospitals benefit financially by earlier discharge of patients with severe illness,[62] freeing up critical care beds for more profitable elective surgical cases.[63] In the UK, it has been estimated that there could be cost savings of 50% per patient per day in managing such patients outside of the ICU.[1] The North of England study determined that prolonged weaning patients occupied 1000 bed days per year in the ICU of the region, with an estimated 12 500 bed days per year across the whole of the UK, with calculated cost savings to the NHS conservatively estimated at £5 million per annum.[64] These data have been supported by more recent UK data, with the potential to reduce intensive care bed occupancy by up to 10% with the establishment of specialist weaning and rehabilitation centres.[65]

Conclusion

Prolonged weaning is a complex and challenging task, which is likely to be more common in the future. Although only a small proportion of all invasively ventilated patients fall into this category, the critical care clinician must prioritize the early identification of such patients, as failure to do so will be detrimental to clinical outcome. Prolonged weaning can be expected in patients with established lung, chest wall, and neuromuscular disease, which will be accompanied by the sequelae of CCI. In addition, it is also likely that obesity-related respiratory failure may contribute to the rise in overall prevalence of such patients. These patients will require personalized weaning and rehabilitation plans, based on their underlying pathological condition as well as their psychological and physiological status by a multidisciplinary team.

References

1 **NHS Modernisation Agency Report.** *Critical care programme. Weaning and long term ventilation.* (2002). NHS Modernisation Agency.

2 **Boles JM, Bion J, Connors A, et al.** Weaning from mechanical ventilation. *Eur Respir J* 2007;**29**:1033–56.

3 **Brochard L, Rauss A, Benito S, et al.** Comparison of three methods of gradual withdrawal from ventilatory support during weaning from mechanical ventilation. *Am J Respir Crit Care Med* 1994;**150**:896–903.

4 **Esteban A, Frutos F, Tobin MJ, et al.** A comparison of four methods of weaning patients from mechanical ventilation. Spanish Lung Failure Collaborative Group. *N Engl J Med* 1995;**332**:345–50.

5 **Krishnan JA, Moore D, Robeson C, Rand CS, Fessler HE.** A prospective, controlled trial of a protocol-based strategy to discontinue mechanical ventilation. *Am J Respir Crit Care Med* 2004;**169**:673–8.

6 **Ely EW, Baker AM, Dunagan DP, et al.** Effect on the duration of mechanical ventilation of identifying patients capable of breathing spontaneously. *N Engl J Med* 1996;**335**:1864–9.

7 **Zilberberg MD, De Wit M, Pirone JR, Shorr AF.** Growth in adult prolonged acute mechanical ventilation: implications for healthcare delivery. *Crit Care Med* 2008;**36**:1451–5.

8 **Zilberberg MD, Luippold RS, Sulsky S, Shorr AF.** Prolonged acute mechanical ventilation, hospital resource utilization, and mortality in the United States. *Crit Care Med* 2008;**36**:724–30.

9 **Penuelas O, Frutos-Vivar F, Fernandez C, et al.** Characteristics and outcomes of ventilated patients according to time to liberation from mechanical ventilation. *Am J Respir Crit Care Med* 2011;**184**:430–7.

10 **Funk GC, Anders S, Breyer MK, et al.** Incidence and outcome of weaning from mechanical ventilation according to new categories. *Eur Respir J* 2010;**35**:88–94.

11 **Cook DJ, Walter SD, Cook RJ, et al.** Incidence of and risk factors for ventilator-associated pneumonia in critically ill patients. *Ann Intern Med* 1998;**129**:433–40.

12 **Safdar N, Dezfulian C, Collard HR, Saint S.** Clinical and economic consequences of ventilator-associated pneumonia: a systematic review. *Crit Care Med* 2005;**33**:2184–93.

13 **Nava S, Rubini F, Zanotti E, et al.** Survival and prediction of successful ventilator weaning in COPD patients requiring mechanical ventilation for more than 21 days. *Eur Respir J* 1994;**7**:1645–52.

14 **Tonnelier A, Tonnelier JM, Nowak E, et al.** Clinical relevance of classification according to weaning difficulty. *Respir Care* 2011;**56**:583–90.

15 **Suh ES, Hart N.** Respiratory failure. *Medicine* 2012;**40**:293–7.

16 **Jubran A, Tobin MJ.** Pathophysiologic basis of acute respiratory distress in patients who fail a trial of weaning from mechanical ventilation. *Am J Respir Crit Care Med* 1997;**155**:906–15.

17 **Watson AC, Hughes PD, Louise Harris M, et al.** Measurement of twitch transdiaphragmatic, esophageal, and endotracheal tube pressure with bilateral anterolateral magnetic phrenic nerve stimulation in patients in the intensive care unit. *Crit Care Med* 2001;**29**:1325–31.

18 **Esteban A, Ferguson ND, Meade MO, et al., and for the Ventila Group.** Evolution of mechanical ventilation in response to clinical research. *Am J Respir Crit Care Med* 2008;**177**:170–7.

19 **Strom T, Martinussen T, Toft P.** A protocol of no sedation for critically ill patients receiving mechanical ventilation: a randomised trial. *Lancet* 2010;**375**:475–80.

20 **Levine S, Nguyen T, Taylor N, et al.** Rapid disuse atrophy of diaphragm fibers in mechanically ventilated humans. *N Engl J Med* 2008;**358**:1327–35.

21 **Sassoon C, Caiozzo VJ.** Bench-to-bedside review: Diaphragm muscle function in disuse and acute high-dose corticosteroid treatment. *Crit Care* 2009;**13**:221.

22 **Schweickert WD, Pohlman MC, Pohlman AS, et al.** Early physical and occupational therapy in mechanically ventilated, critically ill patients: a randomised controlled trial. *Lancet* 2009;**373**:1874–82.

23 **Pohlman MC, Schweickert WD, Pohlman AS, et al.** Feasibility of physical and occupational therapy beginning from initiation of mechanical ventilation. *Crit Care Med* 2010;**38**:2089–94.

24 **Kress JP, Pohlman AS, O'connor MF, Hall JB.** Daily interruption of sedative infusions in critically ill patients undergoing mechanical ventilation. *N Engl J Med* 2000;**342**:1471–7.

25 **Institute For Healthcare Improvement.** *Implement the IHI ventilator bundle (online).* (2011). Available at: http://www.ihi.org/knowledge/Pages/Changes/ImplementtheVentilatorBundle.aspx.

26 **Egerod I, Christensen BV, Johansen L.** Trends in sedation practices in Danish intensive care units in 2003: a national survey. *Intensive Care Med* 2006;**32**:60–6.

27 **Mehta S, Burry L, Cook D, et al.** Daily sedation interruption in mechanically ventilated critically ill patients cared for with a sedation protocol: a randomized controlled trial. *JAMA* 2012;**308**:1985–92.

28 **Macintyre NR, Cook DJ, Ely EW, Jr, et al.** Evidence-based guidelines for weaning and discontinuing ventilatory support: a collective task force facilitated by the American College of Chest Physicians; the American Association for Respiratory Care; and the American College of Critical Care Medicine. *Chest* 2001;**120**:375S–95S.

29 **Esteban A, Frutos F, Tobin MJ, et al.** A comparison of four methods of weaning patients from mechanical ventilation. *N Engl J Med* 1995;**332**:345–50.

30 **Brochard L, Rauss A, Benito S, et al.** Comparison of three methods of gradual withdrawal from ventilatory support during weaning from mechanical ventilation. *Am J Respir Crit Care Med* 1994;**150**:896–903.

31 **Blackwood B, Alderdice F, Burns K, Cardwell C, Lavery G, O'halloran P.** Use of weaning protocols for reducing duration of mechanical ventilation in critically ill adult patients: Cochrane systematic review and meta-analysis. *BMJ* 2011;**342**:c7237.

32 **Rumbak MJ, Newton M, Truncale T, Schwartz SW, Adams JW, Hazard PB.** A prospective, randomized, study comparing early percutaneous dilational tracheotomy to prolonged translaryngeal intubation (delayed tracheotomy) in critically ill medical patients. *Crit Care Med* 2004;**32**:1689–94.

33 **Terragni PP, Antonelli M, Fumagalli R, et al.** Early vs late tracheotomy for prevention of pneumonia in mechanically ventilated adult ICU patients: a randomized controlled trial. *JAMA* 2010;**303**:1483–9.

34 **Pilcher DV, Bailey MJ, Treacher DF, Hamid S, Williams AJ, Davidson AC.** Outcomes, cost and long term survival of patients referred to a regional weaning centre. *Thorax* 2005;**60**:187–92.

35 **Schonhofer B, Euteneuer S, Nava S, Suchi S, Kohler D.** Survival of mechanically ventilated patients admitted to a specialised weaning centre. *Intensive Care Med* 2002;**28**:908–16.

36 **Quinnell TG, Pilsworth S, Shneerson JM, Smith IE.** Prolonged invasive ventilation following acute ventilatory failure in COPD: weaning results, survival, and the role of noninvasive ventilation. *Chest* 2006;**129**:133–9.

37 **Chadwick R, Nadig V, Oscroft NS, Shneerson JM, Smith IE.** Weaning from prolonged invasive ventilation in motor neuron disease: analysis of outcomes and survival. *J Neurol Neurosurg Psychiatry* 2011;**82**:643–5.

38 **Rubini F, Zanotti E, Brigada P, Nava S.** Factors determining the successful weaning of patients with 'difficult weaning'. *Minerva Anestesiol* 1998;**64**:513–20.

39 **Vitacca M, Vianello A, Colombo D, et al.** Comparison of two methods for weaning patients with chronic obstructive pulmonary disease requiring mechanical ventilation for more than 15 days. *Am J Respir Crit Care Med* 2001;**164**:225–30.

40 Bach JR, Saporito LR. Criteria for extubation and tracheostomy tube removal for patients with ventilatory failure. A different approach to weaning. *Chest* 1996;**110**:1566–71.

41 Chatwin M, Ross E, Hart N, Nickol AH, Polkey MI, Simonds AK. Cough augmentation with mechanical insufflation/exsufflation in patients with neuromuscular weakness. *Eur Respir J* 2003;**21**:502–8.

42 Sancho J, Servera E, Vergara P, Marin J. Mechanical insufflation-exsufflation vs. tracheal suctioning via tracheostomy tubes for patients with amyotrophic lateral sclerosis: a pilot study. *Am J Phys Med Rehabil* 2003;**82**:750–3.

43 Goncalves MR, Honrado T, Winck JC, Paiva JA. Effects of mechanical insufflation-exsufflation in preventing respiratory failure after extubation: a randomized controlled trial. *Crit Care* 2012;**16**:R48.

44 Girault C, Daudenthun I, Chevron V, Tamion F, Leroy J, Bonmarchand G. Noninvasive ventilation as a systematic extubation and weaning technique in acute-on-chronic respiratory failure: a prospective, randomized controlled study. *Am J Respir Crit Care Med* 1999;**160**:86–92.

45 Ferrer M, Esquinas A, Arancibia F, et al. Noninvasive ventilation during persistent weaning failure: a randomized controlled trial. *Am J Respir Crit Care Med* 2003;**168**:70–6.

46 Nava S, Ambrosino N, Clini E, et al. Noninvasive mechanical ventilation in the weaning of patients with respiratory failure due to chronic obstructive pulmonary disease. A randomized, controlled trial. *Ann Intern Med* 1998;**128**:721–8.

47 Simonds AK, Elliott MW. Outcome of domiciliary nasal intermittent positive pressure ventilation in restrictive and obstructive disorders. *Thorax* 1995;**50**:604–9.

48 Bourke SC, Tomlinson M, Williams TL, Bullock RE, Shaw PJ, Gibson GJ. Effects of non-invasive ventilation on survival and quality of life in patients with amyotrophic lateral sclerosis: a randomised controlled trial. *Lancet Neurol* 2006;**5**:140–7.

49 Murphy P, Hart N. Who benefits from home mechanical ventilation? *Clin Med* 2009;**9**:160–3.

50 Murphy PB, Brignall K, Moxham J, Polkey MI, Davidson AC, Hart N. High pressure versus high intensity noninvasive ventilation in stable hypercapnic chronic obstructive pulmonary disease: a randomized crossover trial. *Int J Chron Obstruct Pulmon Dis* 2012;**7**:811–18.

51 Murphy PB, Davidson C, Hind MD, et al. Volume targeted versus pressure support non-invasive ventilation in patients with super obesity and chronic respiratory failure: a randomised controlled trial. *Thorax* 2012;**67**:727–34.

52 Borel JC, Tamisier R, Gonzalez-Bermejo J, et al. Noninvasive ventilation in mild obesity hypoventilation syndrome: a randomized controlled trial. *Chest* 2012;**141**:692–702.

53 Gonzalez-Bermejo J, Perrin C, Janssens JP, et al. Proposal for a systematic analysis of polygraphy or polysomnography for identifying and scoring abnormal events occurring during non-invasive ventilation. *Thorax* 2012;**67**:546–52.

54 Janssens JP, Borel JC, Pepin JL. Nocturnal monitoring of home non-invasive ventilation: the contribution of simple tools such as pulse oximetry, capnography, built-in ventilator software and autonomic markers of sleep fragmentation. *Thorax* 2011;**66**:438–45.

55 Adler D, Perrig S, Takahashi H, et al. Polysomnography in stable COPD under non-invasive ventilation to reduce patient-ventilator asynchrony and morning breathlessness. *Sleep Breath* 2012;**16**:1081–90.

56 Drouot X, Roche-Campo F, Thille AW, et al. A new classification for sleep analysis in critically ill patients. *Sleep Med* 2012;**13**:7–14.

57 Kahn JM, Benson NM, Appleby D, Carson SS, Iwashyna TJ. Long-term acute care hospital utilization after critical illness. *JAMA* 2010;**303**, 2253–9.

58 Wise MP, Hart N, Davidson C, et al. Home mechanical ventilation. *BMJ* 2011;**342**:d1687.

59 Needham DM, Colantuoni E, Mendez-Tellez PA, et al. Lung protective mechanical ventilation and two year survival in patients with acute lung injury: prospective cohort study. *BMJ* 2012;**344**:e2124.

60 Camporota L, Hart N. Lung protective ventilation. *BMJ* 2012;**344**:e2491.

61 **Make BJ.** Indications for home ventilation. In: **Robert D, Make BJ, Leger P** (eds.) *Home mechanical ventilation*. Paris: Arnette Blackwell; 1995. pp. 229–40.

62 **Hsia DC, Ahern CA, Ritchie BP, Moscoe LM, Krushat WM.** Medicare reimbursement accuracy under the prospective payment system, 1985 to 1988. *JAMA* 1992;**268**:896–9.

63 **Seneff MG, Wagner D, Thompson D, Honeycutt C, Silver MR.** The impact of long-term acute-care facilities on the outcome and cost of care for patients undergoing prolonged mechanical ventilation. *Crit Care Med* 2000;**28**:342–50.

64 **Robson V, Poynter J, Lawler PG & Baudouin SV.** The need for a regional weaning centre, a one-year survey of intensive care weaning delay in the Northern Region of England. *Anaesthesia* 2003;**58**:161–5.

65 **Lone NI, Walsh TS.** Prolonged mechanical ventilation in critically ill patients: epidemiology, outcomes and modelling the potential cost consequences of establishing a regional weaning unit. *Crit Care* 2011;**15**:R102.

Chapter 50

Models of Rehabilitative Care after Critical Illness

Margaret S. Herridge and Jill I. Cameron

Introduction

Severe critical illness is a traumatic life event for patients and families. Patients acquire new and irreversible disabilities, and carers develop mood disorders. Each has a nagging sense that their lives have been irretrievably altered and that things will never be the same again. New morbidities compromise functional outcome and are costly in both economic and human terms. Interventions to ameliorate these issues will need to be informed by functional outcome and need assessments in patients and caregivers and targeted to specific physical and neuropsychological challenges that are dynamic and will continue to evolve during protracted recovery.

Longitudinal follow-up after ICU and the documentation of the natural history of morbidity after critical illness have helped to underscore the need for a relevant framework to inform interventions and the development of a post-ICU rehabilitation pathway for the survivors, their relatives, and their carers after critical illness. Knowledge of current rehabilitation theory may provide invaluable insights into how tenets from the rehabilitation literature may influence emerging models of care for our critically ill patients and families.

This chapter will highlight the ICF model as a putative rehabilitation construct for patients and families after critical illness. This framework helps to highlight the complexity and interdependence of factors that determine outcome after illness and incorporates multiple facets of the individual experience. The model also serves to emphasize current deficiencies and challenges to the construction, testing, and implementation of interventions for the critically ill patient and family. To assist in the early recognition and stratification of patient groups for testing future rehabilitation interventions, a novel framework of aetiologically neutral clinical phenotypes, with distinct recovery trajectories after critical illness, will be discussed and how these groupings comprise the spectrum of disability after critical illness. Finally, the concept of longitudinal care, incorporating the perspective of changing rehabilitative needs over time and the importance of assisting in transitions of care, will be outlined.

International Classification of Functioning, Disability, and Health (ICF)

The ICF[1] was developed and endorsed by the 54th World Health Assembly in 2001. This framework was highlighted again in 2005 as part of the WHO resolution on 'disability, including prevention, management and rehabilitation' and reinforced a shift in WHO's commitment to mitigating the morbidity associated with different health conditions affecting the international community.

The ICF acknowledges that morbidity and disability are important metrics of health status and provides a unifying framework and standard lexicon to classify health-related states or domains for measurement of health outcome at an individual and population level. The ICF incorporates and emphasizes functional outcome and, in this way, differs significantly from the International Classification of Disease (ICD) which focuses exclusively on disease and its contribution to death. As outlined in Figure 50.1, the ICF consists of three central components, including: body function and structures, activity, and participation. This framework offers a comprehensive and holistic approach to the construction of longitudinal studies and multifaceted interventions for complex patient populations. In light of the emerging data on impaired function and neuropsychological morbidity after critical illness and significant mood disorders sustained by family members, the ICF helps to capture and highlight the interdependence of the myriad of factors that determine outcome.

Any physical dysfunction sustained by an individual is captured by the 'body functions and structures' component of the ICF where any deviation from normal is characterized as impairment. The patients' ability to execute important activities is captured as 'Activity' and highlights the construct of 'activity limitations'. Engagement in different life activities is captured by 'Participation' where 'participation restriction' underscores the difficulties patients may experience when trying to carry out ADLs. The three components of the ICF capture function and disability and are modified by global health, environmental, and personal factors. This framework is quite distinct from QoL models, because the ICF may employ objective functional metrics which may be quantified. This is in contradistinction to many QoL measures which tend to be very personalized and which report function, based on subjective feelings or personal views of satisfaction. For example, the generic SF-36 QoL instrument has been widely used to

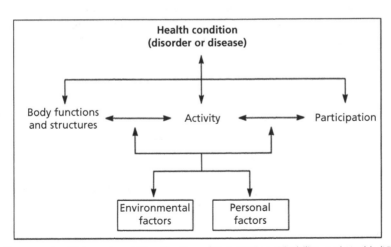

Fig. 50.1 Framework of International Classification of Functioning, Disability, and Health (ICF) by World Health Organization in 2001.

Reproduced from Stucki G, 'International Classification of Functioning, Disability, and Health (ICF): a promising framework and classification for rehabilitation medicine', *American Journal of Physical Medicine and Rehabilitation*, 84, 10, pp. 733–740, copyright 2005, with permission from Wolters Kluwer, Association of Academic Physiatrists and the Asociación Médica Latinoamericana de Rehabilitación (AMLAR).

characterize functional outcomes and to serve as a comparator across different populations. However, it identifies functioning solely in the context of disease and does not incorporate aspects of patient participation or how personal factors or environment influence reported outcome. As a consequence, one may imagine how this limits insights into the specific factors influencing functional disability and how this would fail to assist in the construction of effective rehabilitation interventions to meet those impairments.

The ICF is universal, internationally validated, and integrative and incorporates contextual aspects of the individual and their environment. It offers a lot of value added. The ICF uses a biopsychosocial model that is **aetiologically neutral** and where patients' health and functioning are viewed in the broader context of their person and environment. Its strength is that it encompasses both social and medical elements and is not culturally or age-biased, since it is international in scope. The ICF is a very attractive model for patients and families after critical illness, because it is not driven by the inciting illness but rather by resultant morbidity. After many days in the ICU, the importance of the initial disease state fades and is gradually replaced by the robust and, some might suggest, ubiquitous morbidities of ICUAW and neuropsychological dysfunction. These become the main determinants of long-term morbidity and outcome.

WHO disability assessment schedule, international classification of functioning checklist, and international classification of functioning core sets

As a reference classification system, the ICF is exhaustive and includes over 1400 listed categories. This makes it inclusive, but impractical, as a viable clinical assessment tool. The WHO developed some practical tools relevant for the ICF framework that may also have utility for rehabilitation intervention and outcomes work. These include the generic self-administered WHO Disability Assessment Schedule II (WHODAS II)[2] and the ICF Checklist,[3] and these are focused on the domains of activity and participation. A brief discussion of these follows and helps to highlight how the ICF brings a very unique and comprehensive perspective to models of rehabilitative measures that emphasize many aspects of recovery that have been overlooked to date in models of rehabilitation after critical illness.

WHODAS II

The WHODAS II is a generic and culturally inclusive health status measure that is applicable across a range of educational and cultural backgrounds and includes a 36- and 12-item version comprising six domains, including: understanding and communicating, getting around, self-care, getting along with others, household and work activities, and participation in society. The strength of this measure is its integrative approach with important patient-centred metrics. The disadvantage is that it completely de-emphasizes the disease process and is unable to provide more discrete linkages between disease states and outcome if these are desired.

ICF Checklist

The ICF Checklist is an abbreviated version of the ICF, consisting of 125 second-level categories. All patient-related information from written records, primary respondents, direct observation, family or professional caregiver, or other informants may be used for its completion. It includes inputs from a spectrum of sources and provides an interprofessional evaluation of the patient, her family, and environment and brings this approach to rehabilitation, something that has been lacking in many current models of rehabilitation after critical illness. The barrier to its use is a lengthy completion time which is significantly extended in those patients with multiple impairments, activity limitations, and participation restrictions.

ICF Core Sets

ICF Core Sets have been developed because the ICF Checklist and the WHODAS may be impractical and may not meet the needs of clinicians and researchers focused on patients with specific disease states or those receiving rehabilitation treatment after an acute illness episode. To date, ICF Core Sets have been developed for 12 chronic conditions[4–6] and for acute hospitals and early post-acute rehabilitation facilities.[7]

For each health condition, a Brief ICF Core Set and a Comprehensive ICF Core Set have been established. The Brief ICF Core Set is intended for clinical use and designed to limit categories to be practical but still adequately comprehensive for clinical studies. The categories of the Brief ICF Core Set serve as a minimum data set, intended to be reported in every clinical study, to describe the burden of disease in a comparable way across studies.

The Comprehensive ICF Core Set is intended to guide multidisciplinary assessments in patients with a specified condition and sufficiently inclusive to describe in a comprehensive, multidisciplinary assessment the typical spectrum of problems in functioning of patients with a specific condition. Thus, within the global ICF framework, patient-centred evaluations and both abbreviated and comprehensive tools have been developed and tailored across a spectrum of disease. These may serve as templates for future candidate models of data collection in longitudinal studies after critical illness and the formulation of rehabilitation programmes for patients and families.

A unifying framework of concepts and terminology is of utmost importance for any professional, academic, and scientific field to facilitate and ensure communication and exchange among scientists and practitioners. The ICF framework seems very attractive to critical care practitioners and those engaged in post-ICU rehabilitation, since this is not necessarily restricted by disease although can be made more disease-specific, as outlined previously. The availability of a common framework seems to have particular importance for critical care which is not defined by a specific disease or discrete organ system and which is typically interprofessional, both in research and practice.

Conclusion

Current definitions of rehabilitation have focused on enabling the individual only. Consequently, they have neglected the social perspective recognizing that people with health conditions not only experience disability in relation to impairments, but also in relation to physical, social, and economic barriers of their particular environment. Accordingly, current definitions generally fail to address the immediate environment in the context of the rehabilitation of individuals. As well, they do not explicitly address social policy nor political actions necessary to favourably change the environment for the disabled.

The ICF framework highlights the complexity and interdependence of factors that influence recovery and underscores the myriad factors that need to be considered when designing rehabilitation interventions. It represents a comprehensive and highly relevant construct for making explicit the complex interplay of factors that influence health outcomes and long-term morbidity. Traditional models have based treatment on physical function metrics in isolation and may not have focused or acknowledged that the mechanism of effect may reside with environmental change, e.g in accompanying social supports, patient mood, family caregiver, or more broadly on social or political change.

Challenges to rehabilitative model construction after critical illness

Translational research and rehabilitation after critical illness

There is increasing emphasis on the importance of basic science research and its role in elucidating the molecular aspects of muscle, nerve, and brain injury which constitute the major morbidities after critical illness.[8] It is most likely that body structure and function will be emphasized as the most tangible outcomes for translational work, because the process of translating basic science observations at the molecular, cellular, and system level into rehabilitation treatments is most accessible at the level of the person with limited function and independence. However, it is crucial to be aware of the complex matrix of factors that intersect to create better or worse outcomes during the early and later stages of recovery. Research on therapies that address body structure and function disabilities face the significant challenge of asserting whether a treatment targeted at that level will have an impact on the diverse and complex aspects of participation which are the more typical rehabilitation treatment outcomes.

Treatment and enablement theories

Treatment and enablement theories each contribute a unique perspective and should be included to capture and understand the relationship between a single intervention and its complex downstream consequences on a spectrum of outcomes. These theories have important implications for the timing and capture of target outcome measures for an intervention.

Treatment theory

Treatment theory highlights the way in which a given treatment intervention affects its target. Using ICUAW as an example, the application of early mobility during the ICU stay (**treatment**) may lead to an increase in power and bulk of the muscle (**treatment target**) by suppressing various proteolytic pathways at the muscle molecular level (**treatment mechanism**) Treatment theory will not inform the effect of early mobility on a more distal functional outcome such as walking. The isolated impact of improved muscle strength on the ability to walk will also depend on a variety of other patient factors on which a muscle-directed intervention has no direct impact. These may include: balance and gait, proprioception, cognitive function, mood, and home environment.

Enablement theory

Enablement theory captures the causal interrelationships among variables at different ICF levels. If we use walking ability as one example, enablement theory highlights and dissects the various capacities that need to be operational to ambulate effectively. As an example, these may include visual perception or proprioception (see Figure 50.2). In addition, this theory attempts to parse out the relative contribution of each and its respective role to influence that function. Enablement theory may be summarized as identifying causal contributors and the weight attached to each within the ICF framework. It does not elucidate mechanism.

The spectrum of disability after critical illness comprising different clinical phenotypes

We continue to have a limited understanding of the matrix of factors that promote the development and resolution of muscle, nerve, and brain and their relationship to distal outcomes. As an example, it remains unclear how different risk groups sustain varying degrees of muscle and nerve

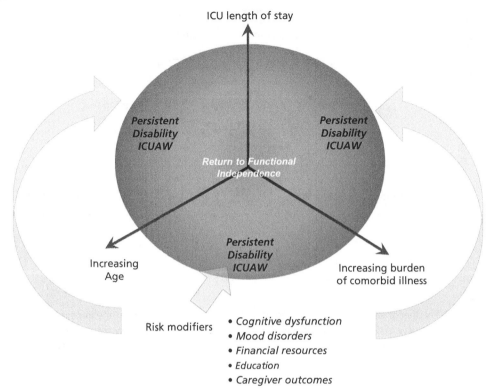

Fig. 50.2 Different clinical phenotypes and the spectrum of disability.

Reprinted with permission of the American Thoracic Society. Copyright © 2014 American Thoracic Society. Batt, Dos Santos, Cameron and Herridge, 2013, *American Journal of Respiratory Critical Care Medicine*, 187, 3, pp. 238–246.

injury and whether early recognition and intervention with early mobility would alter the natural history of the affected organ system. If one looks at the ICF model and construct in Figure 50.3, it is not clear how weakness in isolation will affect the outcomes of driving or return to work. This highlights the need to also target activity and participation, and also economic and personal factors to understand how this complex grouping each contributes to a discrete functional outcome. Risk modification by family or access to expensive resources must be seen as crucial factors to be included in cohort studies and rehabilitation strategies (see Figure 50.2).

Functional disability after critical illness has been described as heterogeneous, but emerging data from recent studies support the hypothesis that the heterogeneity may be organized into discrete phenotypes, with varied risk and recovery after critical illness. It is possible that, by embracing an aetiologically neutral approach, more efficiencies may be realized within rehabilitation programmes, with an understanding of how common patient traits like age, burden of comorbid illness, and ICU length of stay may facilitate the tailoring of programmes to specific patient needs.

The first several months after critical illness are crucial, as many patients have a significant improvement in function.[9–12] There is variability in outcome during this time and evidence to suggest a spectrum of disability across different patient groupings, related to age, burden of comorbid disease, and ICU length of stay. The current outcomes literature suggests that these same factors determine subsequent functional outcome and HRQoL[13–18] and may act as surrogates for muscle and nerve injury and subsequent recovery and health trajectory over time.

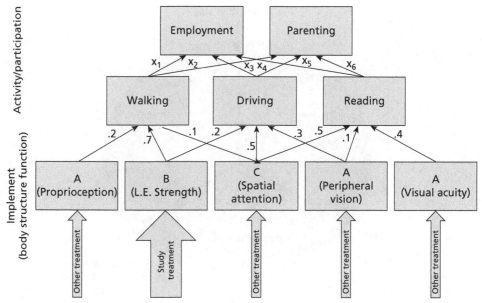

Fig. 50.3 The theoretical relationship among variables in the ICF framework at the impairment (body structure/function) and activity/participation levels. It is important to note how the combination of several variables at the lower level contributes to performance outcomes at the next level. For example, an intervention targeting strength will need to address proprioception and spatial attention in order to effect an improvement in walking outcomes.

Reprinted from *Archives of Physical Medicine and Rehabilitation*, 93, 8, suppl 2, Whyte et al., 'Advancing the evidence base of rehabilitation treatments: a developmental approach', pp. S101–110, copyright 2012, with permission from Elsevier and American Congress of Rehabilitation Medicine.

Type and severity of critical illness, age, and comorbidities

The severe lung injury phenotype has been recognized and robust in the clinical literature for over a decade. Younger patients with severe ARDS and multiorgan dysfunction, who sustain significant ICUAW,[9,12,19–22] may regain functional independence and return to work. In contrast, outcomes in those who are only a decade older, with greater baseline morbidity and who were not working, retired, or disabled at the time of ICU admission were far worse. At 1 year, only 9% of this study sample were alive and functionally independent.[14] These patients were likely to be discharged to a post-acute care facility and incur substantial costs, estimated at $3.5 million per independently functioning survivor at 1 year.[14]

Outcome studies of older patients and those requiring PMV underscore the important impact of age and pre-existing comorbidities. Chelluri and colleagues evaluated factors associated with mortality and QoL in a study sample (median age 65) 1 year after PMV.[22] Survivors had fewer comorbidities, lower severity of illness, and less premorbid functional dependence. In patients receiving MV for ≥14 days, Combes and others showed that age >65 years, poor premorbid cardiac function, immunocompromised status, septic shock at ICU admission, need for RRT in the ICU, and nosocomial septicaemia were associated with death.[23]

In an older patient sample (median age 77), Iwashyna and colleagues observed a lasting reduction in functional outcome after sepsis and a high rate of new functional limitations in those who had no limits prior to their episode of critical illness (mean 1.57 new limitations, 95% CI

0.99–2.15). Those who had compromised ADLs prior to sepsis had an important further reduction in physical and neurocognitive function for at least 8 years after the episode of sepsis, and this altered the patients' ability to live independently.[13]

The impact of increased age on outcomes after critical illness remains somewhat controversial, however. Some report poor survival with advanced age,[24] while others do not.[25,26] Khouli et al.[27] reported on a large sample of patients aged 65 years old and older, and a HRQoL instrument was administered to the patient/proxy at ICU admission and 6 months after hospital discharge. One-third of those 65 years and older died within 6 months of hospital discharge, and risks for death included: number of days during the 30 days before hospitalization that the patient felt their 'physical health was not good', a higher APACHE II score, and chronic pulmonary disease. These authors also found that the oldest survivors (aged 86) had declining HRQoL over time, including more days spent with poor physical and mental health, compared to baseline. Using a national population-based study sample, with an average patient age of almost 80 years, including information on pre-admission functional status, Barnato and others[18] reported that elderly survivors of MV had a marked decline in ADLs and an important reduction in mobility, compared to survivors of hospitalization without MV. There is a prognostic signal in the elderly in terms of the importance of organ reserve, baseline organ dysfunction, and the trajectory of health status prior to critical illness for prediction of subsequent survival, functional status, and HRQoL.

These data would appear to support different groupings of age, degree of comorbid illness and severity of critical illness, and ICU length of stay as distinct clinical phenotypes and potential proxy measures for the degree of muscle and nerve reserve and potential for functional recovery. The collapse of these different risk strata into a single population may account for the notion of heterogeneity in the ICU outcomes literature. Risk modification is a key issue and includes the effects of mood disorders,[20,28] cognitive dysfunction,[29,30] socio-economic status, and the mental and physical health of the caregiver.

More than half of ICU survivors who received long-term MV still required the assistance of a family caregiver 1 year after their critical illness.[22] Provision of this care may have a negative impact on caregivers, including poor HRQoL,[31] PTSD,[32] emotional distress,[33–35] burden,[36] depression,[34] and anxiety.[35] Work from our group reported ARDS survivors' depression and need for high levels of care as important risks for caregivers' depression.[31] Other reports show that caregivers experience more depression and difficulty maintaining valued activities when caring for male ICU survivors with poorer functional status.[33,37,38]

Figure 50.2 depicts a theoretical construct of the risk for, and functional outcomes after, ICUAW. Clinical phenotypes, including younger patients without any comorbidities, older individuals with significant comorbidities, and the chronically critically ill who may have exhausted their muscle and nerve reserve, are outlined. We hypothesize that each of these clinical phenotypes may be associated with different degrees of pre-existing muscle reserve or injury and therefore predisposed to different functional outcomes. This model also highlights the interdependence between patient outcomes and their caregiver's physical and mental health. Socio-economic factors are also included as risk modifiers.

Phase-specific approach to recovery after critical illness

Little is known about the needs of ICU survivors and family caregivers and how these needs interact across the illness and recovery trajectory, especially during inpatient rehabilitation or the first years back in the community. Current work has identified significant information deficits in survivors and family caregivers during acute care hospitalization[39] and the need for psychological care in the community.[40]

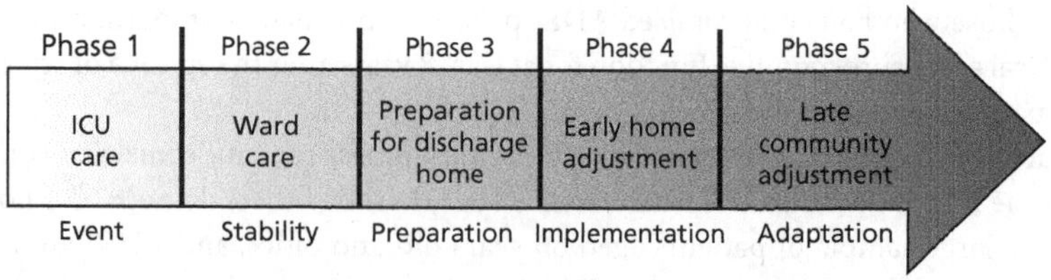

Fig. 50.4 Longitudinal rehabilitative needs and the 'Timing it right' framework.
Reproduced with permission from Jill I. Cameron, PhD.

Timing it right (TIR) framework

Longer-term follow-up and community support are essential for ICU survivors and their family caregivers.[41] When planning interventions, their needs must be addressed across the entire care continuum. To address this, Cameron et al. devised the TIR framework, using the clinical course of stroke as a model of acute illness, to promote an approach to derive and evaluate interventions to meet patients' and family caregivers' needs. This framework has been adapted to critical illness and consists of five phases, including the following: (1) the critical illness event and course of ICU care, (2) phase of stability on the general ward, (3) preparing to return home and to community life, (4) early adjustment in the home, and (5) longer-term adjustment to community living (see Figure 50.4). The premise is that attention to phase-specific needs enhances patient and family preparedness and eases transitions across care environments. The acknowledgement that needs vary across care transitions and over time is a first step to their consideration as part of comprehensive rehabilitation programmes.

Conclusion

Rehabilitation for survivors of critical illness and their families will require a complex and longitudinal intervention, founded on patient and family-centred outcomes. This chapter has argued the need for a validated clinical framework that captures disability for patients and families after critical illness and that incorporates important modifying risks essential to inform the design of future rehabilitation strategies. We also propose a novel construct for aetiologically neutral clinical phenotypes, based on the current literature and with an emphasis on age, burden of comorbid illness, and ICU length of stay. These phenotypes may offer practical and easily recognizable clinical groupings, with similar recovery trajectories for evaluation of different tailored rehabilitation interventions. Finally, we chose to highlight the TIR framework to emphasize a phase-specific approach for longitudinal intervention so that outcomes for patients and families can be optimized across care transitions.

References

1 Stucki G. International Classification of Functioning, Disability, and Health (ICF): a promising framework and classification for rehabilitation medicine. *Am J Phys Med Rehabil* 2005;**84**:733–40.
2 World Health Organization. *WHO Mental Bulletin: a newsletter on noncommunicable diseases and mental health.* Geneva: World Health Organization; 2000.
3 World Health Organization. *ICF Checklist, Version 2.1a, Clinical Form for International Classification of Functioning, Disability and Health.* Geneva, World Health Organization; 2003.

4 **Ustun B, Chatterji S, Kostanjsek N.** Comments from WHO for the Journal of Rehabilitation Medicine Special Supplement on ICF Core Sets. *J Rehabil Med* 2004;**44** Suppl:7–8.

5 **Stucki G, Grimby G.** Applying the ICF in medicine. *J Rehabil Med* 2004;**44** Suppl:5–6.

6 **Cieza A, Ewert T, Ustun TB, Chatterji S, Kostanjsek N, Stucki G.** Development of ICF Core Sets for patients with chronic conditions. *J Rehabil Med* 2004;**44** Suppl:9–11.

7 **Grill E, Ewert T, Chatterji S, Kostanjsek N, Stucki G.** ICF Core Sets development for the acute hospital and early post-acute rehabilitation facilities. *Disabil Rehabil* 2005;**27**:361–6.

8 **Whyte J BA.** Advancing the evidence base of rehabilitation treatments: a developmental approach. *Arch Phys Med Rehabil* 2012;**93**(8 Suppl):S101–10.

9 **Herridge MS, Cheung AM, Tansey CM, et al.** One-year outcomes in survivors of the acute respiratory distress syndrome. *N Engl J Med* 2003;**348**:683–93.

10 **Herridge MS, Tansey CM, Matté A, et al.** Functional disability 5 years after acute respiratory distress syndrome. *N Engl J Med* 2011;**364**:1293–304.

11 **McHugh LG, Milberg JA, Whitcomb ME, Schoene RB, Maunder RJ, Hudson LD.** Recovery of function in survivors of the acute respiratory distress syndrome. *Am J Respir Crit Care Med* 1994;**150**:90–4.

12 **Needham DM, Dennison CR, Dowdy DW, et al.** Study protocol: the Improving Care of Acute Lung Injury Patients (ICAP) study. *Crit Care* 2006;**10**:R9.

13 **Iwashyna TJ, Ely EW, Smith DM, Langa KM.** Long-term cognitive impairment and functional disability among survivors of severe sepsis. *JAMA* 2010;**304**:1787–94.

14 **Unroe M, Kahn JM, Carson SS, et al.** One-year trajectories of care and resource utilization for recipients of prolonged mechanical ventilation: a cohort study. *Ann Intern Med* 2010;**153**:167–75.

15 **de Letter MA, Schmitz PI, Visser LH, et al.** Risk factors for the development of polyneuropathy and myopathy in critically ill patients. *Crit Care Med* 2001;**29**:2281–6.

16 **Hough CL.** Neuromuscular sequelae in survivors of acute lung injury. *Clin Chest Med* 2006;**27**:691–703.

17 **Latronico N, Peli E, Botteri M.** Critical illness myopathy and neuropathy. *Curr Opin Crit Care* 2005;**11**:126–32.

18 **Barnato AE, Albert SM, Angus DC, Lave JR, Degenholtz HB.** Disability among elderly survivors of mechanical ventilation. *Am J Respir Crit Care Med* 2011;**183**:1037–42.

19 **Hopkins RO, Weaver LK, Collingridge D, Parkinson RB, Chan KJ, Orme JF, Jr.** Two-year cognitive, emotional, and quality-of-life outcomes in acute respiratory distress syndrome. *Am J Respir Crit Care Med* 2005;**171**:340–7.

20 **Hopkins RO, Weaver LK, Pope D, Orme JF, Bigler ED, Larson-LOHR V.** Neuropsychological sequelae and impaired health status in survivors of severe acute respiratory distress syndrome. *Am J Respir Crit Care Med* 1999;**160**:50–6.

21 **Dowdy DW, Eid MP, Sedrakyan A, et al.** Quality of life in adult survivors of critical illness: a systematic review of the literature. *Intensive Care Med* 2005;**31**:611–20.

22 **Chelluri L, Im KA, Belle SH, et al.** Long-term mortality and quality of life after prolonged mechanical ventilation. *Crit Care Med* 2004;**32**:61–9.

23 **Combes A, Costa MA, Trouillet JL, et al.** Morbidity, mortality, and quality-of-life outcomes of patients requiring > or = 14 days of mechanical ventilation. *Crit Care Med* 2003;**31**:1373–81.

24 **Somme D, Maillet JM, Gisselbrecht M, Novara A, Ract C, Fagon JY.** Critically ill old and the oldest-old patients in intensive care: short- and long-term outcomes. *Intensive Care Med* 2003;**29**:2137–43.

25 **Chelluri L, Pinsky MR, Donahoe MP, Grenvik A.** Long-term outcome of critically ill elderly patients requiring intensive care. *JAMA* 1993;**269**:3119–23.

26 **Rockwood K, Noseworthy TW, Gibney RT, et al.** One-year outcome of elderly and young patients admitted to intensive care units. *Crit Care Med* 1993;**21**:687–91.

27 **Khouli H, Astua A, Dombrowski W, et al.** Changes in health-related quality of life and factors predicting long-term outcomes in older adults admitted to intensive care units. *Crit Care Med* 2011;**39**:731–7.

28 Jackson JC, Girard TD, Gordon SM, et al. Long-term cognitive and psychological outcomes in the awakening and breathing controlled trial. *Am J Respir Crit Care Med* 2010;**182**:183–91.

29 Ehlenbach WJ, Hough CL, Crane PK, et al. Association between acute care and critical illness hospitalization and cognitive function in older adults. *JAMA* 2010;**303**:763–70.

30 Mikkelsen ME, Christie JD, Lanken PN, et al. The adult respiratory distress syndrome cognitive outcomes study: long-term neuropsychological function in survivors of acute lung injury . *Am J Respir Crit Care Med* 2012;**185**:1307–15.

31 Cameron JI, Herridge MS, Tansey CM, McAndrews MP, Cheung AM. Well-being in informal caregivers of survivors of acute respiratory distress syndrome. *Crit Care Med* 2006;**34**:81–6.

32 Azoulay E, Pochard F, Kentish-Barnes N, et al. Risk of post-traumatic stress symptoms in family members of intensive care unit patients. *Am J Respir Crit Care Med* 2005;**171**:987–94.

33 Van P, Schulz R, Chelluri L, Pinsky MR. Patient-specific, time-varying predictors of post-ICU informal caregiver burden: the caregiver outcomes after ICU discharge project. *Chest* 2010;**137**:88–94.

34 Douglas SL, Daly BJ, Kelley CG, O'Toole E, Montenegro H. Impact of a disease management program upon caregivers of chronically critically ill patients. *Chest* 2005;**128**:3925–36.

35 Pochard F, Darmon M, Fassier T, et al. Symptoms of anxiety and depression in family members of intensive care unit patients before discharge or death. A prospective multicenter study. *J Crit Care* 2005;**20**:90–6.

36 Foster M, Chaboyer W. Family carers of ICU survivors: a survey of the burden they experience. *Scand J Caring Sci* 2003;**17**:205–14.

37 Choi J, Sherwood PR, Schulz R, et al. Patterns of depressive symptoms in caregivers of mechanically ventilated critically ill adults from intensive care unit admission to 2 months postintensive care unit discharge: a pilot study. *Crit Care Med* 2012;**40**:1546–53.

38 Choi J, Donahoe MP, Zullo TG, Hoffman LA. Caregivers of the chronically critically ill after discharge from the intensive care unit: six months' experience. *Am J Crit Care* 2011;**20**:12–22.

39 Nelson JE, Kinjo K, Meier DE, Ahmad K, Morrison RS. When critical illness becomes chronic: informational needs of patients and families. *J Crit Care* 2005;**20**:79–89.

40 Pattison NA, Dolan S, Townsend P, Townsend R. After critical care: a study to explore patients' experiences of a follow-up service. *J Clin Nurs* 2007;**16**:2122–31.

41 Cameron JI, Gignac MA. 'Timing it Right': a conceptual framework for addressing family caregivers' support needs from the hospital to the home. *Patient Educ Couns* 2008;**70**:305–14.

Chapter 51

Post-ICU Rehabilitation

Doug Elliott and Linda Denehy

Introduction

Survival to hospital discharge following a critical illness is relatively similar across the globe. Specifically, it has been shown that survival ranges from 75 to 94% in Europe[1] and 82% in North America.[2] In addition, survival has been documented at 89% for general ICU patients[3] and 78% for those mechanically ventilated in Australia.[4] For some of these survivors, delayed physical,[5] psychological,[6,7] and cognitive recovery[8] is evident. Recent consensus work has identified emerging clinical syndromes and highlighted related practices that require further research across the continuum of critical illness,[9] including:

- ICUAW which results from a combination of the presenting illness (commonly sepsis), treatments and interventions, and bed rest[5,10]

- PICS which encompasses physical, psychological, and cognitive sequelae that persist beyond hospital discharge for patients[11] and their relatives.[12]

Other recent work has explored 'bundles of clinical care' for minimizing the sequelae of ICUAW and delirium, such as the ABCDE approach,[13,14] and interventions specifically focused on cognitive rehabilitation.[15] Specific exercises and mobility activities to minimize physical deconditioning while in ICU include passive stretching and range-of-motion exercises for limbs and joints, positioning, resistive muscle training, aerobic training, muscle strengthening, and ambulation.[16,17] These activities range from in-bed (range of motion, roll, bridge, sitting on edge of bed), standing at the bedside, transfers to and from bed to chair, marching on the spot, and walking.[18,19] These initiatives vary across health systems and are often related to innovations by motivated teams. A detailed description of exercise and early rehabilitation in ICU can be found in Chapters 50 and 52.

The challenge for commencement and continuation of rehabilitation activities in the general wards after ICU discharge relates to the coordination of available resources from the admitting medical teams and other consultants, physiotherapy, and other allied health services. Availability of rehabilitation services for general ICU patients can be influenced by the fiscal context of the health service or system and the demand from other clinical cohorts with defined rehabilitation pathways such as pulmonary, cardiac, stroke, and brain injury.[20] Similarly, the demand for scarce health service outreach or community resources can impact optimal recovery for survivors of a critical illness. Within this context, appropriate, systematic, and timely screening is therefore crucial to identify individuals at risk of physical, psychological, and cognitive sequelae.

This chapter examines the current evidence for post-ICU rehabilitation, for both in-hospital and post-hospital contexts. Initial sections focus on patient engagement with rehabilitation strategies and methodological and pragmatic issues related to measurement of functional recovery.

Post-ICU and post-hospital interventions are also discussed, followed by a description of available resources and support, including the use of evolving technologies.

Measurement of recovery

Once discharged from ICU, patients present with a broad range of functional impairment, often depending on underlying disease processes, premorbid function, time on MV, level of sedation received, length of ICU stay, and current age.[21-23] The acute health care team, particularly physiotherapy, speech and occupational therapists, uses outcome measures to standardize assessments, monitor treatment effectiveness, and improve care quality.[24] However, few measures of function have been specifically designed for the ICU population, with most being drawn from geriatric, neurological, pulmonary, and cardiac rehabilitation cohorts. In most cases, therefore, clinically worthwhile changes for measurement tools specific to ICU populations have not been evaluated or reported.

Measures of function commonly reported in the literature are the 6-minute walk test,[25] shuttle walk test,[26] 10-metre walk test,[27] the short physical performance battery comprising sit to stand; balance; walk speed,[28] and the physical function domain of the SF-36,[29] IADLs,[30] the Timed Up and Go test (TUG),[31] FIM,[32-34] Barthel index,[23,35] handgrip strength,[36,37] and muscle strength using HHD.[38,39] There is a large body of information that describes each of these tests and their clinimetric properties, although few specifically in ICU populations.[40]

With a range of functional abilities in patients in acute care hospital wards, several reports of ceiling and floor effects for these tests are evident. The FIM has demonstrated floor effects in acute populations as a result of low functional status and may not be sensitive to change if ward length of stay is short.[41] Similarly, the TUG and the Barthel index are reported to show both floor and ceiling effects in hospitalized elderly medical patients[42] and patients discharged from ICU.[43] In an observational cohort study of critical care survivors, the shuttle walk test demonstrated an 89% improvement after outpatient rehabilitation, compared with a 58% improvement in the 6-minute walk test.[44] Use of the shuttle walk as an alternative to the 6-minute walk should be examined in future research. To date, no reports have directly related reduced muscle strength to reduced function, so the challenge is to identify a 'package' or bundle of tests that may be suitable for the range in age and ability of post-ICU populations. Development of new tests for different stages of recovery, such as the University of Rochester Acute Care Evaluation, may hold promise.[24] Clearly, establishing the test sensitivity for future research and comparison across studies is important.

Outcome measures after hospital discharge should, in addition, include measures of community-based activity levels,[45] HRQoL, return to work and driving, level of community supports, depression and anxiety, and executive and cognitive function. Several papers report the ongoing deficits in HRQoL up to 5 years after ICU discharge,[46] and review papers present the instrument properties for use to measure outcomes in ICU survivors. Measures, such as HRQoL questionnaires, are commonly utilized, and the generic instrument SF-36 is the most often reported,[47] with supportive clinimetric testing in ICU populations. Other multi-attribute utility instruments, such as the SF6D (derived from the SF-36), EQ-5D, and assessment of quality of life (AQoL),[48] are used to provide additional utility measures for economic analyses. These measures vary in scaling attributes, and small differences can impact cost analyses; more research is required to establish the most appropriate scale for use in ICU survivors. Generic HRQoL instruments also have limitations in the ICU population, as baseline or premorbid measures are difficult to obtain and may be subject to recall bias and response shift. More research into the level of bias in these measures will allow more accurate interpretation of results in the future.

Post-ICU interventions

The current evidence base for practices designed to improve the rehabilitation of patients after ICU discharge is described in this section. There is currently no system-wide approach to recovery and rehabilitation to manage physical, psychological, or cognitive dysfunction,[49] despite some practice guidelines[50] and other resources being available. Most importantly, these guidelines reported that there is currently no evidence defining the optimal timing for initiating rehabilitation and the type of rehabilitation strategy that should be delivered.

Ward-based post-ICU rehabilitation

Contemporary practices for patients discharged from intensive care include ICU liaison services[51,52] and rapid response teams,[53,54] with a focus predominantly on monitoring for clinical deterioration but not developed for delivering rehabilitation activities. This is to manage the 10% of patients who survive to ICU discharge but will die prior to hospital discharge.[55] Screening approaches for identifying relevant patients for rehabilitation during their post-ICU admission may therefore include patients who subsequently die.

Functional decline in older hospitalized medical patients independent of pre-admission illness has been reported.[56] Rehabilitation on acute hospital wards has therefore been advocated to reduce this deconditioning associated with immobility, and functional maintenance programmes have been commenced in some centres to meet this aim.[57] These programmes include group-based rehabilitation in a hospital gymnasium, if possible, as well as increased therapy visits and mobility programmes. However, there is limited evidence of benefit for elderly medical patients on the acute ward receiving multidisciplinary rehabilitation where small or inconclusive increases in discharge to home, reduced hospital stay, and costs were reported.[42] It is, however, interesting to note that the average age of patients in trials that included specific exercise in this systematic review was 78 years, considerably older than the reported age of ICU survivors which is around 60 years.

There is a current lack of evidence on the effects of specific interventions during the post-ICU hospital period, aimed at improving the recovery trajectory and health outcomes for patients with limited physical function. Questions therefore remain regarding the optimal duration, intensity, type, and frequency of interventions.[58] Specific ward-based rehabilitation interventions for ICU survivors are beginning to be investigated, with examples listed in Table 51.1. Impairment in functional ability can be significant for some patients after ICU discharge,[23] and close monitoring and early rehabilitation during this period are recommended. The data detailed in Table 51.1 show the beneficial effect on patient outcome, following an exercise rehabilitation strategy that starts in the ICU and continues to the ward setting.[59] These exercises, commenced in ICU and continued to independence or hospital discharge, began with passive and active protocols and progressed to functional tasks, including balance and transfers before standing and walking.[60] Different physiological exercise strategies were used in another RCT where exercise was prescribed, based on an outcome measure, and progressed in frequency and intensity using a described protocol in order to elicit a training effect.[61] Additionally, exercise was commenced at the highest level possible during the time of intervention. These protocol and progression differences may not be important, as both approaches may result in functional improvements, but highlight the need for detailed description of protocols and more research to refine interventions in the future.

Findings from the remaining studies also indicated the need for further evaluations in this cohort who have significant functional decline after discharge from ICU. These should also include identifying groups who may respond, including a multidisciplinary rehabilitation strategy. Phase one rehabilitation, as applied in other patient cohorts (including COPD and cardiac populations),

Table 51.1 Ward-based intervention studies

Author/design	Sample		Methods	Findings
	Cohort	n		
Van der Schaff (2008)[23]/ observational	MV >48 hours; median MV 6 days; median LOS 7 days	69	Assessments 3–7 days post-ICU discharge: functional status, walking, muscle strength, cognitive function	75% severely dependent for ADLs (Barthel index 0–12), no independent walking for 73%, grip strength reduced in 50%, cognitive impairment in 30%
Salisbury (2010)[103]/ feasibility RCT[a]	For C:I, median MV 12.5:21.5 days; median ICU LOS 16.5:23 days	16	Generic rehabilitation assistant supporting enhanced physiotherapy and nutrition; 3-month follow-up (n = 11)	Higher weekly frequencies of treatments for intervention group— physiotherapy (C:I) 2.6:8.2, dietetics 1.2:4.9; no significant differences for walk tests[b], handgrip dynamometry, fatigue, pain, appetite
Schweikert (2009)[59]/RCT	For C:I, median MV 6.1:3.4 days; median ICU LOS 7.9:5.9 days	104	PT[c] and OT during DIS in ICU and continued post-ICU discharge; 87% of intervention patients	Independent function at hospital discharge was (C:I) 35%:59%; intervention group had shorter duration of delirium—4:2 days, and more VFDs—21.1:23.5 days
Denehy (2012, 2013)[61,69]	For C:I median MV 4.4: 4.1 days; median ICU LOS 7:8	150	PT during ICU continued on the ward as 60 min exercise/day (cardiovascular, strength, and functional exercises)	No significant differences in 6MWT or TUG tests at hospital discharge. HRQoL not assessed

ADLs, activities of daily living; C:I, control: intervention; DIS, daily interruption of sedation; LOS, length of stay; OT, occupational therapy; PT, physiotherapy/physical therapy; RCT, randomized controlled trial; ROM, range of motion; VFD, ventilator-free day.

[a] Service evaluation phase also reported with 24 participants.

[b] Rivermead Mobility Index, TUG, 10-metre walk test, incremental shuttle walk test.

[c] When patient alert and cooperative, active assisted and independent ROM, progressing to bed mobility activities and ADLs.

could be applied to critically ill survivors in the absence of sufficient current evidence.[62] In phase one rehabilitation, an individual plan of care is designed to address deconditioning and promote early discharge with improved levels of function.[24] This rehabilitation commonly involves early physical function and exercise training. For ICU survivors, the addition of cognitive rehabilitation strategies may also be indicated.[15]

Rehabilitation after hospital discharge

Survivors of a critical illness have an almost three times risk of death, compared to the general population, with 5% of survivors dying within 12 months of hospital discharge.[3] For others, functional recovery may be delayed by 12 months or more.[47,63] In a recent observational study of 194 participants from a single centre in Norway, only half had returned to work or study at 1-year follow-up, with the lowest median functioning observed in the post-surgical critical care survivors (PF score of 60/100).[64]

With significant evidence from observational studies, interventions for the post-hospital period, protocols, and study findings are now beginning to be reported. Table 51.2 gives the post-hospital intervention studies. Two reports were for pilot work of multi-component interventions,[15,44] with both demonstrating proof of concept but requiring further evidence of effectiveness with larger sample sizes. Patients in the first study were screened just prior to hospital discharge and enrolled if TUG or TOWER test[65] (executive function screening test for planning and strategic thinking)[15] scores were more than one SD below norm scores.[15]

The only multi-site RCT of a home-based physical rehabilitation programme demonstrated no differences, compared to usual care.[49] While the intervention protocol was conservative for this potentially high-risk cohort in the home setting, working to a level of perceived dyspnoea on moderate to somewhat severe exertion,[66] the intervention was consistent with both exercise programmes in ICU follow-up clinics[67] and with COPD patients.[68] Despite this, the training intensity and frequency may have been inadequate for this cohort of patients who may have acquired significant muscle deconditioning, and activity adherence was not measured objectively.

The most recent study demonstrated no between-group improvements in physical function or HRQoL at 12 months,[69,70] although post hoc examination of the trajectory of improvement in the 6-minute walk test demonstrated improvements in the intervention group, compared to usual care, across time from ICU discharge (unpublished data). The improvements in functional exercise, measured using the 6-minute walk test and TUG test, were not found at hospital discharge despite the exercise programme being a continuum from ICU into the ward and then outpatients. Participant 6-minute walk test results at 12 months were at a level of 65% of healthy controls matched for gender, height, and weight.[71] Disappointingly, only half of the patients returned to the outpatient exercise classes, and only 40% in total completed the programme (defined as greater than 70% of the sessions) which may impact the results, albeit this is relatively consistent with pulmonary rehabilitation completion.[72,73] Further research is needed to investigate the optimal exercise setting post-ICU. These results may be explained, in part, by the differences in physiotherapy usual care in the Australian setting, compared with the US. It is also possible that home-based exercise with carer support or more flexible exercise rehabilitation alternatives may improve adherence to exercise. Given that impairment in physical functioning is considered as the most important sequela of critical illness by patients at 12 months' follow-up,[74] understanding the optimal design and implementation of outpatient rehabilitation is vitally important in future research.

For future research, more in-depth screening, including delirium, muscle strength, activity, and neurocognitive assessment, of patients in the post-ICU period may improve identification of individuals at risk of delayed physical recovery. As well, the rehabilitation outcomes of the combination of cognitive and physical strategies should be studied. Other methodological issues also need to be considered, including motivation and adherence (see Chapter 52), and increasing the intensity, frequency, and training support for any home-based intervention.[49,75] The implementation and evaluation of ICU follow-up clinics [67,76] are described in detail in Chapter 53.

Engagement in recovery

Achieving adherence to exercise strategies is an important aim in most disease populations but particularly in chronic diseases. There is now an increasing awareness and emphasis for individuals to be active partners in the management of their condition.[77] Adherence is defined

Table 51.2 Post-hospital intervention studies

Author/country	Design	Sample n/age	MV (hours)	APACHE II	ICU LOS (median days)	Methods	Findings
Jackson (2012)[15]/US	Single-site feasibility RCT	15/47	I:37; C:115	23	I:2.1; C:5.8	12-week home-based (six visits for cognitive; six televisits for physical)	Improved executive functioning (Tower Test 13.0:7.5; P <0.01) and functional status (FAQ 1:8; P = 0.04)
Elliott (2011)[49]/Australia	Multi-site RCT	161/57	140	19	6	8-week home-based (three visits of 60–90 min; five televisits)	No differences for SF-36 (PF C:I = 41.8:42.6) or 6MWT (116:126 m) at 26 weeks
McWilliams (2009)[44]/UK	Single-site pre/post-intervention only	38/57	264	15	11	6-week outpatient, 2-hour supervised + education, and two unsupervised home-based sessions per week	6MWT 58% increase and ISWT 89% increase at 7 weeks
Denehy (2012, 2013)[61,69]/Australia	Single-site RCT (included ward-based and OP intervention)	150/61	I:105 C:98	19	7.5	8 weeks of 2 x 1 hour supervised sessions: - Cardiovascular - Strength - Functional retraining Daily walking programme given (unsupervised)	No significant difference at 12 months in physical function or HRQoL (SF-36, AQoL) outcomes Improved recovery trajectory for 6MWT in the intervention group (unpublished)

C:I, control: intervention; FAQ, functional activities questionnaire; ICULOS, length of stay in ICU; MV, mechanical ventilation; OP, outpatient; PF, physical function; 6MWT, 6-minute walk test.

as 'the extent to which a person's behaviour . . . corresponds with agreed recommendations from a healthcare provider.' (p. 3).[78] To date there is no gold standard method of measuring adherence,[79] although common measures used include number of sessions attended, measuring daily and weekly activity levels, and number of adverse events.[77] Adherence to physical activity and exercise has been reported in different chronic populations, including diabetes mellitus, osteoarthritis (OA), COPD, and cardiac diseases, although most adherence-based research is focused on medication usage.[77]

Maintenance of new exercise behaviours after rehabilitation ranges from 25% at 3 months to 50% at 6 months in the general population and following cardiac rehabilitation, respectively.[80,81] In pulmonary rehabilitation (PR) 8–50% of referred patients with COPD did not attend outpatient rehabilitation.[72,73] Of those who attended, 10–32% did not complete the programme.[82] In OA, reported strategies to increase exercise adherence are to include supervised and individualized exercise, with self-management education, follow-up exercise sessions, supplementary education materials, such as videos of exercises, and cognitive behavioural techniques.

A significant confounder for ICU populations is that depression is reported to influence attendance at cardiac rehabilitation[83] and non-completion of cardiac[84] and pulmonary rehabilitation.[85] Psychological distress can also affect adherence to treatment advice.[86] In a recent study, depression was reported to be an independent risk factor for physical function impairment in survivors of ALI.[87]

Adherence[78] to health interventions is therefore a complex problem with many theories published that provide a framework for adherence strategies, including the health belief model, the theory of reasoned action, the transtheoretical model (TTM), and the theory of planned behaviour and self-efficacy.[77] As applied to physical activity, TTM defines different stages of readiness to change behaviour from the pre-contemplation (not yet considering exercises) stage through to the maintenance stage (exercising regularly for at least 6 months).[88] It is therefore suggested that interventions matched to the stage of readiness produce better adherence to exercise.[89]

Two psychological techniques motivational interviewing (MI) and CBT have been shown to promote behaviour change and maximize adherence to an exercise regimen.[90,91] MI is a series of patient-centred techniques to help people explore and overcome their ambivalence about change, and thus facilitate behaviour change.[92] Level I evidence demonstrates the efficacy of MI in behaviour change,[90] predominantly in substance use disorders. MI can be effectively performed by practitioners other than clinical psychologists, once trained.[93] CBT is parsimonious with MI techniques and has been used to promote and maintain behaviour change in a wide range of conditions, including physical activity. Given the chronic nature of PICS, adopting these methods as part of a multidisciplinary rehabilitation programme may improve exercise behaviours and maintain improvements for ICU survivors. Involving caregivers and family in these aspects of rehabilitation may also help to improve success.[94]

Resources and support

Some policy guidelines are guiding our evolving practice,[50] although further evaluation and evidence are required. A range of support resources are available and accessible online (see Table 51.3). These materials have generally evolved from local initiatives and practice evaluations and are commonly related to ICU follow-up clinics (see Chapter 53). Further formal evaluations are required to demonstrate the effectiveness of these interventions across a range of settings and health systems.

Table 51.3 Resources to support health care workers, patients, and carers

Title	Description	Structure/sections	Delivery
Mobilization network	Website detailing a network of health professionals, with a focus on early mobilization (http://www.mobilization-network.org), launched 2009	News, meetings, network map, links, publications, media; interactive map lists members across four continents	Website with links to existing resources
Rehabilitation after critical illness	Clinical guideline from NICE (UK), 2009[50] (http://www.nice.org.uk/CG83)	91 pages, with 25 recommendations on screening and assessment, and rehabilitation strategies across the continuum	Website with downloadable and printable guideline and others resources, e.g. rehabilitation care pathway, checklist
ICU recovery manual/ICU rehabilitation manual	A 6-week structured programme from St Helens and Knowsley Hospitals Trust/University of Liverpool	90-page book, supporting weekly reviews of activity record, fitness plan, exercise diary, with specific topics introduced[a] and exercise programme[b]	Study protocol[67] 6-week fitness plan, advice on psychological issues, graded exercise[b]
'ICU steps'	Intensive Care Unit Support Teams for Ex-Patients, a registered charity run by former patients and relatives (http://www.ICUsteps.org), last updated 2011	Support groups, guide, patients and relatives, professionals	Downloadable intensive care guide, a 24-page booklet in a range of languages, with sections on returning home, effects on your body, feelings, eating well[c]
ICAN-UK	Website 'Intensive Care After Care Network' (http://www.i-canuk.co.uk/default.aspx), last updated 2007	Register, literature, national survey, follow-up tools, resources, research, patient area	Website resources for professionals and patients

[a] Short descriptions on specific topics per week: relaxation, 'after intensive care', lifestyle assessment, regular exercise, diet, stress.

[b] Sections on exercises: warm-up/stretching, back and joint, leg and arm strengthening, health heart, and lungs; somewhat hard to hard level of exertion (Borg 13–15/20).

[c] No exercise rehabilitation or psychological training included.

Evolving technologies

Assistive technologies are beginning to be evaluated, including the use of video games, to promote activity whilst the patient is in ICU.[95] These activities could also be used in the post-ICU and post-hospital phases of rehabilitation and provide useful continuity of both interventions and assessments. Current work also includes the use of accelerometers to monitor movement and activities, and the development of sensors and body area networks (BANs)[96] that enable wearable devices and transmission of monitoring data.[97] These data can be physiological, such as heart rate and oxygen saturations, and physical activity, including movement and walking.

Other research has developed a virtual reality device, but with only evaluation in healthy volunteers,[98] and protocols for in-home telerehabilitation.[99] Use of mobile phone technology to monitor and measure outcomes of rehabilitation is growing, and publications describing their use in other chronic diseases are available.[100–102] Development, testing, and use of these applications for telerehabilitation in the PICS cohort also enable equitable access for rural and remote populations, a key pragmatic issue for this cohort.[49]

Conclusion

Improved education of rehabilitation specialists, GPs, and the health community about the ongoing legacy of critical care and PICS is advocated. Development of patient-centred outcomes that are tested in ICU survivors is an urgent requirement in this area. Further research is required that measures the effectiveness of physical and non-physical rehabilitation after ICU discharge. In addition, the amount, type, and timing of intervention and identification of those patients who are most likely to respond to the designated rehabilitation strategy need to be investigated. The use of psychological and technology adjuncts that may motivate individuals and promote long-lasting activity should be included in future work.

References

1 **Azoulay E, Adrie C, De Lassence A, et al.** Determinants of postintensive care unit mortality: a prospective multicenter study. *Crit Care Med* 2003;**31**:428–32.

2 **Levy MM, Rapoport J, Lemeshow S, Chalfin DB, Phillips G, Danis M.** Association between critical care physician management and patient mortality in the intensive care unit. *Ann Intern Med* 2008;**148**:801–9.

3 **Williams TA, Dobb GJ, Finn JC, et al.** Determinants of long-term survival after intensive care. *Crit Care Med* 2008;**36**:1523–30.

4 **Moran JL, Solomon PJ.** Mortality and intensive care volume in ventilated patients from 1995 to 2009 in the Australian and New Zealand binational adult patient intensive care database. *Crit Care Med* 2011;**40**:800–12.

5 **Stevens RD, Dowdy DW, Michaels RK, Mendez-Tellez PA, Pronovost PJ, Needham DM.** Neuromuscular dysfunction acquired in critical illness: a systematic review. *Intensive Care Med* 2007;**33**:1876–91.

6 **Davydow D, Gifford J, Desai S, Needham D, Bienvenu O.** Posttraumatic stress disorder in general intensive care unit survivors: a systematic review. *Gen Hosp Psychiatry* 2008;**30**:421–34.

7 **Griffiths J, Fortune G, Barber V, Young JD.** The prevalence of post traumatic stress disorder in survivors of ICU treatment: a systematic review. *Intensive Care Med* 2007;**33**:1506–18.

8 **Jackson JC, Mitchell N, Hopkins RO.** Cognitive functioning, mental health, and quality of life in ICU survivors: an overview. *Crit Care Clin* 2009;**25**:615–28.

9 **Angus D, Carlet J.** Surviving intensive care: a report from the 2002 Brussels Roundtable. *Intensive Care Med* 2003;**29**:368–77.

10 **Griffiths RD, Hall JB.** Intensive care unit-acquired weakness. *Crit Care Med* 2010;**38**:779–87.

11 **Needham DM, Davidson J, Cohen H, et al.** Improving long-term outcomes after discharge from intensive care unit: report from a stakeholders' conference. *Crit Care Med* 2012;**40**:502–9.

12 **Davidson J, Jones C, Bienvenu O.** Family response to critical illness: postintensive care syndrome-family. *Crit Care Med* 2011;**40**:618–24.

13 **Pandharipande P, Banerjee A, McGrane S, Ely EW.** Liberation and animation for ventilated ICU patients: the ABCDE bundle for the back-end of critical care. *Crit Care* 2010;**14**:157.

14 Vasilevskis EE, Ely EW, Speroff T, Pun BT, Boehm L, Dittus RS. Reducing iatrogenic risks: ICU-acquired delirium and weakness—crossing the quality chasm. *Chest* 2010;**138**:1224–33.

15 Jackson J, Ely EW, Morey MC, et al. Cognitive and physical rehabilitation of intensive care unit survivors: results of the RETURN randomized controlled pilot investigation. *Crit Care Med* 2012;**40**:1088–97.

16 Clini E, Ambrosino N. Early physiotherapy in the respiratory intensive care unit. *Respir Med* 2005;**99**:1096–104.

17 Gosselink R, Bott J, Johnson M, Dean E, Nava S, Norrenberg M. Physiotherapy for adult patients with critical illness: recommendations of the European Respiratory Society and European Society of Intensive Care Medicine Task Force on physiotherapy for critically ill patients. *Intensive Care Med* 2008;**34**:1188–99.

18 Skinner EH, Berney S, Warrillow S, Denehy L. Rehabilitation and exercise prescription in Australian intensive care units. *Physiotherapy* 2008;**94**:220–9.

19 Stiller K, Phillips A. Safety aspects of mobilising acutely ill inpatients. *Physiother Theory Pract* 2003;**19**:19.

20 Morris PE, Herridge MS. Early intensive care unit mobility: future directions. *Crit Care Clin* 2007;**23**:97–110.

21 Dowdy DW, Eid MP, Sedrakyan A, et al. Quality of life in adult survivors of critical illness: a systematic review of the literature. *Intensive Care Med* 2005;**31**:611–20.

22 Herridge M. Long-term outcomes after critical illness: past, present, future. *Curr Opin Crit Care* 2007;**13**:3.

23 van der Schaaf M, Dettling D, Beelen A, Lucas C, Dongelmans D, Nollet F. Poor functional status immediately after discharge from an intensive care unit. *Disabil Rehabil* 2008;**30**:1812–18.

24 DiCicco J, Whalen D. University of Rochester Acute Care Evaluation: development of a new functional outcome measure for the acute care setting. *J Acute Care Phys Ther* 2010;**1**:14–20.

25 Enright P, McBurnie M, Bittner V, et al. The 6-min walk test. A quick measure of functional status in elderly adults. *Chest* 2003;**123**:387–98.

26 Singh SJ, Morgan MD, Scott S, Walters D, Hardman AE. Development of a shuttle walking test of disability in patients with chronic airways obstruction. *Thorax* 1992;**47**:1019–24.

27 Wade DT, Wood VA, Heller A, Maggs J, Langton Hewer R. Walking after stroke. Measurement and recovery over the first 3 months. *Scand J Rehabil Med.* 1987;**19**:25–30.

28 Guralnik JM, Simonsick EM, Ferrucci L, et al. A short physical performance battery assessing lower extremity function: association with self-reported disability and prediction of mortality and nursing home admission. *J Gerontol.* 1994;**49**:M85–94.

29 Ware J. *SF-36 health survey manual and interpretation guide.* Boston, MA: The Medical Outcomes Trust; 1993.

30 Lawton MP, Brody EM. Assessment of older people: self-maintaining and instrumental activities of daily living. *Gerontologist* 1969;**9**:179–86.

31 Podsiadlo D, Richardson S. The timed 'Up & Go': a test of basic functional mobility for frail elderly persons. *J Am Geriatr Soc* 1991;**39**:142–8.

32 Denti L, Agosti M, Franceschini M. Outcome predictors of rehabilitation for first stroke in the elderly. *Eur J Phys Rehabil Med* 2008;**44**:3–11.

33 Granger CV. The emerging science of functional assessment: our tool for outcomes analysis. *Arch Phys Med Rehabil* 1998;**79**:235–40.

34 Kohler F, Dickson H, Redmond H, Estell J, Connolly C. Agreement of functional independence measure item scores in patients transferred from one rehabilitation setting to another. *Eur J Phys Rehabil Med* 2009;**45**:479–85.

35 Novak S, Johnson J, Greenwood R. Barthel revisited: making guidelines work. *Clin Rehabil* 1996;**10**:128–34.

36 **Ali NA, O'Brien JM, Jr, Hoffmann SP, et al.** Acquired weakness, handgrip strength, and mortality in critically ill patients. *Am J Respir Crit Care Med* 2008;**178**:261–8.

37 **Hough CL, Lieu BK, Caldwell ES.** Manual muscle strength testing of critically ill patients: feasibility and interobserver agreement. *Crit Care* 2011;**15**:R43.

38 **Knols RH, Aufdemkampe G, de Bruin ED, Uebelhart D, Aaronson NK.** Hand-held dynamometry in patients with haematological malignancies: measurement error in the clinical assessment of knee extension strength. *BMC Musculoskelet Disord* 2009;**10**:31.

39 **O'Shea SD, Taylor NF, Paratz JD.** A predominantly home-based progressive resistance exercise program increases knee extensor strength in the short-term in people with chronic obstructive pulmonary disease: a randomised controlled trial. *Aust J Physiother* 2007;**53**:229–37.

40 **Elliott D, Denehy L, Berney S, Alison J.** Assessing physical function and activity for survivors of a critical illness: a review of instruments. *Aust Crit Care* 2011;**24**:155–66.

41 **van der Putten JJ, Hobart JC, Freeman JA, Thompson AJ.** Measuring change in disability after inpatient rehabilitation: comparison of the responsiveness of the Barthel index and the Functional Independence Measure. *J Neurol Neurosurg Psychiatry* 1999;**66**:480–4.

42 **de Morton NA, Keating JL, Jeffs K.** Exercise for acutely hospitalised older medical patients. *Cochrane Database Syst Rev* 2007;**1**:CD005955.

43 **Salisbury LG, Merriweather JL, Walsh TS.** Rehabilitation after critical illness: could a ward-based generic rehabilitation assistant promote recovery? *Nurs Crit Care* 2010;**15**:57–65.

44 **McWilliams DJ, Atkinson D, Carter A, Foex BA, Benington S, Conway DH.** Feasibility and impact of a structured, exercise-based rehabilitation programme for intensive care survivors. *Physiother Theory Pract* 2009;**25**:566–71.

45 **Denehy L, Berney S, Whitburn L, Edbrooke L.** Quantifying Physical Activity levels of survivors of intensive care: a prospective observational Study. *Phys Ther* 2012;**92**:1507–17.

46 **Herridge MS, Tansey CM, Matté A, et al.** Functional disability 5 years after acute respiratory distress syndrome. *N Engl J Med* 2011;**364**:1293–304.

47 **Oeyen SG, Vandijck DM, Benoit DD, Annemans L, Decruyenaere JM.** Quality of life after intensive care: a systematic review of the literature. *Crit Care Med* 2010;**38**:2386–400.

48 **Hawthorne G.** Assessing utility where short measures are required: development of the short Assessment of Quality of Life-8 (AQoL-8) instrument. *Value Health* 2009;**12**:948–57.

49 **Elliott D, McKinley S, Alison J, et al.** Health-related quality of life and physical recovery after a critical illness: a multi-centre randomised controlled trial of a home-based physical rehabilitation program. *Crit Care* 2011;**15**:R142.

50 **National Institute for Health and Care Excellence.** *Rehabilitation after critical illness. NICE clinical guideline 83.* London: National Institute for Health and Care Excellence; 2009.

51 **Elliott SJ, Ernest D, Doric AG, et al.** The impact of an ICU liaison nurse service on patient outcomes. *Crit Care Resusc* 2008;**10**:296–300.

52 **Williams TA, Leslie G, Finn J, et al.** Clinical effectiveness of a critical care nursing outreach service in facilitating discharge from the intensive care unit. *Am J Crit Care* 2010;**19**:e63–72.

53 **Hillman K, Chen J, Cretikos M, et al.** Introduction of the medical emergency team (MET) system: a cluster-randomised controlled trial. *Lancet* 2005;**365**:2091–7.

54 **Jones DA, DeVita MA, Bellomo R.** Rapid-response teams. *N Engl J Med* 2011;**365**:139–46.

55 **Moran JL, Bristow P, Solomon PJ, George C, Hart GK.** Mortality and length-of-stay outcomes, 1993–2003, in the binational Australian and New Zealand intensive care adult patient database. *Crit Care Med* 2008;**36**:46–61.

56 **Inouye SK, Acampora D, Miller RL, Fulmer T, Hurst LD, Cooney LM, Jr.** The Yale Geriatric Care Program: a model of care to prevent functional decline in hospitalized elderly patients. *J Am Geriatr Soc.* 1993;**41**:1345–52.

57 Jones C, Lowe A, MacGregor L, Brand C. A randomised controlled trial of an exercise intervention to reduce functional decline and health service utilisation in the hospitalised elderly. *Australasian J Ageing* 2006;**25**:126–33.

58 Denehy L, Elliott D. Strategies for post ICU rehabilitation. *Curr Opin Crit Care* 2012;**18**:503–8.

59 Schweickert WD, Pohlman MC, Pohlman AS, et al. Early physical and occupational therapy in mechanically ventilated, critically ill patients: a randomised controlled trial. *Lancet* 2009;**373**:1874–82.

60 Pohlman MC, Schweickert WD, Pohlman AS, et al. Feasibility of physical and occupational therapy beginning from initiation of mechanical ventilation. *Crit Care Med* 2010;**38**:2089–94.

61 Berney S, Haines K, Skinner EH, Denehy L. Safety and feasibility of an exercise prescription approach to rehabilitation across the continuum of care for survivors of critical illness. *Phys Ther* 2012;**92**: 1524–35.

62 Langer D, Hendriks E, Burtin C, et al. A clinical practice guideline for physiotherapists treating patients with chronic obstructive pulmonary disease based on a systematic review of available evidence. *Clin Rehabil* 2009;**23**:445–62.

63 Cuthbertson B, Roughton S, Jenkinson D, MacLennan G, Vale L. Quality of life in the five years after intensive care: a cohort study. *Crit Care* 2010;**14**:1–12.

64 Myhren H, Ekeberg O, Stokland O. Health-related quality of life and return to work after critical illness in general intensive care unit patients: a 1-year follow-up study. *Crit Care Med* 2010;**38**:1554–61.

65 Delis D, Kaplan E, Kramer J. *Delis-Kaplan Executive Function System (D-KEFS): examiner's manual.* San Antonio, TX: Psychological Corporation; 2001.

66 Borg GA. Psychophysical bases of perceived exertion. *Med Sci Sports Exerc* 1982;**14**:377–81.

67 Jones C, Skirrow P, Griffiths RD, et al. Rehabilitation after critical illness: a randomized, controlled trial. *Crit Care Med* 2003;**31**:2456–61.

68 Maltais F, Bourbeau J, Shapiro S, et al. Effects of home-based pulmonary rehabilitation in patients with chronic obstructive pulmonary disease: a randomized trial. *Ann Intern Med* 2008;**149**:869–78.

69 Denehy L, Skinner E, Edbrooke L, et al. Exercise rehabilitation for patients with critical illness: A randomized controlled trial with 12 months follow up. *Critical Care* 17: R156 doi: 10.1186?cc12835.

70 Denehy L, Berney S, Skinner E, et al. Evaluation of exercise rehabilitation for survivors of intensive care: protocol for a single blind randomised controlled trial. *Open Crit Care Med J* 2008;**1**:39–47.

71 Jenkins S, Cecins N, Camarri B, Williams C, Thompson P, Eastwood P. Regression equations to predict 6-minute walk distance in middle-aged and elderly adults. *Physiother Theory Pract* 2009;**25**: 516–22.

72 Arnold E, Bruton A, Ellis-Hill C. Adherence to pulmonary rehabilitation: a qualitative study. *Respir Med* 2006;**100**:1716–23.

73 Taylor R, Dawson S, Roberts N, Sridhar M, Partridge MR. Why do patients decline to take part in a research project involving pulmonary rehabilitation? *Respir Med* 2007;**101**:1942–6.

74 Agard AS, Egerod I, Tonnesen E, Lomborg K. Struggling for independence: a grounded theory study on convalescence of ICU survivors 12 months post ICU discharge. *Intensive Crit Care Nurs* 2012;**28**:105–13.

75 Herridge MS. The challenge of designing a post-critical illness rehabilitation intervention. *Crit Care* 2011;**15**:1002.

76 Cuthbertson BH, Rattray J, Campbell MK, et al. The PRaCTICaL study of nurse led, intensive care follow-up programmes for improving long term outcomes from critical illness: a pragmatic randomised controlled trial. *BMJ* 2009;**339**:b3723.

77 Jordan JL, Holden MA, Mason EE, Foster NE. Interventions to improve adherence to exercise for chronic musculoskeletal pain in adults. *Cochrane Database Syst Rev* 2010;**1**:CD005956.

78 World Health Organization. *Adherence to long-term therapies: evidence for action.* Geneva: World Health Organization; 2003.

79 **Treuth M.** Applying multiple methods to improve the accuracy of activity assessments. In: Welk G (ed.) *Physical activity assessments for health-related research*. Champaign, IL: Human Kinetics; 2002. pp. 213–26.

80 **Oldridge NB.** Compliance with exercise in cardiac rehabilitation. In: Dishman RK (ed.) *Exercise adherence: its impact on public health*. Champaign, IL: Human Kinetics; 1988. pp. 283–304.

81 **Oldridge NB.** Cardiac rehabilitation services: what are they and are they worth it? *Compr Ther* 1991;**17**:59–66.

82 **Keating A, Lee A, Holland AE.** What prevents people with chronic obstructive pulmonary disease from attending pulmonary rehabilitation? A systematic review. *Chron Respir Dis* 2011;**8**: 89–99.

83 **Glazer KM, Emery CF, Frid DJ, Banyasz RE.** Psychological predictors of adherence and outcomes among patients in cardiac rehabilitation. *J Cardiopulm Rehabil* 2002;**22**:40–6.

84 **Casey E, Hughes JW, Waechter D, Josephson R, Rosneck J.** Depression predicts failure to complete phase-II cardiac rehabilitation. *J Behav Med* 2008;**31**:421–31.

85 **Fan VS, Giardino ND, Blough DK, Kaplan RM, Ramsey SD.** Costs of pulmonary rehabilitation and predictors of adherence in the National Emphysema Treatment Trial. *COPD* 2008;**5**:105–16.

86 **Zarani F, Besharat MA, Sadeghian S, Sarami G.** The effectiveness of the information-motivation-behavioral skills model in promoting adherence in CABG patients. *J Health Psychol* 2010;**15**: 828–37.

87 **Bienvenu OJ, Colantuoni E, Mendez-Tellez PA, et al.** Depressive symptoms and impaired physical function after acute lung injury: a 2-year longitudinal study. *Am J Respir Crit Care Med* 2012;**185**: 517–24.

88 **Prochaska JO, DiClemente CC.** Stages and processes of self-change of smoking: toward an integrative model of change. *J Consult Clin Psychol* 1983;**51**:390–5.

89 **Marcus BH, Simkin LR.** The stages of exercise behavior. *J Sports Med Phys Fitness* 1993;**33**:83–8.

90 **Britt E.** Motivational interviewing in health settings: a review. *Patient Educ Couns* 2004;**53**:147–55.

91 **Marcus BH, Forsyth L.** *Motivating people to be physically active*. Champaign, IL: Human Kinetics; 2009.

92 **Bien TH, Miller WR, Boroughs JM.** Motivational interviewing with alcohol outpatients. *Behavioural Psychother* 1993;**21**:347–56.

93 **Rubak S.** Motivational interviewing: a systematic review and meta-analysis. *Br J Gen Pract* 2005;**55**:305–12.

94 **Davidson J, Jones C, Bienvenu O.** Family response to critical illness: postintensive care syndrome-family. *Crit Care Med* 2012;**40**:618–24.

95 **Kho ME, Damluji A, Zanni JM, Needham DM.** Feasibility and observed safety of interactive video games for physical rehabilitation in the intensive care unit: a case series. *J Crit Care* 2012;**27**:219. e1–6.

96 **Khan JY, Yuce MR, Bulger G, Harding B.** Wireless Body Area Network (WBAN) design techniques and performance evaluation. *J Med Syst* 2012;**36**:1441–57.

97 **Darwish A, Hassanien AE.** Wearable and implantable wireless sensor network solutions for healthcare monitoring. *Sensors (Basel)* 2011;**11**:5561–95.

98 **Van de Meent H, Baken BC, Van Opstal S, Hogendoorn P.** Critical illness VR rehabilitation device (X-VR-D): evaluation of the potential use for early clinical rehabilitation. *J Electromyogr Kinesiol* 2008;**18**:480–6.

99 **Hoenig H, Sanford JA, Butterfield T, Griffiths PC, Richardson P, Hargraves K.** Development of a teletechnology protocol for in-home rehabilitation. *J Rehabil Res Dev* 2006;**43**:287–98.

100 **Dinesen B, Seeman J, Gustafsson J.** Development of a program for tele-rehabilitation of COPD patients across sectors: co-innovation in a network. *Int J Integr Care* 2011;**11**:e012.

101 **Rogante M, Grigioni M, Cordella D, Giacomozzi C.** Ten years of telerehabilitation: a literature overview of technologies and clinical applications. *NeuroRehabilitation* 2010;**27**:287–304.

102 **Vassanyi I, Kozmann G, Banhalmi A, et al.** Applications of medical intelligence in remote monitoring. *Stud Health Technol Inform* 2011;**169**:671–5.

103 **Salisbury LG, Merriweather JL, Walsh TS.** The development and feasibility of a ward-based physiotherapy and nutritional rehabilitation package for people experiencing critical illness. *Clin Rehabil* 2010;**24**:489–500.

Chapter 52

Narratives of Illness and Healing after the ICU

Christina Jones

Introduction

There is a significant difference in the narrative of critical illness reported by the patient, compared with the experience reported by their family, friends, and carers. This chapter will not only explore in detail these differences, but it will also examine the role of health care staff in supporting the patient and family to build a common narrative to improve long-term recovery.

Models of illness

Morse and Johnson[1] proposed an illness model, which takes into account the way the illness affects the sick person and their significant others. It is this aspect of the model that makes it attractive and applicable to patients who are subject to an episode of critical illness. The model defines the illness experience in four stages:

Stage I—stage of uncertainty

In this stage, the first signs of illness become increasingly evident to the individual. There are efforts made by the individual affected to make sense of the symptoms, including an assessment of their seriousness of the condition. Close family and friends also start to notice that the person is ill, and the sick person may volunteer information to them.

Stage II—stage of disruption

The sick person decides that the condition is serious, and they seek medical assistance or, on occasions, the sick person become so ill that independent assessment of the condition is lost and they are hospitalized. The person loses control and becomes totally dependent on their health care workers and their family. The family becomes increasingly concerned for the sick person and openly displays these concerns, as they experience the suffering of the patient. During this early period of critical illness, the relatives are obliged to take over the normal responsibilities of the sick person such as caring for children and dependent elderly relatives.

Stage III—stage of striving to regain self

Stage III is the convalescent phase. The critically ill patient attempts to make sense of the illness and may reflect on reasons for it happening. The sick person may also try to predict the impact of the illness on their life. In addition, the family may try to assist in this process by providing support, direction, and encouragement. The sick person focuses their energy on this task and conserves energy by neglecting other tasks, while family members may aid this process by 'buffering' the patient to protect them from undue stress. This places the patient in a passive role, and, as they regain their strength, they have to negotiate with health care professionals and family members to resume their old responsibilities. A balance has to be struck between the patient and the health care professionals and family members so that the needs of both are met. This is often achieved by the patient setting goals for themselves, while the family polices these goals or modifies them if they feel them not achievable.

Patients who have been through a critical illness report this as the most stressful period of their illness, as they receive reports from health care workers and family of the severity of their illness which often includes the patient being told that, without intensive care support, they may not have survived.[2] This is not surprising, as the patient has minimal recollection of their acute illness, and this is the first phase of the critical illness that the patient has sufficient mental capacity to process the information. Some patients spent considerable time and energy in trying to work through their ICU experience. They actively seek details of their illness from their relatives and friends and from the medical, nursing, and therapy staff. They recount the story to their visitors, reworking it in their minds. This is, in contrast, to the 'buffering' that relatives provide, with the aim of 'protecting' the patient from stress. This may include withholding details of the events, with the premise that 'it is better that they do not know'. This may be confounded by the fact that the relative may be unclear themselves exactly of the nature of the events. Indeed, the stressful situation that they were exposed to at the time may have impaired their understanding of the events, and they may only understand that the patient almost died. Clearly, if the seriousness of the illness is withheld from the patient and the relative refuses to discuss the ICU stay at all, this raises significant concern. In addition, the relatives may be too traumatized themselves to be able to discuss the clinical course during the ICU admission. There is evidence to support this from the ICU support group that was run by the author some years ago. Some of the patients attended the support group by themselves, as they were unable to get their spouse to attend. In particular, the spouse would not tell the patient about their illness or even discuss their feelings.[3] As expected, the most frequent reason given by the relative for this attitude was that they felt that it was better that the patient did not know the severity of their illness, despite the patient requesting the opposite.

Stage IV—stage of regaining wellness

During this stage, the patient regains all their former roles. Specifically, the patient will achieve a full recovery or achieve an acceptance of a lower level of functioning. In this process, the patient relearns to trust in their body, monitors their symptoms, and uses this to set new limits for themselves. Importantly, the family allows the person to regain control.

Making sense of what happened

For many patients, the absence of a story for what brought them into hospital and made them ill enough to need treatment in an ICU is deeply concerning and forces them to question their friends and family to try and fill in the gaps.[4,5] In addition, the lack of a real experience of their illness may put them in conflict with their family who remembers each day and does not want to live the experience again. Family members may actually become overprotective when the patient wants to proceed towards more independence. Some patients report that the recovery phase, in which they learn the extent of their illness and how close they were to death, is the most stressful part of their illness.[6] David Reir, an Israeli sociologist who was admitted to ICU with pneumonia, pieced together his state of mind and experience from a notebook he used to communicate with staff and family, with copies of daily update faxes sent to his family in America.[7] He described his identity as a patient as continually evolving.

> after leaving the ICU for the general medical floor . . . I grew stronger, began to ask lots of questions of doctors, and engaged in keen – if friendly – bargaining with them over things like my date of discharge . . . I tried hard to extract as much information from my physicians as possible without being labelled a troublemaker . . .

For some patients, the aftermath of critical illness fills all aspects of their life; they become overjoyed by life and the love of their family, and their sense of purpose in life seems to be heightened.[8] For others, the frightening delusional memories they recall and replay in their heads mean that their existence is filled with efforts to avoid thinking about their illness and reminders of being in hospital.[9] For the author, her first awareness of this came when trying to set up an ICU support group and having to use a side room in the local public house, because the ICU patients and their families did not want to come back to the hospital.[3]

Narrative theory[10] can be used to make sense of the patients' experience.[11] The first concept is **narrative coherence**; in an illness narrative, the patient, their relatives, and hospital staff all have a part. For some diagnoses, there are known and fixed pathways and parts played by everyone. However, this is not so for critical illness. The patient cannot remember their part, and the family may have been overwhelmed by their role, which can result in conflict between patients and their families (see Table 52.1). The second concept is **narrative closure** where familiarity with the illness is achieved and the understanding of the after-effects understood, and so others are able to understand and support the person. Again, for ICU patients, this is a problem, as even some health care professionals do not understand the critical illness narrative during recovery, let alone the patient and their family. The increasing popularity of websites giving information to ICU patients and their families is to be encouraged, but only where the information has been rigorously gained and tested. Sites, such as Healthtalkonline,[12] which allows sharing of critical illness experiences, have information which is based on good qualitative interviews with patients and their friends and families. These sites allow socialization in order to prevent isolation of both patients and family members. In addition, these sites provides information to families, which allows them to be more supportive as they understand what is 'normal' for ICU patients.

Table 52.1 Conflict between patients and their family

	Patients	**Families and friends**
Narrative for ICU	Absent or fragmentary factual recall May recall delusional memories of hallucinations, nightmares, and paranoid delusions	Recall fear for the patient Remember sitting impotently by the patients' side every day
Explanation for physical condition	Do not understand why they are so weak and unable to do things for themselves Frustrated with the slowness of their recovery and fear this means that they are not getting better	Just grateful to have the patient back with them Overprotective. Do not want the patient to overtire themselves, so try to get them to rest
Returning to family role	Want to return to normal as soon as they can, so try to take back family roles that they are not ready for or have been taken over by another family member	Family members may try to protect the patient by not letting them take back family roles which they feel are too much for them

The final concept is **narrative interdependence**, which refers to the interrelatedness of the narratives of all the individuals involved in the story so, for families, one member's narrative is usually interrelated to the narratives told by other family members. The patients' narrative of critical illness often has no connection to the narrative understood by their family. In addition, the patients' narrative may be fragmentary at best. For all these reasons, our ICU patients and their families need our help to build their illness narrative and the information to be fully informed in their progress following the pathway to recovery.

Delusional memory content

Cognitive approaches to the treatment of auditory hallucinations in schizophrenic patients suggest that the emotional impact of these experiences is influenced by the personal meaning to the individual. Since hallucinations are experiences generated by the patient themselves, then it could be expected that the content will reflect their memories and beliefs. A study looking at the content of delusional memories reported by ICU patients, undertaken prior to and during the Kosovo War (1998 and 1999), found that those patients whose ICU stay occurred during the conflict were significantly more likely to recall experiences that involved themes of war and the military.[13] Those patients who reported themes of war during the period of the Kosovo War were all over the age of 70 and so would have been an age where they could remember the start of the Second World War. Consequently, it could be hypothesized that their experiences of the Second World War meant that the Kosovo War caused them greater concern, and so this was translated into hallucinatory themes of war. Similarly, the patient, whose delusions are discussed in Chapter 21, reported seeing her daughter being sexually abused as part of her ICU experience. The past experience, which influenced her delusional experience, only became clear once she felt she could really trust the author. She revealed that she had been sexually abused as a young child herself and but she had never been able to talk about it to anyone before.

One type of delusion which is fairly common in ICU patients is called a *capgras delusion*. In this delusion, the individual thinks that people around them have been replaced by an identical-looking imposter. In a case study report, one patient reported that all the nurses and most of her family had been replaced by aliens that had the identical appearance of her family, but she knew they were aliens.[14] Her heartfelt, overwhelming fear during this time was that she would be replaced by an alien if she fell asleep. Other patients have since reported being looked after by wax-work or shop dummies. It has been suggested that a defect in the ability to recognize the emotional significance of the face lies at the root of the *capgras delusion* and that there is a more general difficulty in these patients in linking successive episodic memories.[15] This would explain why it is relatively common in ICU patients where sedation and delirium would not allow patients to link different memories over the time of their critical illness. These delusional memories appeared to be the most persistent recollections over time after ICU discharge.[16]

For all patients recovering from critical illness, there is a need for a coherent story about what happened in ICU, but, for those with delusional memories, they need more.[17] They need to be reassured that they are not 'going mad' and that others have experienced the same sort of hallucinations, nightmares, and paranoid delusions. Where the delusions are recalled with great distress, the patients need to be listened to in an empathic and accepting way and encouraged to work through their feelings. This will not happen by chance but has to be planned by the staff looking after them. In helping patients to construct their illness narrative, it is important to remember the key role of the relative and support them to enable clear communication between the patient and their family.

Constructing the illness narrative

The use of ICU diaries, with daily updates by ICU staff on the patients' condition, photographs taken at points of change, and contributions from the family are becoming increasing popular amongst ICU nurses as a means of informing the patient about their illness.[18] The role of the family in the effectiveness of the diary should not be underestimated, for the patient reading the entries of the relatives in the diary can be the most emotional part of going through the diary for the first time as they start to understand the details of their family's experience. This is, however, the first step in the patient appreciating their relatives' narrative and how it clashes with theirs. A grounded theory study looking at patients' and their families' use of diary found that patients used them to fill in the memory gaps for both the ICU stay and their admission to hospital.[19] Diaries have also been found to be helpful to critically injured military personnel to help 'fill in the gaps' in their illness memory, following injury on the battlefield.[20] The timing of going through the diary was found to be important, as the first reading is the most traumatic and the patient needs to be ready to be able to identify with the story and, most importantly, the patient needs to be supported by nursing staff through this process. Most of the patients interviewed in the study had not appreciated the severity of their illness before they went through the diary.

In the recent multicentred RCT of the impact of ICU diaries on new-onset PTSD following critical illness, outlined in Chapter 21, patients were asked to provide feedback on the diaries and detail the support that this approach provided. The majority of the 'diary' intervention patients were very positive about the diary and found benefit from reading it a number of times. In addition, a significant proportion of the patients reported that others had read the diary, including their family, friends, and GP. Although the intervention patients all had a meeting with a nurse to go through their diary, interestingly, only two patients reported that the meeting was helpful in the long term. Forty-nine per cent of patients described reading the text in the diary as the most helpful part, 36% the combination of photographs and text, and 15% just the photographs.[21] For most of the patients, the ability to build a narrative was achieved through the text, but, for some, being able to see they were indeed in the ICU bed was very important in order to personally contextualize and add reality to their illness.

Conclusion

The critical illness narrative is extremely important to the patient during their recovery. Specifically, patients need to understand the cause of their physical weakness and reduced exercise capacity. In addition, this approach helps patients to put delusional memories into context and facilitates with understanding the behaviour of their family. A simple intervention, such as an ICU diary with photographs taken at points of change, is an easy way of supporting patients to build an illness narrative in their journey towards recovery. It also allows the patient to share their relatives' experience and so understand the stress they experienced and potentially be more forgiving of the protective behaviour that the family may demonstrate.

References

1 Morse JM, Johnson JL (eds.). Towards a theory of illness: the illness-constellation model. In: *The illness experience*. California: Sage Publications; 1991. pp. 315–42.

2 Compton P. Critical illness and intensive care: what it means to the client. *Crit Care Nurse* 1991;**11**:50–6.

3 Jones C, Macmillan RR, Griffiths RD. Providing psychological support to patients after critical illness. *Clin Intensive Care* 1994;**5**:176–9.

4 Griffiths RD, Jones C, Macmillan RR. Where is the harm in not knowing? Care after intensive care. *Clin Intensive Care* 1996;7:144–5.

5 Barnett L. Intensive care: an existential perspective. *Therapy Today* 2006;June:33–5.

6 Compton P. Critical illness and intensive care: what it means to the client. *Crit Care Nurse* 1987;11:50–6.

7 Reir D. The missing voice of the critically ill: a medical sociologist's first-person account. *Sociology of Health and Illness* 2000;22:68–93.

8 Papathanassoglou EDE, Patiraki EI. Transformation of self: a phenomenological investigation inot the lived experience of survivors of critical illness. *Nurs Crit Care* 2003;8:13–21.

9 Jones C, Griffiths RD, Humphris GH, PM Skirrow. Memory, delusions, and the development of acute posttraumatic stress disorder-related symptoms after intensive care. *Crit Care Med* 2001;29:573–80.

10 Chatman S. *Story and discourse.* Ithaca, NY: Cornell University Press; 1978.

11 Weingarten K. *Making sense of illness narratives: braiding theory, practice and the embodied life. Working with the stories of women's lives.* Adelaide, Dulwich Centre Publications; 2001.

12 HealthTalkOnline. *Intensive care.* Available at: http://www.healthtalkonline.org/Intensive_care/ (accessed 6 September 2011).

13 Skirrow P, Jones C, Griffiths RD, Kaney S. The impact of current media events on hallucinatory content: The experience of the intensive care unit (ICU) patient. *Br J Clin Psychol* 2002;41:87–91.

14 Jones C, Griffiths RD, Humphris GH. A case of Capgras delusion following critical illness. *Intensive Care Med* 1999;25:1183–4.

15 Hirstein W, Ramachandran VS. Capgras syndrome: a novel probe for understanding the neural representation of the identity and familiarity of persons. *Proc Biol Sci* 1997;264:437–44.

16 Capuzzo M, Valpondi V, Cingolani E, et al. Application of the Italian version of the Intensive Care Unit Memory Tool in the clinical setting. *Crit Care* 2004;8:R48–55.

17 Kiekkas P, Theodorakopoulou G, Spyratos F, Baltopoulos G. Psychological distress and delusional memories after critical care: a literature review. *Int Nurs Rev* 2010;57:288–96.

18 Bäckman CG. Patient diaries in ICU. In: Griffiths RD, Jones C (eds.) *Intensive care aftercare.* Oxford: Butterworth Heinemann; 2002. pp. 125–9.

19 Egerod I, Christensen D, Schwartz-Nielsen KH, Ågård AS. Constructing the illness narrative: a grounded theory exploring patients' and relatives' use of intensive care diaries. *Crit Care Med* 2011;39: 1922–8.

20 Thomas J, Bell E. Lost days—diaries for military intensive care patients. *J R Nav Med Serv* 2011;97:11–15.

21 Jones C, Bäckman C, Capuzzo M, et al., and RACHEL group. Intensive Care diaries reduce new onset PTSD following critical illness: a randomised, controlled trial. *Crit Care* 2010;14:R168.

Chapter 53

ICU Follow-Up Clinics

Shannon L. Goddard and Brian H. Cuthbertson

Introduction

The quality life encountered by the survivors of critical illness is a growing concern in the intensive care community across the world. The traditional focus of critical care practice has been on interventions that improve short-term mortality. However, survivors experience a range of physical and non-physical morbidities after an ICU stay, including impaired physical functioning,[1] cognitive dysfunction,[2–4] depression,[2,3] and sexual dysfunction.[5,6] HRQoL is poor, compared to the general population,[7,8] a problem that persists for at least 5 years after ICU discharge.[9]

A prospective cohort of 126 patients who had undergone PMV in the ICU (median ICU length of stay of 26 days) was followed for 1 year to review health care utilization.[10] The investigators found that this cohort, in addition to having poor health outcomes and a high rate of hospital readmission, had a high level of health care resource utilization. The 1-year cost per patient for care after ICU discharge varied from $6669 for patients living at home to $91 277 for those still managed in the acute care setting. Although these patients were not necessarily representative of the whole general ICU survivorship population, given that long-term ICU morbidity is not just limited to our sickest patients, it could be predicted that many survivors of critical illness would have higher rates of health care utilization after discharge.

With longer-term morbidities reducing the effectiveness of care and ongoing health care utilization and costs being so high, this situation offers a serious threat to the overall effectiveness and cost effectiveness of intensive care management. ICU follow-up clinics have been proposed as a way to follow survivors after they leave hospital, to diagnose and treat various morbidities, both related and unrelated to critical illness, in order to potentially improve the cost effectiveness of care. In fact, in the UK, current guidelines[11] recommend that ICU survivors be followed at 2–3 months after discharge from critical care to be assessed for physical functioning, depression, anxiety, and PTSD, with the intent that referrals be made as appropriate. Interestingly, in the UK, the regional purchasers of health care have been reluctant to fully engage with post-ICU clinics, as the impression from the purchasers is that this service can be provided by the GP, resulting in a patchy distribution of such a service.[12]

Organization of post-ICU follow-up clinics

Goals and outcomes of an ICU follow-up clinic

ICU clinics may have a variety of stated and implicit goals. Historically, the primary aim has been to improve diagnosis and management of chronic conditions common to ICU survivors and to address rehabilitation needs.[13] However, these clinics have also played a role in our understanding of the long-term consequences or critical illness. They may also play an important role in the lives of family members and caregivers.

Organization of ICU follow-up clinics

The majority of experience with ICU follow-up clinics has been from the UK where the practice has become relatively common, although not universal, existing in about 30% of ICUs.[12] The prevalence of these clinics in other parts of the world is unknown, although there are individual reports of clinics in Australia and other countries in Europe. These clinics have generally not been common in North America.

ICU clinics vary widely in terms of their staffing, eligibility for participation, timing and duration of follow-up, use of standardized assessment tools, and the degree to which they provide services or have direct access to referral services. The clinic organization may, in part, be determined by funding models, which differ between centres and countries. Currently, funding for these clinics is minimal and, when present, appears to be somewhat ad hoc, coming from within

Table 53.1 Single-centre descriptions of ICU follow-up clinics

Author (country)	Clinic staffing	Patient eligibility	Clinic timing (after ICU discharge)	Services provided
Kvale (2003) (Norway)[35]	Physician only	Patients who lived within the hospital region	7–8 months	Specialty referral
Engstrom (2008) (Sweden)[19]	Most responsible physician and bedside nurse	ICU stay >72 hours, respiratory care >24 hours	6 months	Visit to the ICU, debriefing about ICU stay, review of ICU diary
Cutler (2003) (UK)[36]	Nurse	ICU stay >5 days	6 months	Post-discharge ICU visit by RN and physician
Daffurn (1994) (Australia)[41]	Nurse and physician	ICU stay >48 hours	3 months	Semi-structured interview, physical examination, medical and other health professional referrals, as needed, and visit to the ICU
Hall-Smith (1997) (UK)[37]	Nurse specialist	ICU stay >5 days	3 months	Interview—research-based clinic
Crocker (2003) (UK)[38]	Nurse, physician, PT, OT	ICU stay >4 days	Ward, 2 and 6 months	ICU visit, speciality referral, medication review, PT/OT assessment
Waldmann (1998) (UK)[39]	Nurse, physician	ICU stay >4 days	2, 6, and 12 months	ICU visit, speciality referral, management of tracheostomy, pulmonary function tests
Sharland (2002) (UK)[40]	Nurse	ICU stay >4 days or referral by ICU staff, ward staff or patient	2, 6, and 12 months	ICU visit, interview, rehabilitation information, speciality referral

PT, physiotherapist; OT, occupational therapist.

existing ICU budgets and appearing to have no formal clinical development or financial plan.[12] In some cases, a home-based rehabilitation programme has run in parallel to the clinic visits.[14,15]

Clinical services provided

In a survey of ICU follow-up clinics in the UK,[12] Griffiths et al. found that just over half were nurse-led clinics, with the rest being physician-led. Approximately one-third of clinics had access to psychotherapy or counselling services, and a similar proportion had access to physiotherapy services. Other speciality services (e.g. otolaryngology, psychiatry) were not commonly available as a routine service.

Depending on the staffing model and resources, ICU clinics may be in a position to directly provide clinical services and information to ICU survivors and their families. They may involve medical consultations, psychosocial support for patients and their families, or consultations and therapy from rehabilitation teams, pharmacists, and other health care professionals. A variety of single-centre descriptive reports of ICU follow-up clinics exist in the literature. These clinics are described in detail in Table 53.1.

Clinics may organize themselves to act as a direct provider of services, such as diagnosis and treatment of ICUAW, or to act as a coordinator of other services and refer the patient to external consultants for management, or some combination of these two. They may also act as a resource for the survivors and their families such as arranging visits to the ICU and providing information and answers to questions the patient may have about their specific experience in the ICU.

Drug management

Drug reconciliation may also be an important role. ICU patients are often taken off regular medications and started on medications to manage temporary acute issues, such as anti-arrhythmics, and may leave the hospital without appropriate reconciliation with pre-admission medications. In fact, ICU patients have a higher risk, compared to other hospitalized patients, of having home medications discontinued and unintentionally not restarted at discharge.[16] Return to ICU follow-up is one potential opportunity to have medication lists reviewed by the ICU pharmacist and/or physician.

Patient-centred outcomes in follow-up clinics

Quantitative evidence

The PRaCTICaL study[15] is the only randomized trial looking specifically at follow-up clinics and their role in patient-centred outcomes. Patients were randomized to a 'usual care' group or to a follow-up programme consisting of a 3-month and 9-month clinic visit with a trained registered nurse, supported by an intensive care physician, and a self-directed manual-based home rehabilitation programme commenced in hospital after ICU discharge. There was no difference found between the two groups in their primary outcome of HRQoL. There was also no difference in any of the preselected secondary outcomes, which included incidence of PTSD (Davidson Trauma Score), depression and anxiety (HADS), satisfaction, and a second measure of HRQoL (EQ-5D).

Another study evaluated the use of a home-based rehabilitation programme in the context of a pre-existing ICU follow-up service.[14] A key difference in this study from the PRaCTICaL study is that both patient groups were followed in an ICU follow-up clinic and the experimental group also received a home-based rehabilitation programme. This study found improved physical function scores on the SF-36, although other clinical outcomes measures were not significantly different and the primary outcome of interest was not clearly specified. The treatment effect in this study is related to the rehabilitation intervention and should not be attributed to the follow-up clinics per se.

A specific intervention which may have effect in long-term outcomes is the use of an ICU diary. A randomized trial, where patients in the intervention group were given a diary in lay language that described their ICU stay, showed no difference in the primary outcome of PTSS score at 3 months. However, in a post hoc analysis, patients in the intervention group were less likely to meet the diagnostic criteria for PTSD.[17] Future studies are required to determine the place of such diaries in practice, and further details of this approach are provided in Chapters 21 and 52.

Qualitative evidence

Other authors have looked qualitatively at the impact of the ICU follow-up clinic on the patient experience and found a positive impact. One UK study of 34 patients from across the UK used thematic coding of narrative and semi-structured interviews to describe the survivor's experience of ICU follow-up clinics.[18] Patients' experiences were generally felt to be positive, and the study authors grouped these experiences into themes of continuity of care, receiving information, having an expert opinion, and having the opportunity to provide feedback to health care providers on their experiences. Of note, this study included interviews with some patients who had been offered ICU follow-up and had chosen not to attend, either because of a feeling of paranoia, their own belief that they did not need the services, or because of geographical constraints. The PRaCTICAL study did not find an improvement in patient satisfaction related to ICU follow-up clinics.[15]

Many ICU patients visit the ICU after discharge, and the follow-up clinic may be a way to formalize the visit and to help patients to use the experience in a positive way. Engstrom et al.[19] performed narrative interviews of nine patients and nine family members from a single ICU in Sweden who participated in post-discharge visits to the ICU. Thematic analysis of these interviews revealed four key roles the clinic played for survivors and their families. First, both participants and families reported 'receiving strength from returning together'. Second, patients, in particular, found that the experience allowed them to 'make sense of the critical illness experience', particularly of the spatial organization of the unit and of the sounds of the equipment. A third theme identified was 'feeling grateful to have survived', and both survivors and family members appreciated the opportunity to meet with the staff who had played a role in their stay. Lastly, patients and family members saw the visits as an 'opportunity to improve care' and to provide feedback on both positive and negative experiences.

Qualitative vs quantitative evidence

Overall, RCT data does not show a benefit to nurse-led follow-up clinics when usual tools for assessing HRQoL, depression, anxiety, and PTSD are used. However, qualitative research of the patients' experience would suggest that patients do have a subjective sense of benefit. A number of possible explanations for this discrepancy exist. First, our tools for measuring these outcomes are poorly validated in this population and therefore may not truly reflect the patient experience. In addition, many of these tools (SF-36, EQ-5D) require the patient to complete a paper survey and rely on self-evaluation of symptoms, which may be difficult in ICU survivors who have experienced cognitive dysfunction. However, it could also be argued that a desire to please the patient's health care providers could lead the participants in qualitative interviews to overstate the achieved health care benefit.

However, the results of this large randomized trial represent the best evidence that we have and should be considered in resource and service planning.[15] Rather than classifying these results as discordant, they may be seen as complementary. Qualitative studies should be seen as hypothesis-generating and providing detailed insight about patients' experience of ICU survivorship. This information can help to instruct us on designing a programme of longitudinal care for ICU survivors.

Support of families and caregivers in follow-up clinics

Not only does an ICU stay have lasting impact on survivors, it can also have a profound impact on the family members or caregivers of those survivors. Azoulay et al. reviewed 284 family members of patients 90 days after either ICU discharge or death and found that nearly one-third had symptoms suggesting increased risk of PTSD,[20] a finding confirmed by other researchers.[21] In informal caregivers of ARDS survivors, symptoms of emotional distress are high and persist to 2 years after hospital discharge.[22] A more recent study of caregivers of ICU survivors showed evidence of depressive symptoms in >30% at 2 months. Even at 12-month follow-up, symptoms persisted in the majority of these caregivers.[23]

With the primary focus of ICU follow-up clinics being patient-related, clinics may not always have reliably targeted the caregivers' and family members' needs and morbidities. Although family members are often encouraged to participate in clinic visits, efforts have not always been directed specifically at the diagnosis or management of their symptoms. In the PRaCTICAL study, although family members were invited to attend the clinic, only about one-third actually chose to attend.[15] Further insight into the reasoning for this approach is provided in Chapter 52. In their qualitative study, Engstrom et al. included nine family members.[19] The family members were not analysed as a separate group, although thematic analysis and comments suggested participation was a positive experience.

In their study of a rehabilitation manual and programme for patients, Jones et al. also looked at and published a separate study of psychological morbidity in caregivers before and after the clinic intervention. They documented PTSD symptoms in 49% of caregivers, symptoms of anxiety in 58–62%, and depression in 22–31% but found no effect of the intervention on any of these symptoms. As noted previously, both groups participated in a follow-up clinic, with the addition of a rehabilitation manual and programme in the intervention group. With the intervention not being specifically directed at caregivers, it is difficult to assess whether a focused intervention in the setting of a follow-up programme would have an impact on caregiver psychological morbidity.

Although one study showed that family members and relatives subjectively report the experience of attending clinic as positive, the psychological burden in this group may require more specific attention. In caregivers who show symptoms of serious psychological morbidity (e.g. depression, PTSD), it may be more appropriate for them to have health care provisions that are separate from that of the ICU survivor.

Promotion of well-being and education of staff members in follow-up clinics

The experience of ICU staff in caring for critically ill patients and their families leads to high levels of burnout, a phenomenon which has been well documented in both nursing staff[24] and physicians.[25] About a quarter of nurses experience symptoms of PTSD[26] and about a third symptoms of severe burnout,[24] although these estimates are based on screening questionnaires for symptoms and do not reflect a formal diagnosis. Some authors have suggested that people suffer less burnout if they feel that their work is valued and important to others. We are unaware of any research that has specifically addressed the psychological morbidity of health care professionals who participate in ICU follow-up clinics. However, one group has completed a thematic analysis of narrative interviews with bedside critical care nurses who participated in ICU follow-up studies.[27] Among other themes, the researchers found that nurses appreciated the experience of 'meeting a healthy person' and also that they saw their participation in the visits as 'a learning experience'.

Other than this one small study, the role of participation in follow-up for ICU staff has not yet been well supported by research which has not looked at the role for other allied health professionals, physicians, or trainees and would not likely be reasonable sole justification for the existence of an ICU follow-up programme. However, if clinics can be proven to be beneficial for patients, it would seem reasonable to include bedside staff in such clinics.

Research-centred approach in follow-up clinics

Outside of the role that outpatient clinics may play in the clinical care of patients, they also have historically been integral to the research programmes that have furthered our understanding of long-term outcomes of critical illness. Large observational studies of physical function, psychiatric morbidity, cognitive function, and HRQoL have changed our understanding of the challenges our patients face after they leave ICU and the hospital.

Long-term outcomes are challenging to study in any population. Critical care is no exception and may be a particular challenge. Attrition may impact on both the power and internal validity of study results, both in cohort studies and clinical trials,[28] if attrition is differentially affected by the exposure or intervention. Furthermore, studies that incorporate prospective long-term follow-up of ICU patients must be powered to account for the reality of high mortality rates in this population.[28] Tansey et al. reviewed strategies that have been successful in other populations of patients as well as their own long-term ARDS cohort[29] and identified the importance of building and maintaining long-term relationships with their patients.

We must continue to follow up patients after they leave the ICU and the hospital, particularly as we embark on important interventional trials. In addition, researchers will need to validate, and possibly develop, tools, such as instruments to study HRQoL, physical and psychiatric morbidity, and cognitive outcomes, to be used in this heterogeneous patient population. Given the importance of building relationships with patients to maintain contact for the duration of the study,[29] ICU follow-up clinics may play an important role in ongoing and future research.

Cost effectiveness of ICU follow-up clinics

It is clear in most countries that health care systems are already stretched and cannot support an unlimited number and scope of interventions. It is important that we evaluate the cost effectiveness of new interventions to ensure that scarce health care resources are justly distributed.

At this time, only the PRaCTICAL study has evaluated the cost effectiveness of ICU follow-up services and found their model not to be cost-effective, which is not surprising given the lack of benefit in terms of QALYs and the increased costs.[15] Other cohort studies have also demonstrated high health care resource utilization[10] and a low accumulation of QALYs in the years after ICU discharge,[9] which threaten the cost effectiveness of future interventions and care. Future studies of ICU follow-up programmes should incorporate a cost effectiveness analysis into their methods. Without a robust financial argument, health care purchasers are unlikely to commission such a service.

Challenges for follow-up clinics

Beyond the current lack of evidence to support their efficacy or cost effectiveness, the implementation and study of follow-up services come with numerous challenges and barriers. A clear challenge is the equitable delivery of these services. For good reason, ICUs are generally concentrated in areas of dense population. In many countries, remote geography and regionalization of ICU care have led to patients being cared for in ICUs far from home. Returning for follow-up visits may represent a significant burden, particularly when family members may have already incurred significant cost and lost income during the ICU stay.

It is not known who the most appropriate clinicians are to provide ICU follow-up services. The default to date has been interested and extremely enthusiastic ICU physicians and nurses, although their training in chronic illness and outpatient medicine can be quite limited, which may limit their ability to offer appropriate care to our patients, despite good intentions. Furthermore, this may not be the best use of the limited and specialized human resource of intensive care physicians and nurses, whose skills may be better used in the ICU itself. There is a risk with follow-up clinics that primary care physicians will be excluded from discussions about long-term morbidities and management. It is clearly essential that clinics work closely with primary care to assure this does not happen. Primary care physicians, in turn, may feel unqualified to manage and coordinate the complex, and sometimes specialized, needs of these patients, such as tracheostomy care, vocal cord dysfunction, neuromuscular disease, and PTSD, among others. In the past, rehabilitation physicians (physiatrists) have often been less involved in the care of these patients, but clearly their wide expertise in rehabilitation medicine could be greatly advantageous to the care of the patient recovering from critical illness.

Measuring the benefit or effect of follow-up services on our patients is challenging. Patients who survive an ICU stay suffer cognitive dysfunction and depression, both of which may interfere with the validity of standard measurement tools for HRQoL and symptoms of anxiety, depression, and PTSD.[30] Also important in evaluating these outcomes is the difficulty in the evaluation of complex multifaceted interventions. Even if a follow-up programme demonstrates efficacy, it may not be clear which elements of the intervention provided benefit, which is important when resources are limited and costs must be contained.

Engaging family members in follow-up, while recognizing their own high levels of psychiatric morbidity, is a further challenge. While family members may subjectively report positive experiences with follow-up clinics,[19] many do not actually attend the clinic.[31] If the role of intensivists in managing the acquired morbidities of ICU survivors is ambiguous, our role in the issues their family members face is even more difficult to identify. Intensivists do not have a health care relationship with family members and do not communicate with their primary care physicians, who may not even know about the critical illness in the family member, let alone be informed about the common challenges facing caregivers of ICU survivors.

Conclusion

Based on the current body of evidence, the use of the commonly used ICU follow-up clinic model may not provide benefit to patients and is not cost-effective. However, this should not reduce the importance of these long-term outcomes or lead us to abandon our patients once they leave the ICU. Through qualitative research, patients themselves and their family members have eloquently vocalized that there are elements of follow-up services that they find subjectively helpful.

Our challenge now is to develop and implement longitudinal models of care that starts on the day a patient enters the ICU and continues once they leave hospital. Our focus should start with the prevention of these morbidities, through earlier initiation of rehabilitation activities[32] and management of delirium,[33] which both impact longer-term outcomes. One intervention that may have benefit in reducing PTSD symptoms is the use of a diary of ICU events kept by health care providers and given to patients after discharge.[17] After ICU and hospital discharge, some have advocated that a follow-up model should include better use of technology, such as telemedicine and electronic health records, to engage and communicate with primary health care providers, inpatient and outpatient rehabilitation facilities, and our patients and their family members.[34] Appropriate use of technology may also help to prevent inequity in service delivery by allowing us to reach out to patients from beyond our immediate urban areas where tertiary ICUs are usually located.

Future research and design of follow-up models should integrate control groups and well-planned outcome analyses, including cost effectiveness. Researchers should also consider carefully the tools we use to assess these outcomes and their validity in ICU survivors, particularly those with cognitive impairment and psychiatric morbidity. Models should be truly longitudinal, beginning with the ICU stay, continuing throughout acute care and beyond to hospital discharge. Communication with primary care physicians and other specialist physicians should continue throughout that time.

References

1 Herridge MS, Tansey CM, Matte A, et al. Functional disability 5 years after acute respiratory distress syndrome. *N Engl J Med* 2011;**364**:1293–304.

2 Adhikari NK, McAndrews MP, Tansey CM, et al. Self-reported symptoms of depression and memory dysfunction in survivors of ARDS. *Chest* 2009;**135**:678–87.

3 Hopkins RO, Weaver LK, Collingridge D, Parkinson RB, Chan KJ, Orme JF, Jr. Two-year cognitive, emotional, and quality-of-life outcomes in acute respiratory distress syndrome. *Am J Respir Crit Care Med* 2005;**171**:340–7.

4 Iwashyna TJ, Ely EW, Smith DM, Langa KM. Long-term cognitive impairment and functional disability among survivors of severe sepsis. *JAMA* 2010;**304**:1787–94.

5 Ulvik A, Kvale R, Wentzel-Larsen T, Flaatten H. Sexual function in ICU survivors more than 3 years after major trauma. *Intensive Care Med* 2008;**34**:447–53.

6 Griffiths J, Gager M, Alder N, Fawcett D, Waldmann C, Quinlan J. A self-report-based study of the incidence and associations of sexual dysfunction in survivors of intensive care treatment. *Intensive Care Med* 2006;**32**:445–51.

7 Dowdy DW, Eid MP, Sedrakyan A, et al. Quality of life in adult survivors of critical illness: a systematic review of the literature. *Intensive Care Med* 2005;**31**:611–20.

8 Graf J, Muhlhoff C, Doig GS, et al. Health care costs, long-term survival, and quality of life following intensive care unit admission after cardiac arrest. *Crit Care* 2008;**12**:R92.

9 Cuthbertson BH, Roughton S, Jenkinson D, MacLennan G, Vale L. Quality of life in the five years after intensive care: a cohort study. *Crit Care* 2010;**14**:R6.

10 Unroe M, Kahn JM, Carson SS, et al. One-year trajectories of care and resource utilization for recipients of prolonged mechanical ventilation: a cohort study. *Ann Intern Med* 2010;**153**:167–75.

11 National Institute for Health and Care Excellence. *Rehabilitation after critical illness.* (2009). London: National Institute for Health and Care Excellence. Available at: http://www.nice.org.uk/CG83.

12 Griffiths JA, Barber VS, Cuthbertson BH, Young JD. A national survey of intensive care follow-up clinics. *Anaesthesia* 2006;**61**:950–5.

13 Griffiths RD, Jones C. *Intensive care aftercare.* 1st ed. Oxford: Butterworth Heinemann; 2002.

14 Jones C, Skirrow P, Griffiths RD, et al. Rehabilitation after critical illness: a randomized, controlled trial. *Crit Care Med* 2003;**31**:2456–61.

15 Cuthbertson BH, Rattray J, Campbell MK, et al. The PRaCTICaL study of nurse led, intensive care follow-up programmes for improving long term outcomes from critical illness: a pragmatic randomised controlled trial. *BMJ* 2009;**339**:b3723.

16 Bell CM, Brener SS, Gunraj N, et al. Association of ICU or hospital admission with unintentional discontinuation of medications for chronic diseases. *JAMA* 2011;**306**:840–7.

17 Jones C, Backman C, Capuzzo M, et al. Intensive care diaries reduce new onset post traumatic stress disorder following critical illness: a randomised, controlled trial. *Crit Care* 2010;**14**:R168.

18 Prinjha S, Field K, Rowan K. What patients think about ICU follow-up services: a qualitative study. *Crit Care* 2009;**13**:R46.

19 Engstrom A, Andersson S, Soderberg S. Re-visiting the ICU Experiences of follow-up visits to an ICU after discharge: a qualitative study. *Intensive Crit Care Nurs* 2008;**24**:233–41.

20 Azoulay E, Pochard F, Kentish-Barnes N, et al. Risk of post-traumatic stress symptoms in family members of intensive care unit patients. *Am J Respir Crit Care Med* 2005;**171**:987–94.

21 Jones C, Skirrow P, Griffiths RD, et al. Post-traumatic stress disorder-related symptoms in relatives of patients following intensive care. *Intensive Care Med* 2004;**30**:456–60.

22 Cameron JI, Herridge MS, Tansey CM, McAndrews MP, Cheung AM. Well-being in informal caregivers of survivors of acute respiratory distress syndrome. *Crit Care Med* 2006;**34**:81–6.

23 Van Pelt DC, Schulz R, Chelluri L, Pinsky MR. Patient-specific, time-varying predictors of post-ICU informal caregiver burden: the caregiver outcomes after ICU discharge project. *Chest* 2010;**137**:88–94.

24 Poncet MC, Toullic P, Papazian L, et al. Burnout syndrome in critical care nursing staff. *Am J Respir Crit Care Med* 2007;**175**:698–704.

25 Embriaco N, Azoulay E, Barrau K, et al. High level of burnout in intensivists: prevalence and associated factors. *Am J Respir Crit Care Med* 2007;**175**:686–92.

26 Mealer ML, Shelton A, Berg B, Rothbaum B, Moss M. Increased prevalence of post-traumatic stress disorder symptoms in critical care nurses. *Am J Respir Crit Care Med* 2007;**175**:693–7.

27 Engstrom A, Soderberg S. Critical care nurses' experiences of follow-up visits to an ICU. *J Clin Nurs* 2010;**19**:2925–32.

28 Rubenfeld GD. Improving clinical trials of long-term outcomes. *Crit Care Med* 2009;**37**(1 Suppl): S112–16.

29 Tansey CM, Matte AL, Needham D, Herridge MS. Review of retention strategies in longitudinal studies and application to follow-up of ICU survivors. *Intensive Care Med* 2007;**33**:2051–7.

30 Seymour DG, Ball AE, Russell EM, Primrose WR, Garratt AM, Crawford JR. Problems in using health survey questionnaires in older patients with physical disabilities. The reliability and validity of the SF-36 and the effect of cognitive impairment. *J Eval Clin Pract* 2001;**7**:411–18.

31 Cuthbertson BH, Rattray J, Johnston M, et al. A pragmatic randomised, controlled trial of intensive care follow up programmes in improving longer-term outcomes from critical illness. The PRACTICAL study. *BMC Health Serv Res* 2007;**7**:116.

32 Schweickert WD, Pohlman MC, Pohlman AS, et al. Early physical and occupational therapy in mechanically ventilated, critically ill patients: a randomised controlled trial. *Lancet* 2009;**373**:1874–82.

33 Girard TD, Jackson JC, Pandharipande PP, et al. Delirium as a predictor of long-term cognitive impairment in survivors of critical illness. *Crit Care Med* 2010;**38**:1513–20.

34 Kahn JM, Angus DC. Health policy and future planning for survivors of critical illness. *Curr Opin Crit Care* 2007;**13**:514–18.

35 Kvale R, Ulvik A, Flaatten H. Follow-up after intensive care: a single center study. *Intensive Care Med* 2003;**29**:2149–56.

36 **Cutler L, Brightmore K, Colqhoun V, Dunstan J, Gay M.** Developing and evaluating critical care follow-up. *Nurs Crit Care* 2003;**8**:116–25.

37 **Hall-Smith J, Ball C, Coakley J.** Follow-up services and the development of a clinical nurse specialist in intensive care. *Intensive Crit Care Nurs* 1997;**13**:243–8.

38 **Crocker C.** A multidisciplinary follow-up clinic after patients' discharge from ITU. *Br J Nurs* 2003;**12**: 910–14.

39 **Waldmann CS.** Intensive care after intensive care. *Curr Anaesthes Crit Care* 1998;**9**:134–9.

40 **Sharland C.** Setting up a nurse-led clinic. In: Griffiths RD, Jones C (eds.) *Intensive care aftercare.* 1st ed. Oxford: Butterworth Heinemann; 2002. pp. 96–113.

41 **Daffurn K, Bishop GF, Hillman KM, Bauman A.** Problems following discharge after intensive care. *Intensive Care Nurs* 1994;**10**:244–51

Index

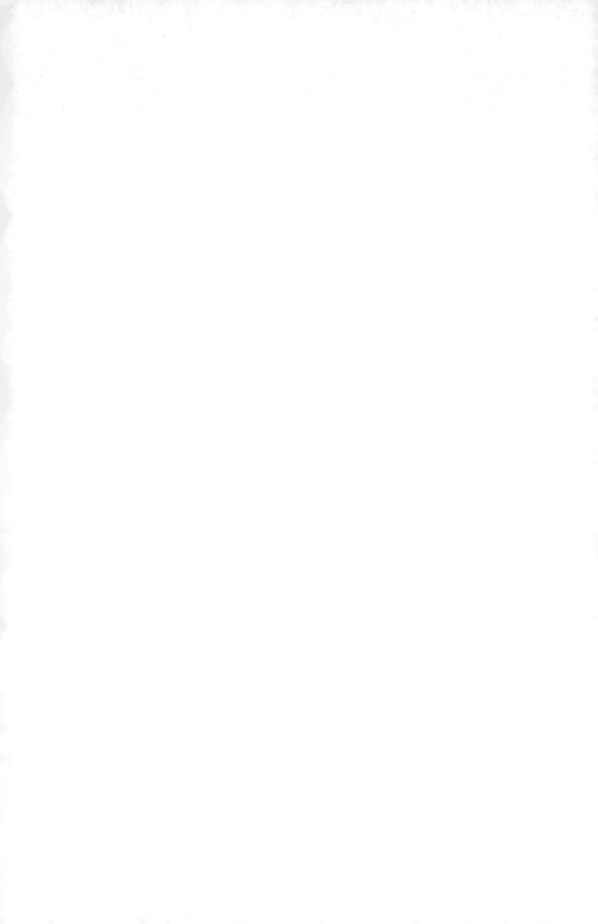